Diagnostic Ultrasonography (Second Series) Test and Syllabus

Thomas L. Lawson, M.D.
Section Chairman

Richard A. Bowerman, M.D.
Beverly G. Coleman, M.D.
Gary M. Kellman, M.D.
William D. Middleton, M.D.

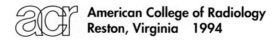
American College of Radiology
Reston, Virginia 1994

Sets Published

Chest Disease
Bone Disease
Genitourinary Tract Disease
Gastrointestinal Disease
Head and Neck Disorders
Pediatric Disease
Nuclear Radiology
Radiation Pathology and
    Radiation Biology
Chest Disease II
Bone Disease II
Genitourinary Tract Disease II
Gastrointestinal Disease II
Head and Neck Disorders II
Nuclear Radiology II
Cardiovascular Disease
Emergency Radiology
Bone Disease III
Gastrointestinal Disease III
Chest Disease III
Pediatric Disease II
Nuclear Radiology III
Head and Neck Disorders III
Genitourinary Tract Disease III

Diagnostic Ultrasound
Breast Disease
Bone Disease IV
Pediatric Disease III
Chest Disease IV
Neuroradiology
Gastrointestinal Disease IV
Nuclear Radiology IV
Magnetic Resonance
Radiation Bioeffects and
    Management
Genitourinary Tract Disease IV
Head and Neck Disorders IV
Pediatric Disease IV
Breast Disease II
Musculoskeletal Disease
Diagnostic Ultrasonography II

Sets in Preparation

Chest Disease V
Gastrointestinal Disease V
Neuroradiology II
Emergency Radiology II
Genitourinary Tract Disease V
Nuclear Radiology V

Note: While the American College of Radiology and the editors of this publication have attempted to include the most current and accurate information possible, errors may inadvertently appear. Diagnostic and interventional decisions should be based on the individual circumstances of each case.

SET 38:
Diagnostic Ultrasonography (Second Series) Test and Syllabus

Editor in Chief
BARRY A. SIEGEL, M.D., Professor of Radiology and Medicine and Director, Division of Nuclear Medicine, Mallinckrodt Institute of Radiology, Washington University School of Medicine, St. Louis, Missouri

Associate Editor
DAVID H. STEPHENS, M.D., Professor of Radiology, Mayo Medical School; Department of Diagnostic Radiology, Mayo Clinic, Rochester, Minnesota

Section Chairman
THOMAS L. LAWSON, M.D., Professor and Chairman, Department of Radiology, Loyola University Chicago, Stritch School of Medicine, Chicago, Illinois

Co-Authors
RICHARD A. BOWERMAN, M.D., Associate Professor of Radiology, University of Michigan Medical Center, Ann Arbor, Michigan
BEVERLY G. COLEMAN, M.D., Professor of Radiology and Obstetrics and Gynecology, and Director of Ultrasound Imaging, University of Pennsylvania Medical Center, Hospital of the University of Pennsylvania, Department of Radiology, Philadelphia, Pennsylvania
GARY M. KELLMAN, M.D., Fairfax Radiological Consultants, Fairfax, Virginia; formerly Director of Ultrasound, Henry Ford Hospital, Detroit, Michigan
WILLIAM D. MIDDLETON, M.D., Associate Professor of Radiology and Chief, Diagnostic Ultrasound, Mallinckrodt Institute of Radiology, Washington University School of Medicine, St. Louis, Missouri

AMERICAN COLLEGE OF RADIOLOGY
PROFESSIONAL SELF-EVALUATION PROGRAM

Publishing Coordinators:	*G. Rebecca Haines and Thomas M. Rogers*
Administrative Assistant:	*Marcy Olney*
Production Editor:	*Sean M. McKenna*
Copy Editors:	*Yvonne Strong*
Text Processing:	*Fusako T. Nowak*
Composition:	*Karen Finkle and Paul Wiegmann*
Index:	*EEI, Inc., Alexandria, Va.*
Lithography:	*Lanman Progressive, Washington, D.C.*
Typesetting:	*Publication Technology Corp., Fairfax, Va.*
Printing:	*John D. Lucas Printing, Baltimore, Md.*

Library of Congress Cataloging-in-Publication Data

Diagnostic ultrasonography test and syllabus / Thomas L. Lawson, section chairman ; [coauthors] Richard A. Bowerman ... [et al.].
   p. cm. — (Professional self-evaluation program; set 38)
   "Committee on Professional Self-Evaluation, Commission on Education, American College of Radiology"—Cover.
   Includes bibliographical references and index.
   ISBN 1-55903-038-0 : $200.00. — ISBN 1-55903-000-3 (series)
   1. Diagnosis, ultrasonographic—Examinations, questions, etc. 2. Diagnosis, ultrasonographic—Outlines, syllabi, etc. I. Lawson, Thomas L. II. Bowerman, Richard A. III. American College of Radiology. Commission on Education. Committee on Professional Self-Evaluation. IV. Series.
   [DNLM: 1. Ultrasonography—examination questions. WN 18 D5378 1994]
   RC78.7.U4M34   1994
   616.07'543'076—dc20
   DNLM/DLC   94-16701
for Library of Congress   CIP

ACR COMMITTEE ON PROFESSIONAL SELF-EVALUATION, COMMISSION ON EDUCATION

Anthony V. Proto, M.D., *Chairman and Associate Editor*

Barry A. Siegel, M.D., *Editor in Chief*

David H. Stephens, M.D., *Associate Editor*

Elias G. Theros, M.D., *Editor Emeritus*

SECTIONS

DIAGNOSTIC ULTRASONOGRAPHY II
Thomas L. Lawson, M.D.,
   Section Chairman
Richard A. Bowerman, M.D.
Beverly G. Coleman, M.D.
Gary M. Kellman, M.D.
William D. Middleton, M.D.

CHEST DISEASE V
Robert H. Choplin, M.D.,
   Section Chairman
Heber M. MacMahon, M.D.
Theresa C. McLoud, M.D.
Nestor L. Müller, M.D.,
   Ph.D.
James C. Reed, M.D.

GASTROINTESTINAL DISEASE V
Dennis M. Balfe, M.D.,
   Section Chairman
Judith L. Chezmar, M.D.
R. Brooke Jeffrey, M.D.
Robert E. Koehler, M.D.
Marc S. Levine, M.D.

NEURORADIOLOGY II
Solomon Batnitzky, M.D.,
   Section Chairman
Edgardo J. C. Angtuaco,
   M.D.
Allen D. Elster, M.D.
Robert R. Lukin, M.D.
Eric J. Russell, M.D.

EMERGENCY RADIOLOGY II
Kent R. Donovan, M.D.,
   Section Chairman
John H. Harris, M.D.
Theodore E. Keats, M.D.
Kathleen A. McCarroll,
   M.D.
Helen C. Redman, M.D.
Myer H. Roszler, M.D.

NUCLEAR RADIOLOGY V
John W. Keyes, Jr., M.D.,
   Section Chairman
Manuel L. Brown, M.D.
Douglas F. Eggli, M.D.
Jeffrey A. Leppo, M.D.
Tom R. Miller, M.D., Ph.D.
Barry A. Siegel, M.D.

GENITOURINARY DISEASE V
N. Reed Dunnick, M.D.,
   Section Chairman
Sachiko T. Cochran, M.D.
Richard H. Cohan, M.D.
Bernard F. King, M.D.
Carl M. Sandler, M.D.

Additional Contributors

CHRISTINE M. DUDIAK, M.D., Assistant Professor of Radiology, Loyola University Chicago Stritch School of Medicine, Chicago, Illinois

PAUL L. GOLDBERG, M.D., Department of Radiology, Edward Hospital, Naperville, Illinois

JILL E. LANGER, M.D., Assistant Professor of Radiology, University of Pennsylvania Medical Center, Hospital of the University of Pennsylvania, Department of Radiology, Philadelphia, Pennsylvania

WALLACE T. MILLER, Jr., M.D., Assistant Professor of Radiology, University of Pennsylvania Medical Center, Hospital of the University of Pennsylvania, Department of Radiology, Philadelphia, Pennsylvania

MARY C. OLSON, M.D., Associate Professor of Radiology, Loyola University Chicago Stritch School of Medicine, Chicago, Illinois

MICHAEL A. SANDLER, M.D., Department of Diagnostic Radiology, Henry Ford Hospital, Detroit, Michigan; Clinical Professor of Radiology, University of Michigan, Ann Arbor, Michigan

CARYL G. SALOMON, M.D., Assistant Professor of Radiology, Loyola University Chicago Stritch School of Medicine, Chicago, Illinois

KAREN J. STUCK, M.D., Department of Diagnostic Radiology, Henry Ford Hospital, Detroit, Michigan

Section Chairman's Preface

This is the second *Diagnostic Ultrasonography Test and Syllabus* in the Professional Self-Evaluation (PSE) program of the American College of Radiology (ACR). This volume was written between the summer of 1991 and the early spring of 1994 and contains "state of the art" images and the most current information on the diagnosis and differential diagnosis of more than 100 diseases and diagnostic entities. Although we could not cover every pertinent topic, we did attempt to choose entities and questions that would focus on the most important issues, new information, or new applications of ultrasonographic imaging.

The first *Diagnostic Ultrasound Test and Syllabus* (1988) contains, by current standards, relatively crude images, many of which were obtained by using static, articulated-arm, gray-scale machines. Most younger radiologists have probably never seen or used this type of equipment. Many recent technical advances have led to dramatic refinements in the sophistication and quality of current ultrasound equipment. Images in the current syllabus demonstrate the marked improvement in spatial resolution of current ultrasound units compared with those available in 1988. Color Doppler ultrasonography was not yet available when the first ultrasonography syllabus was written. In the current syllabus, the application of color Doppler ultrasonography has been extensively explored, with supporting discussion and numerous illustrations.

As in the previous syllabus, the current syllabus stresses the importance of obstetric and gynecologic ultrasonography. Chapters addressing hepatobiliary, pancreatic, and genitourinary disease are also included. New areas covered here include the use of ultrasonography to evaluate patients with AIDS, to examine patients with diseases of the prostate, and to diagnose gastrointestinal abnormalities in the adult. In the latter two instances, these are new applications of ultrasonography that have proven to be clinically useful in the years since the publication of the first ultrasound syllabus.

On behalf of the entire diagnostic ultrasonography committee, I would like to thank G. Rebecca Haines and Thomas M. Rogers from the ACR Publications Department for their help and technical expertise in assembling this volume. This work would not have been completed without their constant attention to detail and frequent reminders concerning overdue chapters! We would also like to thank our two editorial mentors for their skill and abilities in guiding us through this project. We are grateful to Dr. David H. Stephens, the Associate Editor, for his insightful comments and calm approach to difficult situations during occasional tumultuous periods. We would also like to express our deep gratitude to Dr.

Barry A. Siegel, the PSE series Editor in Chief. Barry is an extremely gifted and intelligent man. Even though his own area of radiologic specialty is nuclear medicine, he astounded us all with his vast knowledge and understanding of ultrasonographic techniques and diagnostic criteria. His awesome skills with the English language allowed him to cut through inconsistencies, ambiguous statements, and complex terminology in both the test questions and discussions with apparent ease. His interaction with us, his comments, and his revisions to our manuscripts markedly improved the overall quality of this volume.

Most of all, I would like to acknowledge the invaluable contributions of my fellow committee members: Drs. Richard A. Bowerman, Beverly G. Coleman, Gary M. Kellman, and William D. Middleton. These committee members were chosen for their special interest and expertise in ultrasonography, their proven academic abilities, their strong work ethic, their good humor, and their commitment to teamwork. The latter traits allowed us to collaborate as a congenial, well-coordinated, and highly effective committee.

We sincerely hope the *Diagnostic Ultrasonography (Second Series) Test and Syllabus* will be a valuable teaching and learning aid to our fellow radiologists.

Thomas L. Lawson, M.D.
Section Chairman

Editor's Preface

The last several years have been witness to important advances in the diagnostic applications of ultrasonography. Along with CT and MRI, ultrasonography forms the triumvirate responsible for the ascendancy of cross-sectional anatomic imaging in radiology, and these imaging methods now are central to diagnostic algorithms for diseases of all organ systems. Indeed, an important challenge for the future will be to develop strategies for selecting the best among several methods for approaching a patient with a particular array of signs and symptoms. Ultrasonography's "niche" continues to grow because of technical improvements in image quality and because of sonography's multiplanar capability, its virtual harmlessness (thus, making it ideal for pediatric and obstetrical applications), and its relatively lower technical costs. The addition of Doppler methods to assess vascular anatomy and flow patterns renders sonographic studies ever more definitive.

The current volume, *Diagnostic Ultrasonography (Second Series) Test and Syllabus*, highlights these features of sonographic imaging and provides our readers with an excellent appraisal of the current "state of the art" through in-depth discussions of the individual diagnostic exercises and their accompanying satellite questions.

On perusing this *tour de force*, our readers will surely recognize that all radiologists owe a tremendous debt of gratitude to Dr. Thomas L. Lawson, M.D., and to his principal co-authors, Drs. Richard A. Bowerman, Beverly G. Coleman, Gary M. Kellman, and William D. Middleton. These busy radiologists each gave generously of their considerable expertise and devoted long hours to the creation of this self-evaluation test and the accompanying syllabus. This voluntary effort is a testimonial to their individual and collective devotion to their craft and to the continuing education of all radiologists. Special kudos are due to Tom Lawson, who guided this project with clear vision, superb editorial skills, and a cheerful wit.

Many other individuals contributed to this project in various stages of its evolution. Dr. David H. Stephens, Associate Editor of the Professional Self-Evaluation (PSE) program, brought his own substantial experience to bear in helping to ensure that the test would be both challenging and fair and that the syllabus would be accurate, timely, and clinically relevant. G. Rebecca Haines, along with the publications staff of the American College of Radiology (ACR) she so ably directs, provided the necessary technical and editorial support to turn the Committee's labors into a highly polished finished product. The importance of their contribution cannot be overestimated. Thomas M. Rogers, in particular, is responsible for attention to all of the little editorial details that, taken in aggregate, maintain a high level of quality and consistency in each PSE volume. Dr. Anthony V. Proto, Chairman of the PSE Committee, worked closely with the Editor in Chief to guide the overall program and gently encouraged authors and editors alike to strive for our goals (and keep to our deadlines). Both the ACR Commission of Education, chaired by Dr. Joseph T. Ferrucci, and the Board of Chancellors provide the continuing support and encouragement needed to sustain the PSE program.

The real measure of success of the PSE program is not simply a function of the scientific content or the quality of the syllabi. Rather, our success is best reflected by the continuing endorsement of radiologists, both those in practice and those in training, working in the United States and in many other countries, who "vote" by their participation. This syllabus is the 38th volume in the PSE series, a program sustained over a span of 22 years. We believe that thousands of radiologists have thoroughly enjoyed this approach to continuing education. We keep going because we believe thousands more will want to do so in the future.

Barry A. Siegel, M.D.
Editor in Chief

Diagnostic Ultrasonography (Second Series)

Program Objective

The objective of this program is to provide "state-of-the-art" images and the most current information on the diagnosis and differential diagnosis of more than 100 diseases and diagnostic entities. Once the course is complete, the radiologist will have an in-depth understanding of the use of ultrasonography in obstetrics and gynecology, hepatobiliary, pancreatic, and genitourinary disease, and in the evaluation of patients with AIDS, anomalies of the prostate, and abnormalities of the adult gastrointestinal tract.

CME Credit Award: 25 Credit Hours

The American College of Radiology (ACR) is accredited by the Accreditation Council for Continuing Medical Education to sponsor continuing medical education for physicians.

The ACR designates the following continuing medical education activity as meeting the criteria for up to 25 hours, provided it is completed as designed, and designates this continuing medical education activity for 25 credit hours in Category 1 of the Physician's Recognition Award of the American Medical Association.

The *Diagnostic Ultrasonography (Second Series)* program has been approved for ACR and AMA/PRA Category 1 CME credit for the period from August 1994 through August 1997.

CME Credit Award Process

To receive the Category 1 credit, participants must complete the accompanying *answer sheet* and *evaluation form* and return them to the ACR within 6 months of the date when you purchased the program.

Within 40 days of receipt of the answer sheet and evaluation form, the ACR will provide you with a credit award letter. The letter will indicate your score, the date it was recorded, and a credit award statement. You may also request a report which provides you with a ranking of all the test scores from all the tests completed within the first 6 months of the course. This will allow you to compare your score with those of your peers. To place yourself on the mailing list to receive the report, contact the ACR's Educational Services Division at 1-800-227-5463, ext. 4986.

This CME activity was planned and produced in accordance with the ACCME Essentials. Category 1 CME for this program is not transferable. Only the purchaser may apply for and receive Category 1 credit.

Diagnostic Ultrasonography
(Second Series)
Test

For you to derive the maximum benefit from this program, you should complete the following test, and send your answer sheet to the ACR for scoring, before you proceed to the syllabus.

If for any reason you refer to the syllabus material, or any other references, in answering the questions, please be sure to so indicate when answering Question 118, the first demographic question. Your score will then not be used in developing the norm tables.

CASE 1: Questions 1 through 3

You are shown a longitudinal sonogram of the gallbladder in a 61-year-old woman (Figure 1-1). Additional history is withheld.

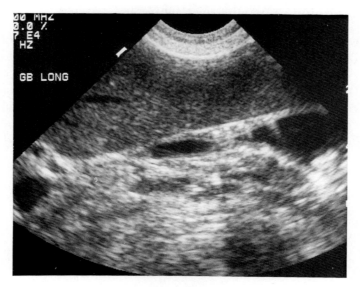

Figure 1-1

1. Which *one* of the following is the MOST likely diagnosis?

    (A) Acute cholecystitis
    (B) Adenomyomatosis
    (C) Gallbladder carcinoma
    (D) Emphysematous cholecystitis
    (E) Porcelain gallbladder

CASE 1 (Cont'd)

QUESTIONS 2 THROUGH 5: MARK YOUR ANSWER SHEET TRUE (T) OR FALSE (F) FOR EACH OF THE RESPONSE CHOICES.

2. Concerning acute cholecystitis,

    F (A) approximately 10% of cases occur without gallstones
    T (B) associated jaundice is most often secondary to Mirizzi's syndrome
    F (C) bacterial infection is important in its pathogenesis
    F (D) it is the most common cause of the wall-echo-shadow complex
    F (E) in a patient with right upper quadrant pain and fever, the presence of gallstones is diagnostic

3. Adenomyomatosis:

    F (A) predisposes to gallbladder carcinoma
    T (B) occurs secondary to chronic inflammation
    T (C) is a common cause of gallbladder polyps
    F (D) is strongly associated with biliary colic
    F (E) cannot be diagnosed by oral cholecystography

4. Concerning emphysematous cholecystitis,

    T (A) it is more common in women than in men
    T (B) ischemia is important in its pathogenesis
    T (C) it nearly always occurs in patients with gallstones
    T (D) mortality is greater than in patients with typical acute cholecystitis
    T (E) it is a potential cause of intraductal pneumobilia

5. Concerning cholesterolosis,

    F (A) it is associated with elevated cholesterol levels in serum
    T (B) it is seen more frequently in women than in men
    T (C) the gallbladder usually appears normal sonographically
    T (D) it predisposes to development of cholesterol stones
    T (E) it is the most common cause of gallbladder polyps

CASE 2: Questions 6 through 9

This 38-year-old woman presented for routine obstetrical ultrasonography. You are shown two axial views of the fetal head (Figure 2-1).

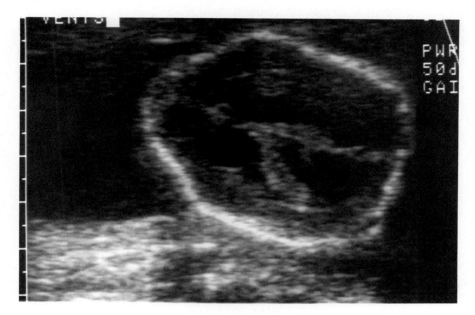

Figure 2-1

6. Which *one* of the following is the MOST likely diagnosis?

   (A) Normal variant
   (B) Dandy-Walker variant
   (C) Trisomy 18
   (D) Arnold-Chiari malformation
   (E) Down's syndrome

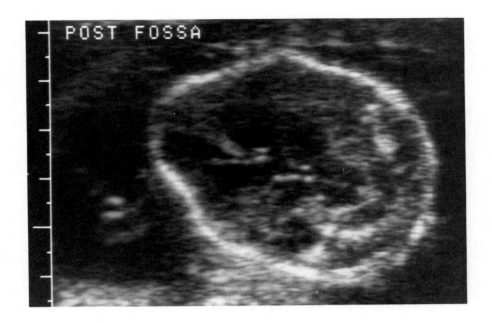

QUESTIONS 7 THROUGH 9: MARK YOUR ANSWER SHEET TRUE (T) OR FALSE (F) FOR EACH OF THE RESPONSE CHOICES.

7. Concerning the Dandy-Walker malformation,

   (A) it is characterized by hypoplasia or aplasia of the cerebellar vermis
   (B) anterolateral splaying of the cerebellar hemispheres is a sonographic feature
   (C) the degree of associated hydrocephalus is greater in patients with the Dandy-Walker variant than in those with the typical Dandy-Walker malformation
   (D) spinal dysraphism with myelomeningocele is the most frequently associated central nervous system anomaly
   (E) affected infants have a better prognosis than do those with the Arnold-Chiari malformation

CASE 2 (Cont'd)

8. Concerning the Arnold-Chiari malformation,

   (A) an elevated concentration of acetylcholinesterase in amniotic fluid is a marker of an open neural tube defect
   (B) the associated hydrocephalus is characterized by enlargement of all ventricles
   (C) it is associated with abnormal calvarial shape developing after 24 weeks gestational age
   (D) it causes enlargement of the cisterna magna
   (E) it causes cerebellar hypoplasia
   (F) both open and closed neural tube defects are associated with the Chiari II malformation

9. Concerning Down's syndrome,

   (A) it is reliably detected on routine prenatal sonography
   (B) it is associated with a low maternal serum α-fetoprotein level
   (C) a nuchal skin fold thickness greater than 6 mm should suggest the diagnosis
   (D) the characteristic sonographic features of associated duodenal atresia are generally not apparent until the third trimester
   (E) central nervous system anomalies are more frequent than in infants with trisomy 18

This 81-year-old man with an abdominal bruit was referred for sonography to rule out an abdominal aortic aneurysm. You are shown a longitudinal sonogram of the left lobe of the liver (Figure 3-1) and a pulsed Doppler waveform obtained from the left portal vein (Figure 3-2).

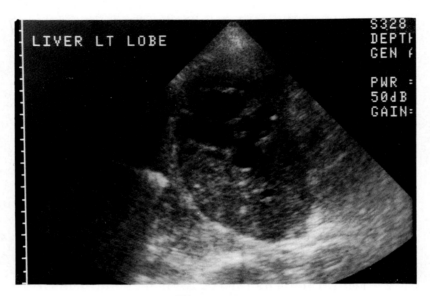

Figure 3-1

10. Which *one* of the following is the MOST likely diagnosis?

    (A) Angiosarcoma
    (B) Tortuous recanalized paraumbilical vein
    (C) Hepatic artery aneurysm
    (D) Arterioportal fistula
    (E) Hypervascular hepatocellular carcinoma

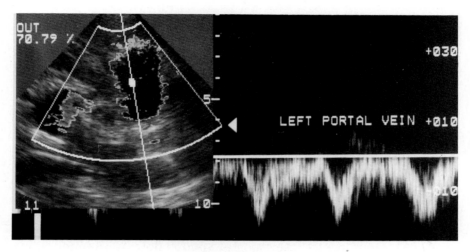

Figure 3-2

QUESTIONS 11 THROUGH 14: MARK YOUR ANSWER SHEET TRUE (T) OR FALSE (F) FOR EACH OF THE RESPONSE CHOICES.

11. Concerning portal hypertension,

(A) the most common type in the United States is intrahepatic

(B) it is one of the causes of the sonographic "parallel-channel sign"

(C) the earliest sonographic sign is flow reversal in the main portal vein

(D) detection of a hypoechoic band in the ligamentum teres is a specific sign

(E) spontaneous splenorenal shunts are the most common portosystemic collaterals detected sonographically

CASE 3 (Cont'd)

12. Concerning hepatic hemodynamics,

    (A) the portal vein normally has minimal or no pulsatility
    (B) in the fasting state, the vascular resistance of the hepatic artery is greater than that of the superior mesenteric artery
    (C) hepatic venous flow is normally bidirectional
    (D) normal portal vein flow velocities are approximately 15 to 20 cm/second
    (E) hepatic venous flow is normally greatest during diastole

13. Concerning portal vein thrombosis,

    (A) inability to detect portal venous flow by Doppler sonography is diagnostic
    (B) the major complication is hepatic infarction
    (C) recanalization is referred to as cavernous transformation
    (D) gray-scale sonography occasionally is normal
    (E) tumor thrombus is generally indistinguishable from bland thrombus

14. Sonographic features of the Budd-Chiari syndrome include:

    (A) caudate lobe hypertrophy
    (B) a monophasic hepatic venous waveform
    (C) hepatic venous to hepatic venous collaterals
    (D) flow reversal in the hepatic vein
    (E) flow reversal in the portal vein

CASE 4: Questions 15 through 19

This 63-year-old woman had a history of Sjögren's syndrome and two lymphomas, first non-Hodgkin's lymphoma and more recently Hodgkin's disease, both of which have been in remission for several years. You are shown a routine follow-up abdominal CT scan (A) and a subsequent transverse renal sonogram (B) (Figure 4-1). The anechoic zone in the near field is a standoff pad.

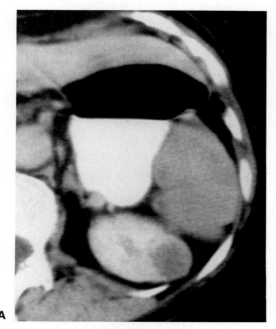

Figure 4-1

15.   Which *one* of the following is the MOST likely diagnosis?

    (A) Lymphoma
    (B) Renal cell carcinoma
    (C) Acute focal pyelonephritis
    (D) Complex renal cyst
    (E) Oncocytoma

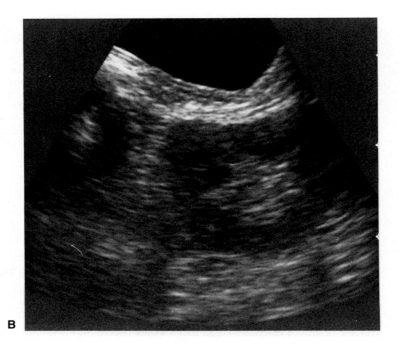

B

QUESTIONS 16 THROUGH 19: MARK YOUR ANSWER SHEET TRUE (T) OR FALSE (F) FOR EACH OF THE RESPONSE CHOICES.

16. Concerning lymphomatous involvement of the kidney,

    (A) it is more commonly due to Hodgkin's disease than to non-Hodgkin's lymphoma

    (B) the pattern of involvement is similar in Hodgkin's disease and non-Hodgkin's lymphoma

    (C) the pattern of multiple bilateral renal masses is most common

    (D) focal lesions exhibit increased through transmission

CASE 4 (Cont'd)

17. Features of renal cell carcinoma include:

    T (A) hypoechoic mass
    F (B) hyperechoic mass
    F (C) solitary metastasis
    T (D) thrombocytosis
    F (E) Budd-Chiari syndrome

18. Concerning complex renal cyst,

    F (A) a fluid-debris level indicates prior hemorrhage
    T (B) enhanced through transmission is occasionally the only
           feature distinguishing it from a solid mass
    F (C) the finding of a single, thin internal septation necessi-
           tates biopsy
    T (D) the finding of thin peripheral calcification necessitates
           biopsy

19. Concerning renal oncocytomas,

    T (A) they arise from the distal renal tubules
    T (B) tumors with similar histology occur in the salivary
           glands
    T (C) most are asymptomatic
    T (D) a central hypoechoic stellate pattern is virtually patho-
           gnomonic
    F (E) they are easily diagnosed by thin-needle biopsy

This 21-year-old man presented with left scrotal pain and swelling. You are shown a longitudinal color Doppler sonogram and a pulsed Doppler waveform of the left hemiscrotum (Figure 5-1).

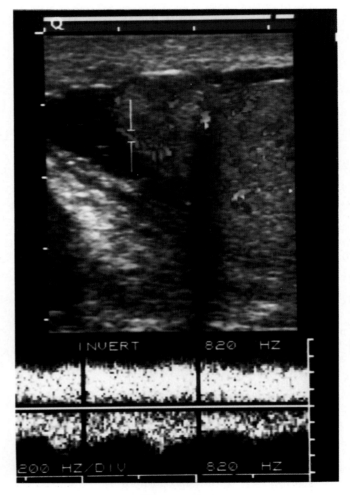

Figure 5-1

20. Which *one* of the following is the MOST likely diagnosis?

(A) Acute testicular torsion
(B) Late testicular torsion
(C) Epididymitis
(D) Adenomatoid tumor
(E) Varicocele

CASE 5 (Cont'd)

QUESTIONS 21 THROUGH 25: MARK YOUR ANSWER SHEET TRUE (T) OR FALSE (F) FOR EACH OF THE RESPONSE CHOICES.

21. Concerning testicular torsion,

    (A) it almost never resolves spontaneously

    (B) if it is reversed between 12 and 24 hours, the likelihood of testicular salvage is >50%

    (C) an associated "bell clapper" deformity is bilateral in most patients

    (D) the epididymis is usually not involved

    (E) it is often preceded by trauma, strenuous exercise, or sexual intercourse

22. Concerning epididymitis,

    (A) it is the most common cause of acute scrotal pain in adults

    (B) it is occasionally isolated to the epididymal tail

    (C) severe cases are occasionally associated with testicular ischemia

    (D) associated peritesticular fluid usually indicates an abscess

23. Concerning testicular tumors,

    (A) they most often present as a painless mass

    (B) most are germ cell tumors

    (C) about 20% are bilateral

    (D) calcification implies a benign histology

    (E) seminomas are avascular or hypovascular

24. Concerning varicoceles,

    (A) most are bilateral

    (B) most are asymptomatic

    (C) most are caused by spermatic vein obstruction

    (D) when they are nonpalpable, repair is not indicated

    (E) venous flow is generally detected only with special maneuvers

CASE 5 (Cont'd)

25. Concerning the normal vascular anatomy of the scrotum,

F (A) the spermatic cord contains three arteries
F (B) intratesticular arteries are not visible on gray-scale sonography
T (C) intratesticular arterial blood flow is directed both toward and away from the mediastinum testis
T (D) centripetal arteries are supplied by capsular arteries
T (E) vascular resistance in the normal testis is high

This 65-year-old man presented with fever and right abdominal pain. You are shown transverse sonograms obtained through the right flank (Figure 6-1).

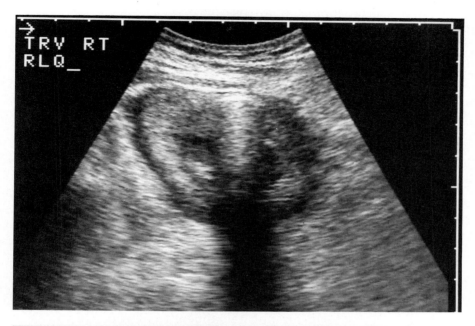

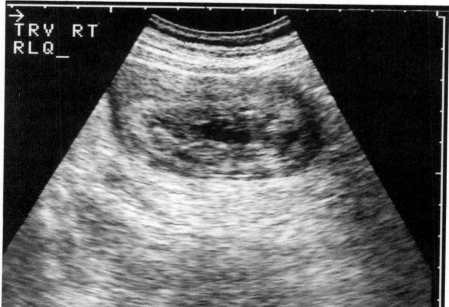

Figure 6-1

26. Which *one* of the following is the MOST likely diagnosis?

    (A) Ischemic colitis
    (B) Periappendiceal abscess
    (C) Mucocele
    (D) Intussusception
    (E) Crohn's disease

QUESTIONS 27 THROUGH 29: MARK YOUR ANSWER SHEET TRUE (T) OR FALSE (F) FOR EACH OF THE RESPONSE CHOICES.

27. Concerning appendicitis,

    (A) the risk of appendiceal perforation is greatest in very young and very old patients
    (B) the highest rate of negative laparotomy for suspected appendicitis occurs in children
    (C) the normal upper limit for appendiceal diameter is 6 mm
    (D) the criteria for normal appendiceal wall thickness in children are the same as those for adults
    (E) free fluid around the cecum is a reliable sonographic sign of perforation

28. Concerning mucocele of the appendix,

    (A) it occurs most commonly in middle-aged to elderly women
    (B) it is due to a benign lesion in approximately 90% of cases
    (C) it generally appears as an anechoic mass in the right lower quadrant
    (D) the presence of wall calcification in a right-lower-quadrant mass should suggest the diagnosis
    (E) pseudomyxoma peritonei is a frequent complication

CASE 6 (Cont'd)

29. Concerning intussusception,

 (A) it is the most common cause of bowel obstruction in patients between 2 months and 5 years of age

 (B) the spontaneous perforation rate is about 5%

 (C) a malignant tumor acts as the lead point in about 75% of adult patients

 (D) it is characterized by a "coiled-spring" appearance on sonograms

 (E) free fluid contraindicates enema reduction

This 33-year-old woman had a maternal α-fetoprotein level in serum elevated three multiples of the mean at 16 weeks gestation. You are shown four images of the fetal head obtained during a fetal sonographic examination performed at 18 weeks gestation (Figure 7-1).

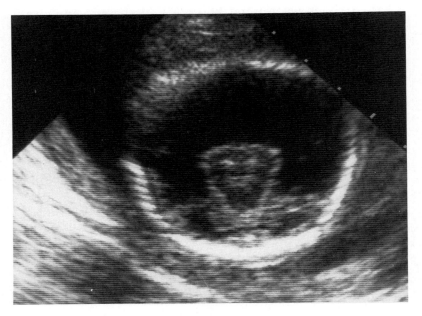

Figure 7-1

30. Which *one* of the following is the MOST likely diagnosis?

    (A) Hydranencephaly
    (B) Porencephaly
    (C) Hydrocephalus
    (D) Semilobar holoprosencephaly
    (E) Agenesis of the corpus callosum

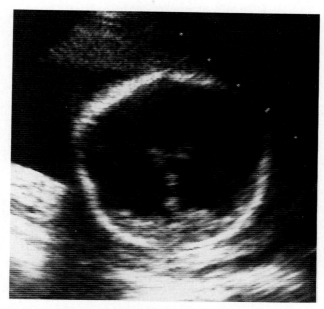

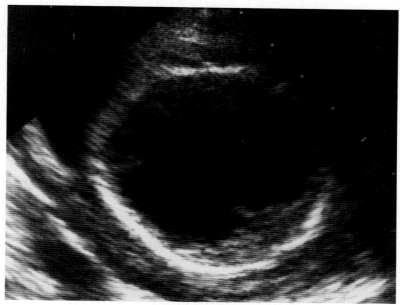

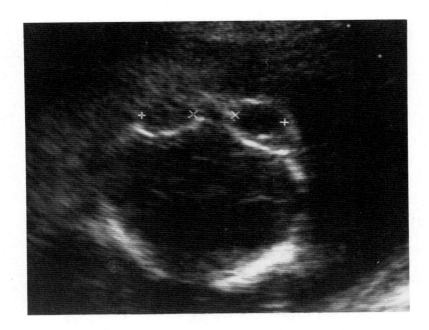

QUESTIONS 31 THROUGH 34: MARK YOUR ANSWER SHEET TRUE (T) OR FALSE (F) FOR EACH OF THE RESPONSE CHOICES.

31. Concerning hydranencephaly,

    T (A) associated anomalies are common

    T (B) the prognosis is uniformly poor

    F (C) macrocephaly is nearly always present *in utero*

    T (D) the presence of a partial falx distinguishes it from holoprosencephaly

    T (E) the absence of infratentorial structures distinguishes it from holoprosencephaly

32. Findings frequently associated with semilobar holoprosencephaly include:

   T (A) absence of the septum pellucidum
   T (B) large dorsal cyst
   T (C) renal dysplasia
   T (D) agenesis of the corpus callosum
   F (E) macrocephaly

33. Concerning holoprosencephaly,

   T (A) the detection of cyclopia or ethmocephaly is diagnostic
   T (B) the absence of facial anomalies excludes the diagnosis of the alobar form
   T (C) trisomy 13 is the most commonly associated chromosomal abnormality
   T (D) it is prognostically important to distinguish the alobar form from the semilobar form
   T (E) most cases are sporadic and clinically unsuspected

34. Concerning sonography of the fetal brain,

   F (A) the ratio of the lateral ventricular width to the hemispheric width is relatively constant throughout gestation
   T (B) the width of the lateral ventricle measured at the level of the atrium is relatively constant throughout gestation
   T (C) a lateral ventricular atrial width greater than 10 mm is considered abnormal
   T (D) the choroid plexus normally fills the entire ventricular width
   F (E) ventriculomegaly is usually an isolated fetal abnormality

CASE 8: Questions 35 through 38

This 60-year-old man was referred for transrectal sonography of the prostate gland because of urinary frequency and postvoid dribbling. You are shown transverse (A) and midline sagittal (B) images (Figure 8-1).

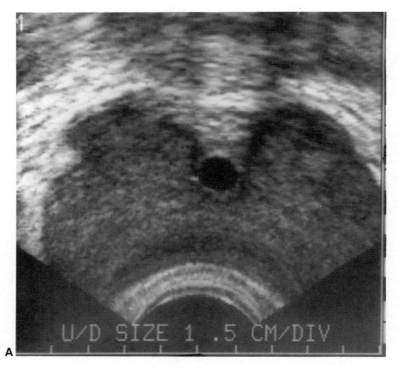

Figure 8-1

35. Which *one* of the following is the MOST likely diagnosis?

    (A) Cystic carcinoma
    (B) Ejaculatory duct cyst
    (C) Prostatic utricle cyst
    (D) Seminal vesicle cyst
    (E) Retention cyst

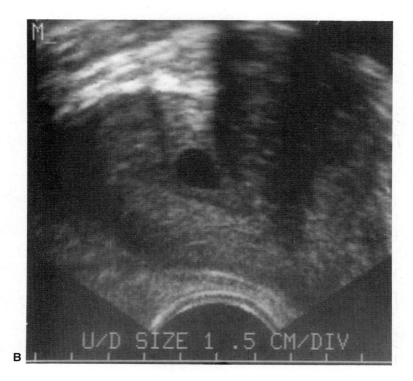

QUESTIONS 36 THROUGH 38: MARK YOUR ANSWER SHEET TRUE (T) OR FALSE (F) FOR EACH OF THE RESPONSE CHOICES.

36.   Concerning carcinoma of the prostate,

   (A) most cases arise within the transition zone of the gland
   (B) it usually appears hypoechoic on sonography
   (C) it frequently contains cystic areas caused by tumor ne-
        crosis
   (D) the sensitivity of transrectal sonography for its detec-
        tion is greater than 90%
   (E) it is accurately staged by transrectal sonography

37. Factors of value in distinguishing cancer of the prostate from benign prostatic hyperplasia include:

   (A) location of the lesion
   (B) presence of urinary retention
   (C) echogenicity of the lesion
   (D) prostate gland volume
   (E) level of prostate-specific antigen in serum

38. Concerning cysts seen on transrectal sonography,

   (A) seminal vesicle cysts are associated with autosomal dominant polycystic disease
   (B) ejaculatory duct cysts are associated with renal agenesis
   (C) ejaculatory duct cysts are associated with hematospermia
   (D) prostatic utricle cysts are associated with cryptorchidism
   (E) prostatic utricle cysts usually contain spermatozoa
   (F) retention cysts are usually associated with ejaculatory pain

This 40-year-old woman complained of vague lower abdominal discomfort. A mass was palpable on pelvic examination. You are shown longitudinal (A) and transverse (B) sonograms of the right pelvis (Figure 9-1).

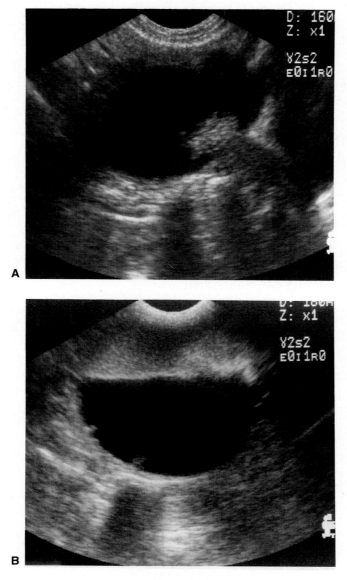

Figure 9-1

CASE 9 (Cont'd)

39. Which *one* of the following is the MOST likely diagnosis?

   (A) Chronic ectopic pregnancy
   (B) Cystic teratoma
   (C) Endometrioma
   (D) Ovarian cystadenocarcinoma
   (E) Appendiceal abscess

QUESTIONS 40 THROUGH 42: MARK YOUR ANSWER SHEET TRUE (T) OR FALSE (F) FOR EACH OF THE RESPONSE CHOICES.

40. Concerning cystic teratoma,

   T (A) it is the most common germ cell tumor
   T (B) the purely cystic form is uncommon
   T (C) it often simulates bowel on sonography
   T (D) the "tip of the iceberg" sign refers to acoustic shadowing from teeth
   T (E) there is a 10% risk of malignant transformation

41. Concerning endometrioma,

   F (A) it is the most common form of endometriosis
   F (B) age is helpful in distinguishing it from cystadenocarci- noma
   F (C) the most common sonographic appearance is a simple cystic mass
   T (D) the ovary is the most common site
   F (E) acoustic shadowing differentiates it from cystic ter- atoma

CASE 9 (Cont'd)

42. Concerning cystadenocarcinomas,

~T~ (A) they arise from the ovarian stroma

~T~ (B) septations and papillary excrescences are typical of both mucinous and serous tumors

~F~ (C) they are the most common cause of simple unilocular ovarian cysts in postmenopausal patients

~F~ (D) they are the most common cause of pseudomyxoma peritonei

~F~ (E) Doppler sonography usually shows abnormally high diastolic flow

This 33-year-old woman has upper abdominal pain. You are shown selected axial (A) and sagittal (B) upper abdominal sonograms and a coronal sonogram through the left flank (C) (Figure 10-1).

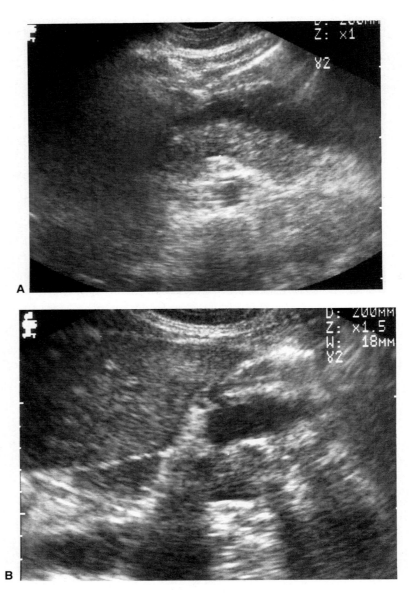

Figure 10-1

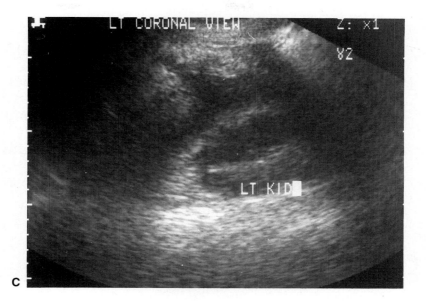

c

43. Which *one* of the following is the MOST likely diagnosis?

    (A) Gastric outlet obstruction
    (B) Acute pancreatitis
    (C) Lymphadenopathy
    (D) Chronic pancreatitis
    (E) Cystic pancreatic neoplasm

QUESTIONS 44 THROUGH 46: MARK YOUR ANSWER SHEET TRUE (T) OR FALSE (F) FOR EACH OF THE RESPONSE CHOICES.

44. Concerning chronic pancreatitis,

    (A) the sonographic finding of pancreatic ductal calcification is diagnostic
    (B) it is associated with characteristic changes in pancreatic parenchymal echogenicity
    (C) it is rarely focal
    (D) it is a progressive disease
    (E) it is rarely caused by gallstones

CASE 10 (Cont'd)

45. Concerning cystic pancreatic neoplasms,

T (A) microcystic adenoma (serous cystadenoma) has virtually no malignant potential

F (B) a specific diagnosis can often be made on the basis of
imaging features alone

T (C) mucinous cystic tumors commonly demonstrate multiple tiny cysts on sonography

T (D) amorphous calcifications are commonly present within
the center of a microcystic adenoma

T (E) the glycogen-rich cytoplasm of the cells lining the cyst
of a microcystic adenoma is a diagnostic feature

46. Concerning carcinoma of the pancreas,

F (A) dilatation of the pancreatic duct is common

F (B) the presence of a pseudocyst effectively excludes the diagnosis

T (C) it most often appears as a focal, relatively hypoechoic
pancreatic mass

F (D) on contrast-enhanced dynamic CT, significant enhancement of the tumor mass is common

F (E) at the time of diagnosis, it is rarely confined to the pancreas

This 72-year-old woman has right upper quadrant pain and jaundice. You are shown transverse (A) and longitudinal (B) right upper quadrant sonograms (Figure 11-1).

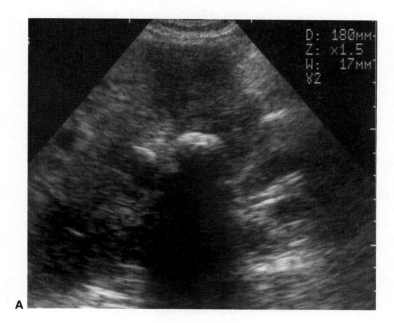

Figure 11-1

47. Which *one* of the following is the MOST likely diagnosis?

(A) Carcinoma of the gallbladder
(B) Hepatocellular carcinoma
(C) Hepatic abscess
(D) Acute cholecystitis
(E) Carcinoma of the hepatic flexure of the colon

CASE 11 (Cont'd)

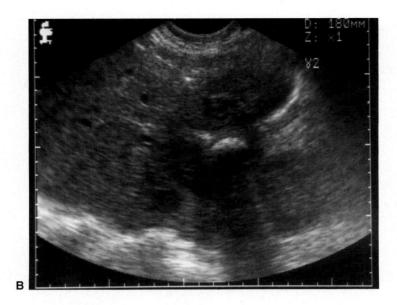

B

QUESTIONS 48 THROUGH 50: MARK YOUR ANSWER SHEET TRUE (T) OR FALSE (F) FOR EACH OF THE RESPONSE CHOICES.

48.   Concerning gallbladder carcinoma,

    T (A)   it is more common in women than in men

    T (B)   it is commonly associated with gallstones

    T (C)   there is an increased incidence in patients with porcelain gallbladder

    F (D)   it frequently obstructs the common bile duct

    T (E)   regional metastases are frequently present at the time of diagnosis

CASE 11 (Cont'd)

49. Concerning hepatic abscess,

    (A) it most commonly appears as an anechoic mass

    (B) its appearance on contrast-enhanced CT is generally diagnostic

    (C) hepatic candidiasis commonly presents as multiple microabscesses

    (D) it is a complication of amebic colitis in about 50% of patients

50. Causes of gallbladder wall thickening include:

    (A) nephrotic syndrome

    (B) constrictive pericarditis

    (C) hepatic veno-occlusive disease

    (D) leukemia

    (E) Kawasaki's disease

You are shown sonograms from two brothers. One is a transverse view of the lower pole of the left kidney in the 31-year-old brother (A), and one is a transverse view of the pancreatic body in the 27-year-old brother (B) (Figure 12-1).

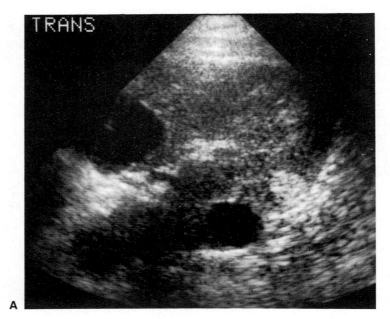

Figure 12-1

51. Which *one* of the following is the MOST likely diagnosis?

(A) Autosomal dominant polycystic disease
(B) Tuberous sclerosis
(C) Acquired cystic disease
(D) von Hippel-Lindau disease
(E) Cystic fibrosis

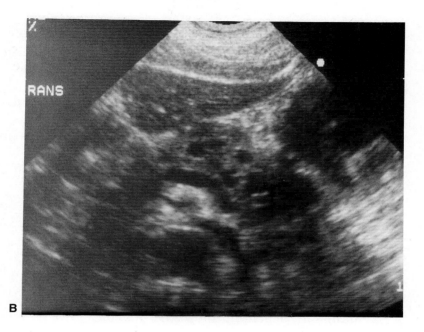

B

QUESTIONS 52 THROUGH 54: MARK YOUR ANSWER SHEET TRUE (T) OR FALSE (F) FOR EACH OF THE RESPONSE CHOICES.

52.   Concerning acquired cystic disease of the kidney,

   (A)   it occurs in patients undergoing either chronic hemodialysis or peritoneal dialysis
   (B)   it occurs in patients with chronic renal disease who are not undergoing dialysis
   (C)   it is usually sonographically apparent within the first year of dialysis
   (D)   cyst hemorrhage is a common complication
   (E)   sonography is more sensitive than CT in detecting solid renal lesions

53. Concerning tuberous sclerosis,

    (A) the classic clinical triad consists of mental retardation, seizures, and cutaneous lesions
    (B) it is associated with atrial myxomas
    (C) pulmonary involvement often results in spontaneous pneumothorax
    (D) associated angiomyolipomas are usually multiple and bilateral
    (E) associated angiomyolipomas occur in about 20% of patients

54. Concerning sporadic renal angiomyolipoma,

    (A) it is a cause of spontaneous perinephric hematoma
    (B) sonography is diagnostic in most patients
    (C) it occurs more frequently in women than in men
    (D) calcification occurs in approximately 20% of patients
    (E) malignant degeneration occurs in about 5% of patients

This 37-year-old gravida 3, para 1 woman underwent obstetric sonography at 23-weeks gestational age because of vaginal bleeding. You are shown longitudinal (A) and transverse (B) images through the lower uterus (Figure 13-1).

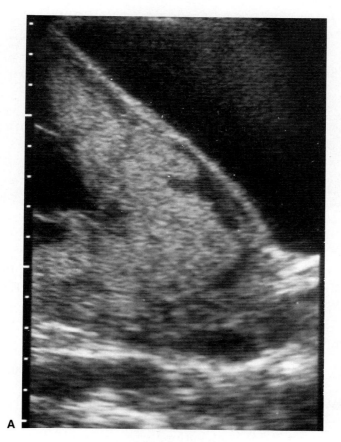

Figure 13-1

55. Which *one* of the following is the MOST likely diagnosis?

    (A) Marginal placenta previa
    (B) Placenta increta
    (C) Subchorionic hemorrhage
    (D) Gestational trophoblastic disease
    (E) Abruptio placentae

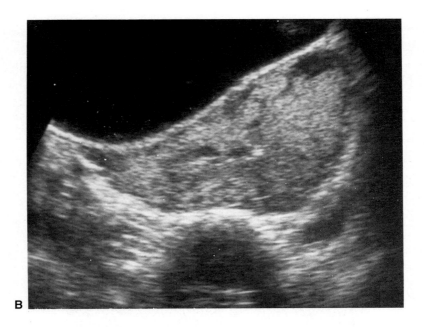

B

QUESTIONS 56 THROUGH 58: MARK YOUR ANSWER SHEET TRUE (T) OR FALSE (F) FOR EACH OF THE RESPONSE CHOICES.

56. Concerning placenta previa,

(A) the presence of a succenturiate lobe can result in a false-positive diagnosis

(B) transvaginal scanning is often necessary for diagnosis in the third trimester

(C) myometrial contractions can cause a false-positive diagnosis in early pregnancy

(D) placenta accreta is rarely associated with it

(E) in most cases of central placenta previa diagnosed in early pregnancy, the placenta migrates to a nonobstructing position by the third trimester

CASE 13 (Cont'd)

57. Concerning pregnancy-related hemorrhage,

    (A) about 50% of women with vaginal bleeding in the first 20 weeks of pregnancy have sonographic evidence of subchorionic hemorrhage

    (B) subchorionic hemorrhage is identified sonographically by its predominantly retroplacental locus

    (C) the sensitivity of sonography for detection of abruptio placentae is lower than 50%

    (D) placenta accreta is a cause of persistent postpartum hemorrhage

    (E) life-threatening hemorrhage is associated with velamentous cord insertion

58. Concerning gestational trophoblastic disease,

    (A) the typical vesicular appearance of a complete hydatidiform mole is usually not sonographically apparent until about 12 weeks

    (B) a normal placenta can be seen in association with a complete hydatidiform mole

    (C) a fetus seen in association with a partial hydatidiform mole usually has a triploid karyotype

    (D) about 50% of patients with a complete hydatidiform mole will develop persistent, invasive, or malignant trophoblastic disease

    (E) bilateral hemorrhagic corpus luteum cysts are seen in about 40% of patients with hydatidiform moles

This 32-year-old HIV-positive man presented for abdominal sonography because of elevated liver enzyme levels. You are shown transverse (A), longitudinal (B), and magnified (C) views of the liver (Figure 14-1).

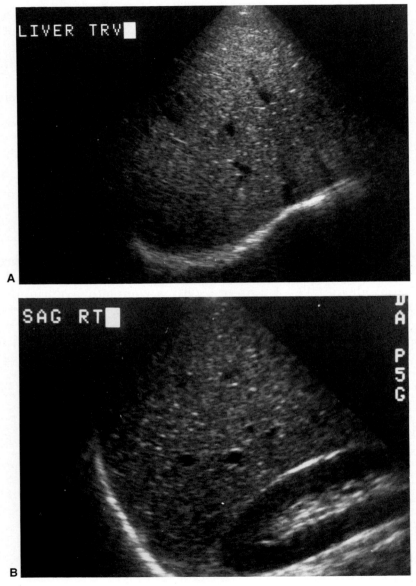

Figure 14-1

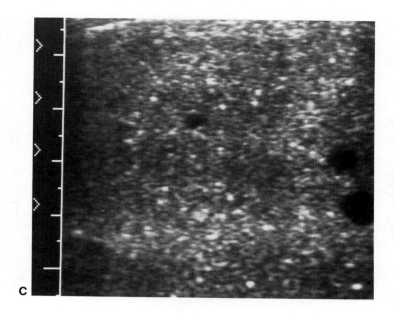

C

59.   Which *one* of the following is the MOST likely diagnosis?

(A)   Lymphoma
(B)   Metastatic Kaposi's sarcoma
(C)   *Pneumocystis carinii* infection
(D)   Peliosis hepatis
(E)   Viral hepatitis

CASE 14 (Cont'd)

QUESTIONS 60 THROUGH 62: MARK YOUR ANSWER SHEET TRUE (T) OR FALSE (F) FOR EACH OF THE RESPONSE CHOICES.

60. Concerning AIDS-related lymphoma,

    T (A) it is associated with Epstein-Barr virus infection
    F (B) it is preceded by progressive generalized lymphadenop-
            athy in most patients
    F (C) it has a predilection for female patients
    F (D) visceral involvement occurs less frequently than it does
            with lymphoma in the general population
    T (E) its sonographic appearance ranges from hypoechoic to
            hyperechoic relative to hepatic parenchyma

61. Concerning AIDS-related Kaposi's sarcoma,

    T (A) its incidence is increasing
    T (B) it occurs predominantly in homosexual patients
    T (C) it is confined to the skin in most patients
    F (D) visceral involvement is easily detected by imaging
            methods
    T (E) hepatic nodules appear hypoechoic on sonography

62. Concerning extrapulmonary *Pneumocystis carinii* infection,

    T (A) it is uncommon
    T (B) most patients with disseminated infection have a his-
            tory of *P. carinii* pneumonia
    T (C) it is characterized pathologically by granuloma forma-
            tion
    F (D) sonography is more sensitive than CT for detection of
            hepatic involvement
    F (E) the sonographic patterns of hepatic and splenic involve-
            ment are different

This 25-year-old pregnant woman underwent obstetric sonography because of a size-date discrepancy. You are shown transverse sonograms of the fetal thorax (A) and upper abdomen (B) and a longitudinal sonogram of the fetal trunk (C) (Figure 15-1).

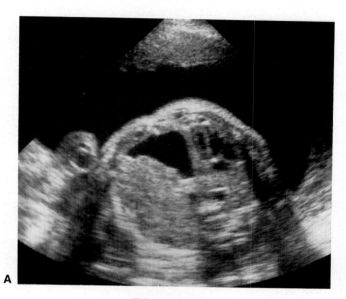

Figure 15-1

63. Which *one* of the following is the MOST likely diagnosis?

   (A) Hydrothorax
   (B) Cystic adenomatoid malformation
   (C) Bronchogenic cyst
   (D) Diaphragmatic hernia
   (E) Asplenia

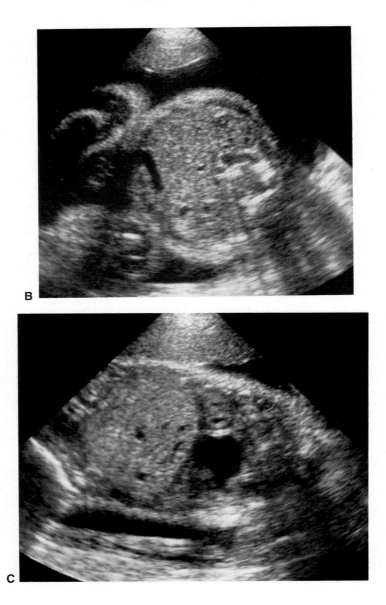

CASE 15 (Cont'd)

QUESTIONS 64 THROUGH 66: MARK YOUR ANSWER SHEET TRUE (T) OR FALSE (F) FOR EACH OF THE RESPONSE CHOICES.

64. Concerning fetal diaphragmatic hernia,

T (A) with a left-sided hernia, the cardiac axis is usually altered so that the apex is directed to the fetal right

T (B) about 30% of fetuses with a prenatal diagnosis will survive

F (C) about 30 to 40% of affected fetuses have an associated structural or chromosomal defect

T (D) early detection (prior to 24 weeks) improves outcome

T (E) there is an 85% mortality rate if polyhydramnios is present

65. Concerning fetal cardiac ultrasonography,

T (A) over 90% of cardiac defects are detected on the four-chamber view

T (B) about 25% of fetuses with a cardiac anomaly detectable on prenatal sonography have a chromosomal abnormality

T (C) pulmonary hypoplasia due to an increased cardiothoracic ratio results from a cardiac abnormality in 75% of cases

F (D) about 50% of fetuses with complete heart block have a structural cardiac defect

T (E) a parallel orientation of the great vessels at the base of the heart is normal

66. Concerning the fetal thorax,

T (A) lung growth continues postnatally with further formation of alveoli

T (B) alveolar growth starts in the early second trimester

T (C) most fetuses with type I (macrocystic) cystic adenomatoid malformation die

T (D) pulmonary hypoplasia is usually secondary to a fetal genitourinary tract anomaly with oligohydramnios

T (E) a unilateral, right-sided pleural effusion is usually secondary to congenital heart disease

This 23-year-old woman presented to the emergency room with a history of pelvic pain and irregular vaginal bleeding. You are shown sagittal (A and B) and coronal (C) transvaginal sonograms of the lower pelvis (Figure 16-1).

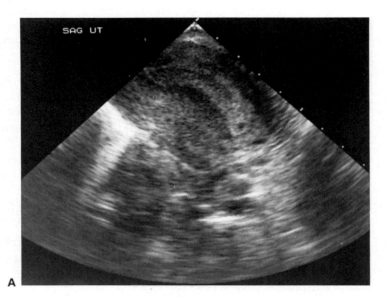

Figure 16-1

67. Which *one* of the following is the MOST likely diagnosis?

   (A) Pelvic inflammatory disease with endometritis
   (B) Ectopic pregnancy
   (C) Early intrauterine gestation with hemorrhagic corpus luteum cyst
   (D) Missed abortion with degenerating products of conception
   (E) Ovarian dermoid

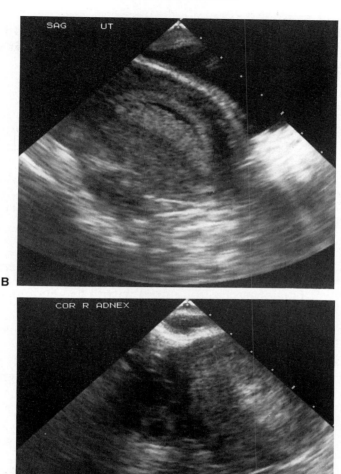

B

C

CASE 16 (Cont'd)

QUESTIONS 68 THROUGH 72: MARK YOUR ANSWER SHEET TRUE (T) OR FALSE (F) FOR EACH OF THE RESPONSE CHOICES.

68. Concerning acute pelvic inflammatory disease,

    T (A) it affects 1% of women between 15 and 39 years of age

    F (B) the "indefinite uterus sign" (poorly defined uterine border) is a specific sonographic sign

    F (C) tubo-ovarian abscesses are commonly unilocular

    T (D) the ovaries are involved in only the most severe cases

    T (E) tubo-ovarian abscess is easily distinguished from appendiceal abscess by transvaginal sonography

69. Concerning the pseudogestational sac of ectopic pregnancy,

    T (A) it is characterized by fluid within the endometrial cavity

    T (B) it can be located within any segment of the uterus

    T (C) it is due to sloughing decidua

    F (D) it has a single surrounding echogenic wall

    T (E) it occurs in approximately 30% of ectopic pregnancies

70. Concerning ectopic pregnancy,

    T (A) transvaginal sonograms usually provide more information than transabdominal scans do

    T (B) a live extrauterine fetus is identifiable sonographically in fewer than 25% of cases

    T (C) isthmic pregnancies tend to rupture latest

    T (D) in a patient with a positive pregnancy test, the finding of particulate cul-de-sac fluid strongly suggests the diagnosis

    T (E) in a patient with a positive pregnancy test, a tubal ring usually represents an unruptured ectopic pregnancy

CASE 16 (Cont'd)

71. Concerning early intrauterine pregnancy,

F (A) threatened abortion occurs in approximately 25% of pregnancies

T (B) embryonic cardiac motion is consistently identifiable on transvaginal scans by 46 menstrual days in all normal gestations

T (C) a disproportionately low serum human chorionic gona-dotropin (β-hCG) level usually indicates incomplete abortion

T (D) most abnormal gestations cease development before a recognizable embryo is formed

F (E) weak choriodecidual echogenicity is a criterion of an abnormal gestational sac

72. Concerning the corpus luteum cysts of pregnancy,

T (A) they form in the ovary at the site of a ruptured follicle

F (B) they are similar in size to follicular cysts

T (C) they are typically both unilocular and unilateral

T (D) they are prone to intermittent hemorrhage and rupture

T (E) most resolve by 6 weeks

This 31-year-old woman was large for dates at 18 weeks gestation. You are shown sonograms of a twin gestation (Figure 17-1). The fetuses are labeled A and B.

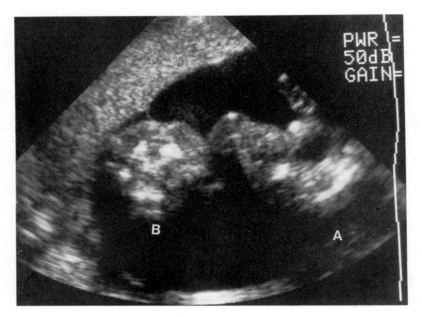

Figure 17-1

73. Which *one* of the following is the MOST likely diagnosis?

   (A) Duodenal atresia in twin A
   (B) Twin-twin transfusion syndrome
   (C) Intrauterine growth retardation in twin B
   (D) Monoamniotic twinning
   (E) Normal twins with idiopathic polyhydramnios

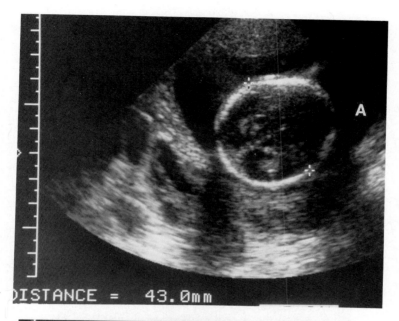

DISTANCE = 43.0mm

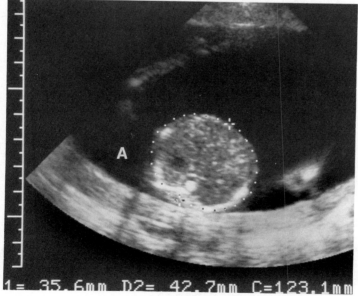

1= 35.6mm D2= 42.7mm C=123.1mm

Figure 17-1 (Continued)

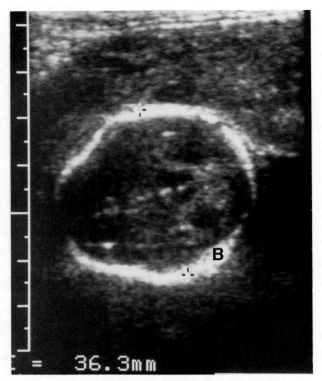

Figure 17-1 (Continued)

QUESTIONS 74 THROUGH 77: MARK YOUR ANSWER SHEET TRUE (T) OR FALSE (F) FOR EACH OF THE RESPONSE CHOICES.

74.   Concerning twin-twin transfusion syndrome,

   (A)   the most common sonographic sign is a discrepancy in amniotic fluid volume between gestational sacs
   (B)   all monozygotic twins are at risk of developing it
   (C)   percutaneous umbilical blood sampling is useful in differentiating it from other causes of a "stuck twin"
   (D)   multiorgan vascular insults occur in both donor and recipient twins

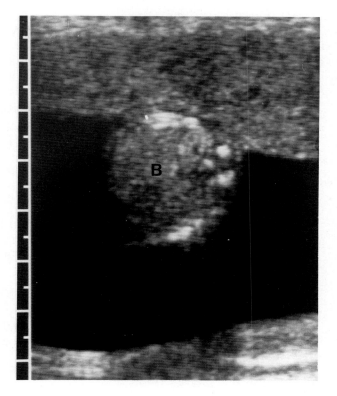

Figure 17-1 (Continued)

75. Concerning intrauterine growth retardation,

   (A) uteroplacental dysfunction accounts for 75% of fetuses that fall below the 10th-percentile weight for gestational age

   (B) the sonographic diagnosis depends on an accurate estimation of gestational age

   (C) the head-to-abdomen circumference ratio is useful for detecting "asymmetric" growth retardation

   (D) the head-to-abdomen circumference ratio is age independent

   (E) the femur length-to-abdomen circumference ratio is useful for detecting "symmetric" growth retardation

   (F) the umbilical artery Doppler waveform shows increased diastolic flow

CASE 17 (Cont'd)

76. Concerning polyhydramnios,

   (A) the most common fetal cause of severe polyhydramnios is a central nervous system abnormality
   (B) when associated with fetal small bowel obstruction, the obstruction is usually proximal
   (C) when present with intrauterine growth retardation, it suggests a congenital anomaly or chromosomal defect
   (D) it is found in about 25% of patients with fetal hydrops

77. Concerning twin gestations,

   (A) dizygotic pregnancies are always dichorionic
   (B) about 10% of dichorionic/diamniotic twins are monozygotic
   (C) with monoamniotic twinning, the fetal mortality is about 20%
   (D) in most cases, the demise of one twin in the first trimester has no untoward effects on the surviving twin
   (E) overall, they are associated with a threefold-greater frequency of fetal anomalies than are singleton pregnancies

This 25-year-old woman underwent routine obstetric sonography at 28 weeks gestation. You are shown transverse images of the fetal upper abdomen (A) and mid-abdomen (B) and a longitudinal image of the fetal trunk (C) (Figure 18-1).

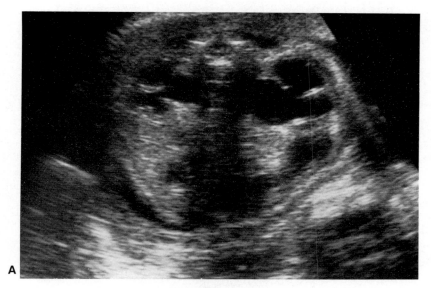

A

Figure 18-1

78. Which *one* of the following is the MOST likely diagnosis?

   (A) Duplication anomaly with obstruction
   (B) Prune belly syndrome
   (C) Multicystic renal dysplasia
   (D) Posterior urethral valves
   (E) Autosomal recessive polycystic disease

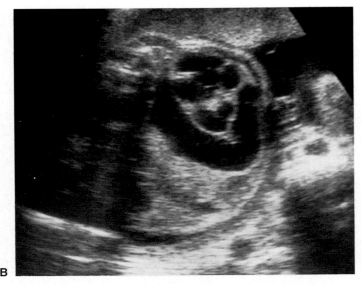

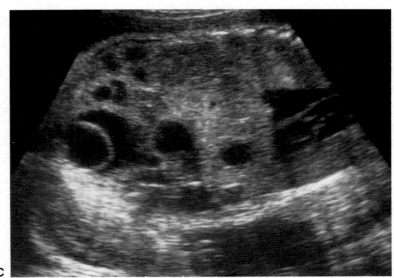

QUESTIONS 79 THROUGH 81: MARK YOUR ANSWER SHEET TRUE (T) OR FALSE (F) FOR EACH OF THE RESPONSE CHOICES.

79.   Concerning fetal hydronephrosis,

   (A)   in the second trimester, the normal renal pelvis measures no more than 5 mm in its anteroposterior dimension
   (B)   ureteropelvic junction obstruction is associated with polyhydramnios
   (C)   fetal interventional therapy for posterior urethral valves should be considered if the amniotic fluid volume is normal
   (D)   ureteropelvic junction obstruction is bilateral in about 20% of cases
   (E)   decompression of the obstruction with formation of urine ascites is a favorable prognostic sign

80.   Concerning fetal renal cystic disease,

   (A)   cystic renal dysplasia is secondary to obstruction in 90% of cases
   (B)   in fetuses with an obstructive uropathy, sonographic detection of renal cysts indicates irreversible cystic renal dysplasia (Potter type IV)
   (C)   about 30% of fetuses with a multicystic dysplastic kidney have a significant contralateral renal anomaly
   (D)   the kidneys in fetuses with autosomal recessive polycystic disease are both large and hypoechoic
   (E)   about 30% of fetuses with trisomy 13 have renal cysts

81.   Concerning fetal renal sonography,

   (A)   the normal range of the ratio of kidney circumference to abdominal circumference is 0.38 to 0.42
   (B)   normal amniotic fluid volume at 14 weeks gestational age excludes bilateral renal agenesis
   (C)   a solid renal mass associated with polyhydramnios is most probably due to a congenital Wilms' tumor
   (D)   about 50% of fetuses with a single umbilical artery have a renal abnormality

CASE 19: Questions 82 through 87

You are shown renal sonograms from four different patients (Figures 19-1 through 19-4). For each of the numbered sonograms listed below (Questions 82 through 85), select the *one* lettered diagnosis (A, B, C, D, or E) that is MOST likely. Each lettered diagnosis may be used once, more than once, or not at all.

82. Figure 19-1
83. Figure 19-2
84. Figure 19-3
85. Figure 19-4

(A) Emphysematous pyelonephritis
(B) Renal tubular acidosis
(C) Oxalosis
(D) Normal kidney
(E) Xanthogranulomatous pyelonephritis

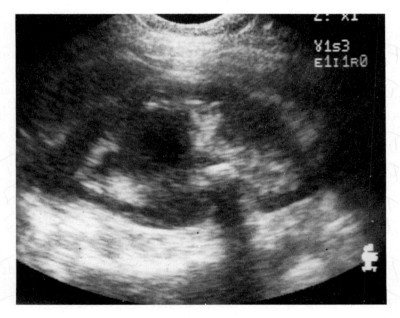

Figure 19-1

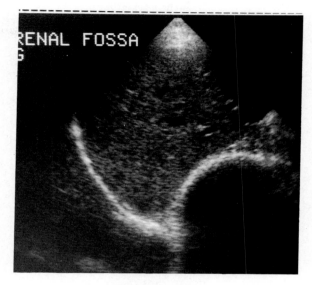

Figure 19-2

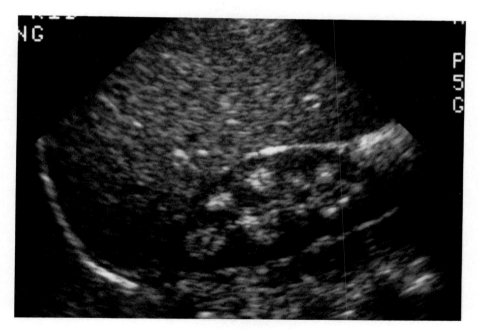

Figure 19-3

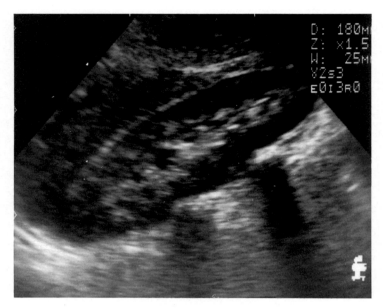

Figure 19-4

QUESTIONS 86 AND 87: MARK YOUR ANSWER SHEET TRUE
(T) OR FALSE (F) FOR EACH OF THE RESPONSE CHOICES.

86.   Concerning renal stones,

   (A)   the presence of acoustic shadowing depends on chemi-
         cal composition
   (B)   they are more accurately detected by sonography than
         by abdominal radiography
   (C)   they are reliably distinguished from pelvic blood clots
         by sonography
   (D)   detection of acoustic shadowing depends on the focal
         zone of the transducer
   (E)   normal renal structures simulate small stones sono-
         graphically

CASE 19 (Cont'd)

87. Concerning xanthogranulomatous pyelonephritis,

T (A) renal sonograms commonly demonstrate renal stones
F (B) most patients are asymptomatic
T (C) it is associated with a syndrome of reversible hepatic dysfunction
F (D) renal involvement is usually focal
F (E) it is frequently associated with renal cell carcinoma

This 35-year-old woman underwent routine obstetric sonography at 22 weeks gestational age. You are shown transverse sonograms of the upper (A) and lower (B) fetal abdomen and of the fetal chest (C) (Figure 20-1).

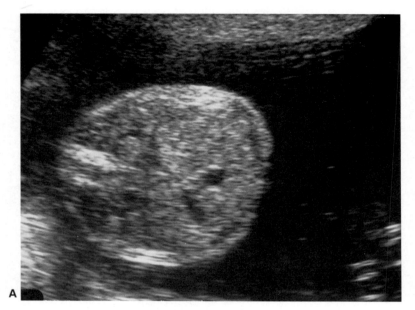

Figure 20-1

88. Which *one* of the following is the MOST likely diagnosis?

(A) Down's syndrome
(B) Beckwith-Wiedemann syndrome
(C) Turner's syndrome
(D) Limb-body wall complex
(E) Trisomy 18

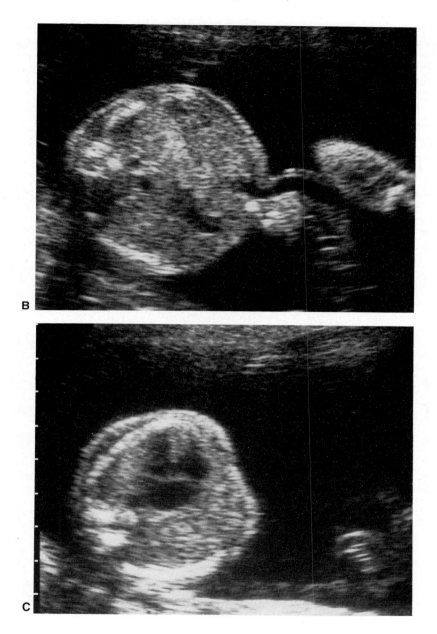

CASE 20 (Cont'd)

QUESTIONS 89 THROUGH 93: MARK YOUR ANSWER SHEET TRUE (T) OR FALSE (F) FOR EACH OF THE RESPONSE CHOICES.

89.   Concerning fetal abdominal wall defects,

   (A)   gastroschisis is frequently associated with genitourinary tract anomalies
   (B)   in up to 60% of cases, omphalocele is associated with other anomalies
   (C)   there is a 40 to 50% chance of an underlying chromosomal defect when an omphalocele is found
   (D)   a small omphalocele containing no liver has a lower probability of an associated chromosomal anomaly than does one containing liver
   (E)   scoliosis is a usual feature of limb-body wall complex

90.   Concerning the fetal anterior abdominal wall,

   (A)   the "mass" due to physiologic midgut herniation is not seen after 12 weeks gestational age
   (B)   an isolated omphalocele has a prognosis similar to that of gastroschisis
   (C)   maternal serum α-fetoprotein levels are higher with a gastroschisis than with an omphalocele
   (D)   typical sonographic features of gastroschisis include a right paraumbilical defect containing bowel but no liver
   (E)   typical sonographic features of omphalocele include a midline mass with a limiting membrane

CASE 20 (Cont'd)

91. Concerning fetal chromosomal abnormalities,

    (A) the risk of trisomy 18 in a fetus with an isolated choroid plexus cyst is 5 to 10%
    (B) karyotyping is indicated following detection of gastroschisis
    (C) chromosomal abnormalities are associated with 15% of early spontaneous abortions
    (D) identification of more than one anomaly increases the probability of a chromosomal abnormality
    (E) the trisomy syndrome most frequently associated with holoprosencephaly is Down's syndrome

92. Concerning Down's syndrome,

    (A) on sonography, affected fetuses usually have short femurs
    (B) about 10% of affected fetuses have duodenal atresia
    (C) it occurs in about 30% of fetuses with duodenal atresia
    (D) it is associated with fetal hydrops
    (E) septal defects are the most frequently imaged cardiac anomalies

93. Concerning fetal hydrops,

    (A) the earliest sonographic finding in the fetus is pericardial fluid
    (B) approximately 30% of cases are of immunologic etiology
    (C) the most common cause of nonimmune hydrops is intrauterine infection
    (D) the presence of associated bilateral cervical cystic hygromas suggests Turner's syndrome
    (E) the mortality rate in fetuses with nonimmune hydrops exceeds 50%

CASE 21: Questions 94 through 100

For each of the numbered normal Doppler waveforms listed below (Questions 94 through 97), select the *one* lettered vessel (A, B, C, D, or E) that is MOST closely associated with it. Each lettered vessel may be used once, more than once, or not at all.

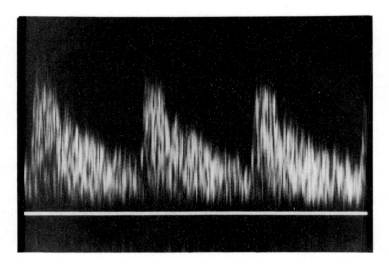

Figure 21-1

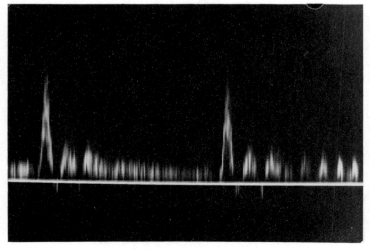

Figure 21-2

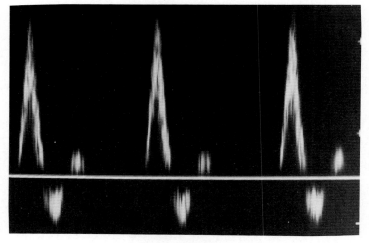

Figure 21-3

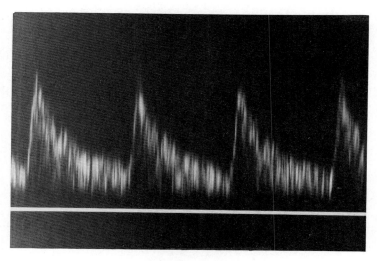

Figure 21-4

(A) External carotid artery
(B) Internal carotid artery
(C) Superficial femoral artery
(D) Renal arcuate artery
(E) Cavernosal artery

QUESTIONS 98 THROUGH 100: MARK YOUR ANSWER SHEET TRUE (T) OR FALSE (F) FOR EACH OF THE RESPONSE CHOICES.

98. Concerning postcatheterization arteriovenous fistulas,

T (A) they occur more frequently after arterial puncture below the femoral bifurcation than after puncture above it
T (B) they are readily detected by gray-scale sonography
T (C) they cause decreased diastolic flow in the proximal femoral artery
T (D) perivascular tissue vibration is a characteristic finding
T (E) venous pulsations are diagnostic

99. Concerning Doppler analysis of the neck vessels,

T (A) bidirectional flow in the vertebral artery is seen occasionally in patients with subclavian or innominate artery stenosis
F (B) gray-scale sonography is more reliable than spectral waveform analysis in detecting a stenosis of less than 50% diameter narrowing
T (C) "externalization" of the common carotid artery waveform occurs with occlusion of the external carotid artery
F (D) the accuracy of Doppler velocity calculations is independent of the Doppler angle
F (E) waveform aliasing can be eliminated by using a higher-frequency transducer

100. Concerning postcatheterization pseudoaneurysm,

T (A) swirling intraluminal blood flow is typical
F (B) "to and fro" blood flow in its neck is typical
F (C) surgical repair is necessary
F (D) it is often indistinguishable from a hematoma by gray-scale sonography
F (E) it generally communicates with the artery via a wide neck

This 51-year-old woman was evaluated by ultrasonography because of elevated liver function tests. You are shown transverse (A) and longitudinal (B) images through the region of the porta hepatis (Figure 22-1).

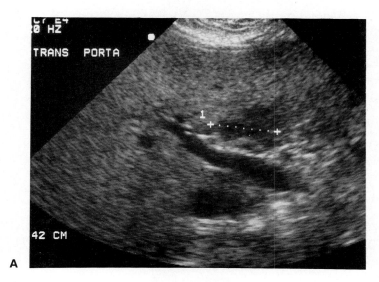

Figure 22-1

101. Which *one* of the following is the MOST likely diagnosis?

    (A) Metastases
    (B) Cavernous hemangioma
    (C) Fatty infiltration
    (D) Focal nodular hyperplasia
    (E) Lymphoma

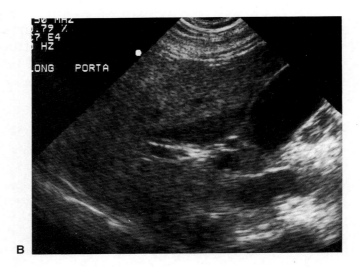

QUESTIONS 102 THROUGH 104: MARK YOUR ANSWER SHEET TRUE (T) OR FALSE (F) FOR EACH OF THE RESPONSE CHOICES.

102. Concerning metastatic disease to the liver,

   (A) calcification occurs most frequently in metastases from colon carcinoma
   (B) target lesions imply a squamous cell origin
   (C) intraoperative sonography is more sensitive than MRI in its detection
   (D) perihepatic ascites is an absolute contraindication to sonographically guided percutaneous biopsy
   (E) sonographic detection of focal lesions in livers that are diffusely heterogeneous as a result of cirrhosis usually indicates regenerating nodules

CASE 22 (Cont'd)

103. Concerning cavernous hemangiomas of the liver,

    (A) they typically exhibit blood flow in multiple vessels on color Doppler ultrasonography

    (B) there is no sex predisposition

    (C) large lesions are easier to characterize sonographically than are small lesions

    (D) scintigraphy with Tc-99m erythrocytes is more sensitive than MRI in detecting them

    (E) in about 25% of cases, percutaneous biopsy results in hemoperitoneum requiring transfusion

104. Concerning fatty infiltration of the liver,

    (A) focal involvement usually has smooth round margins

    (B) focal disease often localizes in the medial segment of the left lobe adjacent to the ligamentum teres

    (C) it increases acoustic attenuation

    (D) focal involvement occasionally simulates hepatic hemangioma

This 19-year-old woman presented with pelvic pain. You are shown transverse (A) and sagittal (B) sonograms of the right ovary (Figure 23-1). The left ovary appeared normal.

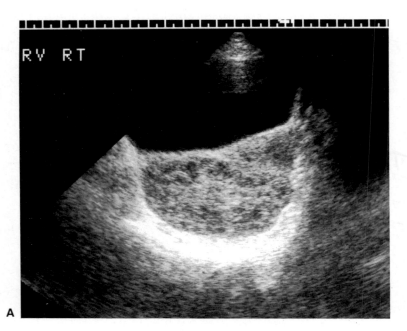

Figure 23-1

105. Which *one* of the following is the MOST likely diagnosis?

(A) Polycystic ovarian disease
(B) Endometrioma
(C) Ovarian torsion
(D) Tubo-ovarian abscess
(E) Hemorrhagic ovarian cyst

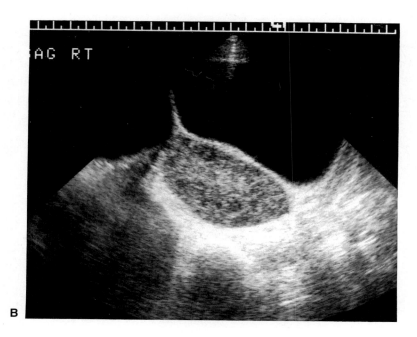

B

QUESTIONS 106 THROUGH 108: MARK YOUR ANSWER SHEET TRUE (T) OR FALSE (F) FOR EACH OF THE RESPONSE CHOICES.

106. Concerning polycystic ovarian disease,

    (A) most patients have the Stein-Leventhal syndrome
    (B) the ovaries are usually normal in size
    (C) it is usually bilateral
    (D) the follicles are usually greater than 1 cm in diameter

107. Concerning ovarian torsion,

    (A) it does not occur in normal ovaries
    (B) it occurs most commonly in prepubertal girls
    (C) the most typical appearance is an enlarged ovary with cortical follicles
    (D) the sonographic appearance is frequently normal
    (E) it is associated with fluid in the cul-de-sac

108. Concerning hemorrhagic ovarian cysts,

(A) most appear as heterogeneous masses
(B) about 20% appear completely anechoic
(C) more than 90% have increased through transmission
(D) they can generally be distinguished from other masses with a similar sonographic appearance by follow-up examination
(E) about 25% of affected patients have recurrent or concomitant ovarian cysts

This 45-year-old man has a history of left-upper-quadrant pain. You are shown left-upper-quadrant longitudinal (A) and transverse (B) sonograms (Figure 24-1).

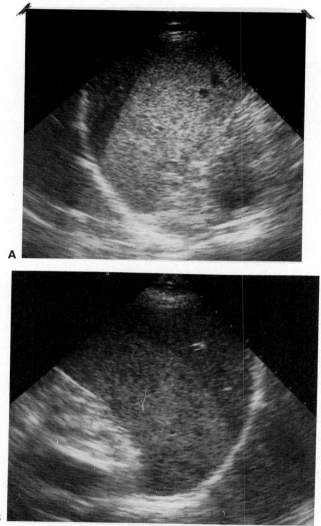

Figure 24-1

109. Which *one* of the following is the MOST likely diagnosis?

    (A) Normal variant
    (B) Splenic subcapsular hematoma
    (C) Left pleural effusion
    (D) Left subphrenic fluid collection
    (E) Splenic infarct

This 30-year-old man has abnormal liver function studies. You are shown a longitudinal sonogram of the porta hepatis (A) and two transverse sonograms of the liver (B and C) (Figure 25-1).

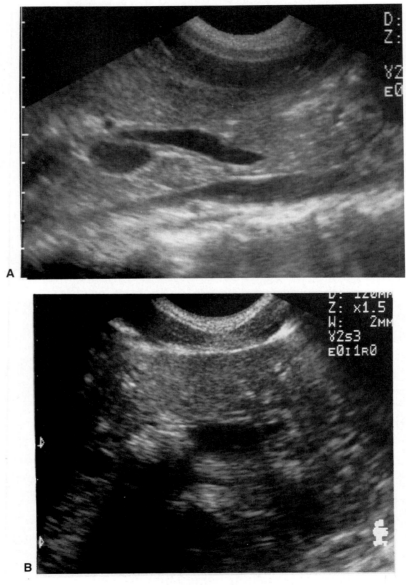

Figure 25-1

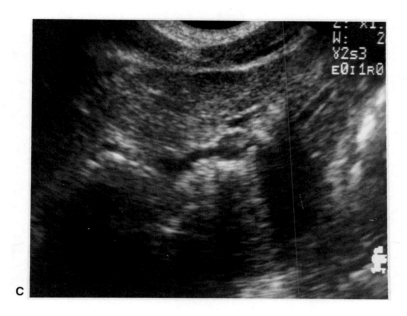

C

110. Which *one* of the following is the MOST likely diagnosis?

   (A) Benign common duct stricture
   (B) Primary sclerosing cholangitis
   (C) Oriental cholangiohepatitis
   (D) AIDS cholangitis
   (E) Choledocholithiasis

QUESTIONS 111 THROUGH 114: MARK YOUR ANSWER SHEET TRUE (T) OR FALSE (F) FOR EACH OF THE RESPONSE CHOICES.

111. Concerning primary sclerosing cholangitis,

   (A) it is associated with an increased risk of bile duct carcinoma
   (B) it is predominantly a disease of middle-aged women
   (C) obstructive jaundice is common
   (D) it is associated with choledocholithiasis
   (E) typically, both extra- and intrahepatic bile ducts are involved

CASE 25 (Cont'd)

112. Concerning Oriental cholangiohepatitis,

T (A) its sonographic diagnosis requires identification of intrahepatic duct stones

T (B) there is disproportionate dilatation of central intrahepatic bile ducts compared with peripheral ducts

F (C) the bile duct stones have the same chemical composition as most gallstones

T (D) it is commonly associated with cholangiocarcinoma

T (E) on sonography, increased periportal echogenicity is typical

113. Concerning AIDS cholangitis,

T (A) sonographically, there is focal nodular thickening of the common bile duct

T (B) dilatation of both intra- and extrahepatic bile ducts is common

T (C) on histologic evaluation, there is characteristic ductal and periportal inflammatory infiltrate

F (D) intrahepatic bile duct stones are common

F (E) it is most commonly caused by *Pneumocystis carinii*

114. Concerning choledocholithiasis,

F (A) the absence of associated acoustic shadowing excludes the diagnosis

T (B) the bile duct system is nearly always dilated

F (C) the sonographic detection rate is about 85%

F (D) it is commonly associated with cholangiocarcinoma

T (E) a fatty meal stimulation test is usually positive with obstructing stones

This 67-year-old woman presented with right upper quadrant pain. You are shown two longitudinal sonograms of the liver (Figure 26-1).

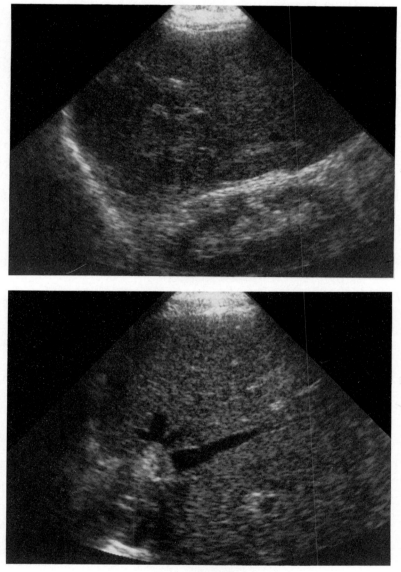

Figure 26-1

CASE 26 (Cont'd)

115. Which *one* of the following is the MOST likely diagnosis?

   (A) Metastasis
   (B) Abscess
   (C) Echinococcosis
   (D) Hepatic adenoma
   (E) Hepatocellular carcinoma

QUESTIONS 116 AND 117: MARK YOUR ANSWER SHEET TRUE (T) OR FALSE (F) FOR EACH OF THE RESPONSE CHOICES.

116. Concerning echinococcosis,

   F (A) no imaging technique can differentiate purely cystic hydatid lesions from simple hepatic cysts
   T (B) suspected echinococcal disease is a contraindication to percutaneous aspiration
   T (C) the brain is the second most frequently affected organ in humans
   T (D) the sonographic features depend on the specific parasite
   T (E) the presence of daughter cysts is pathognomonic

117. Concerning hepatocellular carcinoma,

   T (A) it is the most common neoplasm of the liver
   F (B) measurement of the serum α-fetoprotein level is an accurate screening test
   F (C) hepatic vein involvement is more common than portal vein involvement
   T (D) calcification is most common in the fibrolamellar form
   T (E) underlying cirrhosis limits the ability of both sonography and CT to assess the extent of the tumor

DEMOGRAPHIC DATA QUESTIONS

Please answer all of the questions below. The data you provide will be used to supply information that will allow you to compare your performance on the examination with that of others at similar levels of training and with similar backgrounds, and for purposes of planning continuing education projects. Please answer each question as accurately and as objectively as possible. Please mark the *one* BEST response for each question. Recall, of course, that we do *not* want individual names. Our analyses will reflect only categories and groups; everything will remain completely anonymous, and no attempt will be made to identify any specific individual.

118. The ACR will be evaluating the questions in this examination to determine their degree of difficulty and to determine the success of the examination as an instrument of self-evaluation and continuing education. To assist the ACR, please indicate in which of the following ways you took this examination.

   (A) Used reference materials or read the syllabus portion of this book to assist in answering some portion of the examination
   (B) Did not use reference materials and did not read the syllabus portion of this book while taking the examination

119. How much residency and fellowship training in Diagnostic Radiology have you completed?

   (A) None
   (B) Less than 1 year
   (C) 1 year
   (D) 2 years
   (E) 3 years
   (F) 4 or more years

DEMOGRAPHIC DATA QUESTIONS (Cont'd)

120. When did you finish your residency training in Radiology?

   (A) More than 10 years ago
   (B) 5 to 10 years ago
   (C) 1 to 5 years ago
   (D) Less than 1 year ago
   (E) Not yet completed
   (F) Radiology is not my specialty

121. Have you been certified by the American Board of Radiology in Diagnostic Radiology?

   (A) Yes
   (B) No

122. Have you completed fellowship training in Ultrasonography or Sectional Body Imaging?

   (A) Yes
   (B) No

123. Which one of the categories listed below BEST describes the setting of your practice in the immediate past 3 years? (For residents and fellows, in which one did you or will you spend the major portion of your residency or fellowship?)

   (A) Community or general hospital—less than 200 beds
   (B) Community or general hospital—200 to 499 beds
   (C) Community or general hospital—500 or more beds
   (D) University-affiliated hospital
   (E) Office practice

DEMOGRAPHIC DATA QUESTIONS (Cont'd)

124. In which *one* of the following general areas of Radiology do you consider yourself MOST expert?

    (A) Musculoskeletal radiology
    (B) Chest radiology
    (C) Gastrointestinal radiology
    (D) Genitourinary radiology
    (E) Head and neck radiology
    (F) Neuroradiology
    (G) Breast imaging
    (H) Pediatric radiology
    (I) Cardiovascular radiology
    (J) Other

125. In which *one* of the following radiologic modalities do you consider yourself MOST expert?

    (A) General angiography
    (B) Interventional radiology
    (C) Magnetic resonance imaging
    (D) Nuclear radiology
    (E) Ultrasonography
    (F) Computed tomography
    (G) Radiation therapy
    (H) Other

Diagnostic Ultrasonography
(Second Series)

Table of Contents

The Table of Contents is placed in this unusual location so that the reader will not be distracted by the answers before completing the test. A detailed index of the areas considered in this syllabus is provided (beginning on p. 819) for further reference.

Diagnostic Ultrasonography (Second Series) Syllabus

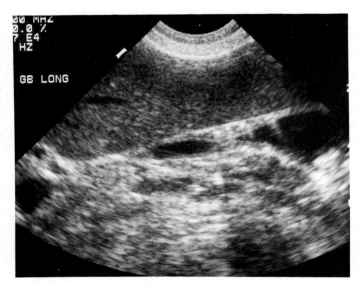

Figure 1-1. You are shown a longitudinal sonogram of the gallbladder in a 61-year-old woman. Additional history is withheld.

Case 1: Adenomyomatosis

Question 1

Which *one* of the following is the MOST likely diagnosis?

(A) Acute cholecystitis
(B) Adenomyomatosis
(C) Gallbladder carcinoma
(D) Emphysematous cholecystitis
(E) Porcelain gallbladder

Figure 1-1 shows focal thickening of the gallbladder wall, resulting in constriction of the lumen and segmentation of the gallbladder into proximal and distal segments (Figure 1-2). The wall thickening involves both the superficial and deep walls. Small, discrete, bright reflectors are present within the thickened gallbladder wall. Short "comet-tail" artifacts (multiple reverberations) are seen arising from several of these bright reflectors and extending into the anechoic gallbladder lumen. The most likely etiology for this constellation of sonographic findings is adenomyomatosis **(Option (B) is correct).**

Acute cholecystitis (Option (A)) and gallbladder carcinoma (Option (C)) can both cause wall thickening, but neither is associated with bright intramural reflectors or with comet-tail artifacts. The focal wall thickening seen in the test patient would also be atypical for acute cholecystitis, which usually causes diffuse wall thickening. Gallbladder cancer is usually more extensive at the time of diagnosis and is usually associated with gallstones (Figure 1-3). Intramural gas can produce a bright reflection from the wall of the gallbladder; therefore, emphysematous cholecystitis (Option (D)) is a consideration. In fact, gas can be associated with a "ring-down" artifact that is very similar to the comet-tail artifacts seen in the test image. However, the ring-down artifact produced by gas is longer and better defined than the comet-tail artifact produced by cholesterol crystals. In addition, emphysematous cholecystitis generally does not produce focal wall thickening. Similarly, porcelain gallbladder (Option (E)) is also unlikely because it does not produce wall thickening

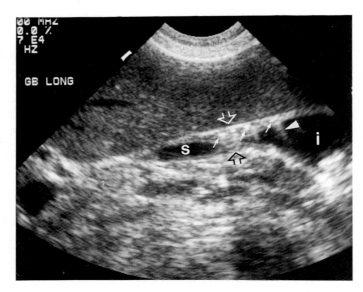

Figure 1-2 (Same as Figure 1-1). Adenomyomatosis. The gallbladder is separated into superior (s) and inferior (i) components by annular segmental wall thickening (open arrows). Several echogenic foci (small arrows) are seen in the thickened portion of the wall; one of these is associated with a short comet-tail artifact (arrowhead).

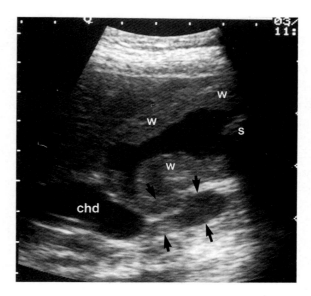

Figure 1-3. Gallbladder carcinoma. A longitudinal sonogram of the gallbladder shows marked wall thickening (w) and extension of tumor into the common bile duct (arrows), resulting in dilatation of the proximal common hepatic duct (chd). A shadowing gallstone (s) is present in the fundus of the gallbladder.

of the magnitude seen in the test image. The calcium deposits in the wall of a porcelain gallbladder should also produce shadowing (Figure 1-4), and this is not seen in the test image.

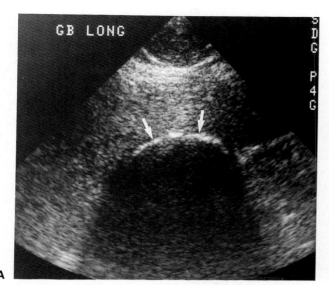

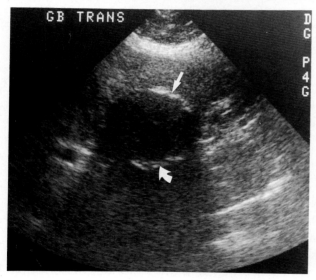

Figure 1-4. Porcelain gallbladder. (A) A longitudinal sonogram of the gallbladder shows a hyperechoic superficial wall (arrows) and dense acoustic shadowing. This might indicate a gallbladder full of stones or a calcified wall. (B) A transverse sonogram also shows the hyperechoic superficial wall (straight arrow) and shadowing from the gallbladder. A portion of the back wall is visualized (curved arrow), indicating lack of complete absorption of sound, as would be expected with a gallbladder full of stones. (C) A coned-down abdominal radiograph shows calcification within the lateral and inferior walls of the gallbladder (arrows).

Pathologically, adenomyomatosis is characterized by hyperplasia of both the mucosal and muscular layers of the gallbladder wall. Outpouchings of mucosa produce characteristic intramural diverticula known as Rokitansky-Aschoff sinuses. The involvement of the gallbladder wall may be diffuse or focal. When it is focal, adenomyomatosis is typically located in the fundus and produces a focal adenomyoma or is annular and is located in the body of the gallbladder (as in the test patient).

Sonographically, the most characteristic finding in patients with adenomyomatosis is that of small, discrete, echogenic foci arising from the

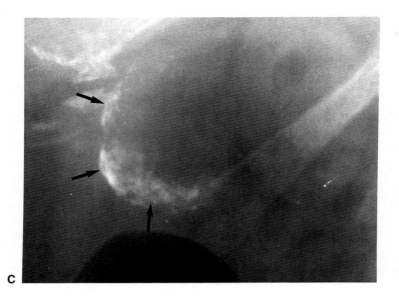

C

gallbladder wall. These result from accumulations of cholesterol crystals within the Rokitansky-Aschoff sinuses. In some cases, sound reverberates (i.e., reflects back and forth) between the superficial and deep surfaces of the cholesterol crystals. With each successive reverberation, some of the sound pulse is transmitted back to the transducer with a time delay equal to the length of time required to travel back and forth in the crystal. The location of a reflector is determined by the length of time taken for sound to travel between it and the transducer; therefore, the sequential delays in transit caused by the internal reverberations result in a series of progressively diminishing echoes located deep to the cholesterol crystal. This has been called a comet-tail artifact and is usually the most dramatic sonographic finding in patients with adenomyomatosis. The comet-tail artifacts generally arise from the superficial wall of the gallbladder but not from the deep wall. This does not indicate preferential involvement of the superficial wall but merely reflects good visualization of the artifact in the anechoic background of bile immediately deep to the superficial wall and poor visualization in the echogenic background of soft tissues deep to the deep wall. Another finding that may be present with adenomyomatosis is diffuse or focal wall thickening. In unusual instances, large Rokitansky-Aschoff sinuses that are filled with bile are identified as cystic spaces in the gallbladder wall.

Question 2

Concerning acute cholecystitis,

(A) approximately 10% of cases occur without gallstones
(B) associated jaundice is most often secondary to Mirizzi's syndrome
(C) bacterial infection is important in its pathogenesis
(D) it is the most common cause of the wall-echo-shadow complex
(E) in a patient with right upper quadrant pain and fever, the presence of gall-stones is diagnostic

The differential diagnosis of acute right upper quadrant pain is rela-tively broad. In addition to acute cholecystitis, it includes inflammatory and neoplastic disease of the liver, right kidney, pancreas, and hepatic flexure. It also includes peptic ulcer disease, hydronephrosis, right lower lobe pneumonia, and even appendicitis and pelvic inflammatory disease. This wide range of possible causes often makes it difficult to establish the correct diagnosis clinically. In fact, when acute cholecystitis is sus-pected clinically, it turns out to be the correct diagnosis in only about 25% of patients. As a result, diagnostic imaging has become important in helping to establish a definitive diagnosis.

Acute cholecystitis is most frequently caused by obstruction of the cystic duct by a gallstone. Persistent secretion of mucus causes gall-bladder distension and increased intraluminal pressure, and it may ulti-mately reduce venous outflow and arterial inflow. With persistent obstruction of the cystic duct, the gallbladder wall initially becomes thickened as a result of edema and infiltration of inflammatory cells and may ultimately become gangrenous and perforate. Bacterial infection is often present in patients with acute cholecystitis, but it is not believed to play a significant role in the etiology of the disorder **(Option (C) is false).** However, gallbladder infections may be important in some of the complications of cholecystitis. The most commonly involved organisms are gram-negative aerobes such as *Escherichia coli* and *Klebsiella*, *Enter-obacter*, and *Proteus* species. The course of therapy of patients with acute cholecystitis varies somewhat from institution to institution and also varies depending on the patient's clinical condition. In most centers, patients are admitted for intravenous hydration and antibiotics. This generally results in resolution of the patient's symptoms and allows for nonemergent surgery to be performed later.

Cholecystitis not associated with gallstones (i.e., acalculous cholecys-titis) is a much less common form and accounts for approximately 5 to 10% of cases **(Option (A) is true).** The etiology of acalculous cholecysti-tis is probably multifactorial and includes ischemia, gallbladder wall infection, direct chemical toxicity, and cystic duct obstruction. Acalculous cholecystitis occurs after severe trauma or burns, major surgery, or prolonged total parenteral nutrition or in patients with severe underlying illnesses.

There is considerable controversy about the roles of ultrasonography and hepatobiliary scintigraphy in the evaluation of patients with suspected cholecystitis. Sonography is recommended as the initial imaging test by many authorities (and by a practice guideline of the American College of Physicians) for several reasons. As mentioned above, most patients with acute right upper quadrant pain do not have acute cholecystitis, and sonography is more likely to point to an alternative diagnosis than is scintigraphy. Sonography can also effectively exclude the diagnosis by identifying a normal, stone-free gallbladder. Sonography is more prone to false-positive diagnoses of acute cholecystitis than is scintigraphy, but most of these occur in patients with gallstones and symptomatic chronic cholecystitis. These patients generally require cholecystectomy anyway, and so the practical impact of misclassifying them as acute cholecystitis is minimal. In fact, in their 1985 study, Ralls et al. showed that the positive predictive value of sonography for diagnosing conditions that require cholecystectomy is 99%.

Perhaps the most compelling argument for the use of ultrasonography as the initial imaging modality is the emerging popularity and widespread use of laparoscopic cholecystectomy. With laparoscopic techniques, it is very important for the surgeon to have preoperative information about the size of the gallbladder and the stones, the status of the gallbladder wall, and the presence of associated fluid collections. In addition to evaluating the gallbladder, it is very important to obtain good preoperative anatomic information about the pancreas, liver, and right kidney because these organs are difficult to inspect laparoscopically. Sonography provides these types of information, whereas hepatobiliary scintigraphy does not.

It is also important to know whether biliary obstruction is present, because obstruction is usually due to choledocholithiasis (Figure 1-5) and, in most cases, can be effectively treated preoperatively by endoscopic stone removal and sphincterotomy. Mirizzi's syndrome is a very uncommon cause of biliary obstruction or jaundice in patients with acute cholecystitis **(Option (B) is false).** It is due to compression of the common hepatic duct by cystic duct stones and occurs when the cystic duct runs in a common sheath with the common hepatic duct. Mirizzi's syndrome can be suggested by ultrasonography (Figure 1-6), but cholangiography is usually required to make a definitive diagnosis.

Scintigraphy should be reserved for patients in whom sonography is equivocal. The individual sonographic signs of acute cholecystitis are nonspecific, and hence scintigraphy can be a very valuable means of

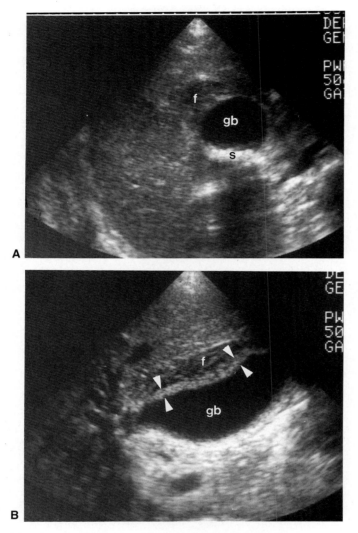

Figure 1-5. Acute cholecystitis and choledocholithiasis. (A) A transverse sonogram shows multiple small gallstones (s) and a fluid collection (f) adjacent to the gallbladder (gb). (B) A longitudinal sonogram shows thickening of the gallbladder wall (arrowheads) and an elliptical fluid collection (f) between the gallbladder (gb) and liver. (C) A longitudinal sonogram of the common duct shows two shadowing intraluminal stones (arrows) within a dilated duct (d).

establishing or excluding the diagnosis unequivocally. Scintigraphy can also provide valuable information about acute biliary obstruction before the development of ductal dilatation by demonstrating delayed transit of the tracer into the small bowel.

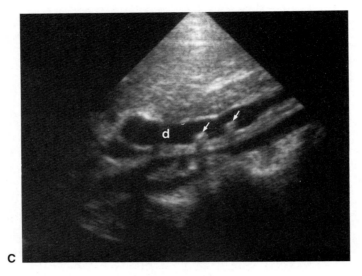

Figure 1-5 (Continued)

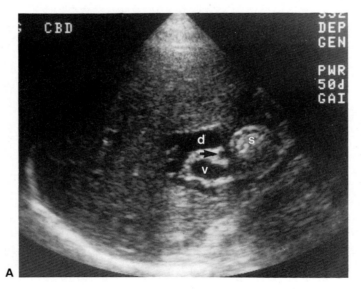

Figure 1-6. Mirizzi's syndrome. (A) A longitudinal sonogram shows a dilated common hepatic duct (d) anterior to the portal vein (v) and right hepatic artery (arrow). A wall-echo-shadow complex (s) at the level of the obstruction is due to a stone in the neck of the gallbladder. (B) Endoscopic retrograde cholangiopancreatography (ERCP) shows marked intrahepatic ductal dilatation due to a smooth extrinsic compression on the common hepatic duct (arrows). The combination of the ERCP and sonographic findings establishes the diagnosis of Mirizzi's syndrome.

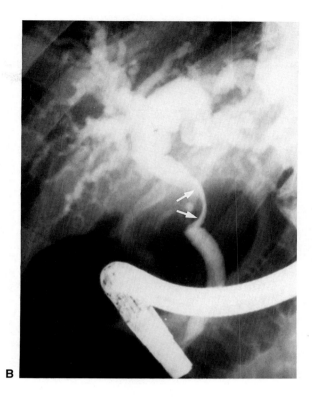

B

Five sonographic findings are used in establishing the diagnosis of acute cholecystitis: gallstones, gallbladder wall thickening, gallbladder enlargement, pericholecystic fluid collections, and focal tenderness directly over the gallbladder. The more of these findings that are present, the more likely the patient is to have acute cholecystitis. It is important to realize, however, that all of these signs are not seen in all patients (Table 1-1). Just as important, these individual signs by themselves are not specific (Table 1-2). For instance, gallstones are a common incidental finding in patients who present with right upper quadrant pain and fever due to nonbiliary causes **(Option (E) is false).** In fact, it is estimated that 10% of the general population have gallstones and that only 20% of these individuals will ever develop biliary symptoms.

The detection of focal tenderness located directly over the gallbladder is referred to as a positive sonographic Murphy's sign; it has a reported sensitivity of 63 to 94% and a reported specificity of 85 to 94% in the diagnosis of acute cholecystitis. Therefore, it is important to compress the abdomen with the transducer and determine the location of maximal tenderness. A convincingly positive sonographic Murphy's sign is strong evidence for the diagnosis of acute cholecystitis. Likewise, a

Table 1-1: Predictive values of multiple sonographic criteria for diagnosis of acute cholecystitis[a]

Sonographic findings	Predictive value (%)
Positive	
Stones and positive Murphy's sign	90
Stones and thickened gallbladder wall	94
Stones, positive Murphy's sign, and thickened gallbladder wall	92
Negative	
No stones and negative Murphy's sign	97
No stones and normal gallbladder wall	98
No stones, negative Murphy's sign, and normal gallbladder wall	99

[a] Adapted with permission from Ralls et al. [14]. Data were obtained from a patient population with a 62% prevalence of acute cholecystitis.

Table 1-2: Analysis of single sonographic criteria for diagnosis of acute cholecystitis[a]

Sonographic findings	Sensitivity (%)	Specificity (%)	PPV (%)	NPV (%)
Stones	83–98	52–77	86	96
Positive Murphy's sign	75–94	85–87	88	72
Thickened gallbladder wall	45–72	76–88	84	56

[a] Adapted from studies by Laing et al. [10] and Ralls et al. [14], in which the prevalence of acute cholecystitis was 35 and 62%, respectively. PPV = positive predictive value; NPV = negative predictive value.

negative sonographic Murphy's sign is strong evidence against acute cholecystitis. However, patients with gangrenous cholecystitis may not exhibit a positive Murphy's sign, because of altered gallbladder innervation (Figure 1-7). Additionally, in some patients, assessment for Murphy's sign may be equivocal or the sign may not be evaluable, e.g., in patients who are unresponsive or when the gallbladder is positioned deep to the ribs or is surrounded by ascites and is not compressible.

Thickening of the gallbladder wall (≥ 3 mm) is present in most patients with acute cholecystitis (Figure 1-5). Unfortunately, it can also

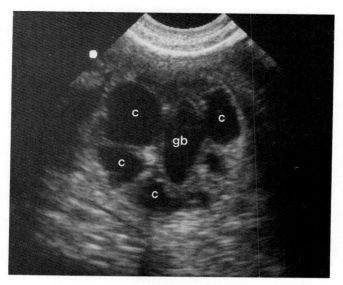

Figure 1-7. Gallbladder necrosis in a patient with nonspecific abdominal symptoms and a negative sonographic Murphy's sign. A transverse sonogram of the gallbladder (gb) shows marked thickening of the gallbladder wall with multiple large cystic spaces (c) in the wall. A gallstone impacted in the neck of the gallbladder was seen on other views.

be caused by a large number of other conditions. These include liver dysfunction, congestive heart failure, hypoalbuminemia, hepatitis, renal disease, portal hypertension, lymphatic obstruction, and adjacent inflammatory processes such as peptic ulcer disease and pancreatitis. It was originally hoped that the appearance of the thickened gallbladder wall would be useful in distinguishing acute cholecystitis from nonbiliary abnormalities. Specifically, it was reported that the finding of irregular striated sonolucencies in the thickened gallbladder wall was a specific sign of acute cholecystitis. Unfortunately, this has not proven to be the case (Figure 1-8).

The final sonographic sign of acute cholecystitis is pericholecystic fluid collections, which occur in up to 25% of patients. Most of these collections are seen between the gallbladder and the liver (Figure 1-5), but some are within the wall (Figures 1-7 and 1-9) or loculated within the peritoneal cavity (Figure 1-10). Pericholecystic fluid collections indicate an increased risk of gallbladder perforation, so their detection is important and implies that more urgent surgical intervention is generally required.

The wall-echo-shadow complex occurs in patients with a contracted gallbladder full of stones. Extending from superficial to deep along the

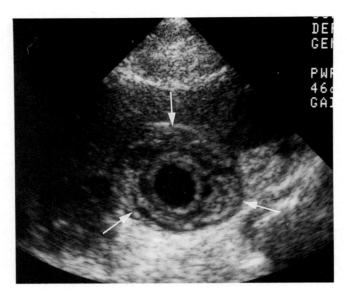

Figure 1-8. Congestive heart failure causing thickening of the gallbladder wall. A transverse sonogram of the gallbladder shows marked wall thickening (arrows) with irregular, striated intramural sonolucencies. This patient had no right upper quadrant signs or symptoms and no gallstones.

axis of the ultrasound beam, it consists of an echogenic arc (representing the interface between the gallbladder and liver), a hypoechoic arc (representing the gallbladder wall itself), a second echogenic arc (representing the leading edge of either a single large stone or multiple smaller stones), and an acoustic shadow (Figure 1-11). It is a sign of cholelithiasis but, in most cases, is associated with chronic and not acute cholecystitis **(Option (D) is false).**

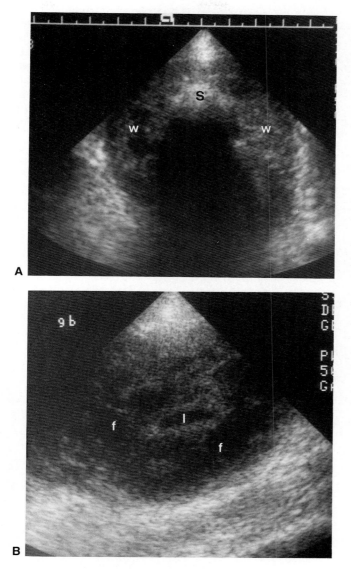

Figure 1-9. Intramural gallbladder abscess. (A) A transverse sonogram of the mid-gallbladder shows a large shadowing stone (s) surrounded by a markedly thickened wall (w). (B) A transverse sonogram of the upper gallbladder shows a contracted lumen (l) and complex intramural fluid (f).

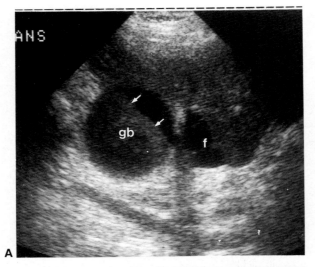

A

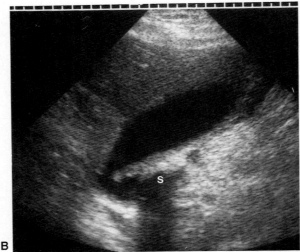

B

Figure 1-10 (left). Pericholecystic fluid. (A) A transverse sonogram shows the
gallbladder (gb) with an
intraluminal sludge-bile
level (arrows) and an adjacent pericholecystic fluid collection loculated within the
peritoneal cavity (f). (B) A
longitudinal sonogram
shows a gallstone (s) im-
pacted in the gallbladder
neck. Pus was aspirated
from the gallbladder during
percutaneous cholecys-
tostomy.

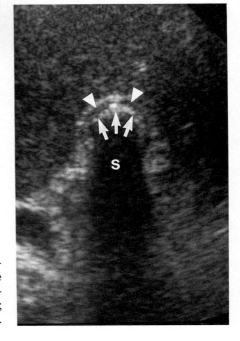

Figure 1-11 (right). Contracted gallbladder full of stones. A transverse
sonogram shows a typical wall-echo-
shadow complex (s). Arrowheads = wall;
arrows = echo; s = shadow.

16

Question 3

Adenomyomatosis:

(A) predisposes to gallbladder carcinoma
(B) occurs secondary to chronic inflammation
(C) is a common cause of gallbladder polyps
(D) is strongly associated with biliary colic
(E) cannot be diagnosed by oral cholecystography

Jutras first used the term "hyperplastic cholecystoses" in 1960. The seven entities he originally included in this classification were adenomatosis, myomatosis, cholesterolosis, neuromatosis, fibromatosis, elastosis, and lipomatosis. Currently, it is believed that the pathologic differences are sufficient to justify only two distinct entities. These are cholesterolosis and adenomyomatosis (a combination of adenomatosis and myomatosis). There is also sentiment in favor of eliminating the term "hyperplastic cholecystoses" since there is little similarity between adenomyomatosis and cholesterolosis on either a pathologic or radiologic basis. Adenomyomatosis occurs in three forms: diffuse, annular (segmental), and focal. The focal form is usually isolated to the fundus in the form of a sessile, polypoid mass with a central umbilication (Figures 1-12 and 1-13). This mass is often referred to by the misnomer "adenomyoma." It is well described and might be referred to as a gallbladder "polyp," but it is not a common cause of gallbladder polyps **(Option (C) is false)**. The annular form is illustrated in the test image (Figures 1-1 and 1-2). It consists of a circumferential zone of wall thickening that compartmentalizes the gallbladder into two segments, which communicate via a narrowed lumen. The diffuse form of adenomyomatosis results in variable thickening of both the mucosal and muscular layers of the gallbladder wall (Figure 1-14).

Potential causes of adenomyomatosis include increased intraluminal pressure, narrowing of the distal common bile duct, and excessive neuromuscular activity. However, all of these are unproven, and the true etiology of adenomyomatosis is unknown. Nonetheless, it is well established that adenomyomatosis is not caused by an inflammatory process **(Option (B) is false).** When inflammation coexists with adenomyomatosis, it is usually secondary to the presence of gallstones.

In addition to adenomyomatosis, gallbladder carcinoma is an important entity in the differential diagnosis of focal gallbladder wall thickening or gallbladder wall masses. In sonograms of most patients with adenomyomatosis, the characteristic comet-tail artifacts allow this disease to be distinguished from carcinoma. However, in some patients a firm distinction may not be possible. In such cases, oral cholecystography

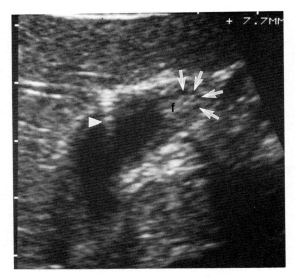

Figure 1-12 (left). Fundal adenomyomatosis. A longitudinal sonogram shows a focal area of wall thickening in the fundus of the gallbladder (f). Several bile-filled Rokitansky-Aschoff sinuses are seen as small intramural cysts (arrows). A typical comet-tail artifact (arrowhead) is seen arising from the superficial wall.

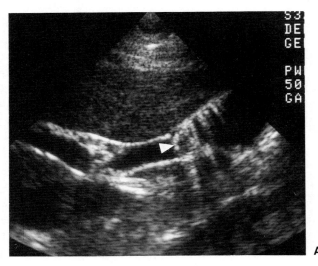

A

Figure 1-13 (right). Focal adenomyomatosis. (A) A longitudinal sonogram demonstrates a focal mass (arrowhead) near the neck of the gallbladder, as well as several adjacent comet-tail artifacts. (B) An upright oral cholecystogram shows multiple layering stones (solid arrows) and a mass (open arrow) with central umbilication near the neck of the gallbladder.

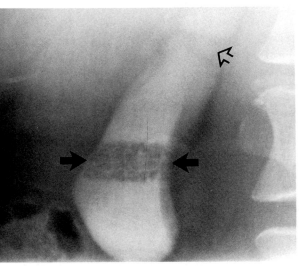

B

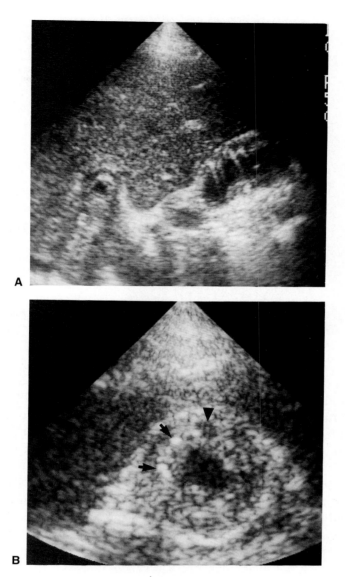

Figure 1-14. Diffuse adenomyomatosis. (A) A longitudinal sonogram shows diffuse thickening of the gallbladder wall and multiple comet-tail artifacts. (B) A magnified transverse sonogram shows concentric uniform wall thickening with several Rokitansky-Aschoff sinuses. One of the sinuses is filled with bile and appears cystic (arrowhead), and several sinuses are filled with crystalline material and appear echogenic (arrows).

may be helpful because it can identify the characteristic Rokitansky-Aschoff sinuses (Figure 1-15) and thus establish a definitive diagnosis of adenomyomatosis **(Option (E) is false).**

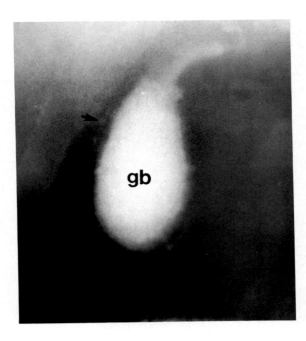

Figure 1-15. Diffuse adenomyomatosis. An oral cholecystogram shows numerous contrast-filled Rokitansky-Aschoff sinuses (arrows) adjacent to the opacified gallbladder lumen (gb).

The clinical significance of adenomyomatosis is somewhat unclear. In many individuals without biliary symptoms, it is identified as an incidental finding **(Option (D) is false).** In fact, the test patient was being evaluated for a renal mass and had no right upper quadrant symptoms. In patients with biliary symptoms, there is often coexistent cholelithiasis, and it is likely that the stones (rather than the adenomyomatosis) are producing the symptoms. Management of such patients should be directed toward treating the stones rather than the adenomyomatosis. Occasionally, patients with adenomyomatosis have symptoms consistent with biliary colic, but they have no associated stones. Cholecystectomy frequently relieves the symptoms in such patients, and therefore surgery is probably justified. It is important to realize, however, that adenomyomatosis is not premalignant and does not predispose to gallbladder carcinoma **(Option (A) is false).** Therefore, cholecystectomy should not be performed for fear of neoplasm. The only exception to this is in the occasional patient with a gallbladder wall abnormality in whom the diagnosis of adenomyomatosis is not firmly established by either ultrasonography or oral cholecystography. In such a patient, the possibility of gallbladder carcinoma must be considered and surgery may be necessary.

Question 4

Concerning emphysematous cholecystitis,

(A) it is more common in women than in men
(B) ischemia is important in its pathogenesis
(C) it nearly always occurs in patients with gallstones
(D) mortality is greater than in patients with typical acute cholecystitis
(E) it is a potential cause of intraductal pneumobilia

Emphysematous cholecystitis is an unusual form of acute cholecystitis that is believed to be caused by gallbladder ischemia **(Option (B) is true)** with development of superinfection by gas-forming organisms, most commonly *Clostridium* species, *E. coli*, streptococci, and other intestinal organisms. Unlike most other gallbladder abnormalities, emphysematous cholecystitis occurs more frequently in men than in women **(Option (A) is false).** Presumably, this is related to a higher incidence of vascular disease in the male population. The predominant role of ischemia in the pathogenesis of emphysematous cholecystitis is also probably the reason why approximately 30% of patients develop this disorder without associated cholelithiasis **(Option (C) is false).** Traditionally, emphysematous cholecystitis is diagnosed by abdominal radiographs, which show gas in the lumen or wall of the gallbladder. However, many patients are evaluated by sonography before abdominal radiographs are taken, and it is therefore important to recognize the sonographic appearance of emphysematous cholecystitis. Gas is a very strong reflector and therefore appears as a very bright echo. Like gas within loops of bowel, gas in the gallbladder generally produces a "dirty" shadow, unlike the "clean" shadow of gallstones or gallbladder wall calcification. Gas often produces a ring-down artifact that appears as a streak of high-level echoes within the envelope of the sonic shadow (Figure 1-16). This occurs because fluid trapped between small bubbles of gas resonates when it is excited by the sound beam, and this resonating fluid acts as an independent sound transmitter. Gallstones, gallbladder wall calcification, and cholesterol crystals do not produce this type of artifact. At times, gas may produce a comet-tail type of artifact or an acoustic shadow similar to that produced by cholesterol crystals or gallstones. In such cases the mobile, nondependent nature of gas helps to distinguish it from stones or cholesterol. Occasionally, sonography is equivocal and abdominal radiographs are required. In some patients, gas within the gallbladder lumen can pass through the cystic duct and produce intraductal pneumobilia (Figure 1-17) **(Option (E) is true).**

The prognosis of emphysematous cholecystitis is significantly worse than that of gallstone-induced cholecystitis, with an estimated mortality

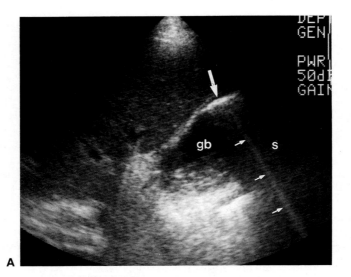

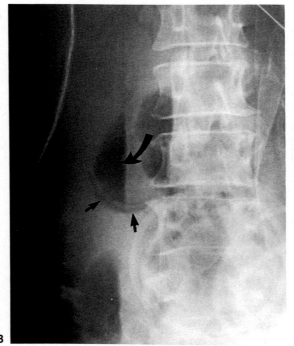

Figure 1-16. Emphysematous cholecystitis. (A) A longitudinal sonogram of the gallbladder (gb) shows a bright reflection from the nondependent portion of the lumen (long arrow). There is an associated shadow (s) and a characteristic ringdown artifact (short arrows), confirming that the nondependent reflections are due to gas. (B) A left lateral decubitus abdominal radiograph shows gas in the gallbladder wall (straight arrows) and lumen (curved arrow).

of 15% versus <5%. The mortality from emphysematous cholecystitis remains 15% regardless of the patient's age, whereas the mortality from gallstone-induced cholecystitis is only 1% in patients less than 60 years old. This marked difference in prognosis in younger patients, in whom coexistent disease is minimized, truly indicates the greater lethal poten-

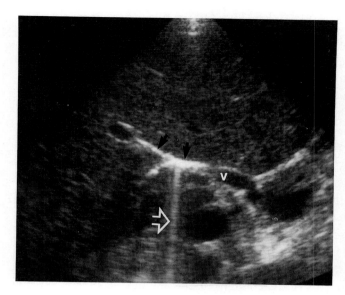

Figure 1-17. Pneumobilia. An oblique sonogram of the porta hepatis shows a bright linear reflection (black arrows) adjacent to the portal vein (v). This represents gas in the bile duct. A typical ring-down artifact (open arrow) is seen emanating from the gas.

tial of emphysematous cholecystitis **(Option (D) is true).** In addition, 75% of patients with emphysematous cholecystitis experience gangrene and 20% of gallbladders are perforated at the time of surgery. This represents 30-fold and 5-fold increases in the incidences of these respective complications when compared with those in typical acute cholecystitis.

Question 5

Concerning cholesterolosis,

    (A) it is associated with elevated cholesterol levels in serum
    (B) it is seen more frequently in women than in men
    (C) the gallbladder usually appears normal sonographically
    (D) it predisposes to development of cholesterol stones
    (E) it is the most common cause of gallbladder polyps

Cholesterolosis is an abnormality consisting of deposition of cholesterol precursors, cholesterol esters, and triglycerides in the wall of the gallbladder. The abnormal lipid is initially found in macrophages in the tips of mucosal villi. As the villi distend, this frequently results in a macroscopic appearance of small yellow nodules scattered on a background of reddened hyperemic mucosa, resulting in the term "strawberry gallbladder." In the planar variety of cholesterolosis, which accounts for most cases, the nodules remain small (<1 mm) and cause the mucosal surface to appear granular. This form is generally not detectable by either sonography or oral cholecystography **(Option (C) is true).** In some cases, the nodules become larger and form focal or multifocal polypoid masses. This polypoid form of cholesterolosis is much less common than the planar form. However, because cholesterolosis itself is so common (10% of gallbladders removed for stones have cholesterolosis), cholesterol polyps account for the vast majority of gallbladder polyps that are seen sonographically **(Option (E) is true).** Pathologically, cholesterol polyps are devoid of stromal or glandular elements and thus differ from other types of gallbladder polyps such as adenomas or papillomas.

As with adenomyomatosis, the etiology of cholesterolosis is unknown. It may be related to increased absorption of cholesterol from the bile by the gallbladder or to increased hepatic synthesis of cholesterol precursors. However, it is not related to obesity, elevated cholesterol levels in serum **(Option (A) is false),** atherosclerosis, or diabetes. In addition, it does not appear to be related to the formation of cholesterol stones **(Option (D) is false),** and, unlike cholelithiasis, its incidence is equal in men and women **(Option (B) is false).**

Sonographically, cholesterol polyps appear as nonmobile, nonshadowing masses adjacent to the gallbladder wall (Figure 1-18). They are usually multiple on pathologic examination, but it is not uncommon to identify only the single largest polyp on sonography. Most cholesterol polyps are less than 5 mm in diameter, and it is quite uncommon for them to grow larger than 1 cm.

Gallbladder polyps are relatively common, and so it is important to have a rational strategy for dealing with them. As mentioned above, the vast majority of polyps are cholesterol polyps, and these require no further evaluation or treatment. Gallbladder adenomas, gallbladder papillomas, and polypoid gallbladder carcinoma are almost always single; therefore, the finding of multiple polyps makes the diagnosis of cholesterol polyps even more likely. The one exception to this is in patients with malignant melanoma, since this tumor has a tendency to metastasize to the gallbladder and can appear as multiple polyps. In addition to multiplicity, polyp size is useful in determining management. Unlike cholesterol polyps, polypoid cancers are almost always larger than 1 cm. Therefore, it is reasonable to ignore all solitary polyps that are <5 mm in size. Polyps between 5 mm and 1 cm should be monitored to ensure stability. If such a polyp enlarges, cholecystectomy is probably warranted. Solitary polyps that are >1 cm in size when initially discovered should be considered potentially malignant and should probably be removed. If the patient is a poor surgical candidate, the polyps should be monitored closely by ultrasonography.

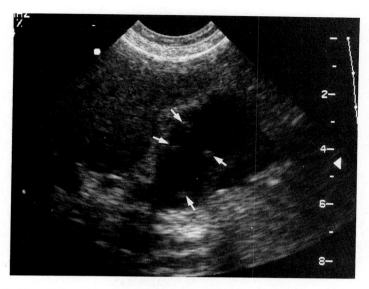

Figure 1-18. Polypoid cholesterolosis. A longitudinal sonogram shows several nonshadowing nodules (arrows) adjacent to the dependent and nondependent walls of the gallbladder.

The other major consideration when a nonshadowing filling defect is identified adjacent to the gallbladder wall is tumefactive sludge. Sludge normally layers out and produces a characteristic bile-sludge layer on sonography, but tumefactive sludge is very thick and viscous and appears mass-like. It can be distinguished from a polyp or gallbladder tumor by documenting motion or a change in shape as the patient changes position (Figure 1-19). Occasionally, tumefactive sludge does not move during the course of a sonographic examination. In such cases, a follow-up examination several days later is usually effective in documenting motion or a change in the shape of the mass.

William D. Middleton, M.D.

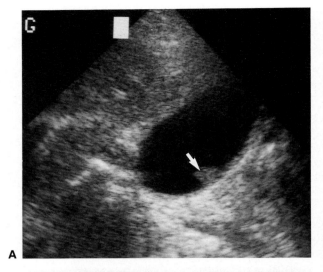

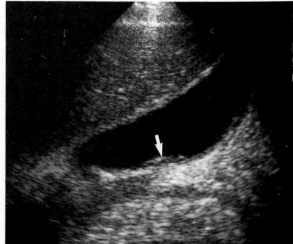

Figure 1-19. Sludge. (A) A longitudinal sonogram in the supine position shows a non-shadowing nodule (arrow) adjacent to the gallbladder wall. This appearance is similar to that of the polyps shown in Figure 1-15. (B) A longitudinal sonogram in the upright position shows a change in shape of the mass (arrow). On real-time viewing, motion could also be observed, confirming that this was thick mobile sludge and not a polyp.

SUGGESTED READINGS

ADENOMYOMATOSIS

1. Berk RN, van der Vegt JH, Lichtenstein JE. The hyperplastic cholecystoses: cholesterolosis and adenomyomatosis. Radiology 1983; 146:593–601
2. Cover KL, Slasky BS, Skolnick ML. Sonography of cholesterol in the biliary system. J Ultrasound Med 1985; 4:647–653
3. Fowler RC, Reid WA. Ultrasound diagnosis of adenomyomatosis of the gallbladder: ultrasonic and pathological correlation. Clin Radiol 1988; 39:402–406

4. Jutras JA. Hyperplastic cholecystoses. AJR 1960; 83:795–827
5. Kidney M, Goiney R, Cooperberg PL. Adenomyomatosis of the gallbladder: a pictorial exhibit. J Ultrasound Med 1986; 5:331–333
6. Lafortune M, Gariépy G, Dumont A, Breton G, Lapointe R. The V-shaped artifact of the gallbladder wall. AJR 1986; 147:505–508
7. Raghavendra BN, Subramanyam BR, Balthazar EJ, Horii SC, Megibow AJ, Hilton S. Sonography of adenomyomatosis of the gallbladder: radiologic-pathologic correlation. Radiology 1983; 146:747–752
8. Rice J, Sauerbrei EE, Semogas P, Cooperberg PL, Burhenne HJ. Sonographic appearance of adenomyomatosis of the gallbladder. J Clin Ultrasound 1981; 9:336–337

ACUTE CHOLECYSTITIS

9. Cohan RH, Mahony BS, Bowie JD, Cooper C, Baker ME, Illescas FF. Striated intramural gallbladder lucencies on US studies: predictors of acute cholecystitis. Radiology 1987; 164:31–35
10. Laing FC, Federle MP, Jeffrey RB, Brown TW. Ultrasonic evaluation of patients with acute right upper quadrant pain. Radiology 1981; 140:449–455
11. Marton KI, Doubilet P. How to image the gallbladder in suspected cholecystitis. Ann Intern Med 1988; 109:722–729
12. Marton KI, Doubilet P, et al. How to study the gallbladder. Ann Intern Med 1988; 109:752–754
13. Raghavendra BN, Feiner HD, Subramanyam BR, et al. Acute cholecystitis: sonographic-pathologic analysis. AJR 1981; 137:327–332
14. Ralls PW, Colletti PM, Lapin SA, et al. Real-time sonography in suspected acute cholecystitis. Prospective evaluation of primary and secondary signs. Radiology 1985; 155:767–771
15. Ralls PW, Halls J, Lapin SA, Quinn MF, Morris UL, Boswell W. Prospective evaluation of the sonographic Murphy sign in suspected acute cholecystitis. JCU 1982; 10:113–115
16. Takada T, Yasuda H, Uchiyama K, Hasegawa H, Asagoe T, Shikata J. Pericholecystic abscess: classification of US findings to determine the proper therapy. Radiology 1989; 172:693–697
17. Teefey SA, Baron RL, Bigler SA. Sonography of the gallbladder: significance of striated (layered) thickening of the gallbladder wall. AJR 1991; 156:945–947

EMPHYSEMATOUS CHOLECYSTITIS

18. Blaquiére RM, Dewbury KC. The ultrasound diagnosis of emphysematous cholecystitis. Br J Radiol 1982; 55:114–116
19. Hunter ND, Macintosh PK. Acute emphysematous cholecystitis: an ultrasonic diagnosis. AJR 1980; 134:592–593
20. Mentzer RM Jr, Golden GT, Chandler JG, Horsley JS III. A comparative appraisal of emphysematous cholecystitis. Am J Surg 1975; 124:10–15
21. Nemcek AA Jr, Gore RM, Vogelzang RL, Grant M. The effervescent gallbladder: a sonographic sign of emphysematous cholecystitis. AJR 1988; 150:575–577

22. Parulekar SG. Sonographic findings in acute emphysematous cholecystitis. Radiology 1982; 145:117–119

CHOLESTEROLOSIS

23. Grieco RV, Bartone NF, Vasilas A. A study of fixed filling defects in the well-opacified gallbladder and their evolution. AJR 1963; 90:844–853
24. Koga A, Watanabe K, Fukuyama T, Takiguchi S, Nakayama F. Diagnosis and operative indications for polypoid lesions of the gallbladder. Arch Surg 1988; 123:26–29
25. Ochsner SF. Solitary polypoid lesions of the gallbladder. Radiol Clin North Am 1966; 4:501–510
26. Price RJ, Stewart ET, Foley WD, Dodds WJ. Sonography of polypoid cholesterolosis. AJR 1982; 139:1197–1198
27. Ruhe AH, Zachman JP, Mulder BD, Rime AE. Cholesterol polyps of the gallbladder: ultrasound demonstration. JCU 1979; 7:386–388

Notes

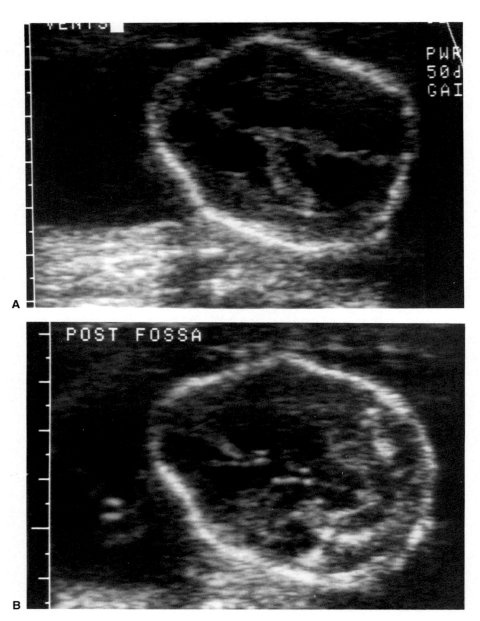

Figure 2-1. This 38-year-old woman presented for routine obstetrical ultrasonography. You are shown two axial views of the fetal head.

Case 2:   Arnold-Chiari Malformation

Question 6

Which *one* of the following is the MOST likely diagnosis?

(A) Normal variant
(B) Dandy-Walker variant
(C) Trisomy 18
(D) Arnold-Chiari malformation
(E) Down's syndrome

A transventricular view of the fetal head (Figure 2-1A) shows dilatation of the lateral ventricle, with the atrium measuring 14 mm (Figure 2-2A). The choroid plexus is dangling within the dependent far-field ventricle, with the posterior portion of the choroid lying against the lateral wall. The shape of the fetal head is abnormal, showing a concave contour to the frontal bones, the "lemon sign." Figure 2-1B is a sonogram at the level of the fetal cerebellum; it shows that the normal anatomy of the posterior fossa is distorted (Figure 2-2B). The fluid space of the cisterna magna between the cerebellum and inner margin of the occipital bone is effaced. In addition, the cerebellar hemispheres are wrapped around the posterior aspect of the midbrain, resulting in the "banana sign." The findings of hydrocephalus, the lemon sign, effacement of the cisterna magna, and the banana sign are most probably due to the Arnold-Chiari (Chiari II) malformation as a result of an open neural tube defect **(Option (D) is correct).** The associated lumbar myelomeningocele (Figure 2-3) in this fetus is not shown in the test images.

The lemon sign has been described as a normal variant (Option (A)) in about 1% of normal fetuses. The frontal contour is usually linear in these variants (Figure 2-4A) rather than biconcave, as seen in the test images. Often the lemon shape in the normal variants is best seen at the base of the cranium, lower than with the true lemon sign. In normal fetuses, no intracranial abnormality should be identified. The normal ventricular width should not exceed 9 to 10 mm. The normal cisterna magna outlining the bilobed cerebellum is identified as a posterior fossa

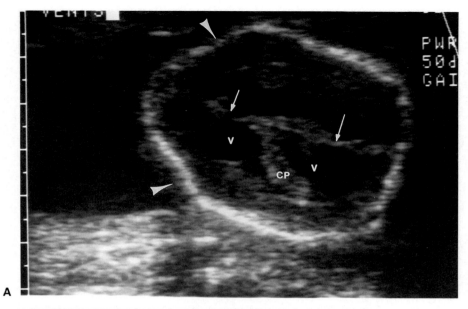

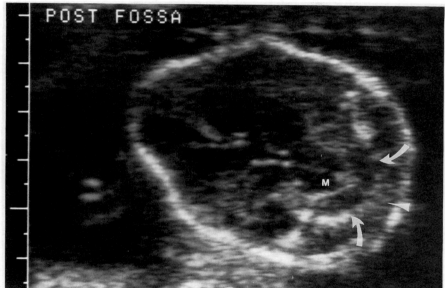

Figure 2-2 (Same as Figure 2-1). Arnold-Chiari malformation with mye-lomeningocele. (A) A transventricular axial sonogram through the fetal head shows a "dangling" choroid plexus (CP) within a dilated lateral ven-tricle (V). The arrows indicate the midline falx. A lemon sign is also dem-onstrated, with a concave frontal contour to the fetal head (arrowheads). (B) A transcerebellar sonogram shows the cerebellar hemispheres (ar-rows) wrapped around the midbrain (M). The fluid-filled cisterna magna should be identified at this level; however, in this case the space is filled with echoes (arrowhead). The lemon-shaped head is also apparent at this level.

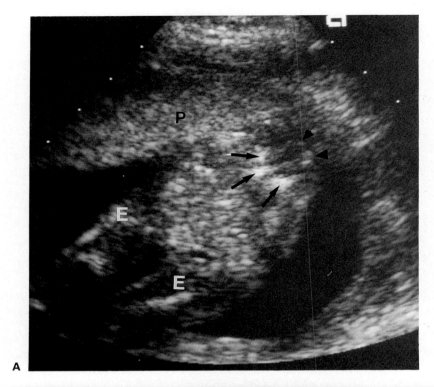

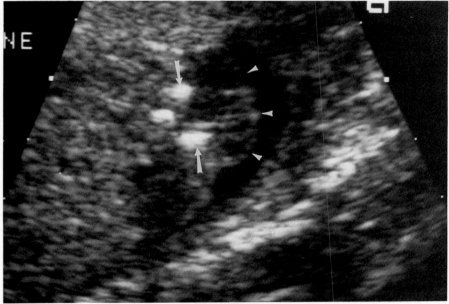

Figure 2-3. Same patient as in Figures 2-1 and 2-2. Arnold-Chiari malformation with myelomeningocele. (A) A transverse sonogram at the level of the lumbosacral spine shows the three ossification centers of the spine (arrows). The posterior two elements are splayed, and there is an associated myelomeningocele sac (arrowheads). P = placenta; E = extremities. (B) A zoomed axial sonogram of the lumbar region shows splaying of the dorsal ossification centers (arrows). A small myelomeningocele sac is better seen (arrowheads).

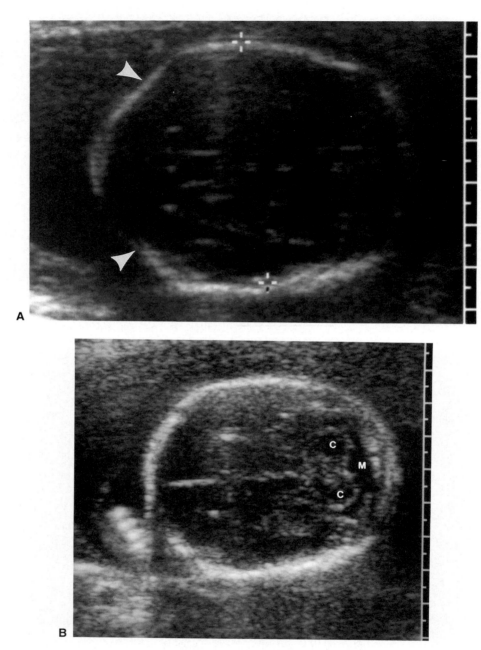

Figure 2-4. Normal-variant lemon sign. (A) A transventricular sonogram shows straightening of the frontal contour of the calvarium (arrowheads). (B) A transcerebellar sonogram demonstrates normal cerebellar hemispheres (C) and a normal cisterna magna (M). This confirms that this lemon shape is a normal variant.

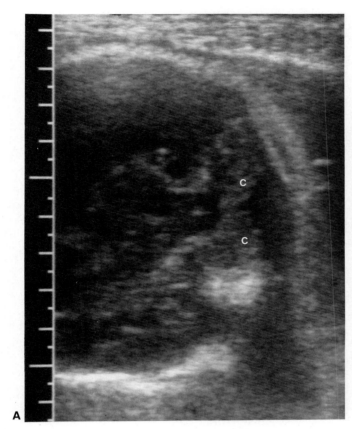

Figure 2-5. Dandy-Walker variant. (A) A transcerebellar sonogram through the superior cerebellum shows normally shaped cerebellar hemispheres (C). (B) A more caudal sonogram shows an enlarged cisterna magna (CM) with an anterior funnel-shaped fluid extension to the posterior aspect of the midbrain (arrowhead). This represents a small ventricular cyst with vermian aplasia.

fluid structure (Figure 2-4B). The presence of the hydrocephalus and abnormal posterior fossa in the test images makes normal variant an unlikely diagnosis.

The Dandy-Walker variant (Option (B)) is a less-severe form of the Dandy-Walker malformation. Sonography of fetuses with this anomaly shows a small fourth ventricle cyst with mild vermian dysplasia (Figure 2-5). On transcerebellar views, enlargement of the cisterna magna associated with a normal to mildly enlarged posterior fossa would be expected, the opposite of the findings in the test images. Mild hydrocephalus may be seen with the Dandy-Walker variant, but the lemon sign is not a feature. Therefore, Dandy-Walker variant is not a likely diagnosis.

Trisomy 18 (Option (C)) is one of the most common chromosomal defects associated with multiple malformations. The most common abnormalities include skeletal, cardiovascular, and gastrointestinal malformations; craniofacial abnormalities; and intrauterine growth retardation.

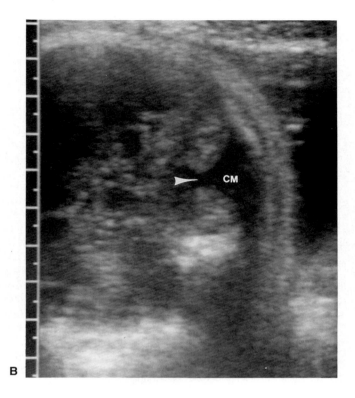

B

Central nervous system (CNS) defects, including choroid plexus cysts, hydrocephalus, spina bifida, and a large cisterna magna (Figure 2-6), have been described. The findings in the test images could be associated with a spina bifida defect of trisomy 18, but other abnormalities are not seen that support the diagnosis. The Arnold-Chiari malformation occurs as an isolated defect more commonly than trisomy 18 does; therefore, trisomy 18 is not the most likely diagnosis.

Hydrocephalus is not commonly associated with Down's syndrome (trisomy 21) (Option (E)). Increased nuchal skin thickening has been reported as a potential sign of trisomy 21, with reported sensitivities ranging from 9 to 38%; this should be identified on transcerebellar views (Figure 2-7). The lack of skin thickening in the test images, as well as the weak association of trisomy 21 and hydrocephalus, militates against the diagnosis of Down's syndrome.

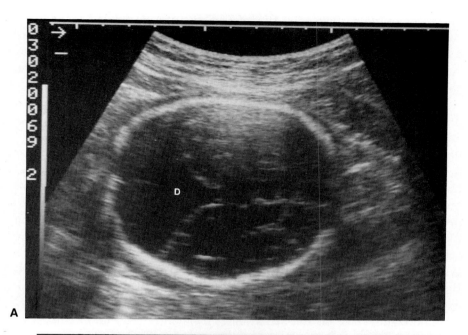

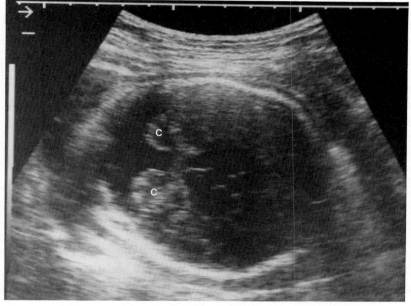

Figure 2-8. Dandy-Walker malformation. (A) A transaxial sonogram shows that the posterior fossa is enlarged and has been replaced by a large, triangular fluid collection typical of a Dandy-Walker malformation (D). (B) A sonogram at a different level shows anterolateral splaying of the cerebellar hemispheres (C) and fluid separating the hemispheres as a result of vermian aplasia.

measurement is performed at the level of the inferior portion of the third ventricle at approximately 10 to 15° of transducer inclination from the canthomeatal line. Greater degrees of transducer inclination can spuriously increase the dimension of the cisterna magna as a result of the oblique or near-coronal imaging of the cisterna magna.

The differential diagnosis of Dandy-Walker malformation includes a prominent but normal cisterna magna, trisomy 18, and retrocerebellar arachnoid cyst. In the study by Barkovich et al., patients with a prominent but normal cisterna magna had no enlargement of the posterior fossa and no evidence of vermian hypoplasia. The enlargement of the cisterna magna was largely the result of degenerative diseases of the CNS and associated atrophy. In a recent study by Nyberg et al. of sonographic findings in fetuses with trisomy 18, a large cisterna magna was found in 9 of 47 fetuses (19%) (see Figure 2-6). Retrocerebellar arachnoid cysts are typically round rather than having the funnel shape of the Dandy-Walker malformation. They are asymmetric rather than midline in location, and they compress but do not communicate with the fourth ventricle.

The Dandy-Walker malformation is frequently associated with CNS and extra-CNS anomalies. It is associated with hydrocephalus in approximately 70% of cases. Agenesis of the corpus callosum is the most common associated anomaly (14 to 19% of cases) (Figure 2-9); others include lipomas, aqueductal stenosis, and nonspecific gyral abnormalities. Spinal dysraphism and myelomeningocele are infrequent **(Option (D) is false)**. Extra-CNS anomalies have been noted in 25 to 43% of infants with Dandy-Walker malformation. The most common anomalies include polydactyly, cardiac defects, renal malformations, and facial anomalies. The frequency of chromosomal defects is uncertain because of the small number of reported cases. Chromosomal analysis is suggested for all fetuses identified with the Dandy-Walker malformation.

The natural history of fetuses with the Dandy-Walker malformation is also not well known. An overall mortality rate of 12 to 50% has been reported in the neurosurgical literature. In a 1988 series by Nyberg et al., the mortality rate (71%) in infants with the Dandy-Walker malformation was greater than that previously observed in other types of fetal hydrocephalus (63%), excluding holoprosencephaly and encephaloceles. The mortality is directly dependent on the presence and severity of extra-CNS anomalies. The functional outcome for survivors varies, with subnormal intelligence (IQ <83) manifested in 41 to 71% **(Option (E) is false)**.

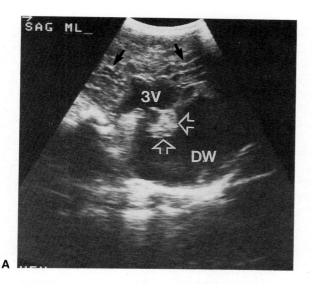

A

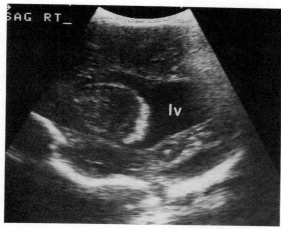

B

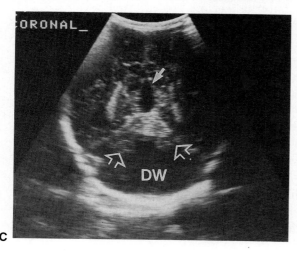

C

Figure 2-9. Neonate with agenesis of the corpus callosum and Dandy-Walker variant. (A) A midline sagittal image shows Dandy-Walker cyst (DW) and hypoplastic cerebellum (open arrows). There is no identifiable corpus callosum or cingulate gyrus. Medial gyri and sulci are radially oriented (solid arrows). 3V = third ventricle. (B) A parasagittal image shows a dilated lateral ventricle (lv) with the occipital horn most severely affected (colpocephaly). (C) A coronal image shows a Dandy-Walker cyst (DW) and hypoplastic cerebellum (open arrows). The third ventricle (solid arrow) is dilated and elevated. There is no identifiable corpus callosum.

Question 8

Concerning the Arnold-Chiari malformation,

(A) an elevated concentration of acetylcholinesterase in amniotic fluid is a marker of an open neural tube defect

(B) the associated hydrocephalus is characterized by enlargement of all ventricles

(C) it is associated with abnormal calvarial shape developing after 24 weeks gestational age

(D) it causes enlargement of the cisterna magna

(E) it causes cerebellar hypoplasia

(F) both open and closed neural tube defects are associated with the Chiari II malformation

The Chiari II malformation is a complex of anomalies involving almost all parts of the neural axis. The hallmark of the malformation is dysgenesis of the hindbrain manifested by a caudally displaced fourth ventricle and brain stem, with cerebellar tonsillar and vermian herniation through the foramen magnum. This is almost always associated with spina bifida, and nearly 80 to 90% of fetuses have hydrocephalus.

The prevalence of spina bifida differs in different parts of the world, with differing rates among races and an apparent east-west gradient ranging from a high prevalence in Great Britain to a low incidence on the west coast of Canada. The risk of neural tube defect (NTD) rises to 20 to 30 per 1,000 in families with a previous child with NTD, but most cases occur in families with no history of such abnormality. Screening tests to improve the detection of fetuses with these defects have become available.

α-Fetoprotein (AFP) is a glycoprotein produced by the fetal liver. Some AFP enters the amniotic fluid via fetal urine, and a small amount crosses the placenta to the maternal serum. Normal AFP levels in both amniotic fluid and maternal serum vary with the gestational age. Maternal serum AFP (MS-AFP) and amniotic fluid AFP levels are increased in fetuses with NTDs that are not covered by skin. However, an elevated MS-AFP level is not specific for NTD but can occur as a result of conditions such as multifetal pregnancy, misdated pregnancy, fetal death, and placental aberrations leading to fetomaternal transfusion and anomalies such as gastroschisis, omphalocele, and congenital nephrosis. Amniotic fluid AFP is a fairly reliable diagnostic screening tool for the detection of NTDs, although the mixture of fetal blood and amniotic fluid can prevent an accurate interpretation.

An assay for amniotic fluid acetylcholinesterase was developed in the early 1980s and is now used as a complementary test to AFP detection. Acetylcholinesterase originates in the tissues of the brain or spinal cord.

Its concentration in amniotic fluid is less influenced by fetal blood than is the level of AFP, and it can be interpreted independently of the gestational age. In the series by Milunsky and Sapirstein, high AFP and acetylcholinesterase activity were detected in all cases of open NTDs. The absence of acetylcholinesterase activity in the presence of a high AFP level correctly reclassified 89% of pregnancies as normal. A false-positive result of 11% was observed in fetuses with a normal oucome but high AFP values and acetylcholinesterase activity. Although the acetylcholinesterase assay is not free of false-positive results, it is useful as an adjunct to AFP when amniotic fluid is admixed with fetal blood; an elevated concentration is a marker for open NTDs **(Option (A) is true).**

Sonography has also become an important adjunct to the evaluation of women with increased MS-AFP levels. Sonography is performed, often in conjunction with amniocentesis, to permit detection of spina bifida before the time of fetal viability. Utilizing current technology and the sonographic signs described below, recent studies have shown a sensitivity of 91 to 100% in affected fetuses, leading to the suggestion by Benacerraf and others that a normal sonogram in the setting of an elevated MS-AFP level may obviate amniocentesis, a procedure with a reported fetal loss rate of 0.5 to 1%. This remains controversial, however.

Filly et al. have recommended a practical method for evaluation of the fetal cranium, which can help identify CNS anomalies in 95% of cases. The fetal cranium should be evaluated at three levels: transventricular, transthalamic, and transcerebellar. The atrium of the lateral ventricle is imaged on the transventricular view (Figure 2-10A). Unlike other parts of the lateral ventricles, which change during rapid cerebral growth, the diameter of the ventricular atrium remains constant throughout the second and third trimesters. The landmark for the atrium is the glomus of the choroid plexus. The atrial diameter is measured perpendicular to the long axis of the ventricle across the most posterior portion of the glomus and should not exceed 10 mm.

The transthalamic view is the standard plane for measuring the biparietal diameter and head circumference. The cavum septi pellucidi, frontal horns of the lateral ventricles, and Sylvian cisterns are also identified at this level (Figure 2-10B).

At the level of the cerebellum, both the shape of the cerebellar hemispheres and the size of the cisterna magna should be evaluated. The diameter of the normal cisterna magna is between 2 and 11 mm. Within the cisterna magna, echogenic lines or cystic structures are occasionally identified. These were previously thought to represent the straight sinus but have now been shown to be either normal subarachnoid septa or dural folds of the falx cerebelli. The normal cerebellum has a bilobed configuration, with the lateral hypoechoic hemispheres separated by a slightly more echogenic midline vermis (Figure 2-11).

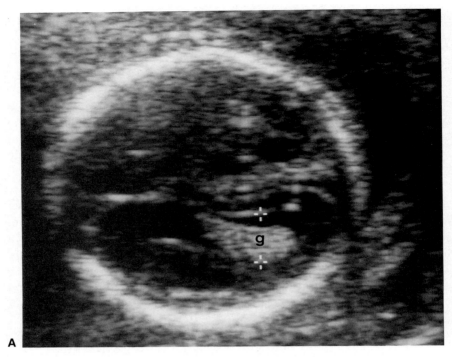

A

Figure 2-10. Normal cranial sonogram in a 20-week-old fetus. (A) The correct level at which to measure lateral ventricular diameter is at the atrium, which is marked by the glomus of the choroid plexus (g). The medial atrial wall (top cursor) is a better specular reflector than the lateral wall (bottom cursor), although the dependent edge of the glomus also marks the position of the lateral wall. The cursors should be positioned perpendicular to the long axis of the atrium at the lumenal margins. (B) A transthalamic view shows the diamond-shaped hypoechoic thalamus-hypothalamus complex (t) separated by an echogenic midline slitlike structure, the third ventricle. The anterior horn of the dependent lateral ventricle (v) and the cavum septi pellucidi (between arrows) are identified.

In the fetus being evaluated for possible spina bifida, the sonographic findings most useful for diagnosis are (1) direct visualization of the dysraphic spinal defect, (2) soft tissue features of a myelomeningocele (a sac or disruption of the overlying integument), and (3) identification of associated cranial abnormalities. The cranial findings are present because of the nearly universal association of an open myelomeningocele with the Chiari II malformation.

The cranial abnormalities associated with the Chiari II malformation are characteristic. Approximately 80% of fetuses with an open

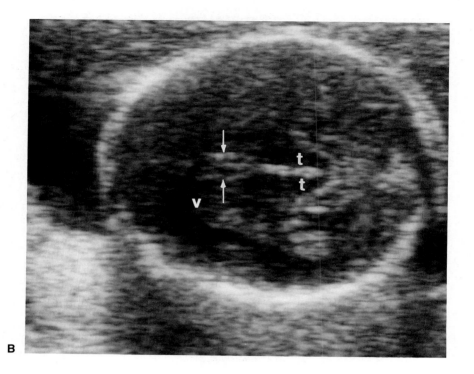

B

myelomeningocele have hydrocephalus by 24 weeks gestation. The lateral ventricles are enlarged with the occipital horns often disproportionately larger than the frontal horns; although the third ventricle is often enlarged, compression by an associated enlargement of the massa intermedia may cause the third ventricle to appear only slightly larger than normal. The fourth ventricle is effaced and elongated rather than dilated **(Option (B) is false).** A characteristic calvarial shape has also been identified in these fetuses. The frontal contour is concave or flattened instead of being convex; the resultant calvarial shape has become known as the lemon sign. The lemon sign is best imaged at the transventricular level prior to 24 weeks gestation **(Option (C) is false).** The abnormal shape may be related to low intraspinal pressure, which causes deformity of the relatively malleable frontal bones. With increasing maturation, the calvarium becomes stronger and more resistant to pressure changes. It has been alternatively theorized that the lemon sign results from a mesenchymal dysplasia of the cranium, the same process giving rise to the craniolacunae frequently associated with NTDs. The lemon sign invariably resolves by 34 weeks.

In the 1988 study by Nyberg et al., prior to 24 weeks gestational age the lemon sign had a sensitivity of 93%, a specificity of 99%, a positive-

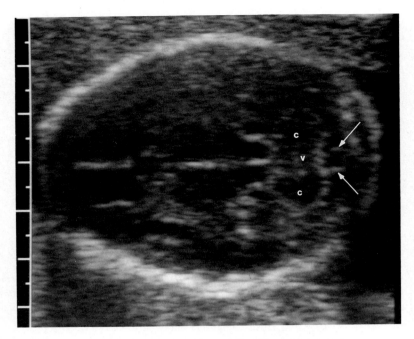

Figure 2-11. Normal fetal sonogram demonstrating cisterna magna septa. Echogenic structures in the cisterna magna create the appearance of a cyst (arrows). These were previously thought to be the straight sinus but have since been shown to represent either normal subarachnoid septa or dural folds of the falx cerebelli. The normal cerebellar contour is shown, with the hypoechoic cerebellar hemispheres (c) separated by the slightly more echogenic vermis (v).

predictive value of 81%, and a negative-predictive value of 99.5% for spina bifida. These numbers suggest that the absence of a lemon sign in association with spina bifida prior to 24 weeks is unusual. A small number of normal fetuses (about 1%) have a lemon sign. In these cases, however, the frontal contour is linear rather than concave and the appearance is often created at the base of the skull. If normal ventricular size and a normal posterior fossa can be demonstrated, it is likely that the linear contour is a normal variant. The lemon sign, while most commonly associated with the Chiari II malformation, can also be seen with other fetal anomalies, even in the absence of a myelomeningocele. Ball et al. have reported examples associated with encephalocele, Dandy-Walker malformation and encephalocele, thanatophoric dysplasia, cystic hygroma, diaphragmatic hernia and agenesis of the corpus callosum, fetal hydronephrosis, and umbilical vein varix with two-vessel cord.

The evaluation of the posterior fossa is important since 15 to 20% of fetuses with open myelomeningoceles have normal ventricular size. If only transventricular and transthalamic views were obtained in these fetuses, significant CNS abnormalities would be missed. Two important signs have been described in the posterior fossa in association with spina bifida as a result of the associated Arnold-Chiari malformation and the downward displacement of the cerebellum and fourth ventricle. The effacement of the cisterna magna is the more sensitive sign, being present in 95% of cases **(Option (D) is false).** The posterior fossa is shallow, and the cerebellar hemispheres are often hypoplastic **(Option (E) is true).** In about 57% of cases, the cerebellar hemispheres lose their normal bilobed shape and are wrapped around the brain stem, resulting in the banana sign (Figure 2-2B). The banana sign is considered to be a more severe abnormality than effacement of the cisterna magna.

Assessing the different cranial findings can provide important information about the likelihood of spina bifida. The presence of a lemon sign in conjunction with ventricular dilatation and/or obliteration of the cisterna magna is highly suspicious for spina bifida, regardless of the spinal findings. The reported cases of a normal cisterna magna and spina bifida have involved closed defects, either skin-covered meningocele or lipomyelomeningocele, which are not associated with the Chiari II malformation **(Option (F) is false).**

Anomalies associated with spina bifida can be categorized as (1) neuromuscular deformities resulting from the spinal defect itself, (2) additional CNS anomalies, and (3) extra-CNS anomalies. Neuromuscular anomalies include foot deformities, primarily clubfoot, and hip dislocation. CNS malformations, other than hydrocephalus, include holoprosencephaly, agenesis of the corpus callosum, and, rarely, Dandy-Walker malformation. Tethered cord, diastematomyelia, intraspinal lipoma, and dermoid cysts are also commonly associated with myelomeningocele. Extra-CNS anomalies involve a wide range of organs (face, kidneys, gastrointestinal tract, thorax, and extremities).

The physical and intellectual disabilities of infants with spina bifida vary considerably. Three factors contributing to the eventual outcome are location and extent of the spinal defect, open versus closed defect, and the presence or absence of hydrocephalus. Motor deficits are worse in infants with proximal and/or open spinal defects than in those with distal and closed defects. Normal ambulation can be expected for only 23% of infants with open defects compared with 70% of those with closed defects.

Hindbrain dysfunction is a serious complication of treated myelomeningocele. Symptoms include pain at the base of the neck and skull, nystagmus, weakness in the upper extremities, hypotonia, and spasticity. Up to one-third of patients with hindbrain dysfunction will die of this complication, usually as a result of respiratory failure. Symptomatic patients require surgical decompression of the brain stem.

Question 9

Concerning Down's syndrome,

<ul style="list-style:none">
<li>(A) it is reliably detected on routine prenatal sonography</li>
<li>(B) it is associated with a low maternal serum α-fetoprotein level</li>
<li>(C) a nuchal skin fold thickness greater than 6 mm should suggest the diagnosis</li>
<li>(D) the characteristic sonographic features of associated duodenal atresia are generally not apparent until the third trimester</li>
<li>(E) central nervous system anomalies are more frequent than in infants with trisomy 18</li>
</ul>

Improved prenatal detection of Down's syndrome (trisomy 21) is an important goal of modern genetic evaluation. Although newborns with Down's syndrome have several physical characteristics that are readily identified by physical examination, the antenatal sonographic diagnosis is not readily made **(Option (A) is false).** The association between advanced maternal age and Down's syndrome is well known. However, mothers aged 35 and over account for only 20 to 25% of all liveborn infants with Down's syndrome, and most mothers have no known clinical risk factors. In recent years, significant effort has been directed to the improved recognition of these pregnancies.

In 1984, an association between low MS-AFP levels and trisomy 21 was reported **(Option (B) is true).** Low MS-AFP levels have been shown to be present in approximately 20% of women younger than 35 years whose fetuses have Down's syndrome. Recent research has been directed at increasing the detection rate of Down's syndrome by using the AFP profile. The profile uses three biochemical markers in maternal serum, AFP, serum estriol, and human chorionic gonadotropin, which provide independent risk data concerning Down's syndrome. The use of these three markers offers the advantage of tripling the number of cases of Down's syndrome detected in fetuses of women younger than 35 years. A screen-positive result with an AFP profile indicates a patient-specific risk of at least 1 in 270 for carrying a fetus affected with Down's syndrome. The AFP profile usually identifies 5 to 7% of pregnancies as screen positive. In these cases, sonography is performed to confirm gestational dating. If results remain positive after a check of dating, then the woman is offered genetic counseling regarding the risk of Down's syndrome and an amniocentesis for chromosome and amniotic fluid AFP testing.

The increasing use of routine sonography in the second trimester has stimulated interest in identifying anomalies that are readily reproducible and associated with Down's syndrome. Benacerraf et al. reported the potential value of nuchal skin fold thickness greater than 6 mm as a sign of Down's syndrome **(Option (C) is true).** The thickness should be measured at the level of the cisterna magna on axial views through the cerebellum (Figure 2-7). Measurement in the sagittal plane can be erroneous because of changes in thickness with flexion and extension of the fetal neck. Other authors have confirmed this association with reported sensitivities from 9 to 38% and a positive-predictive value of 8% for identifying Down's syndrome.

In the review of prenatal sonographic findings in fetuses with Down's syndrome by Nyberg et al., the anomalies most frequently detected before 20 weeks gestation were cystic hygromas, nuchal fold thickening, and hyperechogenic bowel. Cystic hygromas can appear similar to nuchal fold thickening (Figure 2-12), and there is speculation that nuchal thickening may result from a cystic hygroma that has resolved. Identification of a nuchal ligament separating two distinct cystic spaces is characteristic of a cystic hygroma. Cystic hygromas indicate the highest risk of a chromosomal abnormality of any malformation and are associated with an underlying chromosomal defect in 75% of cases when karyotyping is successful. Turner's syndrome accounts for 80% of cases, and trisomies 18 and 21 make up most of the remainder. Cystic hygromas are seen less frequently in the third trimester than in the second trimester, reflecting their high natural intrauterine mortality rate.

Hyperechogenic bowel was observed in 7% of fetuses with trisomy 21 in the series by Nyberg et al. This appeared as an unusually prominent, echogenic mass in the lower abdomen. The cause of this finding is uncertain, but it is hypothesized that a decreased transit time of amniotic fluid predisposes to inspissated, echogenic meconium. This hypothesis is supported by an association between chromosomal abnormalities and decreased levels of intestinal microvillar enzymes in the amniotic fluid. Unfortunately, the echogenic bowel is nonspecific and can also be seen in fetuses with cystic fibrosis and in normal fetuses.

The bowel anomaly most frequently associated with Down's syndrome is duodenal atresia. Approximately 5% of fetuses with Down's syndrome have duodenal atresia, and 30 to 40% of all fetuses with duodenal atresia prove to have trisomy 21. Duodenal atresia should be detected uniformly by sonography after 24 weeks gestation because the atresia is a complete obstruction that results in a classic "double bubble" finding, usually in conjunction with polyhydramnios. Duodenal atresia is not

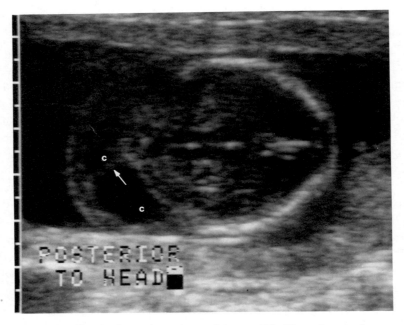

Figure 2-12. Cystic hygroma in a fetus with Down's syndrome. The appearance of the cystic hygroma can be confused with nuchal fold thickening (see Figure 2-6). However, a cystic hygroma tends to have a greater fluid component, and a nuchal ligament (arrow) can be identified. This midline septation is typically outlined by bilateral cysts (c) and attaches at the posterior neck; it represents the most specific sign for a cystic hygroma.

usually detectable before 24 weeks, presumably because the fetus swallows relatively little amniotic fluid **(Option (D) is true).** The diagnosis might be suggested before 20 weeks if there is mild dilatation of the duodenum without polyhydramnios.

CNS anomalies are less frequent in fetuses with trisomy 21 than in those with trisomies 18 and 13 **(Option (E) is false).** Mild cerebral ventricular dilatation has been reported; this is probably a nonobstructive dilatation related to decreased brain mass or to brain atrophy. However, there is no single anomaly that is suggestive of trisomy 21 as holoprosencephaly is for trisomy 13. Cardiovascular malformations are common in fetuses with Down's syndrome, although they are frequently missed on routine sonography.

The utility of screening for femur length shortening in fetuses with Down's syndrome remains controversial. Initial reports by Lockwood et al. and Benacerraf et al. in 1987 proposed that a ratio of measured to expected femur length of 0.91 or lower indicated Down's syndrome with a sensitivity of 40%, specificity of 95%, and positive-predictive value of 3.1%. However, other investigators in other centers have not been able to reproduce this high correlation. In the series by Nyberg et al., 14% of fetuses with Down's syndrome had short femur lengths, although 6.1% of fetuses with normal karyotypes also had a ratio of 0.91 or less. The maximum positive-predictive value for a high-risk population (prevalence of Down's syndrome, 1:250) was only 0.93%, and that for a low-risk population (prevalence of Down's syndrome, 1:700) was 0.33%. Nyberg et al. concluded that although fetuses with Down's syndrome are more likely to have short femur lengths than are chromosomally normal fetuses, the data did not support determination of short femur length by itself as a screening test for trisomy 21. When used in conjunction with other risk factors, however, it might help to predict which mothers are at risk and should undergo further evaluation by genetic amniocentesis. In this regard, Benacerraf et al. have proposed a sonographic scoring index incorporating several findings associated with Down's syndrome. These include nuchal fold thickening, a major structural defect, short femur, short humerus, and renal pyelectasis. Other skeletal abnormalities include hypoplasia of the middle phalanx of the fifth digit with an inward curve (clinodactyly). This is seen in 60% of infants with Down's syndrome, but it can be difficult to image. Similarly, prenatal detection of the simian crease has been described but is also technically difficult and time-consuming.

Karen J. Stuck, M.D.
Gary M. Kellman, M.D.

SUGGESTED READINGS

ARNOLD-CHIARI MALFORMATION

1. Ball RH, Filly RA, Goldstein RB, Callen PW. The lemon sign: not a specific indicator of meningomyelocele. J Ultrasound Med 1993; 12:131–134
2. Benacerraf BR. Should patients with elevated levels of maternal serum alpha-fetoprotein always undergo amniocentesis? Radiology 1993; 188:17–18
3. Benacerraf BR, Stryker J, Frigoletto FD Jr. Abnormal US appearance of the cerebellum (banana sign): indirect sign of spina bifida. Radiology 1989; 171:151–153
4. Campbell J, Gilbert WM, Nicolaides KH, Campbell S. Ultrasound screening for spina bifida: cranial and cerebellar signs in a high-risk population. Obstet Gynecol 1987; 70:247–250
5. Filly RA, Callen PW, Goldstein RB. Alpha-fetoprotein screening programs: what every obstetric sonologist should know. Radiology 1993; 188:1–8

6. Filly RA, Cardoza JD, Goldstein RB, Barkovich AJ. Detection of fetal central nervous system anomalies: a practical level of effort for a routine sonogram. Radiology 1989; 172:403–408

7. Filly RA, Goldstein RB, Callen PW. Fetal ventricle: importance in routine obstetric sonography. Radiology 1991; 181:1–7

8. Furness ME, Barbary JE, Verco PW. Fetal head shape in spina bifida in the second trimester. JCU 1987; 15:451–453

9. Goldstein RB, La Pidus AS, Filly RA, Cardoza J. Mild lateral cerebral ventricle dilatation *in utero*: clinical significance and prognosis. Radiology 1990; 176:237–242

10. Goldstein RB, Podrasky AE, Filly RA, Callen PW. Effacement of the fetal cisterna magna in association with myelomeningocele. Radiology 1989; 172:409–413

11. Knutzon RK, McGahan JP, Salamat MS, Brant WE. Fetal cisterna magna septa: a normal anatomic finding. Radiology 1991; 180:799–801

12. Mahony BS, Callen PW, Filly RA, Hoddick WK. The fetal cisterna magna. Radiology 1984; 153:773–776

13. Milunsky A, Sapirstein VS. Prenatal diagnosis of open neural tube defects using the amniotic fluid acetylcholinesterase assay. Obstet Gynecol 1982; 59:1–5

14. Nicolaides KH, Campbell S, Gabbe SG, Guidetti R. Ultrasound screening for spina bifida: cranial and cerebellar signs. Lancet 1986; 2:72–74

15. Nyberg DA, Mack LA. The spine and neural tube defects. In: Nyberg DA, Mahony BS, Pretorius DH (eds), Diagnostic ultrasound of fetal anomalies. Chicago: Year Book; 1990:160–182

16. Nyberg DA, Mack LA, Hirsch J, Mahony BS. Abnormalities of fetal cranial contour in sonographic detection of spina bifida: evaluation of the "lemon" sign. Radiology 1988; 167:387–392

17. Nyberg DA, Mack LA, Hirsch J, Pagon RO, Shepard TH. Fetal hydrocephalus: sonographic detection and clinical significance of associated anomalies. Radiology 1987; 163:187–191

18. Penso C, Redline RW, Benacerraf BR. A sonographic sign which predicts which fetuses with hydrocephalus have an associated neural tube defect. J Ultrasound Med 1987; 6:307–311

19. Pretorius DH, Kallman CE, Grafe MR, Budorick NE, Stamm ER. Linear echoes in the fetal cisterna magna. J Ultrasound Med 1992; 11:125–128

20. Robbin M, Filly RA, Fell S, et al. Elevated levels of amniotic fluid alphafetoprotein: sonographic evaluation. Radiology 1993; 188:165–169

DANDY-WALKER MALFORMATION

21. Barkovich JA, Kjos BO, Norman D, Edwards MS. Revised classification of posterior fossa cysts and cystlike malformations based on the results of multiplanar MR imaging. AJR 1989; 153:1289–1300

22. Fitz CR. Disorders of ventricles and CSF spaces. Semin US CT MR 1988; 9:216–230

23. Harlow CL, Hay TC, Rumack CM. The pediatric brain. In: Rumack CM, Wilson SR, Charboneau JW (eds), Diagnostic ultrasound. Chicago: Mosby-Year Book; 1991:2:1018–1024

24. Kollias SS, Ball WS, Prenger EC. Cystic malformation of the posterior fossa: differential diagnosis clarified through embryologic analysis. RadioGraphics 1993; 6:1211–1231

25. Kramer D, Nyberg DA, Mahony BS, Resta R, Luthy DA, Hickok DE. Prenatal sonographic findings of trisomy 18: a review of 40 cases. J Ultrasound Med 1992; 11:S39

26. Nyberg DA, Cyr DR, Mack LA, Fitzsimmons J, Hickok D, Mahony BS. The Dandy-Walker malformation prenatal sonographic diagnosis and its clinical significance. J Ultrasound Med 1988; 7:65–71

27. Nyberg DA, Kramer D, Resta RG, et al. Prenatal sonographic findings of trisomy 18: review of 47 cases. J Ultrasound Med 1993; 12:103–113

28. Russ PD, Pretorius DH, Johnson MJ. Dandy-Walker syndrome: a review of fifteen cases evaluated by prenatal sonography. Am J Obstet Gynecol 1989; 161:401–406

29. Sato Y, Kao SC, Smith WL. Radiologic manifestations of anomalies of the brain. Radiol Clin North Am 1991; 29:179–194

DOWN'S SYNDROME

30. Benacerraf BR, Cnann A, Gelman R, Laboda LA, Frigoletto FD Jr. Can sonographers reliably identify anatomic features associated with Down syndrome in fetuses? Radiology 1989; 173:377–380

31. Benacerraf BA, Neuberg D, Bromley B, Frigoletto FD Jr. Sonographic scoring index for prenatal detection of chromosomal abnormalities. J Ultrasound Med 1993; 11:449–458

32. Benacerraf BR, Gelman R, Frigoletto FD Jr. Sonographic identification of second-trimester fetuses with Down's syndrome. N Engl J Med 1987; 317:1371–1376

33. Benacerraf BR, Laboda LA, Frigoletto FD. Thickened nuchal fold in fetuses not at risk for aneuploidy. Radiology 1992; 184:239–242

34. Cuckle H, Wald N, Quinn J, Royston P, Butler L. Ultrasound fetal femur length measurement in the screening for Down's syndrome. Br J Obstet Gynecol 1989; 96:1373–1378

35. LaFollette L, Filly RA, Anderson R, Golbus MS. Fetal femur length to detect trisomy 21. A reappraisal. J Ultrasound Med 1989; 8:657–660

36. Lockwood C, Benacerraf B, Krinsky A, et al. A sonographic screening method for Down syndrome. Am J Obstet Gynecol 1987; 157:803–808

37. Nyberg DA. Intra-abdominal anomalies. In: Nyberg DA, Mahony BS, Pretorius DH (eds), Diagnostic ultrasound of fetal anomalies. Chicago: Year Book; 1990:355–363

38. Nyberg DA, Resta RG, Hickok DE, Hollenbach KA, Luthy DA, Mahony BS. Femur length shortening in the detection of Down syndrome: is prenatal screening feasible? Am J Obstet Gynecol 1990; 162:1247–1252

39. Nyberg DA, Resta RG, Luthy DA, Hickok DE, Mahony BS, Hirsch JH. Prenatal sonographic findings of Down syndrome: review of 94 cases. Obstet Gynecol 1990; 76:370–377

40. Persutte WH. Second trimester hyperechogenicity in the lower abdomen of two fetuses with trisomy 21: is there a correlation? JCU 1990; 18:425–428

40. Romero R, Ghidini A, Costigan K, Touloukian R, Hobbins JC. Prenatal diagnosis of duodenal atresia: does it make any difference? Obstet Gynecol 1988; 71:739–741

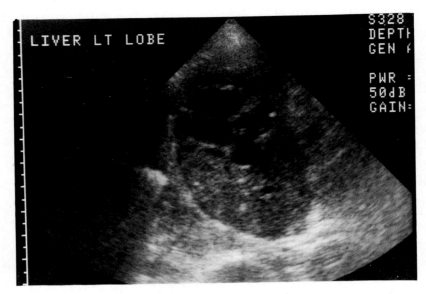

Figure 3-1

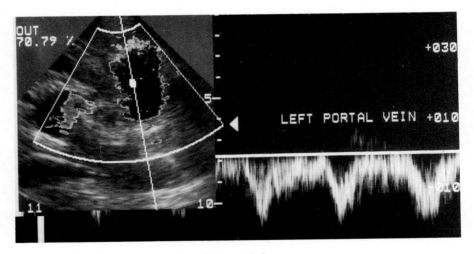

Figure 3-2

Figures 3-1 and 3-2. This 81-year-old man with an abdominal bruit was referred for sonography to rule out an abdominal aortic aneurysm. You are shown a longitudinal sonogram of the left lobe of the liver (Figure 3-1) and a pulsed Doppler waveform obtained from the left portal vein (Figure 3-2).

Case 3: Arterioportal Fistula

Question 10

Which *one* of the following is the MOST likely diagnosis?

(A) Angiosarcoma
(B) Tortuous recanalized paraumbilical vein
(C) Hepatic artery aneurysm
(D) Arterioportal fistula
(E) Hypervascular hepatocellular carcinoma

Figure 3-1 shows a multicystic-appearing mass in the left lobe of the liver. Figure 3-2 shows that the left portal vein has blood flow below the baseline, representing reversed (hepatofugal) flow. Additionally, the waveform from the left portal vein is pulsatile and in fact appears arterial in nature. This constellation of findings is consistent with an arterioportal fistula between the left hepatic artery and the left portal vein **(Option (D) is correct).** Imaging of the mass itself by color Doppler ultrasonography confirmed that the "multicystic mass" was actually a collection of dilated and tortuous vessels with abundant internal blood flow (Figure 3-3).

Arterioportal fistulas can be acquired or congenital. Acquired fistulas are usually due to penetrating hepatic trauma (stab wounds, liver biopsy, or surgical trauma). They can also result from rupture of a hepatic artery aneurysm into an adjacent portal vein. When they are large enough, they can cause portal hypertension. Like arteriovenous fistulas elsewhere in the body, arterioportal fistulas cause increased flow velocities and flow volumes in the supplying and draining vessels. This eventually causes vessel enlargement and tortuosity. Arterioportal fistulas are almost always associated with turbulent blood flow and may therefore result in a bruit, as in the test patient.

Primary hepatic neoplasms such as angiosarcoma (Option (A)) or hepatocellular carcinoma (Option (E)) can be extremely vascular, can have extensive arteriovenous shunting, and can invade the portal veins. Hepatocellular carcinoma (hepatoma) in particular is noted for its arteri-

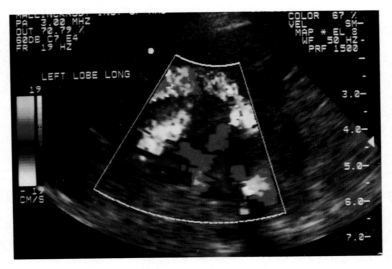

Figure 3-3. Same patient as in Figures 3-1 and 3-2. Arterioportal fistula. A longitudinal color Doppler sonogram of the left lobe of the liver confirms that the multicystic mass is a vascular malformation.

oportal shunting and its portal vein invasion. In fact, case reports have indicated that tumor thrombus in the portal vein secondary to hepatocellular carcinoma can result in an arterial waveform arising from within the portal vein. However, both angiosarcoma and hepatocellular carcinoma are solid tumors, and although associated hemorrhage and necrosis occasionally produce cystic regions, these tumors do not appear as purely cystic or multicystic lesions. It would also be quite uncommon for a hepatic neoplasm to cause a bruit that could be mistaken for an abdominal aortic aneurysm on physical examination.

Recanalized paraumbilical vein (Option (B)) is a common portosystemic shunt that occurs in the setting of portal hypertension. It is located in the ligamentum teres at the junction of the medial and lateral segments of the left lobe of the liver. It is supplied by the left portal vein and shunts blood from the left portal vein into abdominal wall varices (Figure 3-4). With long-standing portal hypertension, the paraumbilical vein may become quite large and tortuous and could conceivably result in an appearance similar to that seen in Figure 3-1. However, since the recanalized paraumbilical vein is supplied by the left portal vein, it is associated with antegrade flow in the left portal vein. It also would not explain an arterialized portal vein waveform.

Intrahepatic arterial aneurysms (Option (C)) are rare but do occur. Uncomplicated hepatic artery aneurysms result from atherosclerosis and

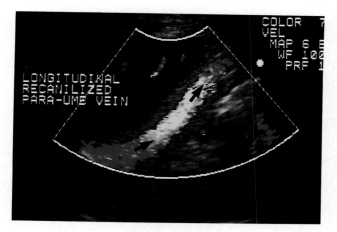

Figure 3-4. Recanalized paraumbilical vein. A longitudinal color Doppler image through the left lobe of the liver at the site of the ligamentum teres shows a large recanalized paraumbilical vein with blood flow directed away from the liver (arrows).

appear as a unilocular cystic mass on gray-scale imaging. As with other types of aneurysms, they generally have a swirling pattern of blood flow on color Doppler images (Figure 3-5). When they are large, they can contain mural thrombus. The multicystic appearance in Figure 3-1 is not consistent with an aneurysm. In addition, an uncomplicated hepatic artery aneurysm would not explain the reversed flow or the arterialized waveform in the left portal vein. As mentioned above, a ruptured hepatic artery aneurysm that communicates with the portal vein is a potential cause of an acquired arterioportal fistula and therefore could have an appearance similar to the one shown in Figure 3-1.

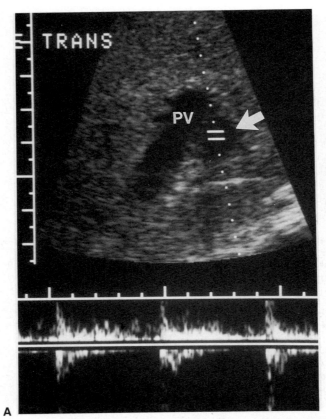

Figure 3-5. Hepatic artery aneurysm. (A) A transverse sonogram and pulsed Doppler waveform show the Doppler sample volume within a cystic structure (arrow) adjacent to the left portal vein (PV). Pulsatile arterial flow is confirmed on pulsed Doppler, documenting that the cystic structure communicates with the hepatic artery. (B) A transverse color Doppler image shows the typical swirling pattern of blood flow in the aneurysm (arrows). PV = portal vein.

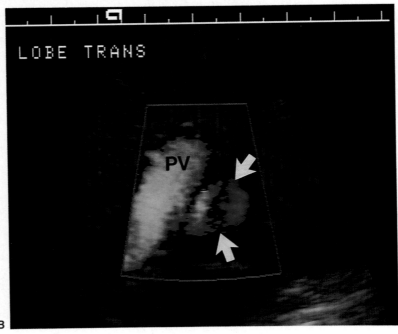

Question 11

Concerning portal hypertension,

    (A) the most common type in the United States is intrahepatic
    (B) it is one of the causes of the sonographic "parallel-channel sign"
    (C) the earliest sonographic sign is flow reversal in the main portal vein
    (D) detection of a hypoechoic band in the ligamentum teres is a specific sign
    (E) spontaneous splenorenal shunts are the most common portosystemic collaterals detected sonographically

Portal hypertension is defined as a portal pressure of >10 mm/Hg. It can be classified in a number of ways depending on (1) whether there is increased portal venous flow versus increased resistance to portal venous flow or (2) whether the underlying abnormality is prehepatic versus intrahepatic versus posthepatic. Intrahepatic causes can be further subdivided into those that are presinusoidal versus postsinusoidal. In the United States, the most common cause of portal hypertension is cirrhosis, which is classified as intrahepatic **(Option (A) is true).**

To understand cirrhosis and portal hypertension, it is important to remember the microscopic vascular anatomy of the hepatic lobule. This is displayed in Figure 3-6. Hepatocytes are arranged in radial columns centered around the central draining vein. Between the columns of hepatocytes are the sinusoids. Blood flow from the hepatic arteries and the portal veins drains into the sinusoids, mixes, and then drains into the central vein, which ultimately drains into larger venules and then into the major branches of the hepatic veins. Peripheral portal triads are positioned around the edge of the hepatic lobule. In addition to draining directly into the sinusoids, hepatic arteries and portal veins supply a plexus around the biliary ductules. Anastomoses exist between the portal vein and hepatic arteries at the level of the sinusoids and the biliary plexus. These anastomoses allow for shunting of hepatic arterial flow into the portal vein when resistance to hepatic venous outflow is elevated.

In patients with alcoholic cirrhosis, hepatocellular death is followed by the generation of fibrous tissue, which replaces the sinusoids and distorts the central veins. Development of regenerating nodules also compresses hepatic venous outflow. The result is an increased resistance to hepatic venous outflow and thus to portal venous inflow. Initially, elevation of portal pressure allows for maintenance of portal vein flow volumes. However, as the process becomes more advanced, resistance to portal flow becomes equal to resistance to flow in portal systemic collaterals and a portion of portal flow begins to be shunted away from the liver. Hepatic arterial flow increases and partially compensates for the

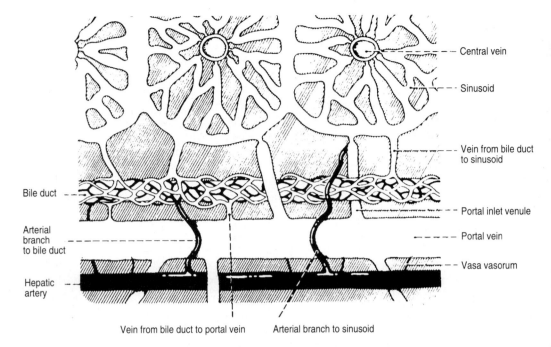

Figure 3-6. Microvascular anatomy of the liver. Branches from the portal vein drain into the sinusoids, and other branches communicate with the peribiliary plexus. Hepatic artery branches supply the sinusoids, the peribiliary plexus, and the vasa vasorum of the portal vein. Anastomoses between the hepatic artery and portal vein exist at the level of the sinusoids and the peribiliary plexus. (Adapted with permission from Cho and Lunderquist [4].)

decreased portal venous flow. This can result in dramatic enlargement of the intrahepatic arteries until they are equal in size to the adjacent portal vein, thus producing the "parallel-channel sign" (Figure 3-7A) **(Option (B) is true).** Doppler analysis in such cases will document that both channels are vascular and will exclude biliary dilatation as the source of the parallel-channel sign (Figure 3-7B).

In patients with more-advanced cirrhosis, resistance to flow through the sinusoids and hepatic veins becomes so great that hepatic arterial flow exits the liver via arterial portal shunting, thus converting the portal vein into an outflow vessel for the liver. Development of retrograde (hepatofugal) flow in the portal vein often starts as a focal process in the more severely cirrhotic segments of the liver. Therefore, isolated flow reversal may be seen in either the left or right portal vein. With progressive disease, flow reverses even in the main portal vein. Flow reversal in

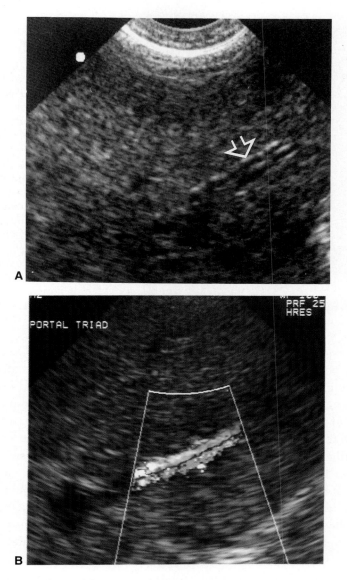

Figure 3-7. Enlarged hepatic artery simulating intrahepatic biliary ductal dilatation. (A) An oblique view of the left lobe of the liver shows two peripheral parallel channels (open arrow). (B) A color Doppler view shows that both channels contain blood flow. The anterior vessel is an enlarged hepatic artery with normally directed blood flow. The posterior vessel is a portal vein with reversed blood flow due to portal hypertension.

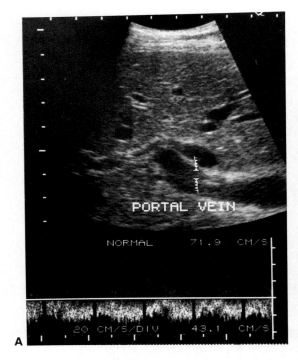

Figure 3-8. Helical flow in the main portal vein. (A) A pulsed Doppler waveform from the main portal vein shows flow below the baseline. Taken by itself, this would indicate hepatofugal flow in the main portal vein and severe portal hypertension. (B) A color Doppler view of the portal vein shows that there is antegrade flow in the portal vein. The area of flow reversal is focal and is due to a helical pattern of flow at the curve in the portal vein.

the main portal vein indicates advanced disease and is one of the late sonographic signs of portal hypertension **(Option (C) is false).** When determining flow direction in the main portal vein, it is important to realize that a normal portal vein may have helical flow patterns that can appear as reversed flow if color Doppler is not available (Figure 3-8).

The diagnosis of portal hypertension can be suggested sonographically when there is portal vein enlargement, splenomegaly, and ascites. Unfortunately, splenomegaly and ascites are nonspecific abnormalities and the portal vein diameter is so variable that specific measurements have not been sufficiently well established to allow the diagnosis of portal hypertension. Therefore, the hallmark for sonographic detection of portal hypertension is identification of portosystemic collaterals.

Sonographically, the easiest collateral to detect is the recanalized paraumbilical vein. It appears as a variably sized anechoic tubular channel running in the ligamentum teres between the medial and lateral segments of the left lobe (Figures 3-9 and 3-10). It communicates with the left portal vein and provides hepatofugal drainage into abdominal wall vessels. Aneurysmal dilatation of the recanalized paraumbilical vein occasionally occurs and may appear as a cystic mass in the left lobe of the liver (Figure 3-11). Hepatofugal venous flow detected in any hypoechoic

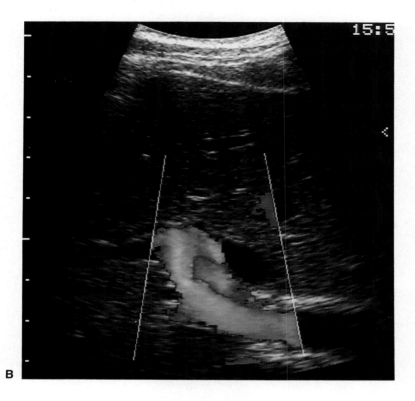

B

or anechoic band within the ligamentum teres is a specific sign of portal hypertension. However, in some normal individuals, a thin (i.e., ≤2 mm) anechoic or hypoechoic cord without Doppler-detectable flow (or with arterial flow) is seen in the ligamentum teres. This should not be confused with a recanalized paraumbilical vein and is not indicative of portal hypertension **(Option (D) is false)**.

Enlarged, tortuous veins can be seen in the splenic hilum in patients with portal hypertension. Unfortunately, similar-appearing venous enlargement can be seen in patients with splenomegaly from other causes or in patients with splenic vein thrombosis. If a direct splenorenal or splenoretroperitoneal collateral is identified (Figure 3-12), the diagnosis of portal hypertension can be made with more certainty. However, spontaneous splenorenal shunts are relatively uncommon and can be difficult to detect sonographically **(Option (E) is false)**.

The coronary (left gastric) vein is another important portosystemic collateral since it is responsible for the formation of esophageal varices. It arises near the portosplenic confluence and ascends to the gastroesophageal junction. When the coronary vein is small, it generally can

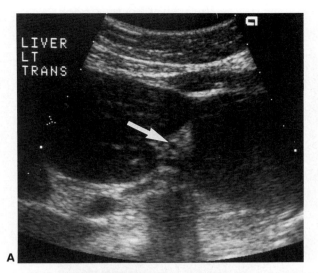

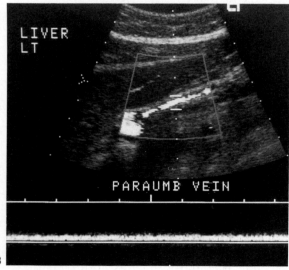

Figure 3-9. Small recanalized paraumbilical vein. (A) A transverse view of the left lobe of the liver shows a 2-mm anechoic circular structure in the fat of the ligamentum teres (arrow). (B) A longitudinal view and a pulsed Doppler waveform confirm that this is a small recanalized paraumbilical vein with flow away from the liver.

be detected only by color Doppler sonography. Determination that blood flows away from the portosplenic confluence confirms that the flow is abnormal (Figure 3-13). As the coronary vein enlarges further, it becomes detectable on gray-scale sonography as a tortuous tubular vessel with reversed venous flow (Figure 3-14). With marked enlargement, it can appear as a multicystic mass deep to the left lobe of the liver (Figure 3-15). Other collaterals, which are seen less frequently, are short gastric veins, pericholecystic veins, retroperitoneal veins, and mesenteric veins.

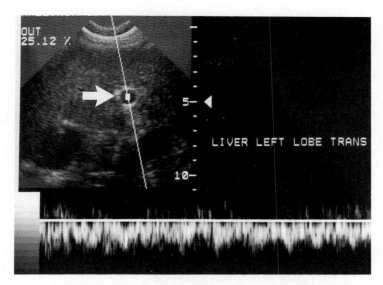

Figure 3-10. Large recanalized paraumbilical vein. A transverse view of the left lobe shows a large anechoic circular structure (arrow) in the expected location of the ligamentum teres. The pulsed Doppler waveform from this structure confirms that it is venous.

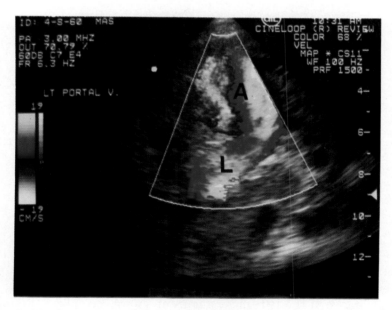

Figure 3-11. Aneurysm of the paraumbilical vein. A transverse view of the left portal vein (L) demonstrates communication with a large aneurysm of the paraumbilical vein (A). The swirling pattern of flow in the aneurysm is typical.

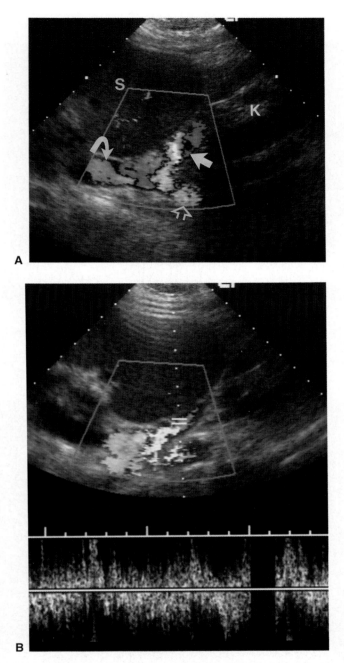

Figure 3-12. Spontaneous splenorenal shunt. (A) A transverse color Doppler image of the left upper quadrant shows the spleen (S) and left kidney (K). The renal vein (straight arrow) is enlarged and communicates with a large collateral vein (curved arrow) that could be traced to the splenic hilum. Another retroperitoneal collateral (open arrow) is seen arising from the renal vein. (B) A pulsed Doppler waveform from the renal vein shows turbulent venous flow.

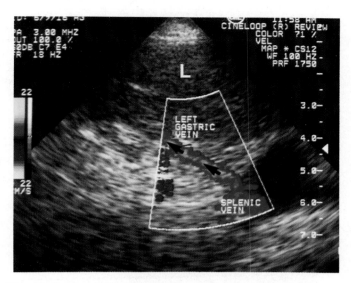

Figure 3-13. Coronary vein in a patient with esophageal varices. A longitudinal view of the epigastrium, using the left lobe of the liver (L) as a window, shows a small coronary vein (left gastric vein) arising from the splenic vein. This vein was not visualized on gray-scale sonography. Color Doppler sonography shows that coronary blood flow is reversed (arrows) and is traveling away from the splenic vein and toward the esophagus.

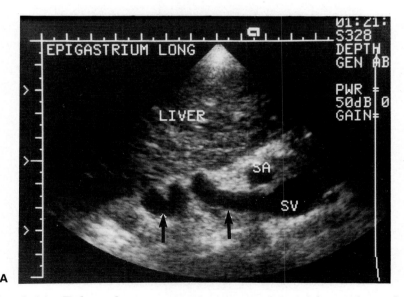

Figure 3-14. Enlarged coronary vein in a patient with esophageal varices. (A) A longitudinal view of the epigastrium, using the liver as a window, shows a large coronary vein (arrows) arising from the splenic vein (SV). The splenic artery (SA) is seen adjacent to the splenic vein. (B) A pulsed Doppler waveform from the coronary vein shows that the venous flow is away from the splenic vein.

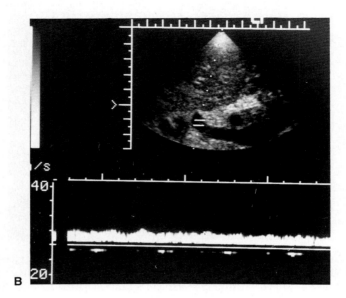

B

Figure 3-14 (Continued)

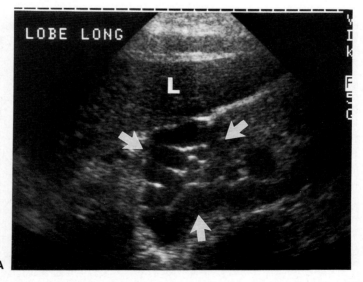

A

Figure 3-15. Enlarged coronary vein producing a pseudomass. (A) A longitudinal view of the epigastrium shows a multicystic-appearing mass (arrows) deep to the left lobe of the liver (L). (B) A longitudinal color Doppler view confirms that the mass is made up of a localized group of enlarged, tortuous vessels.

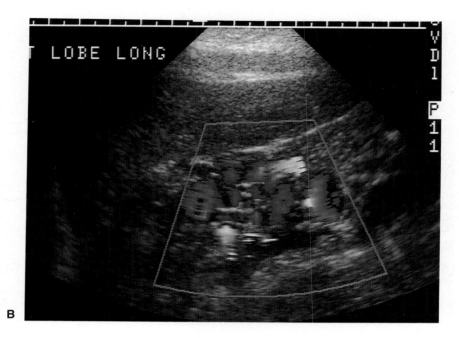

B

Question 12

Concerning hepatic hemodynamics,

(A) the portal vein normally has minimal or no pulsatility
(B) in the fasting state, the vascular resistance of the hepatic artery is greater than that of the superior mesenteric artery
(C) hepatic venous flow is normally bidirectional
(D) normal portal vein flow velocities are approximately 15 to 20 cm/second
(E) hepatic venous flow is normally greatest during diastole

Like the pulmonary circulation, the hepatic circulation has a dual blood supply, consisting of the portal vein and hepatic artery. Normally, 75% of hepatic blood flow is delivered via the portal vein and the remainder is delivered via the hepatic artery. Arterial flow to the liver is similar to that to other parenchymal organs such as the spleen and kidneys. Vascular resistance is low, and therefore Doppler waveforms of the hepatic artery demonstrate broad systolic peaks and high levels of diastolic flow throughout the cardiac cycle. This low-resistance arterial profile in the hepatic artery applies to both the fasting and nonfasting states. The normal superior mesenteric artery, on the other hand, demonstrates a high-

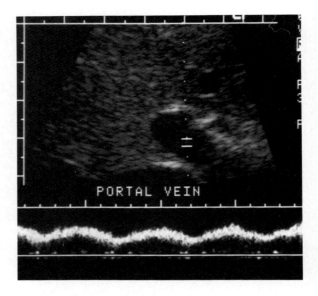

Figure 3-16. Normal portal venous flow. Mild portal vein pulsatility is present.

resistance pattern during fasting when the bowel is at rest **(Option (B) is false)** and converts to a low-resistance pattern only after eating.

The portal blood flow is driven by a constant pressure gradient between the portal vein and systemic veins. In normal patients, this results in a monophasic waveform on Doppler sonography that has minimal if any pulsatility (Figure 3-16) **(Option (A) is true).** When pulsations are present in the portal vein, the minimum velocity should remain antegrade and should measure at least one-half to two-thirds the maximum velocity. In normal individuals, portal vein flow velocities average approximately 15 to 20 cm/second **(Option (D) is true).**

With increased right atrial pressure due to congestive heart failure, sinusoidal congestion develops and pressure fluctuations related to the cardiac cycle can be transmitted into the portal vein. In many individuals with congestive heart failure, this results in a conversion of portal venous flow to a markedly pulsatile pattern. Tricuspid regurgitation can contribute to and worsen abnormal portal vein pulsatility. However, right-sided heart failure can cause portal vein pulsatility without associated tricuspid regurgitation. Portal vein pulsatility (defined as a minimum velocity of less than one-half to two-thirds the maximum velocity) is not very sensitive for detection of elevated right atrial pressures; however, it is relatively specific. Therefore, passive congestion of the liver as a result of right-sided heart disease should be suspected when portal vein pulsatility is detected (Figure 3-17). Since this can explain abnormal liver function tests, abdominal pain, and hepatomegaly, it is worth-

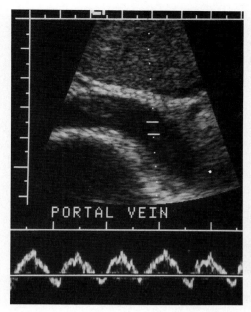

Figure 3-17. Pulsatile portal vein due to congestive heart failure. A longitudinal view of the portal vein and a pulsed Doppler waveform show marked portal vein pulsatility with some flow below the baseline.

while to obtain portal venous waveforms on patients being evaluated for these reasons.

Unlike the portal vein, the hepatic veins normally do exhibit a pulsatile pattern with periods of antegrade and retrograde flow, reflecting changes in the right atrium **(Option (C) is true).** The normal hepatic venous waveform is shown in Figure 3-18. During right atrial contraction, there is a brief cessation of hepatic venous flow and, in most cases, an actual reversal of flow. As the right atrium expands, there is a rapid forward flow out of the hepatic veins and into the right atrium. As the right atrium becomes progressively filled, forward flow out of the hepatic veins slows and may even stop or transiently reverse. Then, as the tricuspid valve opens, there is a second surge of hepatic venous flow in a forward direction into the right atrium. This second forward pulse ceases with right atrial contraction, and the cycle then repeats. In normal individuals, the first forward pulse, which occurs during cardiac systole, is larger than the second pulse, which occurs during diastole **(Option (E) is false).** The systolic pulse decreases and the diastolic pulse increases during deep inspiration, and the opposite changes occur during expiration. In addition, hepatic vein pulsatility can be dampened and even completely eliminated in normal individuals during performance of a Valsalva maneuver. If hepatic venous pulsations are not detected during quiet respiration, cirrhosis should be considered. In fact, loss of hepatic

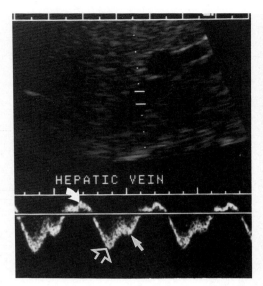

Figure 3-18 (left). Normal hepatic venous flow. A Doppler waveform shows the typical flow reversal during right atrial contraction (curved arrow) followed by rapid antegrade flow during atrial filling (open arrow). A second small antegrade pulse (straight solid arrow) occurs after the tricuspid valve opens.

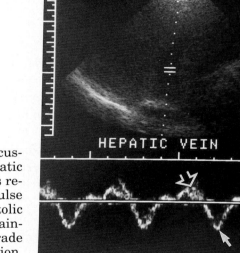

Figure 3-19 (right). Tricuspid regurgitation. A hepatic venous waveform shows reversal of the systolic pulse (open arrow). The diastolic pulse (solid arrow) maintains an antegrade direction.

vein pulsatility correlates with more severe functional impairment in cirrhotic patients. Tricuspid insufficiency can also alter the hepatic venous waveform. With right ventricular systole, regurgitant flow into the right atrium elevates right atrial pressure, and this pressure elevation is transmitted to the hepatic veins, resulting in a decrease or reversal of the systolic pulse (Figure 3-19).

Question 13

Concerning portal vein thrombosis,

(A) inability to detect portal venous flow by Doppler sonography is diagnostic
(B) the major complication is hepatic infarction
(C) recanalization is referred to as cavernous transformation
(D) gray-scale sonography occasionally is normal
(E) tumor thrombus is generally indistinguishable from bland thrombus

Portal vein thrombosis can be caused by a number of underlying processes. Portal hypertension with resulting sluggish or static flow is a common etiology, as is metastatic disease to the liver. Other causes include inflammatory or infectious diseases such as inflammatory bowel disease, appendicitis, diverticulitis, and pancreatitis. Hypercoagulable states such as pregnancy and polycythemia vera are also predisposing causes, as are primary hepatic tumors (especially hepatocellular carcinoma) and trauma.

Portal vein thrombosis is the most common type of prehepatic portal hypertension. Like other forms of portal hypertension, its major complications are bleeding esophageal varices, ascites, splenomegaly, and hypersplenism. Because of the dual blood supply to the liver, hepatic infarction is uncommon **(Option (B) is false)**. In fact, liver function tests and liver biopsies are often normal in patients with isolated portal vein thrombosis.

Portal vein thrombosis can have a variety of appearances on grayscale sonography. In most cases, thrombus appears more echogenic than the adjacent nonclotted portal vein. Therefore, when thrombosis is focal, it appears as an echogenic filling defect in the portal vein lumen (Figure 3-20). When it is diffuse, it appears as an abnormally echogenic portal vein and can be difficult to distinguish from artifactual echoes that sometimes occur in the portal vein lumen. If color Doppler sonography demonstrates flow throughout the lumen, the internal echoes must be artifactual. The portal vein is often enlarged in patients with diffuse portal vein thrombosis (Figure 3-21).

In some patients, portal vein thrombosis is extremely hypoechoic or even anechoic and can completely mimic a patent portal vein on grayscale sonography (Figure 3-22) **(Option (D) is true)**. Again, Doppler sonography can be useful in documenting the presence or absence of flow. If flow is detected in the portal vein lumen, thrombosis is effectively excluded. When no flow is detected and the gray-scale appearance is not definitive for thrombosis, one must consider both hypoechoic or anechoic thrombosis and extremely slow flow. Before diagnosing portal vein thrombosis under such circumstances, one must maximize Doppler sen-

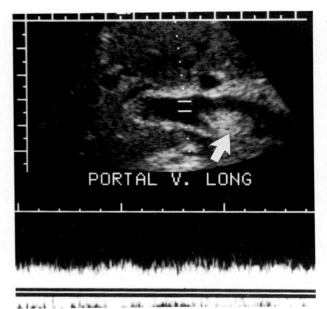

Figure 3-20 (left).
Focal nonocclusive portal vein thrombosis. A longitudinal view shows an echogenic thrombus (arrow) in the portal vein lumen. The pulsed Doppler waveform confirms that antegrade venous flow is maintained across this nonoccluding thrombus.

Figure 3-21 (right).
Complete portal vein thrombosis. A longitudinal view of the portal vein (arrows) shows portal vein enlargement and intraluminal echogenicity similar to that of hepatic parenchyma. No flow was detected on Doppler analysis.

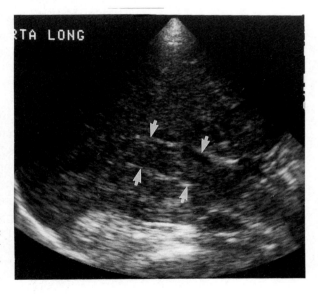

sitivity. This is done by using a low Doppler scale, low wall filter, high color priority setting, large sample volume, appropriate transducer frequency, and as many sound pulses per line of information as possible while maintaining an acceptable frame rate. In addition, a view should be found such that the flow is oriented as much as possible either directly toward or directly away from the transducer. Even when these parame-

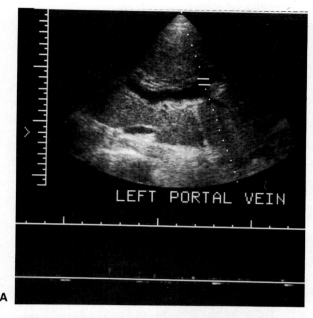

A

LEFT PORTAL VEIN

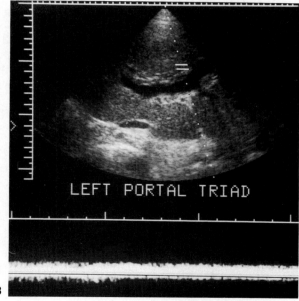

B

LEFT PORTAL TRIAD

Figure 3-22. Anechoic portal vein thrombosis. (A) A transverse view of the portal vein bifurcation shows an anechoic, normal-appearing lumen. The pulsed Doppler waveform from the left portal vein shows no detectable blood flow. (B) A pulsed Doppler waveform from the left periportal region shows antegrade venous flow from a small periportal collateral.

ters are all appropriately adjusted, very slow portal vein flow may not be detected. Portal venous flow tends to be slow when flow is converting from antegrade to retrograde (Figure 3-23). Tessler et al. have recently shown that the positive-predictive value of a Doppler diagnosis of portal

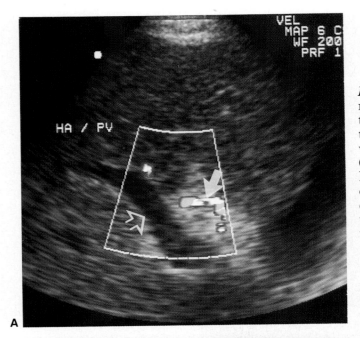

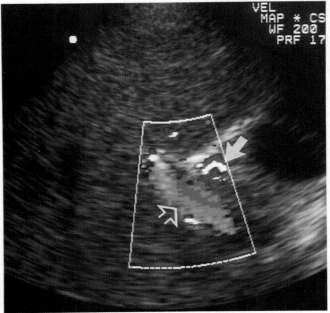

Figure 3-23. Slow flow mimicking portal vein thrombosis. (A) A longitudinal color Doppler view of the portal vein (open arrow) shows low-level intraluminal echoes consistent with either artifacts or thrombosis. No flow was detected in the portal vein on Doppler sonography, and the diagnosis of portal vein thrombosis was incorrectly made. Arterial flow was readily detected in the adjacent hepatic artery (solid arrow). (B) A longitudinal color Doppler view obtained 3 weeks later with identical technical parameters again shows flow in the hepatic artery (solid arrow) and now also shows retrograde flow in a widely patent portal vein (open arrow). This suggests that flow was probably changing from antegrade to retrograde at the time of the original examination and that the resulting sluggish flow (in either direction) was too slow to be detected.

vein thrombosis is approximately 62%, with the false-positive results occurring in the setting of very slow portal venous flow **(Option (A) is false).** Therefore, if a thrombus is not seen on gray-scale sonography and

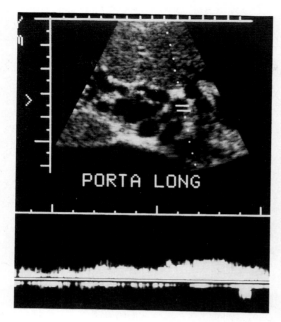

Figure 3-24. Cavernous transformation of the portal vein. A longitudinal view of the porta hepatis shows multiple tortuous veins in the expected location of the portal vein. A normal portal vein was not identified. The pulsed Doppler waveform shows antegrade venous flow within these periportal collaterals.

flow is not detected by Doppler sonography, other studies should be performed before a definitive diagnosis of portal vein thrombosis is made.

In some patients, portal vein thrombosis is accompanied by development of periportal collaterals that travel in the porta hepatis and within the intrahepatic portal triads. This is referred to as cavernous transformation of the portal vein. This nomenclature is somewhat confusing since it does not actually refer to recanalization of the portal vein **(Option (C) is false)** but rather to the development of periportal collateral veins. Sonographically, cavernous transformation is usually detected as tortuous venous channels anterior to the main portal vein at the level of the porta hepatis and adjacent to the intrahepatic portal vein branches (Figure 3-24). In some instances, the periportal venous collaterals are too small to be detected on gray-scale sonography but do produce a detectable Doppler signal (Figure 3-22).

In addition to bland thrombus, the portal vein can be invaded by adjacent tumors, resulting in tumor thrombosis. In most cases, tumor thrombus is similar in appearance to bland thrombus **(Option (E) is true).** If vessels can be detected within the thrombus by duplex or color Doppler sonography, the diagnosis of tumor thrombosis is very strongly suggested (Figure 3-25).

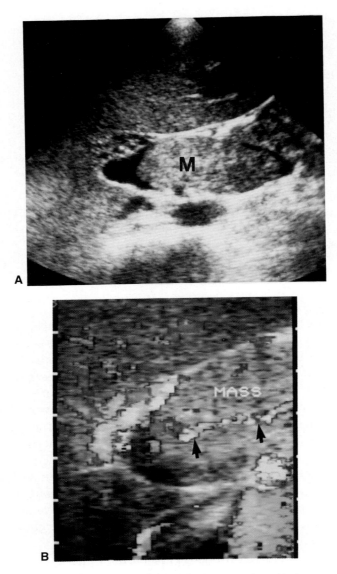

Figure 3-25.   Tumor thrombus in the portal vein. (A) A transverse view
of the portal vein shows a large intraluminal mass (M). (B) A transverse
color Doppler view shows internal vascularity (arrows) within the mass,
confirming that the mass represents tumor thrombus rather than bland
thrombus. The primary cancer in this patient was an islet cell tumor.

Question 14

Sonographic features of the Budd-Chiari syndrome include:

(A) caudate lobe hypertrophy
(B) a monophasic hepatic venous waveform
(C) hepatic venous to hepatic venous collaterals
(D) flow reversal in the hepatic vein
(E) flow reversal in the portal vein

Budd-Chiari syndrome refers to obstruction of hepatic venous outflow. It can occur at a number of levels ranging from the small hepatic venules (hepatic veno-occlusive disease) to the major hepatic veins (hepatic vein thrombosis) to the inferior vena cava (inferior vena caval membranes). Budd-Chiari syndrome can be idiopathic or can be due to such predisposing factors as hypercoagulable states, trauma, neoplasm, and pregnancy. Clinically, patients often present with ascites, hepatomegaly, and abdominal pain when the obstruction is acute. Chronic Budd-Chiari syndrome is often associated with complications of cirrhosis and portal hypertension.

Sonographically, Budd-Chiari syndrome is characterized by a number of abnormalities. Its separate venous drainage into the inferior vena cava means that the caudate lobe is often spared (Figure 3-26) and thus undergoes marked hypertrophy **(Option (A) is true).** Changes due to associated cirrhosis, such as left lobe enlargement, right lobe atrophy, and parenchymal heterogeneity, are also frequently present. In some patients, the cause of Budd-Chiari syndrome, such as tumor thrombosis or inferior vena caval membranes, can be visualized. In others, the hepatic veins and inferior vena cava merely appear compressed or tortuous.

A number of abnormalities of hepatic vein flow are characteristic of Budd-Chiari syndrome. Because of the outflow obstruction, the hepatic veins are isolated from the right atrium so that normal hepatic vein pulsatility is lost and a monophasic pattern is seen (Figure 3-27) **(Option (B) is true).** However, it is important to realize that monophasic hepatic venous flow can also be seen in patients with cirrhosis (Figure 3-28) and, as mentioned above, can be produced artificially by the Valsalva maneuver. Therefore, additional, more specific abnormalities should be sought before diagnosing Budd-Chiari syndrome solely on the basis of a monophasic hepatic vein waveform.

The blockage of hepatic vein outflow means that collateral pathways must develop in patients with Budd-Chiari syndrome. The most frequently visualized sonographically is intrahepatic hepatic-vein-to-hepatic-vein collaterals **(Option (C) is true).** Hepatic-vein-to-subcapsular-systemic-vein collaterals can also be visualized in some cases. In both

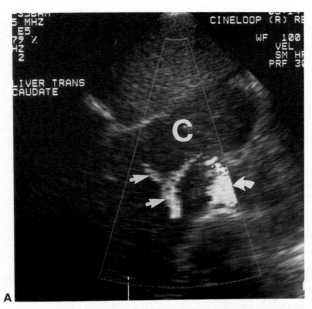

A

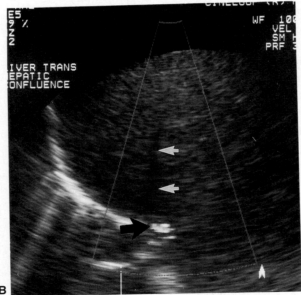

B

Figure 3-26. Idiopathic Budd-Chiari syndrome. (A) A transverse color Doppler view (reproduced in gray scale) shows marked enlargement of the caudate lobe (C). Patent caudate lobe veins (straight arrows) drain directly into the vena cava. The curved arrow indicates the aorta. (B) A transverse color Doppler view (reproduced in gray scale) through the superior aspect of the liver shows lack of flow in a barely detectable hepatic vein (white arrows) but detectable flow in the inferior vena cava (black arrow).

instances, it is possible to detect reversal of hepatic vein flow (Figure 3-27) in the vein draining to the collateral **(Option (D) is true).** In addition, because Budd-Chiari syndrome is a cause of portal hypertension, it should not be surprising that portal vein flow reversal (Figure 3-29) is a frequent feature of Budd-Chiari syndrome **(Option (E) is true).** Other

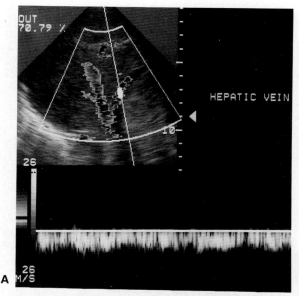

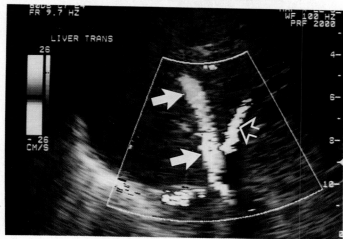

Figure 3-27. Budd-Chiari syndrome due to inferior vena cava tumor thrombus. (A) A transverse view and pulsed Doppler waveform show decreased pulsatility in hepatic venous flow. (B) A transverse color Doppler view near the confluence shows reversed flow (color coded red) in a patent hepatic vein (solid arrows). Normal flow (color coded blue) is seen in an adjacent hepatic vein (open arrow).

signs of portal hypertension such as portosystemic collaterals are also sonographic features of the Budd-Chiari syndrome.

William D. Middleton, M.D.

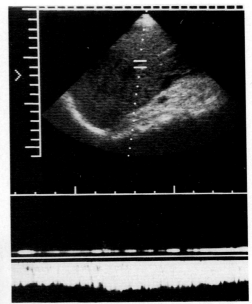

Figure 3-28 (right). Nonpulsatile hepatic venous flow due to cirrhosis. A longitudinal view of the liver and a pulsed Doppler waveform from a hepatic vein show nonpulsatile flow. This patient had no clinical evidence of Budd-Chiari syndrome, and the inferior vena cava and hepatic veins were widely patent by Doppler analysis.

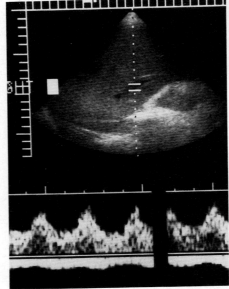

Figure 3-29 (left). Veno-occlusive disease. A longitudinal view and a pulsed Doppler waveform through a right portal triad show hepatic arterial flow above the baseline. Portal venous flow should be in the same direction (i.e., above the baseline) but is instead reversed owing to the veno-occlusive disease and is seen below the baseline.

SUGGESTED READINGS

GENERAL

1. Becker CD, Cooperberg PL. Sonography of the hepatic vascular system. AJR 1988; 150:999–1005
2. Koslin DB, Berland LL. Duplex Doppler examination of the liver and portal venous system. J Clin Ultrasound 1987; 15:675–686
3. Ralls PW. Color Doppler sonography of the hepatic artery and portal venous system. AJR 1990; 155:517–525

PORTAL HYPERTENSION

4. Cho KJ, Lunderquist A. The peribiliary vascular plexus: the microvascular architecture of the bile duct in the rabbit and in clinical cases. Radiology 1983; 147:357–364
5. Gibson PR, Gibson RN, Ditchfield MR, Donlan JD. A comparison of duplex Doppler sonography of the ligamentum teres and portal vein with endoscopic demonstration of gastroesophageal varices in patients with chronic liver disease or portal hypertension, or both. J Ultrasound Med 1992; 11:327–331
6. Gibson RN, Gibson PR, Donlan JD, Clunie DA. Identification of a patent paraumbilical vein by using Doppler sonography: importance in the diagnosis of portal hypertension. AJR 1989; 153:513–516
7. Goyal AK, Pokharna DS, Sharma SK. Ultrasonic measurements of portal vasculature in diagnosis of portal hypertension. A controversial subject reviewed. J Ultrasound Med 1990; 9:45–48
8. Lafortune M, Marleau D, Breton G, Viallet A, Lavoie P, Huet PM. Portal venous system measurements in portal hypertension. Radiology 1984; 151:27–30
9. Moriyasu F, Nishida O, Ban N, et al. "Congestion index" of the portal vein. AJR 1986; 146:735–739
10. Mostbeck GH, Wittich GR, Herold C, et al. Hemodynamic significance of the paraumbilical vein in portal hypertension: assessment with duplex US. Radiology 1989; 170:339–342
11. Subramanyam BR, Balthazar EJ, Madamba MR, Raghavendra BN, Horii SC, Lefleur RS. Sonography of portosystemic venous collaterals in portal hypertension. Radiology 1983; 146:161–166
12. Vilgrain V, Lebrec D, Menu Y, Scherrer A, Nahum H. Comparison between ultrasonographic signs and the degree of portal hypertension in patients with cirrhosis. Gastrointest Radiol 1990; 15:218–222

HEPATIC HEMODYNAMICS

13. Abu-Yousef MM. Duplex Doppler sonography of the hepatic vein in tricuspid regurgitation. AJR 1991; 156:79–83
14. Abu-Yousef MM. Normal and respiratory variations of the hepatic and portal venous duplex Doppler waveforms with simultaneous electrocardiographic correlation. J Ultrasound Med 1992; 11:263–268
15. Abu-Yousef MM, Milam SG, Farner RM. Pulsatile portal vein flow: a sign of tricuspid regurgitation on duplex Doppler sonography. AJR 1990; 155:785–788
16. Bolondi L, LiBassi S, Gaiani S, et al. Liver cirrhosis: changes of Doppler waveform of hepatic veins. Radiology 1991; 178:513–516
17. Duerinckx AJ, Grant EG, Perrella RR, Szeto A, Tessler FN. The pulsatile portal vein in cases of congestive heart failure: correlation of duplex Doppler findings with right atrial pressures. Radiology 1990; 176:655–658
18. Hosoki T, Arisawa J, Marukawa T, et al. Portal blood flow in congestive heart failure: pulsed duplex sonographic findings. Radiology 1990; 174:733–736

PORTAL VEIN THROMBOSIS

19. Atri M, de Stempel J, Bret PM, Illescas FF. Incidence of portal vein thrombosis complicating liver metastasis as detected by duplex ultrasound. J Ultrasound Med 1990; 9:285–289
20. Kauzlaric D, Petrovic M, Barmeir E. Sonography of cavernous transformation of the portal vein. AJR 1984; 142:383–384
21. Miller VE, Berland LL. Pulsed Doppler duplex sonography and CT of portal vein thrombosis. AJR 1985; 145:73–76
22. Tessler FN, Gehring BJ, Gomes AS, et al. Diagnosis of portal vein thrombosis: value of color Doppler imaging. AJR 1991; 157:293–296
23. Van Gansbeke D, Avni EF, Delcour C, Engelholm L, Struyven J. Sonographic features of portal vein thrombosis. AJR 1985; 144:749–752
24. Weltin G, Taylor KJ, Carter AR, Taylor CR. Duplex Doppler: identification of cavernous transformation of the portal vein. AJR 1985; 144:999–1001

BUDD-CHIARI SYNDROME

25. Brown BP, Abu-Yousef M, Farner R, LaBrecque D, Gingrich R. Doppler sonography: a noninvasive method for evaluation of hepatic venocclusive disease. AJR 1990; 154:721–724
26. Grant EG, Perrella R, Tessler FN, Lois J, Busuttil R. Budd-Chairi syndrome: the results of duplex and color Doppler imaging. AJR 1989; 152:377–381
27. Hosoki T, Kuroda C, Tokunaga K, Marukawa T, Masuike M, Kozuka T. Hepatic venous outflow obstruction: evaluation with pulsed duplex sonography. Radiology 1989; 170:733–737
28. Menu Y, Alison D, Lorphelin JM, Valla D, Belghiti J, Nahum H. Budd-Chiari syndrome: US evaluation. Radiology 1985; 157:761–764
29. Ralls PW, Johnson MB, Radin DR, Boswell WD Jr, Lee KP, Halls JM. Budd-Chiari syndrome: detection with color Doppler sonography. AJR 1992; 159:113–116
30. Stanley P. Budd-Chiari syndrome. Radiology 1989; 170:625–627

Notes

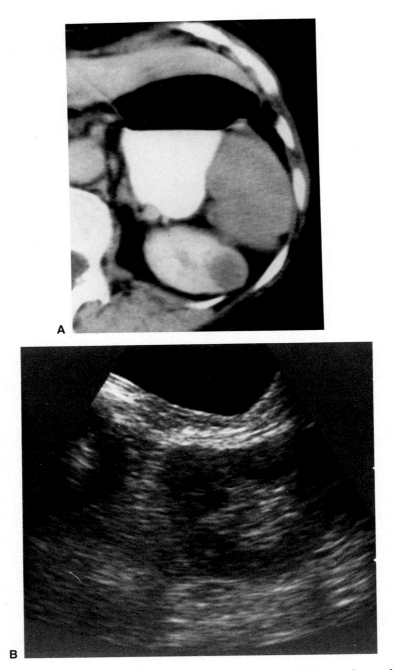

Figure 4-1. This 63-year-old woman had a history of Sjögren's syndrome and two lymphomas, first non-Hodgkin's lymphoma and more recently Hodgkin's disease, both of which have been in remission for several years. You are shown a routine follow-up abdominal CT scan (A) and a subsequent transverse renal sonogram (B). The anechoic zone in the near field is a standoff pad.

Case 4:   Renal Cell Carcinoma

Question 15

Which *one* of the following is the MOST likely diagnosis?

(A) Lymphoma
(B) Renal cell carcinoma
(C) Acute focal pyelonephritis
(D) Complex renal cyst
(E) Oncocytoma

Figure 4-1A is a contrast-enhanced CT scan on which a small hypoattenuating mass in the upper pole of the left kidney was serendipitously discovered. Figure 4-1B is a transverse sonogram that reveals a contour deformity along the lateral aspect of the kidney. Closer examination shows a solid mass that is isoechoic with the adjacent normal kidney and compresses and displaces the more hypoechoic medullary pyramid (Figure 4-2).

In view of the test patient's history, lymphomatous involvement of the kidney (Option (A)) must be given strong consideration. Hodgkin's disease very rarely involves the kidneys. Of the 29 cases of renal involvement by lymphoma in the Duke University tumor registry between 1979 and 1990, only 1 represented Hodgkin's disease. Non-Hodgkin's lymphoma more commonly involves the kidneys, with a reported 33% frequency at autopsy in patients with disseminated disease. However, Hodgkin's disease was the more recent lymphoma in the test patient, and it is unlikely that the non-Hodgkin's lymphoma would recur, given an intervening malignancy. Solitary renal masses account for only 5% of cases of lymphomatous involvement of the kidneys. Renal lymphomas are most commonly sonographically hypoechoic rather than isoechoic, as seen in the test image. Therefore, for all these reasons, lymphoma is an unlikely diagnosis for the mass in the test patient.

Renal cell carcinoma is the most common malignancy of the kidney and accounts for the majority of solitary renal masses. These tumors are also most often isoechoic relative to renal parenchyma, although they

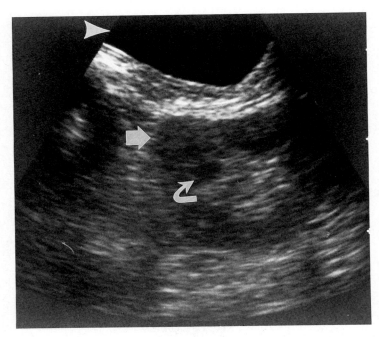

Figure 4-2 (Same as Figure 4-1B). Small renal cell carcinoma. A transverse sonogram of the upper pole of the left kidney as imaged from the left flank was obtained. The mass (straight arrow) is isoechoic to renal parenchyma and compresses the more hypoechoic medullary pyramid (curved arrow). The anechoic zone in the near field (arrowhead) is a standoff pad.

can range from hyperechoic to hypoechoic. Without the distracting history of two previous lymphomas, this would be the obvious choice. The medical history is often helpful in narrowing the differential diagnosis of a renal mass. However, as the test case illustrates, care must be taken in avoiding overemphasis on history. Renal cell carcinoma is the most likely etiology for the mass in the test patient **(Option (B) is correct).**

Acute focal pyelonephritis (Option (C)) is a focal bacterial infection that simulates a mass lesion. This has been known previously by a plethora of names: focal bacterial nephritis, acute focal bacterial nephritis, lobar nephritis, lobar nephronia, renal cellulitis, renal phlegmon, and renal carbuncle. Because of the ambiguity and confusion these terms produced, it is now recommended that they be eliminated from radiology reports and be replaced by the term "acute focal pyelonephritis."

Acute focal pyelonephritis is usually a poorly marginated oval or round mass, hypoechoic to renal parenchyma (Figure 4-3). However, it

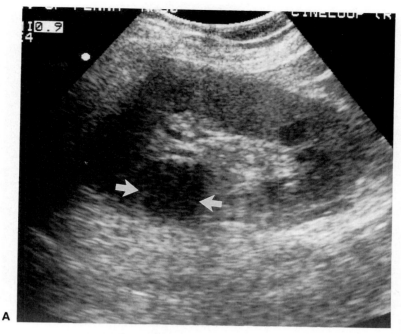

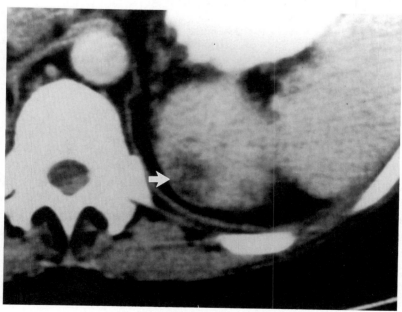

Figure 4-3. Acute focal pyelonephritis. (A) A longitudinal sonogram of the kidney of this 42-year-old woman with fever and flank pain demonstrates a hypoechoic region in the medial upper pole (arrows). (B) An enhanced CT scan reveals a similar indistinct area of decreased attenuation (arrow). This combination of history and radiologic findings is quite characteristic of acute focal pyelonephritis.

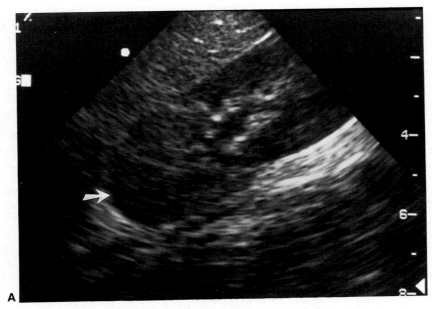

A

Figure 4-4. Acute focal pyelonephritis. This 7-year-old boy presented with fever and an abdominal mass. (A) A sonogram of the abdomen revealed a horseshoe kidney (not demonstrated) with a large, slightly hyperechoic mass involving the right upper pole (arrow) seen on this sagittal image. The mass is relatively more echogenic than renal parenchyma, an unusual feature for acute focal pyelonephritis. (B) A postcontrast CT scan shows a mass in the upper pole with decreased attenuation relative to renal parenchyma. The mass, originally thought to be a Wilms' tumor, resolved with oral antibiotic therapy.

can be isoechoic or hyperechoic to renal parenchyma (Figure 4-4). If left untreated, focal pyelonephritis can develop into a frank abscess. Focal pyelonephritis is most often discovered because of symptoms of fever, flank pain, and other signs of urinary tract infection. The test patient was asymptomatic, and the incidental discovery of acute focal pyelonephritis would be very unusual.

The sonographic criteria for a simple cyst are lack of internal echoes; smooth, well-defined, echogenic back wall; round or oval shape; and enhanced through transmission. A complex cyst (Option (D)) is characterized by one or more of the following features: the presence of internal echoes, one or more septa, a thick wall, calcification, or a solid component such as a mural nodule. The lesion in the test patient could represent a high-density cyst on the CT scan (Figure 4-1A), but the absence of enhanced through transmission and the poor wall definition in the sonographic study (Figure 4-1B) exclude this diagnosis. Enhanced through

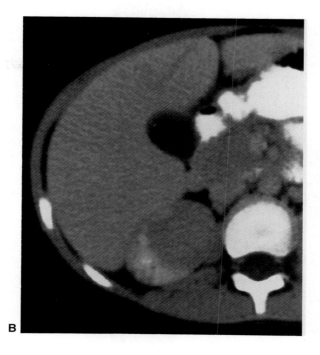

B

transmission is the major sonographic criterion that differentiates a complex cyst from a hypoechoic solid mass. In a single image, enhanced through transmission is not always apparent, since it depends on the gain setting and the angle of insonation. Therefore, real-time examination with close scrutiny for the presence of enhanced through transmission should be performed to exclude a complex cyst during evaluation of a renal mass. Care must also be exercised that a homogeneous tumor with faint or equivocal enhanced through transmission not be mistaken for a complex cyst. Aspiration should be performed in any questionable cases.

Oncocytoma (Option (E)) is an unusual tumor of the proximal renal tubules. It is often found incidentally and occurs more frequently in men than in women (1.7 to 1). The age distribution for oncocytoma and renal cell carcinoma is similar, with a peak incidence in the sixth and seventh decades. Oncocytomas are usually isoechoic to renal parenchyma and could resemble the mass detected in the test image (Figure 4-1B). They are typically homogeneous and sharply marginated on sonograms and CT scans. A central stellate scar, usually hypoechoic on sonograms and with low attenuation on CT, is often seen in larger tumors and can be a distinguishing feature. However, the central scar is rarely seen in smaller tumors, of similar size to the mass in the test case. Small renal

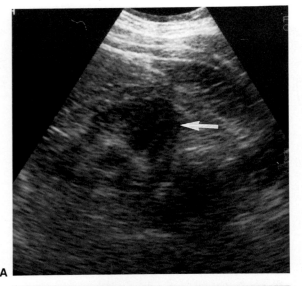

A

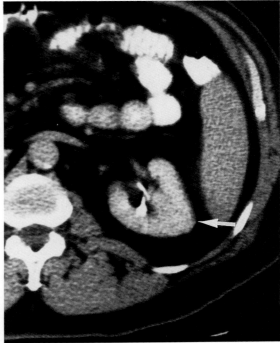

B

Figure 4-5. Column of Bertin. (A) A transverse sonogram of the left kidney from the flank demonstrates a geographic hypoechoic region in the lateral aspect of the kidney (arrow). (B) A CT scan of the left kidney in the same region demonstrates normal medullary and cortical tissue without mass lesion (arrow).

cell carcinomas and oncocytomas can appear identical; however, since renal cell carcinoma is so much more common, oncocytoma must be considered a less likely diagnosis.

Two other mass lesions that might have been considered in the differential diagnosis of a small asymptomatic renal mass are a prominent

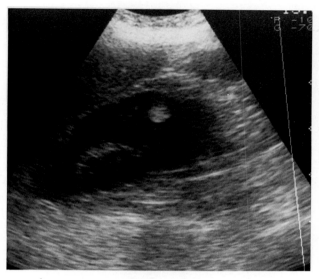

Figure 4-6. Small angiomyolipoma. A longitudinal sonogram of the right kidney demonstrates a small hyperechoic mass in the inferior pole. The lesion's echogenicity is similar to that of the renal sinus fat as well as the surrounding perinephric fat. This appearance is characteristic of an angiomyolipoma, a lesion that quite frequently is found incidentally. Unfortunately, some renal cell carcinomas are echogenic, and therefore CT or MRI is suggested to prove the fatty nature of the mass.

column of Bertin and an angiomyolipoma. A column of Bertin is a "double layer" of renal cortex that extends between two pyramids and is formed by the fusion of adjacent renal lobes (renunculi) during development of the fetal kidney. It does not deform the contour of the kidney. On ultrasonography, a prominent column of Bertin can appear as an isoechoic or slightly hypoechoic masslike area in the region of the medulla (Figure 4-5). The lesion in the test patient is clearly cortical with compression of the underlying renal pyramid; therefore, it cannot represent a column of Bertin.

Angiomyolipoma is a benign neoplasm of the kidney most commonly seen in women over 40 years of age. In 10% of cases angiomyolipomas are associated with tuberous sclerosis, and they are typically bilateral, multiple, and small when seen in patients with this disease. The vast majority of angiomyolipomas contain sufficient fat to appear densely echogenic on sonograms. Therefore, the lesion in the test patient would be very unlikely to represent an angiomyolipoma. Most angiomyolipomas are small, asymptomatic, and incidentally discovered during cross-

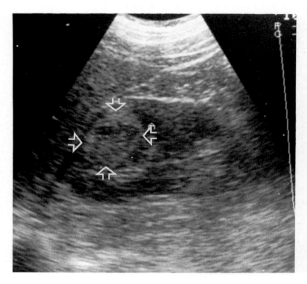

Figure 4-7. Hyperechoic renal cell carcinoma. A slightly heterogeneous hyperechoic mass (arrows) is seen in the superior pole of the right kidney. This lesion could be confused with an angiomyolipoma, although most often the latter is even more echogenic.

sectional imaging (Figure 4-6). Larger angiomyolipomas can present with flank pain or gross hematuria because of spontaneous hemorrhage. The hyperechogenic appearance of angiomyolipomas, although characteristic, is not pathognomonic; rarely, renal cell carcinomas are hyperechoic (Figure 4-7). Therefore, a hyperechogenic mass detected by sonography should be evaluated by CT or MRI to demonstrate the fatty nature of the mass definitively and thereby prove that it is an angiomyolipoma (Figure 4-8).

A hypoechoic region that superficially resembles a fluid-filled bladder is seen in the near field of the test patient's sonogram (Figure 4-1B). This appearance is caused by a standoff pad, which is made of a solid aqueous gelatinous material that allows for minimal impedance of the sound waves generated by the ultrasound transducer (Figure 4-9). The maximal resolution of the ultrasound transducer is in the intermediate field, at the focal length of the transducer. Some transducers have variable focal lengths, but the very near field is still poorly imaged. The standoff pad is used to raise the transducer away from the skin surface and thereby maximize the spatial resolution of the structures just beneath the skin surface. This was necessary in the test case because of the patient's thin body habitus and the superficial location of her mass. In a sonogram of the test patient without the use of this pad, the mass was undetected because of its small size and isoechoic character (Figure 4-10). A higher-frequency transducer can also increase the spatial resolution of objects in the near field, but it does so at the expense of decreasing

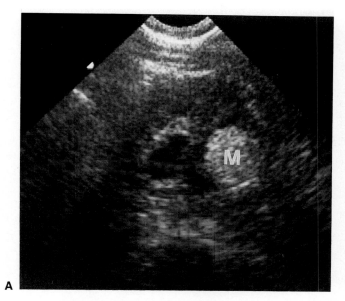

A

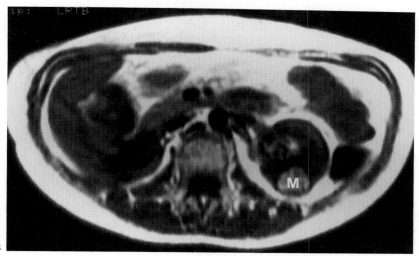

B

Figure 4-8. Angiomyolipoma. (A) A uniformly hyperechoic mass (M) is seen in the interpolar region of the left kidney in this transverse sonogram. This is characteristic, although not diagnostic, of an angiomyolipoma. (B) A T1-weighted MR image shows the mass (M) to be hyperintense, confirming the fatty nature of this angiomyolipoma.

the field of view. This would have made it difficult to determine the relationship of the mass to the remainder of the kidney in the test patient.

The test case emphasizes the difficulty in detecting small, low-contrast objects by sonography. Amendola et al. demonstrated that sonography was only 67% sensitive for the detection of renal cell carcinomas less than 3 cm in diameter. In particular, it is more difficult to image the left kidney than the right kidney because of the absence of the acoustic window provided by the liver. Vallancien et al. have estimated that 16% of tumors that would be detected in the right kidney are missed in the

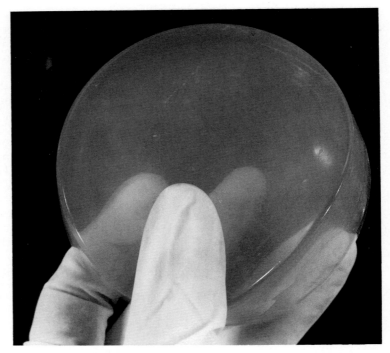

Figure 4-9. Standoff pad. This is one type of standoff pad. It is made of a solid, aqueous, gelatinous material designed to maximize sound transmission. It raises the transducer away from the skin surface, thereby moving the focal zone to a more superficial region of the patient.

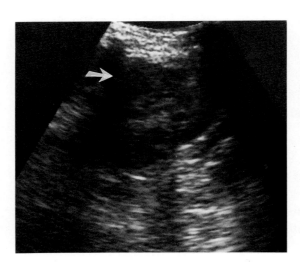

Figure 4-10. Same patient as in Figures 4-1 and 4-2. In this transverse sonogram of the test patient prior to the use of the standoff pad, the renal cell carcinoma (arrow) is virtually indistinguishable from the normal renal parenchyma. Note the great increase in detail on the images in which the standoff pad was used (Figures 4-1B and 4-2).

left kidney. The test case also emphasizes that the very near field is often less optimally imaged than deeper structures and that special maneuvers may be required to evaluate this region adequately. Lastly, it points out the danger of using sonography as a screening method for renal masses, since small isoechoic lesions can easily be overlooked.

Question 16

Concerning lymphomatous involvement of the kidney,

   (A) it is more commonly due to Hodgkin's disease than to non-Hodgkin's lymphoma
   (B) the pattern of involvement is similar in Hodgkin's disease and non-Hodgkin's lymphoma
   (C) the pattern of multiple bilateral renal masses is most common
   (D) focal lesions exhibit increased through transmission

The various types of lymphoma each have their distinct clinical and pathologic features, but, in general, they can be divided into two broad categories: Hodgkin's disease and non-Hodgkin's lymphoma. Hodgkin's disease has a characteristic anatomic distribution and nodal progression. It usually involves the cervical and supraclavicular lymph nodes (60 to 80% of patients), followed by the mediastinal, paracardiac, and para-aortic lymph nodes and spleen. It is distinctly uncommon for Hodgkin's disease to skip a nodal group in this caudal progression. Only 10% of patients present with isolated subdiaphragmatic disease, such as inguinal or abdominal adenopathy, without disease above the diaphragm. At the time of initial diagnosis, extranodal disease, except for involvement of the spleen and bone marrow, is rare. During recurrences, nodal involvement is still the most common manifestation, although extranodal involvement occurs more frequently than in the initial disease course.

Non-Hodgkin's lymphoma is more likely to involve extranodal sites both at initial presentation and during recurrences. It is also more likely to involve extra-axial lymph nodes such as the axillary or mesenteric nodes. Renal involvement is more common both at presentation and during recurrences in patients with non-Hodgkin's lymphoma than in those with Hodgkin's disease **(Option (A) is false).** Isolated renal involvement without other evidence of disease was shown to be uncommon in a large autopsy series reported by Richmond et al. in 1962. However, more recent data from the Duke tumor registry have revealed that renal involvement by lymphoma was seen without associated abdominal adenopathy in 48% of cases. The high frequency of isolated renal involvement in the Duke study probably reflects the high proportion of patients with recurrent disease in their study. Also, autopsy data select for far-advanced disease, which commonly involves multiple sites, as reflected

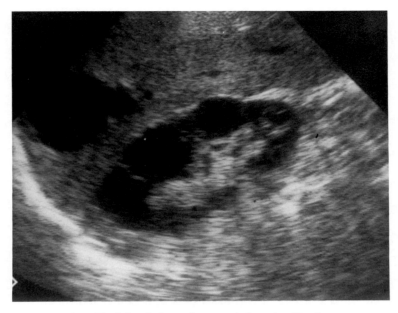

Figure 4-11. Non-Hodgkin's lymphoma. A longitudinal sonogram of the right kidney reveals several nearly anechoic masses in the kidney and a similar mass in the liver. Faint through transmission suggests that these may be cystic. These proved to be multiple foci of lymphoma. The indistinct borders of the masses are unusual for cysts and suggest the possibility of lymphoma.

in the data of Richmond et al. Antemortem detection of renal involvement is uncommon, being seen in only 0.5 to 8.3% of patients. Primary renal lymphoma is extremely rare, and therefore the diagnosis of lymphoma is usually known before the detection of renal abnormalities by imaging procedures. Renal involvement by lymphoma rarely produces symptoms referable to the urinary tract, although flank pain, hematuria, or a palpable mass has been described in some cases. Death from renal involvement is rare, being reported in only 0.5% of patients.

Despite differences in the extrarenal pattern of disease, Hodgkin's disease and non-Hodgkin's lymphoma have a similar appearance when they involve the kidneys **(Option (B) is true).** Its uniform histologic character, without tissue planes to reflect the ultrasound beam, means that lymphoma generally produces homogeneous and hypoechoic masses. Lymphomas occasionally appear entirely anechoic, but this is exceedingly rare with the newer real-time transducers (Figure 4-11). Lymphomas generally demonstrate little if any increased transmission of sound **(Option (D) is false).** In addition, the infiltrative nature of lymphoma means that margins are typically indistinct, lacking a sharply

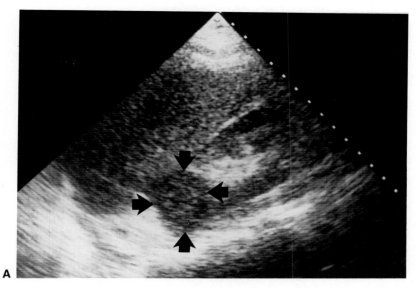

A

Figure 4-12. Non-Hodgkin's lymphoma. (A) A longitudinal sonogram of the right kidney demonstrates an isoechoic mass (arrows) in the superior pole. (B) A slightly hypoechoic mass is seen in the interpolar region of the left kidney (arrow). Multiple other masses were demonstrated bilaterally in this woman with widespread non-Hodgkin's lymphoma.

defined wall. These last features help to distinguish lymphoma from complicated cysts (Figure 4-11).

The most common appearance for renal lymphoma is as multiple hypoechoic masses, usually bilateral in distribution **(Option (C) is true)** (Figure 4-12). This is due to hematogenous dissemination of tumor, not to lymphatic spread. This pattern has been seen in autopsy and radiologic series in 59 to 77% of cases. This form of renal involvement is most readily diagnosed by imaging procedures. In adults the differential diagnosis of multiple, bilateral, hypoechoic renal masses is limited primarily to lymphoma, multiple cysts, and metastasis. Usually, there is an antecedent history of lymphoma to suggest the diagnosis.

The second most common form of renal involvement is direct extension from contiguous retroperitoneal masses; this is seen in 11 to 28% of patients. Lymphoma can also appear as a solitary hypoechoic mass (3 to 7% of patients). The differential diagnosis in this setting includes renal cell carcinoma, renal adenoma, acute focal pyelonephritis, abscess, and complex renal cyst. Diffuse renal lymphomatous infiltration is reported to occur in 6 to 10% of patients (Figure 4-13). Renal infiltration by lymphoma may go undetected by sonography or CT, as reflected in the

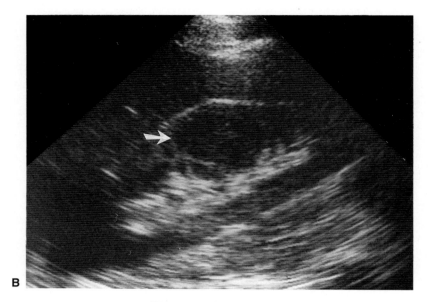

B

Figure 4-12 (Continued)

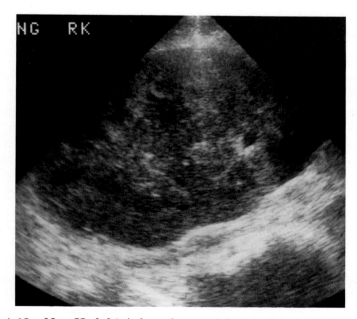

Figure 4-13. Non-Hodgkin's lymphoma. A longitudinal sonogram shows that the right kidney is markedly enlarged with an irregular lobulated contour and distortion of the normal renal architecture. This was proven to be due to lymphomatous infiltration.

higher frequency of autopsy-proven involvement compared with ante-mortem-detected involvement. The kidneys usually maintain a smooth contour despite the multinodular parenchymal invasion. Increased size of one or both kidneys may be a clue to diffuse infiltration by lymphoma. In addition to direct renal involvement, patients with lymphoma can have hydronephrosis secondary to ureteral obstruction by enlarged retroperitoneal lymph nodes and renovascular hypertension secondary to compression of the renal vascular pedicle.

Question 17

Features of renal cell carcinoma include:

(A) hypoechoic mass
(B) hyperechoic mass
(C) solitary metastasis
(D) thrombocytosis
(E) Budd-Chiari syndrome

Renal cell carcinoma, or hypernephroma, is the most common renal malignancy in adults. It is most commonly seen in patients between 50 and 70 years old. The "classic" triad of renal cell carcinoma—flank pain, gross hematuria, and palpable renal mass—is now seen in only 4 to 9% of cases. However, any individual feature of the triad is present in about 65% of cases. Constitutional symptoms such as weight loss, fever, and malaise are also common, and approximately 35% of patients have no symptoms referable to the urinary tract. Approximately 9% of patients present with symptoms or signs of metastatic disease such as bone pain or pulmonary nodules on a chest radiograph. Rarely, renal cell carcinomas produce humoral substances giving rise to various paraneoplastic syndromes, including erythrocytosis or hypercalcemia. Thrombocytosis is not a known complication **(Option (D) is false)**. Increasingly, renal cell carcinoma is an unsuspected finding on cross-sectional imaging done for other reasons, and, as in the test patient, the masses are often small and the prognosis is probably better than that for symptomatic patients.

At one time, it was thought that all nonfatty, solid renal masses less than 3 cm in diameter were benign adenomas. However, there is abundant recent evidence that many solid masses less than 3 cm are small renal cell carcinomas. Several authors, including Amendola et al. and Foster et al., have noted difficulty in distinguishing hyperdense cysts from renal cell carcinomas because enhancement characteristics on CT are not always reliable for very small masses. Sonography is extremely

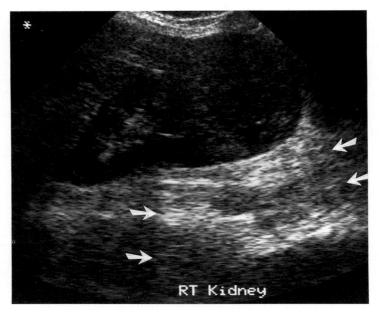

Figure 4-14. Renal cell carcinoma. A longitudinal sonogram demonstrates a large isoechoic renal cell carcinoma engulfing the inferior one-third of the right kidney. Note the increased through transmission below the mass (arrows). Increased through transmission is a property of homogeneous structures. This is most commonly seen with cysts, but it can be seen with uniform solid masses.

useful in this situation to prove the cystic or solid nature of the lesion, as in the test patient.

On sonography, about 85% of renal cell carcinomas appear as a mass that is isoechoic relative to renal parenchyma (Figures 4-14 and 4-15). However, they can also be either hypoechoic or hyperechoic **(Options (A) and (B) are true)** (Figure 4-7). Large renal cell carcinomas are usually somewhat heterogeneous, and therefore, although they are predominantly isoechoic, they can be differentiated from surrounding renal parenchyma. The mass itself often has an irregular or lobulated contour and may be partially calcified (Figure 4-15). Distortion of the contour of the kidney or intrarenal structures, as in the test patient, can help in the detection of small tumors.

In evaluating a potential renal cell carcinoma, the radiologist should attempt to define the stage of the lesion, because of the importance of stage in determining the prognosis of the tumor. Stage I renal cell carcinomas are confined within the renal capsule, without evidence of spread to regional lymph nodes or distant organs. Stage II lesions have ex-

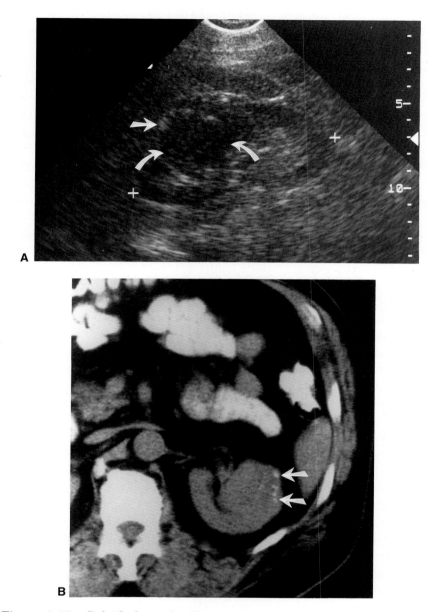

Figure 4-15. Calcified renal cell carcinoma. (A) A longitudinal sonogram shows a heterogeneous mass (curved arrows) in the interpolar region of the right kidney (cursors). The bright echoes near the periphery of the mass suggest regions of dystrophic calcification (straight arrow). (B) A noncontrast CT scan confirms the presence of dystrophic calcification (arrows).

tended through the renal capsule but remain within the confines of Gerota's fascia. A lesion can directly involve the ipsilateral adrenal gland and still be classified as stage II. Stage III lesions are those with local spread of tumor either intravascularly via the renal veins or inferior vena cava (stage IIIA) or to regional lymph nodes (stage IIIB) or both (stage IIIC). Intravascular growth of tumor is a known feature of renal cell carcinoma and can extend as tumor thrombus into the right atrium. When a tumor extends beyond the juncture of the inferior vena cava and hepatic veins, obstruction of the venous outflow of the liver can occur, resulting in Budd-Chiari syndrome **(Option (E) is true).**

When a tumor extends locally beyond the confines of Gerota's fascia, it is classified as stage IVA. Gerota's fascia is not seen on sonograms, and therefore stage II and stage IVA tumors cannot be differentiated during the sonographic examination. When there is surrounding neoplastic or inflammatory process, Gerota's fascia is often seen by CT. For this reason and others, CT is the preferred imaging modality for the clinical staging of renal cell carcinoma.

Stage IVB tumors are those with metastases to distant organs. The liver, bones, lungs, contralateral adrenal, and contralateral kidney, in order of frequency, are the most common sites of metastasis from renal cell carcinoma. Metastasis can be seen at the time of initial presentation or can be detected decades later following a long disease-free period. Solitary metastasis, particularly to lung or bone, is also a known feature of renal cell carcinoma and occurs in about 3% of patients **(Option (C) is true).** Bone metastases are often very expansile and mimic aneurysmal bone cysts.

Because CT is the preferred method for staging renal cell carcinoma, most tumors detected by sonography will be unexpected findings. When a solid renal mass is encountered in a sonographic examination, it should be assumed that it potentially represents a renal cell carcinoma and therefore should be staged as thoroughly as possible. This staging includes surveys of the liver, adrenals, and contralateral kidney to look for metastases; a review of the retroperitoneum for lymphadenopathy; and, if possible, Doppler or color flow sonography of the ipsilateral renal vein and inferior vena cava to look for venous extension of tumor.

Prognosis is most dependent on tumor stage and histologic grade. It is also affected by tumor size, host resistance, and the number of primary tumors. The 5-year survival rates have been reported to be 67, 51, 33, and 13% for stage I, II, III, and IV tumors, respectively, in a recent analysis. A similar report of histologic grade revealed 5-year survivals of 63, 48, 27, and 15% for grades 1 through 4, respectively.

The evaluation of a renal mass depends on the clinical situation in which it is found. In most adults without known malignancy, a nonfatty, isolated, solid renal mass will be a renal cell carcinoma. A small percentage (approximately 5%) of these masses will be benign adenomas. Unfortunately, needle biopsy is sometimes unable to distinguish renal carcinoma from renal adenomas because of sampling error and the pleomorphic nature of renal cell carcinomas, which can have regions indistinguishable from benign adenomas.

However, in individuals with a known extrarenal malignancy, needle biopsy is indicated to attempt to distinguish between a primary renal tumor and metastasis. It was thought in the past that needle biopsy was contraindicated in patients with possible renal cell carcinomas because of the potential for the tumor to be spread along the needle tract. This has been shown to happen only rarely and should not deter the radiologist from performing a needle biopsy of a renal mass in situations in which it will alter subsequent management of the patient.

Question 18

Concerning complex renal cyst,

(A) a fluid-debris level indicates prior hemorrhage
(B) enhanced through transmission is occasionally the only feature distinguishing it from a solid mass
(C) the finding of a single, thin internal septation necessitates biopsy
(D) the finding of thin peripheral calcification necessitates biopsy

A high-quality sonographic examination is the most reliable method of evaluating renal cysts. The most important feature of cysts is the presence of enhanced through transmission, and in some instances this is the only feature that indicates that a renal mass is cystic **(Option (B) is true).** However, the presence of increased through transmission must be searched for carefully because it is not always easily detected. Improper gain setting, angle of insonation, and positioning of the focal zone of the transducer can obscure the presence of through transmission. Unfortunately, very homogeneous solid masses occasionally produce increased through transmission, and therefore, although all cysts produce enhanced through transmission, not all masses that produce enhanced through transmission are cysts (Figure 4-14).

The feature that most commonly distinguishes a complex cyst from a simple cyst is the presence of internal echoes. These echoes can be produced by the high protein content of the cyst fluid or by the presence of blood or pus. In some instances, persistent echoes are due to technical factors such as a deep-seated position of the lesion, proximity to the renal sinus structures, or morbid obesity.

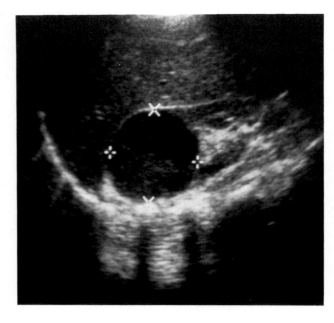

Figure 4-16. Infected renal cyst. A longitudinal sonogram of the right kidney demonstrates a complicated cyst (cursors) in the upper pole in this febrile patient. There is a fluid-debris level within the cyst.

Abscesses often can be distinguished from cysts with hemorrhagic or proteinaceous contents by the presence of thick walls and the characteristic clinical history of fever and flank pain. However, both abscesses and hemorrhagic cysts can have fluid-fluid or fluid-debris levels, caused by the separation of their more cellular and more fluid elements **(Option (A) is false)** (Figure 4-16). Cysts with proteinaceous contents do not usually contain fluid-fluid levels.

The further evaluation of cysts with internal echoes depends on the clinical situation. If the cyst is thought to represent an abscess, needle aspiration is required to confirm the diagnosis and percutaneous drainage may be necessary for adequate treatment. If the patient is asymptomatic and internal echoes are the only complex feature of a cyst, a dedicated CT scan of the kidney should be performed and should include both pre- and postcontrast images. If the cyst has well-defined margins and a smooth thin wall, does not enhance after contrast agent administration, and contains water density material (0 to 20 HU), it meets the CT criteria for a simple cyst. In this situation, the presence of internal echoes on the sonogram was probably caused by artifact, either secondary to improper machine settings (gain, location of the focal zone, power, etc.) or due to the body habitus of the patient. If all criteria except the last (water density material) are met, the most likely diagnosis is a cyst with high-density contents, and careful follow-up is usually sufficient to exclude malignancy. If there are other complex features (and especially a

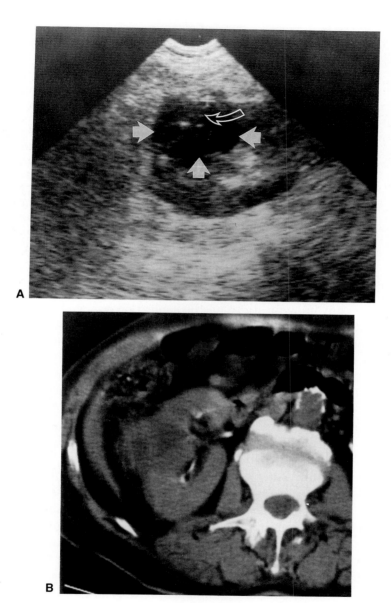

Figure 4-17. Complex cystic lesion due to a renal abscess. (A) A transverse sonogram of the right kidney demonstrates a mixed-echogenicity mass (straight arrows) in the interpolar region. Note the increased through transmission, indicating its partial cystic character. However, there are areas of the wall superiorly that appear more solid (curved arrow). Therefore, this mass requires invasive evaluation. (B) A postcontrast CT scan again demonstrates an interpolar mass. Note the soft tissue stranding in the perinephric fat. This constellation of features is most suggestive of a renal abscess, although a renal cell carcinoma can have a similar appearance.

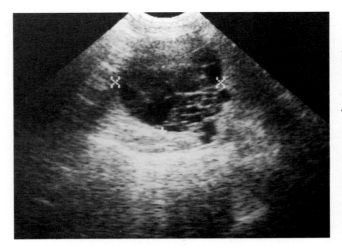

Figure 4-18. Multiseptated renal cyst. This complex cyst (cursors) projected exophytically off of the inferior pole of the left kidney. Extensive through transmission is seen. Numerous septations, seen as echogenic lines, are present within the cyst.

thick wall) on any imaging study, needle aspiration or open biopsy is necessary to exclude malignancy (Figure 4-17). Thick walls can occur but are not commonly seen in cysts with hemorrhagic or proteinaceous contents. They are a typical feature of abscesses and can also be seen in centrally necrotic neoplasms, particularly renal cell carcinomas. The presence of thick walls is an ominous finding and requires invasive evaluation, either thin-needle aspiration or open biopsy. CT and sonographic examinations often provide complementary information, and in certain instances the combination of the two imaging studies is necessary to confirm the benign nature of a complex cyst.

Septations within a cyst can be thin or thick, single or multiple (Figure 4-18). Sonography is the most reliable means of demonstrating septa and will often reveal septa missed by CT (Figure 4-19). Multiple thin septations in a complex cyst are probably due to the conglomeration of multiple, closely placed simple cysts. Previous hemorrhage or infection can also result in internal septations. A multiseptated renal cyst in a child is most probably a multilocular cystic nephroma. This is a benign neoplasm with multiple epithelium-lined cysts separated by a thin myxomatous stroma. Usually there are no renal elements, except for a few deformed nephrons, within the mass of cysts. The remainder of the kidney is usually deformed by the presence of the cystic mass. Unfortunately, renal cell carcinoma occasionally presents as a unilocular or multicystic mass. The more masslike the abnormality and the more irregular the cysts, the more likely it is to be a renal cell carcinoma (Figure 4-20). When the individual locules of the multiloculated cyst have the features of simple cysts with sharply defined walls, thin septations, and absence of internal echoes and there is no significant solid component to the cyst, it is more

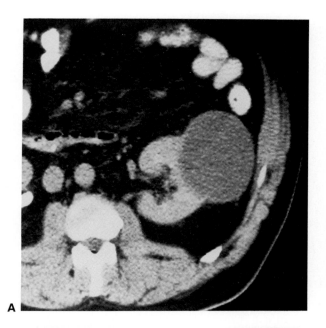

A

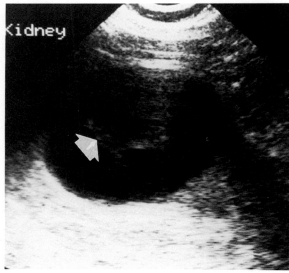

B

Figure 4-19. Papillary cystadenocarcinoma. (A) A CT scan of the left kidney demonstrates a relatively uniform cyst. (B) A sonogram of the same mass reveals that the mass contains a thick septation (arrow) that was not seen on the CT scan. Thick septations are a worrisome finding and raise the possibility of a malignancy, a finding unsuspected on the CT scan.

likely to be a benign complicated cyst. Under these circumstances, CT of the kidney is often useful to confirm the low likelihood of malignancy. If both CT and sonography suggest a benign lesion, follow-up scans should be performed. A lack of change over time further excludes malignancy. If the features of a cystic lesion change on subsequent imaging in any

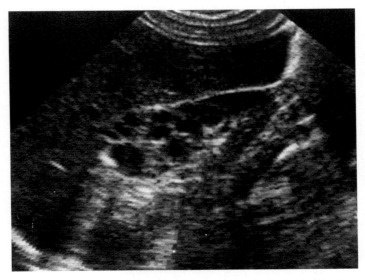

Figure 4-20. Cystic renal cell carcinoma. A longitudinal sonogram shows a complex cystic mass in the interpolar region of the right kidney. Note the multiple thick septa. This must be considered a neoplasm until proven otherwise, and establishing a tissue diagnosis is essential. The multilocular features of this mass are suggestive of a multilocular cystic nephroma. However, this proved to be a renal cell carcinoma. (Reprinted with permission from Coleman BG, Arger PH, Pollack HM, Banner M, Grossman RA. Contrast medium pooling in cystic renal carcinoma: CT findings. J Comput Assist Tomogr 1984; 8:1208–1210.)

patient being monitored, a more invasive evaluation, such as cyst aspiration, is usually necessary. In certain situations, it is also prudent to perform a needle aspiration to confirm a diagnosis of benign cyst.

A solitary thin septation, defined as less than 1 mm thick, is a benign finding. In most instances this probably represents a fibrous band caused by prior hemorrhage within the cyst. If this is the only feature that makes a cyst complex, no further evaluation is required in most instances **(Option (C) is false).** Only in situations where there is clinical concern for a renal malignancy should additional evaluation be considered.

The management of a calcified cyst is somewhat controversial. Daniel et al., in a review of 2,709 renal masses, discovered 111 masses that were visibly calcified on abdominal radiographs. Those with central or irregular calcifications had a high probability of malignancy. Of 19 masses with thin peripheral curvilinear calcification, 4 were renal cell carcinomas. This has been used to justify the belief that a mass with any

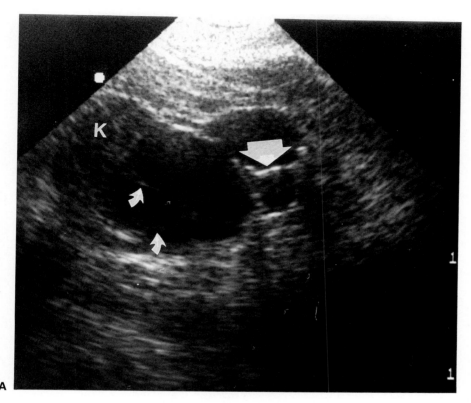

A

Figure 4-21. Complicated renal cyst. (A) A transverse sonogram of the left kidney (K), as imaged from the left flank, reveals a complicated cyst. Multiple thin septations (curved arrows) are seen, as are several regions of septal calcification (thick arrow). Increased through transmission is also identified. (B) A CT scan at the level of the kidneys again identifies a multiseptated cyst with calcified septa (arrow). This cyst has been monitored for over 1 year without change.

form of calcification is potentially a renal cell carcinoma. However, Daniel et al. did not have the advantages of cross-sectional imaging. More recently, Bosniak and Aronson et al. have argued that if (1) the calcification is thin and present in the wall or septa, (2) there is no associated soft tissue mass, (3) the center of the mass is of water density, and (4) no portion of the wall enhances, the cyst can be considered benign. These CT criteria can be extrapolated to sonographic criteria to include both (1) and (2) above, as well as (3) no internal echoes and (4) walls less than 1 mm thick. With strict adherence to these criteria, either comparison CT or follow-up sonography should be sufficient to exclude a renal malignancy **(Option (D) is false)** (Figure 4-21).

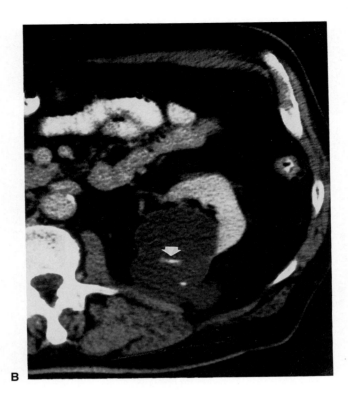

B

Question 19

Concerning renal oncocytomas,

    (A) they arise from the distal renal tubules
    (B) tumors with similar histology occur in the salivary glands
    (C) most are asymptomatic
    (D) a central hypoechoic stellate pattern is virtually pathognomonic
    (E) they are easily diagnosed by thin-needle biopsy

Renal oncocytoma, also known as proximal tubular adenoma with oncocytic features, is a specific variety of renal adenoma with a characteristic histologic appearance of large epithelial cells with granular eosinophilic cytoplasm. Renal oncocytomas are derived from the cells of the proximal renal tubules **(Option (A) is false).** Histologically similar tumors occur in the adrenal, salivary, thyroid, and parathyroid glands **(Option (B) is true).** Most oncocytomas are histologic grade I tumors

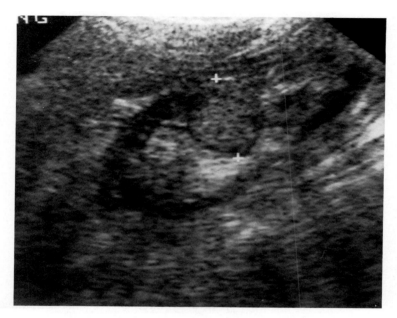

Figure 4-22. Small oncocytoma. A sonogram of the right kidney demonstrates a well-defined mass (cursors) that is slightly echogenic relative to renal parenchyma in the interpolar region. The absence of through transmission indicates that this is a solid lesion. This is a nondescript mass with a differential diagnosis similar to that of the test lesion. Histologic examination following nephrectomy demonstrated this to be an oncocytoma.

(no evidence of necrosis, mitoses, or nuclear anaplasia). To date, none of these neoplasms has been shown to metastasize. A few oncocytomas are histologic grade II neoplasms (they exhibit moderate anaplasia). In the Mayo Clinic series of grade II oncocytomas, 4 of 28 patients died of metastatic disease. Not infrequently, renal cell carcinoma has regions of the tumor that histologically resemble oncocytomas; that is, they have "oncocytic features." Therefore, oncocytoma and renal cell carcinoma cannot be distinguished on the basis of a needle biopsy because of the sampling error inherent in that procedure **(Option (E) is false)**.

Oncocytomas are unusual renal neoplasms that are most often asymptomatic and are incidentally detected during evaluation for other problems **(Option (C) is true)**. Occasional symptoms such as flank pain, hematuria, hypertension, or palpable flank mass can lead to the discovery of the oncocytoma. Approximately 5% of renal tumors preoperatively suspected to be renal cell carcinomas are in fact oncocytomas.

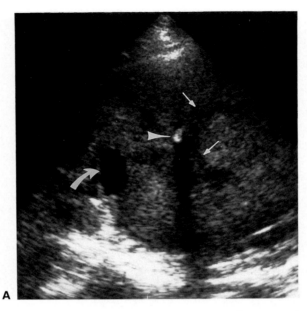

A

Figure 4-23. Large oncocytoma. (A) A sonographic examination of the right kidney demonstrates a large mass with a central hypoechoic stellate region (straight arrows). This appearance is characteristic of an oncocytoma with a central scar and is more often seen in a larger tumor, as in this case. An area of calcification with shadowing is seen within the central scar (arrowhead). There is also dilatation of the renal collecting system, seen as an anechoic region (curved arrow). (B) A postcontrast CT scan demonstrates the diminished enhancement of the central scar.

An oncocytoma most commonly appears on sonography as a well-defined homogeneous isoechoic mass (Figure 4-22). The presence of a hyperechoic central stellate scar is a clue to the diagnosis of oncocytoma. Unfortunately, the central scar is demonstrated by sonography in only about 25% of oncocytomas, usually the larger masses (Figure 4-23). Also, a renal cell carcinoma can have a central scar exactly mimicking that seen in an oncocytoma. Thus, this sign is neither sensitive nor specific **(Option (D) is false).** CT demonstrates a central scar in about 33% of oncocytomas, and MRI can also show the central scar. The classic angiographic feature, the spoke wheel pattern of vascularity, is seen in only 25% of cases. Arteriovenous shunting is uncommon in patients with oncocytoma but is commonly seen in patients with renal cell carcinoma. Unfortunately, renal cell carcinoma can mimic the angiographic, sonographic, CT, and MR features of oncocytoma. Therefore, to date, there is no method short of open biopsy for definitively distinguishing an oncocy-

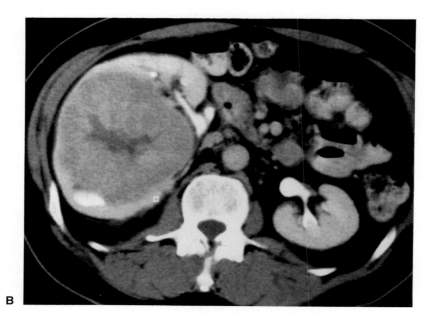

B

toma from a renal cell carcinoma. However, if an oncocytoma is suspected on the basis of imaging characteristics, kidney-sparing surgery
might be considered in certain clinical situations.

Wallace T. Miller, Jr., M.D.
Beverly G. Coleman, M.D.

SUGGESTED READINGS

RENAL CELL CARCINOMA

1. Amendola MA, Bree RL, Pollack HM, et al. Small renal cell carcinomas: resolving a diagnostic dilemma. Radiology 1988; 166:637–641
2. Benson MA, Haaga JR, Resnick MI. Staging renal carcinoma. What is sufficient? Arch Surg 1989; 124:71–73
3. Charboneau JW, Hattery RR, Ernst EC III, James EM, Williamson B Jr, Hartman GW. Spectrum of sonographic findings in 125 renal masses other than benign simple cyst. AJR 1983; 140:87–94
4. Coleman BG, Arger PH, Mintz MC, Pollack HM, Banner MP. Hyperdense renal masses: a computed tomographic dilemma. AJR 1984; 143:291–294
5. Foster WL Jr, Roberts L Jr, Halvorsen RA Jr, Dunnick NR. Sonography of small renal masses with indeterminant density characteristics on computed tomography. Urol Radiol 1988; 10:59–67

6. Levine E. Malignant renal parenchymal tumors in adults. In: Pollack HM (ed), Clinical urography. Philadelphia: WB Saunders; 1990:1216–1291
7. Levine E, Huntrakoon M, Wetzel LH. Small renal neoplasms: clinical, pathologic, and imaging features. AJR 1989; 153:69–73
8. McClennan BL. Oncologic imaging. Staging and follow-up of renal and adrenal carcinoma. Cancer 1991; 67:1199–1208
9. Vallancien G, Torres LO, Gurfinkel E, Veillon B, Brisset JM. Incidental detection of renal tumours by abdominal ultrasonography. Eur Urol 1990; 18:94–96

RENAL LYMPHOMA

10. Bakemeier RF, Zajurs G, Cooper RA, Rubin P. The malignant lymphomas. In: Rubin P (ed), Clinical oncology: a multidisciplinary approach. Rochester, NY: American Cancer Society; 1983:346–369
11. Carrasco CH, Richli WR, Lawrence D, Katz RL, Wallace S. Fine needle aspiration biopsy in lymphoma. Radiol Clin North Am 1990; 28:879–883
12. Carroll BA, Ta HN. The ultrasonic appearance of extranodal abdominal lymphoma. Radiology 1980; 136:419–425
13. Charnsangavej C. Lymphoma of the genitourinary tract. Radiol Clin North Am 1990; 28:865–877
14. Cohan RH, Dunnick NR, Leder RA, Baker ME. Computed tomography of renal lymphoma. J Comput Assist Tomogr 1990; 14:933–938
15. Hartman DS, Davis CJ Jr, Goldman SM, Friedman AC, Fritzsche P. Renal lymphoma: radiologic-pathologic correlation of 21 cases. Radiology 1982; 144:759–766
16. Heiken JP, McClennan BL, Gold RP. Renal lymphoma. Semin US CT MR 1986; 7:58–66
17. Richmond J, Sherman RS, Diamond HD, Craver LF. Renal lesions associated with malignant lymphomas. Am J Med 1962; 32:184–207
18. Shirkhoda A, Staab EV, Mittelstaedt CA. Renal lymphoma imaged by ultrasound and gallium-67. Radiology 1980; 137:175–180

ONCOCYTOMA

19. Goiney RC, Goldenberg L, Cooperberg PL, et al. Renal oncocytoma: sonographic analysis of 14 cases. AJR 1984; 143:1001–1004
20. Lieber MM, Tomera KM, Farrow GM. Renal oncocytoma. J Urol 1981; 125:481–485
21. Quinn MJ, Hartman DS, Friedman AC, et al. Renal oncocytoma: new observations. Radiology 1984; 153:49–53
22. Williamson B Jr. Benign neoplasms of the renal parenchyma. In: Pollack HM (ed), Clinical urography. Philadelphia: WB Saunders; 1990:1193–1215

ACUTE FOCAL PYELONEPHRITIS

23. Lee JK, McClennan BL, Melson GL, Stanley RJ. Acute focal bacterial nephritis: emphasis on gray scale sonography and computed tomography. AJR 1980; 135:87–92

24. Rosenfield AT, Glickman MG, Taylor KJ, Crade M, Hodson J. Acute focal bacterial nephritis (acute lobar nephronia). Radiology 1979; 132:553–561

COMPLEX RENAL CYSTS

25. Aronson S, Frazier HA, Baluch JD, Hartman DS, Christenson PJ. Cystic renal masses: usefulness of the Bosniak classification. Urol Radiol 1991; 13:83–90
26. Bosniak MA. The current radiological approach to renal cysts. Radiology 1986; 158:1–10
27. Daniel WW Jr, Hartman GW, Witten DM, Farrow GM, Kelalis PP. Calcified renal masses. A review of ten years experience at the Mayo Clinic. Radiology 1972; 103:503–508
28. Hartman DS. Cysts and cystic neoplasms. Urol Radiol 1990; 12:7–10
29. Pollack HM, Banner MP, Arger PH, Peters J, Mulhern CB Jr, Coleman BG. The accuracy of gray-scale renal ultrasonography in differentiating cystic neoplasms from benign cysts. Radiology 1982; 143:741–745

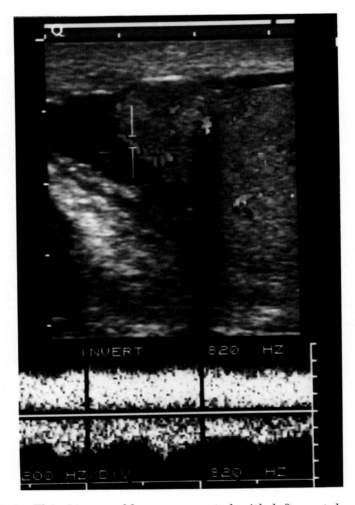

Figure 5-1. This 21-year-old man presented with left scrotal pain and swelling. You are shown a longitudinal color Doppler sonogram and a pulsed Doppler waveform of the left hemiscrotum.

Case 5:   Epididymitis

Question 20

Which *one* of the following is the MOST likely diagnosis?

(A) Acute testicular torsion
(B) Late testicular torsion
(C) Epididymitis
(D) Adenomatoid tumor
(E) Varicocele

In adults who present with acute scrotal pain and swelling, the major clinical considerations are epididymitis and testicular torsion. On a statistical basis, epididymitis is more likely to occur in an older patient and is more likely to be associated with fever and pyuria. Unfortunately, these statistical differences in large patient populations are not useful when dealing with an individual patient. In addition, the marked scrotal tenderness associated with both conditions often hinders the physical examination of the scrotum. The result of these limitations is that epididymitis cannot be distinguished from torsion, even by experienced urologic surgeons, in approximately 50% of cases. Therefore, imaging becomes important.

Figure 5-1 shows the upper pole of the testis and the head of the epididymis. There is readily detectable flow in the testis. The head of the epididymis is slightly enlarged, and there is readily detectable flow in the epididymis. In normal individuals, flow in the head of the epididymis is impossible or extremely difficult to detect with current color Doppler equipment. Therefore, the test image illustrates a hypervascular epididymal head. The Doppler waveform from the head of the epididymis shows low-resistance arterial flow below the baseline and detectable venous flow above the baseline. All of these findings are characteristic of epididymitis **(Option (C) is correct).**

Acute testicular torsion (Option (A)) differs dramatically from epididymitis on color Doppler sonography. In most cases, there is complete absence of detectable flow in the testis and the epididymis. Therefore, the readily detectable flow in both of these structures in the test image makes acute testicular torsion extremely unlikely. If torsion is not reversed, the affected testis will infarct. This is referred to as late or missed torsion (Option (B)); it causes a decrease in the echogenicity of the testis on gray-scale imaging and an inflammatory hyperemia in the peritesticular tissues. As with acute torsion, late torsion should not have detectable testicular flow, so it should not be a consideration in the test patient.

Adenomatoid tumors (Option (D)) are benign neoplasms of the epididymis. They are the most common epididymal tumor; however, epididymal tumors in general are very rare. The color Doppler sonographic appearance of adenomatoid tumors of the epididymis has not been described because they are so rare. Conceivably, they could be hypervascular and could explain all of the findings in Figure 5-1. However, on a statistical basis alone, adenomatoid tumor would be a very unlikely diagnosis in the test patient. In addition, it would be unusual for an adenomatoid tumor to present with scrotal pain. Therefore, this is not a likely diagnosis.

A varicocele (Option (E)) is a vascular abnormality that occurs in the peritesticular region and might therefore be considered in the differential diagnosis of the test patient. However, the dilated veins of a varicocele do not involve the head of the epididymis. The Doppler waveform is also inconsistent with a varicocele because a varicocele is a purely venous abnormality and so no arterial flow should be seen on the Doppler waveform. Therefore, the findings in Figure 5-1 are not consistent with a varicocele.

Question 21

Concerning testicular torsion,

(A) it almost never resolves spontaneously
(B) if it is reversed between 12 and 24 hours, the likelihood of testicular salvage is >50%
(C) an associated "bell clapper" deformity is bilateral in most patients
(D) the epididymis is usually not involved
(E) it is often preceded by trauma, strenuous exercise, or sexual intercourse

Testicular torsion annually affects approximately 1 in 4,000 males below the age of 25. It occurs most frequently in the neonatal and peripubertal age groups. In the neonatal period, torsion is usually extravaginal and occurs without associated anatomic anomalies. It is believed to be due to overall laxity of the scrotal tissues in the neonatal period. In the older age group, testicular torsion is referred to as intravaginal and is associated with an abnormal development of the tunica vaginalis known as the "bell clapper" deformity. This anomaly is caused by a tunica vaginalis that completely surrounds the testis, the epididymis, and the inferior aspect of the spermatic cord so that these structures are freely suspended in the scrotal sac like a clapper in a bell. Torsion occurs when the testis rotates and the spermatic cord twists on itself. This produces obstruction of the venous outflow and eventually reduction of the arterial inflow to the testis and epididymis **(Option (D) is false).** The bell clapper deformity is bilateral in most cases **(Option (C) is true),** and so surgical correction of a testicular torsion should also include a contralateral orchiopexy. When this is not done, the frequency of subsequent contralateral torsion may be as high as 40%. The presence of a bell clapper deformity predisposes to testicular torsion at any age. Presumably, the rapid growth of the testes at puberty results in a peak incidence in this age group.

In many cases, torsion is believed to be initiated by forceful contraction of the cremasteric muscles, which presumably retract and rotate the testis. Therefore, activities that cause a cremasteric response, such as trauma, strenuous exercise, or sexual intercourse, precede torsion in approximately 50 to 60% of cases **(Option (E) is true).** It is important to remember the association between trauma and torsion since most post-traumatic scans are performed to exclude hemorrhage and testicular fracture rather than torsion. Torsion can also develop during sleep. This is presumably due to cremasteric contraction associated with nocturnal activation of the sexual response.

The primary presenting symptom in patients with acute testicular torsion is scrotal pain, although some patients complain primarily of abdominal or inguinal pain. As many as one-half of patients with testicular torsion will relate previous similar episodes of testicular pain, which presumably were due to torsion that resolved spontaneously **(Option (A) is false).** Nausea and vomiting can also accompany acute testicular torsion.

On physical examination, scrotal tenderness, edema, and erythema are almost universal findings. Retraction of the testis and a horizontal lie of the testis are uncommon findings but are more reliable in distinguishing torsion from epididymitis. Fever is present in approximately 15% of patients, and 30 to 50% have an elevated leukocyte count. Urinalysis is usually normal, although an abnormal urinalysis does not exclude the diagnosis.

Rapid surgical correction of testicular torsion is critical to prevent permanent testicular damage. Animal studies have shown that both the duration and degree of torsion are important in predicting testicular via-

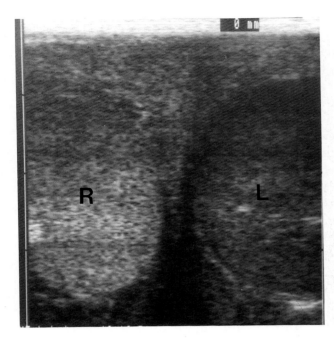

Figure 5-2. Late left testicular torsion. A transverse view of the scrotum shows normal echogenicity of the asymptomatic right testis (R). The left testis (L) is markedly decreased in echogenicity. This patient had been treated for presumed epididymitis, and sonography was requested when the symptoms did not resolve after 36 hours. At surgery, the testis was infarcted.

bility. There is no identifiable histologic change in dogs with 90° torsion, even over prolonged periods. However, 50% of canine testes suffer irreversible damage after 2 days of 180° torsion and undergo complete necrosis after 24 hours of 360° torsion. Williamson has shown that irreversible testicular damage in humans can occur as early as 4 hours when the torsion is tight. Between 4 and 10 hours, the chance of salvaging an affected testis becomes progressively more remote. After 10 hours of symptoms, most testes with torsion are no longer viable **(Option (B) is false)** and some of those that appear viable at surgery will subsequently become atrophic. Although the likelihood of infarction increases with the duration of torsion, some patients with mild degrees of torsion will have viable testes despite prolonged delays in treatment. Therefore, it is not possible to set a time limit beyond which surgery is not indicated.

Gray-scale sonography is capable of detecting a number of abnormalities in patients with acute testicular torsion. In dogs, the testes become enlarged and hypoechoic within 1 hour after complete ligation of the spermatic cord or 720° of cord twisting. Slight increases in testicular and epididymal size and decreases in echogenicity have been reported in humans who have had torsion for less than 6 hours; however, these changes generally do not occur until later (Figure 5-2). The changes in testicular morphology may be accompanied by scrotal skin thickening

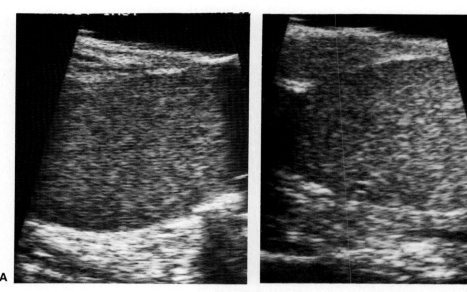

A

B

Figure 5-3. Acute left testicular torsion. The patient had symptoms for 6 hours. (A) A longitudinal view of the normal right testis shows normal homogeneous echogenicity. (B) A longitudinal view of the torsed left testis shows a normal homogeneous echogenicity symmetric with the right side.

and reactive hydroceles. Unfortunately, these findings are very nonspecific and are frequently encountered in patients with epididymitis. In addition, gray-scale sonography can be completely normal in the critical early stages of torsion (Figure 5-3).

Color Doppler ultrasonography, on the other hand, is almost always abnormal in patients with acute testicular torsion. In the vast majority of cases, testicular perfusion decreases to a level so low that the testis appears completely avascular on color Doppler sonograms (Figure 5-4). This appearance is almost pathognomonic for testicular ischemia (from either torsion or vascular obstruction of other etiologies) provided that the Doppler technical parameters have been optimized for detection of low-velocity, low-volume testicular blood flow. Proper adjustment of parameters can be confirmed by noting readily detectable flow in the contralateral testis. In patients with partial torsion (<360°), blood flow to the testis can be detectable but diminished when compared with the normal side (Figure 5-5). With time, an inflammatory response develops in the peritesticular soft tissues; this can be detected as hypervascularity on color Doppler sonography (Figure 5-6).

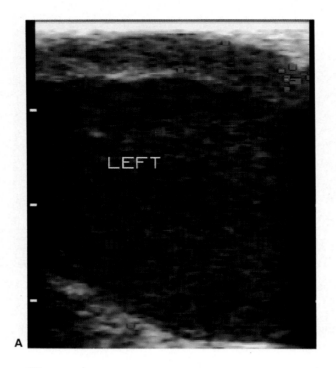

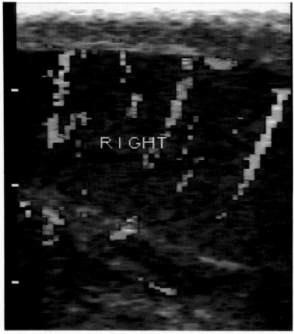

Figure 5-4. Acute left testicular torsion. The patient had symptoms for 4 hours. (A) A longitudinal color Doppler view of the left testis shows no detectable testicular blood flow. (B) A longitudinal color Doppler view of the right testis shows readily detectable intratesticular blood flow.

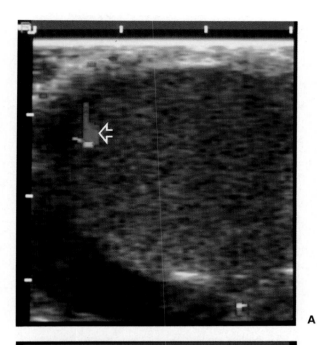

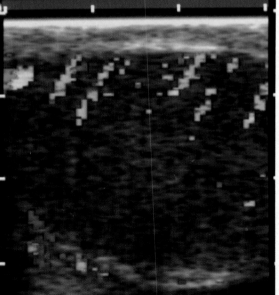

Figure 5-5. Partial (180°) right testicular torsion. (A) A longitudinal color Doppler view of the right testis shows a single small vessel (arrow) in the upper pole. The remainder of the testis has no detectable blood flow. (B) A longitudinal color Doppler view of the left testis shows readily detectable intratesticular blood flow. (Reprinted with permission from Middleton et al. [10].)

The sensitivity of color Doppler sonography in detecting torsion in adults has been well documented; the combined results from multiple studies indicate a sensitivity of >95%. However, potential limitations do

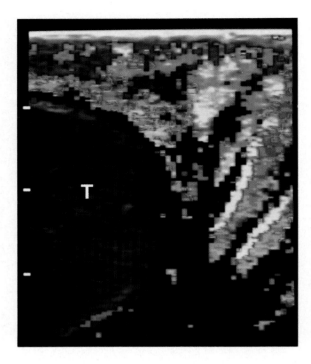

Figure 5-6. Late left testicular torsion. A color Doppler image shows markedly increased peritesticular blood flow and no detectable flow in the testis (T). (Reprinted with permission from Middleton et al. [10].)

exist. Lack of detectable blood flow occurs only if torsion is present at the time of the color Doppler examination. Therefore, intermittent torsion or torsion that has recently resolved can have normal-appearing blood flow. In fact, if the torsion has recently been reversed, a postischemic hyperemia can be present, and this can mimic the appearance of epididymoorchitis. In such patients, urgent surgery is not necessary. Nonetheless, they are at risk for developing persistent torsion in the future. Therefore, when the clinical scenario strongly suggests intermittent torsion, elective scrotal exploration and orchiopexy should be considered despite a negative color Doppler examination. Fortunately, this is uncommon.

The relative value of color Doppler sonography and scintigraphy has not been extensively studied. One comparative study in a primarily adult patient population has indicated that color Doppler sonography is slightly more accurate than scintigraphy in distinguishing torsion from other causes of acute scrotal pain. In the pediatric patient population, color Doppler sonography is more difficult, particularly for evaluating small prepubertal testes. However, even in children color Doppler sonography appears to be as effective as scintigraphy. The structural information available and the lack of radiation make sonography the preferred way of evaluating both adult and pediatric patients with suspected torsion, provided that the low-flow sensitivity is adequate. However, scintigraphy remains an accurate means of evaluating acute scrotal pain and should be used at least in situations in which it can be performed and interpreted more rapidly than color Doppler sonography. It should also be used when experience with color Doppler sonography is limited or when there is doubt about the sonographic diagnosis. Regardless of which modality is preferred, it is important to realize that imaging of any type should be avoided if it will cause a delay in treatment of a patient with a high clinical suspicion of testicular torsion.

Question 22

Concerning epididymitis,

(A) it is the most common cause of acute scrotal pain in adults
(B) it is occasionally isolated to the epididymal tail
(C) severe cases are occasionally associated with testicular ischemia
(D) associated peritesticular fluid usually indicates an abscess

It is estimated that 634,000 men per year seek medical attention because of epididymitis or epididymo-orchitis. Epididymitis is the most common cause of acute scrotal pain in adults **(Option (A) is true).** *Chlamydia trachomatis* and *Neisseria gonorrhoeae* are the most common etiologic organisms in men younger than 35 years, and *Escherichia coli* and *Proteus mirabilis* are the most common in older men. In approximately 20% of cases, no organism can be cultured. Infection of the scrotal contents is believed to result primarily from bladder and prostate infections that spread via the vas deferens. Hematogenous spread and lymphatic spread also occur but are believed to be much less common.

Most scrotal inflammatory processes start in the epididymis, but they frequently spread to the testis. Isolated orchitis is usually viral in origin and occurs much less frequently than epididymo-orchitis. If not treated appropriately, any of these conditions can progress to abscess or pyocele formation.

Most cases of epididymo-orchitis occur in men older than 20 years of age. However, approximately 20% occur in younger men and boys. Fifteen percent of men with epididymo-orchitis have experienced a previous similar episode. The onset of pain is as likely to be acute as gradual. Urinary tract symptoms occur in only 7% of patients. On physical examination, tenderness and swelling are almost always noted in the epididymis, testis, or both. Fever is present in one-third of patients, and pyuria is present in approximately one-half.

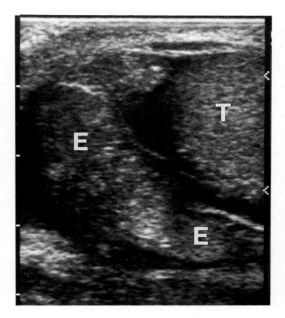

Figure 5-7. Epididymitis. A longitudinal view of the testis (T) and epididymal head and body (E) shows marked enlargement and decreased echogenicity of the epididymis.

The overlap in signs and symptoms between epididymitis and testicular torsion means that it may be difficult to distinguish between the two conditions clinically. Therefore, it is not uncommon for patients with epididymitis to be referred for sonography to exclude torsion or associated complications such as abscess formation.

On gray-scale sonography, epididymitis usually appears as an enlarged and hypoechoic epididymis (Figure 5-7). When the testis is involved, it generally enlarges and becomes hypoechoic as well. In some patients, extensive involvement of periepididymal soft tissues and cord structures makes the epididymis itself difficult to visualize. Instead, a complex mass with both hyper- and hypoechoic components is seen in the expected location of the epididymis (Figure 5-8). Reactive hydroceles are common and do not indicate abscess formation in most cases **(Option (D) is false).** When a hydrocele contains gas, multiple internal echoes, or thick septations, superimposed infection and pyocele formation should be considered (Figure 5-9).

On color Doppler ultrasonography, the hallmark of scrotal inflammatory disease is hypervascularity of the involved structure. As mentioned above, with current color Doppler equipment it is generally not possible to detect blood flow in the normal epididymis. Therefore, whenever intraepididymal vessels are seen, they should be considered abnormal. In the future, improvements in color Doppler sensitivity may make it possible

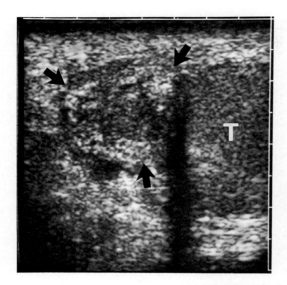

Figure 5-8. Epididymitis. A longitudinal view of the upper scrotum shows a heterogeneous mass (arrows) situated above the testis (T) and in the expected position of the epididymal head.

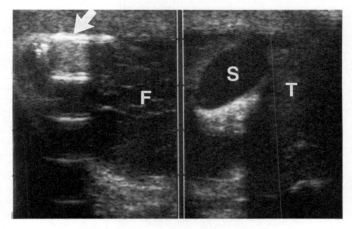

Figure 5-9. Gas-containing pyocele. A composite longitudinal view of the superior aspect of the scrotum shows the upper pole of the testis (T) and a spermatocele (S) in the epididymal head. A complex fluid collection (F) with multiple internal echoes and septations is seen superior to the spermatocele. A highly echogenic collection of gas (arrow) is seen in the nondependent portion of the pyocele. Multiple reverberation artifacts are present deep to the gas collections.

to detect normal epididymal vascularity. Currently, it is possible to detect flow in normal scrotal wall vessels, and these should not be confused with intraepididymal vessels.

Epididymitis is usually diffuse, but in approximately 20% of cases the involvement is focal. Isolated involvement of the tail occurs in

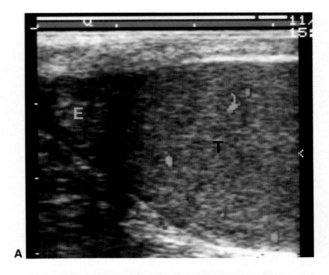

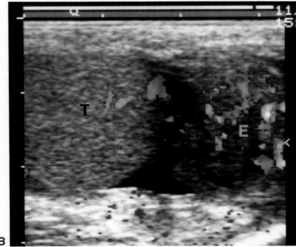

Figure 5-10. Epididymitis isolated to the tail of the epididymis. (A) A longitudinal color Doppler view of the upper scrotum demonstrates flow in the testis (T) but no detectable flow in the head of the epididymis (E). This is normal. (B) A longitudinal view of the lower scrotum shows enlargement, decreased echogenicity, and marked hypervascularity of the tail of the epididymis (E). In this case, the epididymis contains more detectable vessels than the adjacent testis (T).

approximately 10% of cases **(Option (B) is true).** Therefore, it is important to visualize the entire structure carefully to detect focal areas of hypervascularity (Figure 5-10). In addition, in some patients with epididymitis the gray-scale appearance is normal and the only indication of an underlying inflammatory disorder is the hypervascularity visualized on color Doppler sonography.

In patients with more advanced epididymitis, the inflammatory process often spreads to the testis and produces orchitis (Figure 5-11). This appears as enlargement and decreased echogenicity of the testis on gray-scale sonography and as hypervascularity on color Doppler sonography.

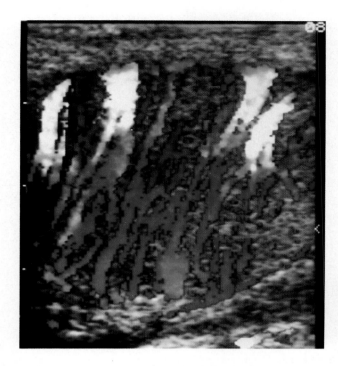

Figure 5-11. Orchitis. A longitudinal color Doppler view of the testis shows marked hypervascularity.

Since vessels should normally be detected in the testis, increased vascularity is best appreciated by comparing images of the affected side with images of the contralateral side.

Interestingly, severe cases of epididymitis can also be associated with decreased testicular blood flow **(Option (C) is true).** This occurs because of obstruction of testicular venous outflow by the swelling around the epididymis. As with venous outflow obstruction of other organs, this causes increased resistance to arterial inflow and can even produce diastolic flow reversal in intratesticular arteries (Figure 5-12). If the resulting ischemia is prolonged, the testis can infarct just as in patients with testicular torsion.

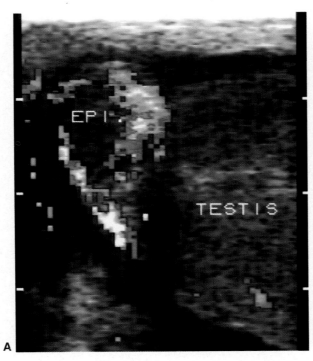

Figure 5-12. Epididymitis with testicular ischemia. (A) A longitudinal color Doppler view through the upper pole of the testis and the head of the epididymis (EPI) shows multiple epididymal vessels, indicative of hyperemia. (B) A waveform from the epididymal head shows abnormal low-resistance arterial flow above the baseline and detectable venous flow below the baseline. (C) A waveform from an intratesticular artery shows essentially no effective blood flow through the testis, with antegrade systolic flow being negated by retrograde diastolic flow.

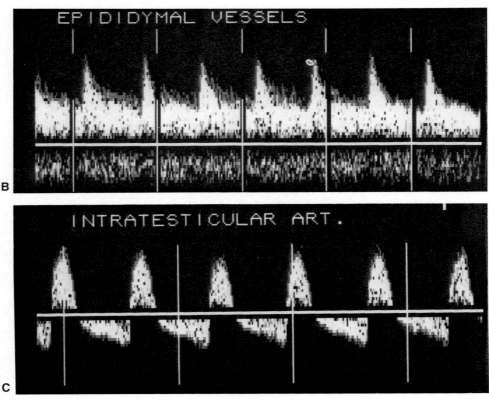

Question 23

Concerning testicular tumors,

    (A) they most often present as a painless mass
    (B) most are germ cell tumors
    (C) about 20% are bilateral
    (D) calcification implies a benign histology
    (E) seminomas are avascular or hypovascular

Testicular carcinoma is the most common malignant tumor in young men. Approximately 2,500 new cases are diagnosed each year in the United States. The overall incidence is 2 to 3 per 100,000 men per year, but between the ages of 15 and 32 years the incidence is twice as high.

A testicular tumor most often presents as a painless mass in the testis **(Option (A) is true).** Approximately 10% of patients have metastatic disease on initial presentation. Occasionally, patients first complain of scrotal pain, and the workup is directed toward epididymo-orchitis or torsion. In addition, it is not unusual for patients to first become aware of a mass after an episode of trauma. Therefore, it is important to consider neoplasms in any patient who presents with acute scrotal symptoms.

Approximately 95% of primary testicular tumors are of germ cell origin **(Option (B) is true).** Stromal cell neoplasms such as Sertoli and Leydig cell tumors do occur but are rare. Approximately 8% of patients have bilateral testicular tumors at presentation or eventually develop a contralateral tumor **(Option (C) is false).** Seminomas are the most common type of germ cell tumor, accounting for approximately 40 to 50% of the total. They tend to occur in a slightly older patient population than do other testicular tumors. Seminomas are frequently divided into classic, anaplastic, and spermatocytic types. The classic seminoma has an excellent prognosis because of its marked radiosensitivity. Anaplastic seminomas carry a worse prognosis but fortunately account for only 10% of all seminomas. Spermatocytic seminomas are named for their production of spermatocytes. They are the least aggressive of the seminomas and tend to occur in older patients. They also tend to be bilateral more often than do classic seminomas. Seminomas are the most likely testicular tumor to occur in a pure form, but approximately 10 to 15% contain other germ cell elements. In such cases, the more aggressive nonseminomatous elements determine the biologic behavior of the tumor.

The most aggressive type of germ cell neoplasm is the embryonal cell tumor, which, in its pure form, is relatively rare, accounting for <10% of lesions. Embryonal cell tumor elements are the most common components in mixed germ cell tumors, which make up approximately 50% of all testicular tumors. Teratomas make up another 10% of testicular tumors. In adults, testicular teratomas can be histologically mature and well differentiated yet metastasize widely. In children, however, they are regarded as benign tumors. Teratocarcinoma is a confusing name used in the past for tumors composed of both teratoma and embryonal cell carcinoma. It is not used to distinguish malignant teratomas from benign teratomas. Choriocarcinoma occurs in the setting of mixed tumors but, like embryonal cell carcinoma, is rarely seen in the pure form. It has a much greater tendency to metastasize hematogenously than do other testicular tumors, which usually spread via lymphatics. Testicular choriocarcinoma has a much worse prognosis than the histologically equivalent germ cell tumor encountered in women.

In elderly patients, primary testicular tumors are less common than metastatic disease, lymphoma, and leukemic infiltration. The most common primary tumor to metastasize to the testis is prostatic carcinoma. Others include lung, kidney and gastrointestinal tract tumors, and melanoma. Leukemic infiltration of the testis frequently occurs when the patient is otherwise in remission. This is believed to be due to a blood-gonad barrier to chemotherapy drugs, which allows the testis to serve as a sanctuary for the disease.

Sonography is capable of detecting almost all testicular tumors, including nonpalpable lesions in patients who present with metastatic disease. It is also very accurate at distinguishing intratesticular from extratesticular masses. Hence, sonography is widely employed to evaluate scrotal masses.

Most palpable scrotal masses are extratesticular; the most common extratesticular masses are spermatoceles and epididymal cysts. A spermatocele results from obstruction of the epididymal ducts and is filled with fluid containing spermatozoa. The lesion arises from the head of the epididymis and can become large and multilobulated. When a spermatocele enlarges, it obscures the head of the epididymis. An epididymal cyst is less common, contains clear serous fluid, and can occur anywhere along the course of the epididymis. In general, cystic lesions of the epididymis are extremely common, occurring in at least 30% of the population. Spermatoceles and epididymal cysts both appear cystic on sonography (Figure 5-13). Epididymal tumors are extremely uncommon and are usually benign; adenomatoid tumors of the epididymis are the most frequent. In general, all extratesticular masses, either cystic or solid, can be considered benign with a high degree of certainty.

Intratesticular masses are somewhat more problematic. Certainly, any solid intratesticular mass should be considered malignant until proven otherwise. Unfortunately, a number of benign lesions can mimic tumors. These include hemorrhage, contusion, atrophy (Figure 5-14), focal orchitis (Figure 5-15), infarcts (Figure 5-16), and benign tumors.

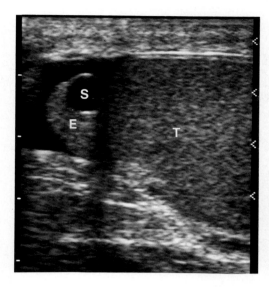

Figure 5-13 (left). Spermatocele. A longitudinal view of the
upper pole of the testis (T) and
head of the epididymis (E)
shows a small spermatocele (S)
arising from the epididymal
head.

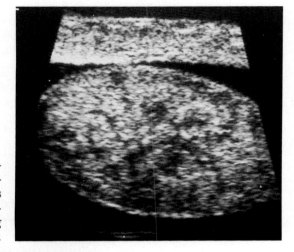

Figure 5-14 (right). Testicular atrophy. A longitudinal view of the testis shows
diffuse heterogeneity simulating an infiltrating
tumor.

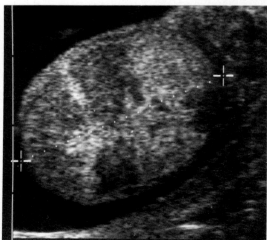

Figure 5-15 (left). Multifocal orchitis. A longitudinal
view of the testis shows
multiple hypoechoic le-
sions simulating testicular
neoplasia.

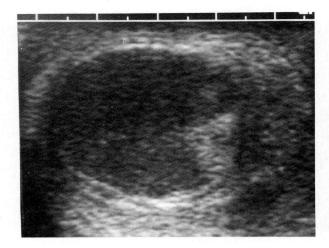

Figure 5-16. Testicular infarct. A longitudinal view of the testis demonstrates a large hypoechoic lesion involving most of the testis. This was an evolving infarct that occurred following a hernia repair.

Whenever an intratesticular mass is detected sonographically, a survey of the retroperitoneum, particularly at the level of the kidneys, should be performed to evaluate for metastatic lymphadenopathy. If enlarged nodes are seen, malignancy can be diagnosed with some assurance. On the other hand, if there is no evidence of lymphadenopathy and there is strong clinical evidence to suggest a diagnosis other than tumor, immediate surgical exploration can be replaced by periodic sonographic follow-up. If a lesion fails to improve or resolve with therapy, surgery should be performed. Even with this approach, sonography cannot prevent an occasional orchiectomy for benign lesions.

Cystic lesions of the testis can also be benign or malignant. Benign testicular cysts occur in up to 10% of the population. They are more common in the elderly and tend to occur in the region of the mediastinum. Most benign intratesticular cysts satisfy all sonographic criteria of a cyst and are nonpalpable on physical examination (Figure 5-17). Most cystic neoplasms are palpable and appear complex sonographically (i.e., they contain internal echoes, solid components, calcifications, or thick septations) (Figure 5-18). Other unusual cystic lesions include cysts of the tunica albuginea and tubular ectasia of the rete testes. Tunica albuginea cysts are benign lesions that present as small, very firm, easily palpable peripheral testicular masses on physical examination. On sonography, they appear as benign cysts centered on the tunica albuginea (Figure 5-19). Tubular ectasia of the rete testes is most commonly seen in older men and is not palpable. It is usually bilateral but can be symmetric. It appears as an elongated hypoechoic zone composed of a multitude of variably sized cystic structures replacing the mediastinum testis (Figure 5-20).

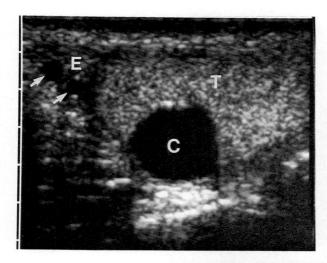

Figure 5-17 (left).
Benign testicular
cyst. A longitudinal
view of the testis (T)
shows a large intrat-
esticular cyst (C). Two
small spermatoceles
(arrows) are present
in the head of the epi-
didymis (E).

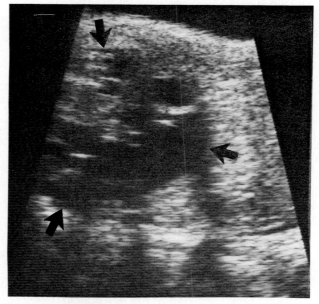

Figure 5-18 (right).
Cystic teratoma. A
longitudinal view of
the upper pole of the
testis shows a com-
plex cystic mass (ar-
rows). This appear-
ance is quite
different from a sim-
ple cyst, and this
mass was easily
palpable.

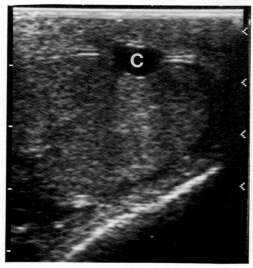

Figure 5-19 (left). Tunica albuginea cyst. A transverse
view of the testis shows a simple cyst (C) centered on the tunica albuginea. This lesion was
palpable and firm on physical
examination.

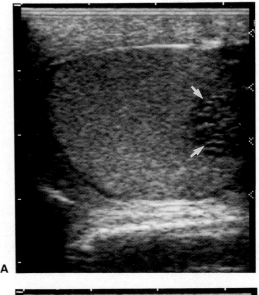

A

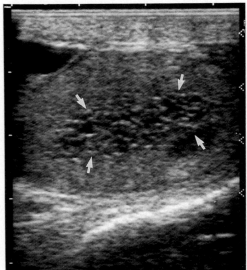

B

Figure 5-20. Tubular ectasia of the rete testis. (A) A transverse view of the testis shows a hypoechoic mass consisting of multiple small cysts replacing the mediastinum (arrows). (B) A longitudinal view shows that the lesion (arrows) is elongated similar to the normal mediastinum.

Sonography is not capable of distinguishing the different types of testicular tumors in an individual patient, but some general sonographic patterns have been described. Seminomas are usually homogeneous hypoechoic masses (Figure 5-21). They rarely contain calcifications or cystic changes. Nonseminomatous germ cell tumors tend to be heterogeneous and frequently contain cystic changes (Figure 5-22). Calcifications occur in 20 to 35% of nonseminomatous germ cell tumors (Figure 5-23)

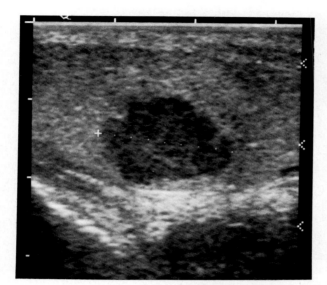

Figure 5-21 (left).
Seminoma. A longitudinal view shows a homogeneous, hypoechoic mass with well-defined margins.

Figure 5-22 (right).
Mixed germ cell tumor. A longitudinal view of the lower pole of the testis shows a complex cystic mass (arrows) consisting of teratoma and embryonal cell carcinoma.

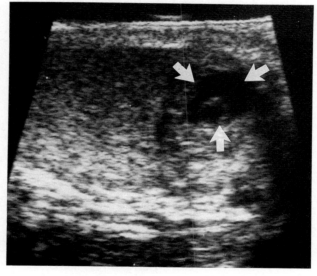

and do not imply a benign histology **(Option (D) is false).** Lymphoproliferative diseases are usually hypoechoic but can be diffuse or focal, unilateral or bilateral, or homogeneous or heterogeneous (Figures 5-24 and 5-25). Involvement of the epididymis is variable.

Color Doppler sonographic analysis of lesion vascularity adds little useful information beyond that provided by the gray-scale image and the clinical history in patients with suspected testicular tumors. Detection of tumor vessels and hypervascularity depends more on tumor size than on

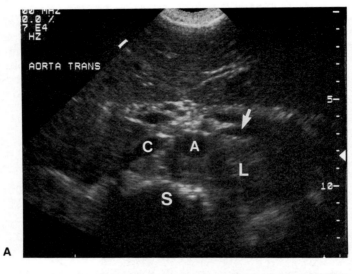

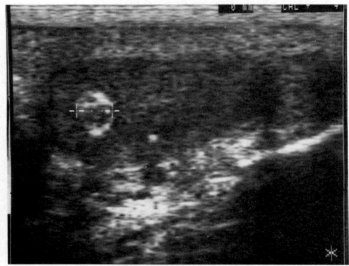

Figure 5-23. Metastatic teratoma. (A) A transverse view of the upper abdomen performed to evaluate the kidneys in a patient with back pain shows marked left para-aortic lymphadenopathy (L) displacing the left renal vein (arrow) anteriorly and separating the aorta (A) and inferior vena cava (C) away from the spine (S). This is the typical pattern of spread of a left testicular tumor. (B) A longitudinal view of the left testis shows a 4-mm peripherally calcified lesion (cursors) that was nonpalpable. Pathologically, this was a benign-appearing teratoma and scar tissue.

tumor type. Most tumors less than 1.6 cm in size are hypovascular, whereas larger tumors (including seminomas) are hypervascular when

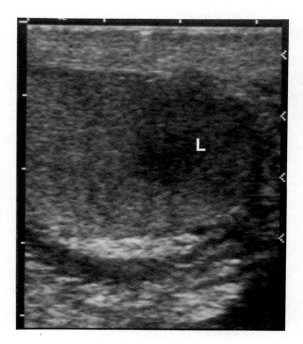

Figure 5-24 (left). Testicular lymphoma. A longitudinal view of the testis shows a poorly marginated hypoechoic lymphomatous mass (L) in the lower pole of the testis.

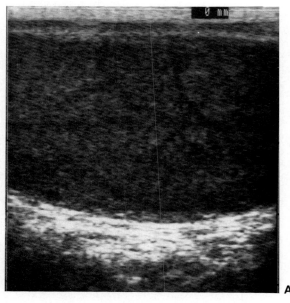

Figure 5-25 (right and on following page). Leukemia infiltration. (A) A longitudinal view of the symptomatic testis shows enlargement and diffuse homogeneously decreased echogenicity. (B) A longitudinal view of the normal contralateral testis for comparison.

A

compared with normal testicular parenchyma **(Option (E) is false)** (Figure 5-26).

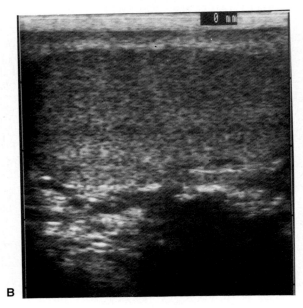

B

Figure 5-25 (Continued)

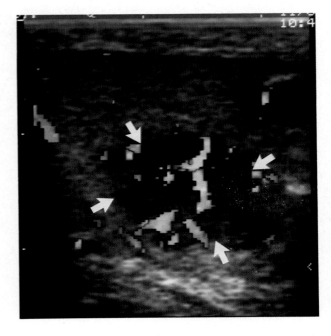

Figure 5-26. Hypervascular seminoma. A transverse color Doppler view of the testis shows a hypoechoic mass (arrows) that is hypervascular compared with the normal testicular parenchyma.

Question 24

Concerning varicoceles,

(A) most are bilateral
(B) most are asymptomatic
(C) most are caused by spermatic vein obstruction
(D) when they are nonpalpable, repair is not indicated
(E) venous flow is generally detected only with special maneuvers

Venous outflow from the testis drains into the pampiniform plexus, which in turns drains into the internal spermatic vein (also called the testicular vein). In normal individuals, valves in the internal spermatic vein limit the hydrostatic pressure that can develop in the vein and ensure that venous flow can progress only in the cephalic direction. When these valves are incompetent, hydrostatic pressure in the spermatic vein increases and the vessels of the pampiniform plexus dilate. These dilated veins are referred to as varicoceles. Incompetent or congenitally absent valves cause the vast majority of varicoceles. Spermatic vein obstruction is a very uncommon cause **(Option (C) is false).** Most varicoceles (80 to 90%) are isolated to the left side, for many reasons **(Option (A) is false).** The left spermatic vein is longer than the right and can function as a larger hydrostatic column. In addition, the right spermatic vein drains at an oblique angle into the low-pressure inferior vena cava, whereas the left spermatic vein drains at a right angle into the higher-pressure left renal vein. Compression of the left renal vein as it passes between the superior mesenteric artery and the aorta may also elevate renal vein pressure even further and contribute to the development of left-sided varicoceles. Varicoceles are bilateral in 10 to 15% of patients. Isolated right-sided varicoceles are quite uncommon. When they occur, the possibility of an obstructing retroperitoneal tumor or situs inversus should be considered.

Varicoceles can cause pain, but most are asymptomatic and are detected incidentally or during a workup for infertility **(Option (B) is true).** The relationship between varicoceles and infertility is controversial and poorly understood. Most experts in infertility believe that varicoceles are at least potential causes of infertility because (1) varicoceles are frequently associated with abnormal testicular histology and semen analysis; (2) semen analysis does improve in some patients after varicocele repair; and (3) varicoceles are more common in infertile men than in the general population.

The pathophysiology of infertility in patients with varicoceles is not established. Proposed etiologies include increased scrotal and testicular temperature, stagnation of testicular blood flow with resulting hypoxia,

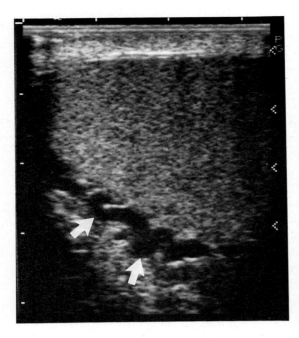

Figure 5-27. Varicocele. A longitudinal view of the upper pole of the testis shows a dilated, tortuous peritesticular vein (arrows).

reflux of toxic renal or adrenal metabolites, and alteration in the hypothalamic-pituitary-gonadal axis. It is clear, however, that in some men even nonpalpable varicoceles can be associated with infertility and that their repair can result in spermatologic improvements **(Option (D) is false).** Because of this, it is important to identify asymptomatic, nonpalpable varicoceles in infertile patients.

On gray-scale sonography, varicoceles appear as dilated and tortuous venous channels (Figure 5-27). They are usually best visualized superior and/or lateral to the testis. When large, they can extend posterior and inferior to the testis. The upper limit of normal diameter for peritesticular veins is 2 to 3 mm.

On color Doppler ultrasonography, reflux of venous flow can be identified when patients perform a Valsalva maneuver or stand upright (Figure 5-28). In general, venous flow within varicoceles is too slow to be detected unless these maneuvers are performed **(Option (E) is true).**

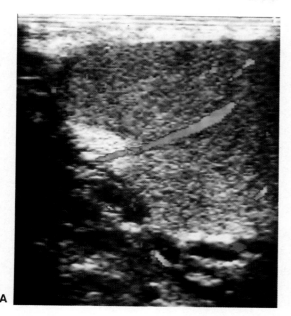

A

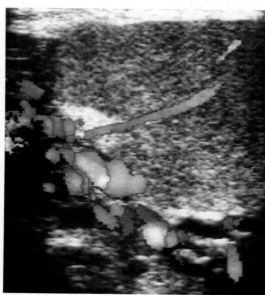

B

Figure 5-28. Varicocele.
(A) A transverse color Doppler view shows prominent peritesticular veins posterior to the testis. Blood flow in these veins is too slow to be detected when the patient is at rest. (B) A transverse view, obtained while the patient performed a Valsalva maneuver, shows increased venous flow in the varicocele as a result of venous reflux down the spermatic vein and into the varicocele.

Question 25

Concerning the normal vascular anatomy of the scrotum,

    (A) the spermatic cord contains three arteries
    (B) intratesticular arteries are not visible on gray-scale sonography
    (C) intratesticular arterial blood flow is directed both toward and away from the mediastinum testis
    (D) centripetal arteries are supplied by capsular arteries
    (E) vascular resistance in the normal testis is high

The testicular arteries arise from the aorta just inferior to the level of the renal arteries. They descend in the retroperitoneum and enter the ipsilateral spermatic cord at the deep inguinal ring. Within each spermatic cord, the testicular artery is accompanied by the cremasteric artery, which is a branch of the inferior epigastric artery, and the deferential artery, which is a branch of the vesicular artery **(Option (A) is true).** Anastomoses between these three vessels do exist; however, the testicular artery supplies primarily the testis, whereas the deferential and cremasteric arteries supply primarily the epididymis and vas deferens, and the peritesticular tissues, respectively (Figure 5-29).

After entering the scrotum, the testicular artery runs along the posterior aspect of the testis and may branch before entering the testis. In some individuals, the testicular artery, or a large branch of the testicular artery, penetrates the mediastinum and travels completely through the testicular parenchyma to the surface opposite the mediastinum. This is referred to as a transmediastinal artery. Anatomic studies performed in the mid-1900s and early color Doppler studies indicated that transmediastinal arteries were unusual normal variants occurring in fewer than 20% of testes. However, with improvements in sensitivity, these arteries are now being seen more frequently and probably occur in approximately 50% of testes (Figure 5-30). In most testes only a single transmediastinal artery is identified, but in some testes they are multiple. Although most intratesticular arteries are not visible by gray-scale sonography, the transmediastinal artery frequently can be seen as a thin hypoechoic band running through the testicular parenchyma (Figure 5-31) **(Option (B) is false).**

After traversing the testicular parenchyma, transmediastinal arteries supply arterial branches that travel just deep to the tunica albuginea in a layer called the tunica vasculosa. These arteries are referred to as capsular arteries. In individuals who do not have a transmediastinal artery, the capsular arteries are supplied directly from the testicular artery (Figure 5-32).

17. Gooding GA, Leonhardt W, Stein R. Testicular cysts: US findings. Radiology 1987; 163:537–538
18. Hamm B, Fobbe F, Loy V. Testicular cysts: differentiation with US and clinical findings. Radiology 1988; 168:19–23
19. Heiken JP, Balfe DM, McClennan BL. Testicular tumors: oncologic imaging and diagnosis. Int J Radiat Oncol Biol Phys 1984; 10:275–287
20. Horstman WG, Melson GL, Middleton WD, Andriole GL. Testicular tumors: findings with color Doppler US. Radiology 1992; 185:733–737
21. Leung ML, Gooding GA, Williams RD. High-resolution sonography of scrotal contents in asymptomatic subjects. AJR 1984; 143:161–164
22. Lupetin AR, King W III, Rich P, Lederman RB. Ultrasound diagnosis of testicular leukemia. Radiology 1983; 146:171–172
23. Nochomovitz LE, DeLa Torre FE, Rosai J. Pathology of germ cell tumors of the testis. Urol Clin North Am 1977; 4:359–378
24. Phillips G, Kumari-Subaiya S, Sawitsky A. Ultrasonic evaluation of the scrotum in lymphoproliferative disease. J Ultrasound Med 1987; 6:169–175
25. Schwerk WB, Schwerk WN, Rodeck G. Testicular tumors: prospective analysis of real-time US patterns and abdominal staging. Radiology 1987; 164:369–374
26. Silverberg E. Cancer in young adults (ages 15 to 34). CA Cancer J Clin 1982; 32:32–42
27. Steinfeld AD. Testicular germ cell tumors: review of contemporary evaluation and management. Radiology 1990; 175:603–606
28. Tackett RE, Ling D, Catalona WJ, Melson GL. High resolution sonography in diagnosing testicular neoplasms: clinical significance of false positive scans. J Urol 1986; 135:494–496

VARICOCELE

29. Dubin L, Amelar RD. Varicocele. Urol Clin North Am 1978; 5:563–572
30. Gonda RL Jr, Karo JJ, Forte RA, O'Donnell KT. Diagnosis of subclinical varicocele in infertility. AJR 1987; 148:71–75
31. Marsman JW. Clinical versus subclinical varicocele: venographic findings and improvement of fertility after embolization. Radiology 1985; 155:635–638
32. McClure RD, Hricak H. Scrotal ultrasound in the infertile man: detection of subclinical unilateral and bilateral varicoceles. J Urol 1986; 135:711–715
33. McClure RD, Khoo D, Jarvi K, Hricak H. Subclinical varicocele: the effectiveness of varicocelectomy. J Urol 1991; 145:789–791
34. Pryor JL, Howards SS. Varicocele. Urol Clin North Am 1987; 14:499–513
35. Wolverson MK, Houttuin E, Heiberg E, Sundaram M, Gregory J. High-resolution real-time sonography of scrotal varicocele. AJR 1983; 141:775–779

NORMAL TESTICULAR VASCULAR ANATOMY

36. Fakhry J, Khoury A, Barakat K. The hypoechoic band: a normal finding on testicular sonography. AJR 1989; 153:321–323
37. Harrison RG. The distribution of the vasal and cremasteric arteries to the testis and their functional importance. J Anat 1949; 83:267–282

38. Harrison RG, Barclay AE. The distribution of the testicular artery (internal spermatic artery) to the human testis. Br J Urol 1948; 20:57–66
39. Kormano M, Suoranta H. An angiographic study of the arterial pattern of the human testis. Anat Anz 1971; 128:69–76
40. Middleton WD, Bell MW. Further observations on normal testicular vascular anatomy with emphasis on the transmediastinal artery. Radiology (submitted for publication)
41. Middleton WD, Thorne DA, Melson GL. Color Doppler ultrasound of the normal testis. AJR 1989; 152:293–297

Notes

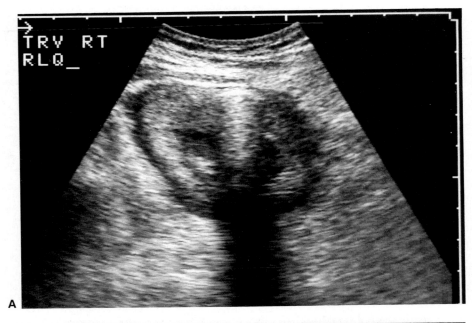

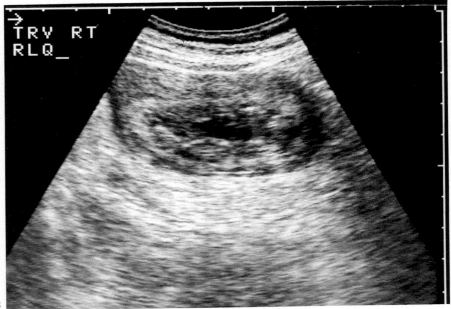

Figure 6-1. This 65-year-old man presented with fever and right abdominal pain. You are shown transverse sonograms obtained through the right flank.

Case 6:   Ischemic Colitis

Question 26

Which *one* of the following is the MOST likely diagnosis?

(A) Ischemic colitis
(B) Periappendiceal abscess
(C) Mucocele
(D) Intussusception
(E) Crohn's disease

Figures 6-1A and B are transverse views of the right abdomen show-ing a thick-walled tubular structure. The tubular nature of the mass sug-gests that it represents a bowel loop; the location along the right flank is most consistent with the ascending colon. The thickened wall has a con-centric-ring appearance consisting of alternating hypoechoic and hyper-echoic rings that correspond to the different histologic layers of the bowel wall (Figure 6-2). This has been termed the "gut signature" or "target pattern" and provides further evidence that the mass represents a bowel loop. Up to five layers can be observed (see Table 6-1), although fewer are seen in the test images. In addition, Figures 6-1A and 6-2A show a linear hyperechoic focus in the bowel wall that produces a reverberating ("dirty") shadow, indicating the presence of gas. Of the options listed, is-chemic colitis is by far the most likely to produce a thickened bowel wall containing intramural gas in an elderly man **(Option (A) is correct).**

Ischemic colitis is one of the most common disorders of the large intestine in elderly patients. More than 90% of patients are over 60 years of age, and the disease rarely occurs in patients under age 45. Most patients have associated medical problems such as cardiovascular dis-ease or diabetes mellitus. The disease is less commonly associated with arrhythmias, shock, sepsis, hypovolemic conditions, hemoglobinopathies, hypercoagulable states, vasculitides, aortic aneurysms, obstructing col-orectal masses, and the use of various drugs (cocaine, ergots, vaso-pressin, and oral contraceptives). Iatrogenic surgical causes include aor-toiliac reconstruction and abdominoperineal resection, both of which can

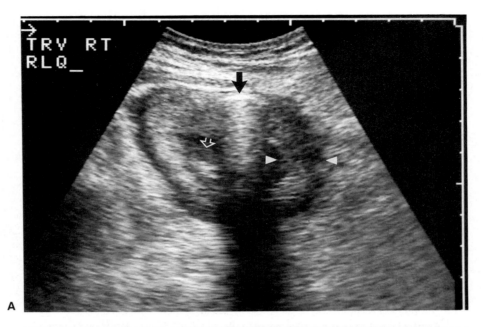

A

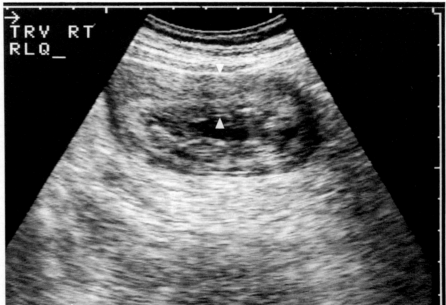

B

Figure 6-2 (Same as Figure 6-1). Ischemic colitis. Transverse sonograms of the right abdomen show the thick wall (between arrowheads) of the ascending colon. The hyperechoic layer represents the submucosa, and the outer hypoechoic layer corresponds to the muscularis propria. Where visible, the inner hypoechoic layer represents the mucosa. There is gas in the outer layer of the bowel wall (black arrow), which produces dirty shadowing. Thumbprinting (open arrow) impinges on the lumen.

result in occlusion of the inferior mesenteric artery. However, there is no consistent relationship between occlusion of a major mesenteric artery and development of ischemic colitis. Many patients with such occlusions do not develop this disease, whereas many patients with ischemic colitis have patent major mesenteric arteries. Therefore, the patency of smaller vessels and the efficiency of collateral circulation are clearly important factors in determining which patients develop ischemic colitis.

The splenic flexure has been emphasized as the most vulnerable site for development of ischemic colitis because this region represents the watershed zone between the superior and inferior mesenteric arterial circulations and because the marginal artery of Drummond is at its greatest distance from the bowel wall. The disease more frequently involves the left half of the colon; however, any segment from cecum to rectosigmoid can be involved. Involvement is usually segmental. Low-flow states generally result in longer segments of involvement than do embolic causes.

The clinical presentation of ischemic colitis is variable and depends on the degree and duration of vascular occlusion, the efficiency of collateral circulation, and the extent of secondary bacterial invasion. Clinical manifestations range from mild reversible injury to frank gangrene and perforation. The classic presentation consists of sudden onset of crampy abdominal pain, tenderness over the involved segment, transient peritonitis, fever, and increased leukocyte count. The patient may report similar previous episodes. Rectal bleeding is common but is rarely massive. Vomiting is uncommon. In approximately half of the patients, symptoms abate over 24 to 48 hours with clinical, endoscopic, and radiographic evidence of healing within 2 weeks (Figure 6-3). Approximately one-third of patients have a more protracted course, resulting in colonic stricture. The remaining patients develop gangrene of the colon, and perforation follows within hours. Poor prognostic signs are persistent peritonitis, increasing temperature or leukocyte count, and development of ileus and shock. Barium enema is contraindicated in patients with suspected gangrenous colitis.

Radiologic abnormalities may be absent in patients with bowel ischemia or, when present, may be nonspecific. Reported findings have included bowel dilatation, bowel wall thickening, intramural gas, portal or mesenteric venous gas, and mesenteric artery thrombosis. Bowel ischemia is characterized by submucosal edema and hemorrhage, resulting in the classic wall thickening and "thumbprinting" seen in association with this disease. These changes can be appreciated on abdominal radiographs, barium enema, sonography (Figure 6-3A), or CT (Figure 6-3B). Barium enema can also show superficial ulcerations that mimic a segmental ulcerative colitis-type pattern. The presence of gas in the bowel wall suggests a severe insult but can still be seen in patients with

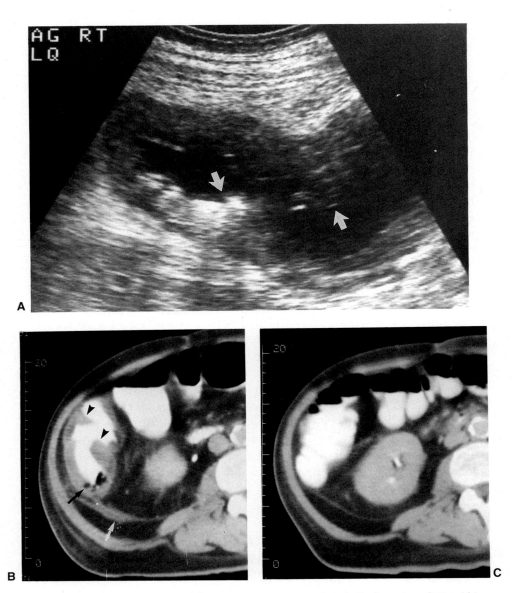

Figure 6-3. Same patient as in Figures 6-1 and 6-2. Ischemic colitis. (A) A longitudinal section of the ascending colon shows the thickened wall with thumbprinting and intramural gas (arrows). (B) A CT scan shows diffuse wall thickening with thumbprinting (arrowheads), intramural gas (black arrow), and adjacent fascial thickening (white arrow). (C) A CT scan obtained 2 weeks later shows resolution of findings, consistent with reversible ischemia.

Table 6-1: Correlation of sonographic and histologic layers of the gut wall from the lumen outward[a]

Sonography	Histology
Echogenic	Superficial mucosa ± Luminal content/mucosal interface
Hypoechoic	Deep mucosa, including muscularis mucosa
Echogenic	Submucosa + Submucosa/muscularis propria interface
Hypoechoic	Muscularis propria
Echogenic	Serosa + Subserosal fat + marginal interface

[a] Adapted from Wilson [70].

reversible disease (Figure 6-3B and C). Gas in the portal venous system generally indicates a poor outcome. An unusual manifestation of colon ischemia is pyocolon, which represents a dilated, thin-walled, aperistaltic segment containing pus and mucosal debris. This can be confused with an abscess by CT or sonography. The passage of a colon cast should suggest this diagnosis.

Periappendiceal abscess (Option (B)) is a complication of appendicitis. Appendicitis can be diagnosed sonographically by demonstrating a thickened, noncompressible tubular structure in the expected region of the appendix. The wall of the appendix contains the same layers as other portions of the gut and therefore can have a typical "gut signature" (Table 6-1 and Figure 6-4). However, the abnormality in the test patient is too great in diameter and occupies too large an area to represent even an enlarged appendix. A periappendiceal abscess could appear as a thick-walled cystic mass and might contain gas (Figure 6-5); however, the uniform nature of the concentric rings observed in the test images would not be expected.

Mucocele of the appendix (Option (C)) is a cystic mass that represents a dilated appendiceal lumen caused by abnormal accumulation of mucin. It usually appears on images as an ovoid cystic mass in the expected region of the appendix (Figure 6-6). Curvilinear or punctate wall calcification can occur and strongly suggests the diagnosis of mucocele (Figure 6-7). The findings in the test patient of a tubular mass with a gut signature would not be the expected appearance of a mucocele. In addition, although the nature of the shadowing may not always enable differentiation of gas and calcification, the dirty shadowing emanating

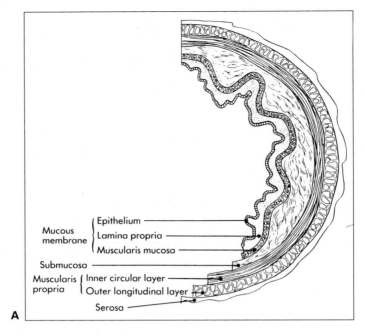

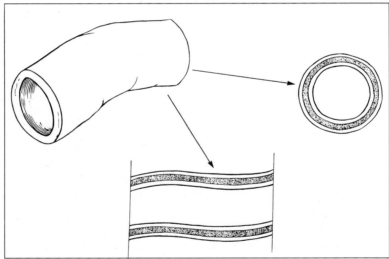

Figure 6-4. Sonographic gut signature. (A) A diagram of the histologic layers. (B) A diagrammatic representation of gut signature in the transverse and longitudinal planes shows five alternating hyperechoic and hypoechoic layers. See Table 6-1 for additional description. (C) A longitudinal sonogram of the appendix (between arrowheads) in a patient with simple acute appendicitis shows the five sonographic layers. The arrow indicates the hyperechoic interface between the lumen and the mucosa. There is an appendicolith (a) within the lumen. (D) A transverse sonogram of the appendix (arrows) shows the same findings. (Panels A and B are reprinted with permission from Wilson [70].)

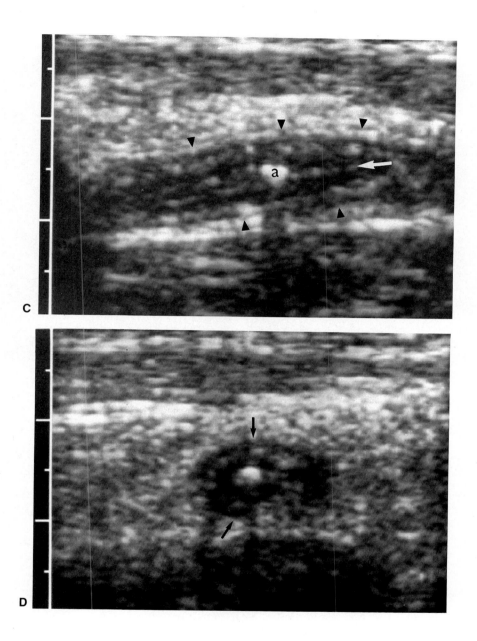

C

D

from the hyperechoic focus in the bowel wall is more suggestive of the former. Finally, mucocele has a strong female predilection. Therefore, mucocele is not the most likely diagnosis.

Intussusception (Option (D)) occurs most commonly in the terminal ileum but frequently progresses into the colon; therefore, it is commonly observed in the same region as the findings in the test images. The sonographic findings of intussusception are often quite characteristic and have been described as having a "target" or "doughnut" appearance when

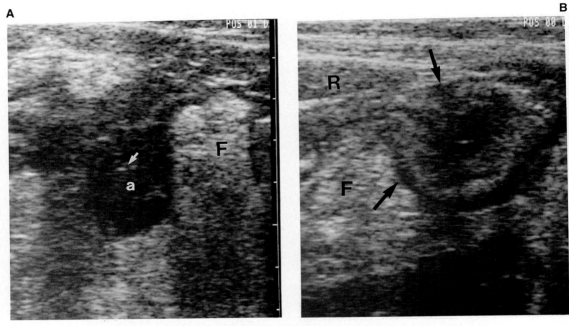

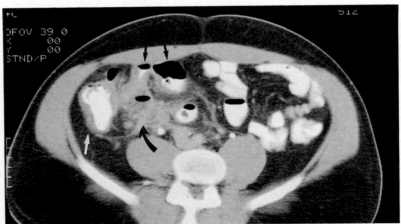

Figure 6-5. Acute appendicitis with periappendiceal abscess. (A) The abscess (a) appears as a hypoechoic mass containing bright echoes corresponding to gas (arrow). Through transmission is seen posterior to the abscess, and hyperechoic fat (F) is present along its anteromedial margin. The appendix is not visible. (B) The inflammatory process results in thickening of the small bowel wall (arrows) posterior to the rectus abdominus muscle (R). Note the characteristic gut signature that distinguishes it from an abscess. F = fat. (C) A CT scan obtained the same day shows the abscess (curved black arrow) and thickened small bowel (straight black arrows) with intervening fat. The wall of the cecum is also thickened (white arrow).

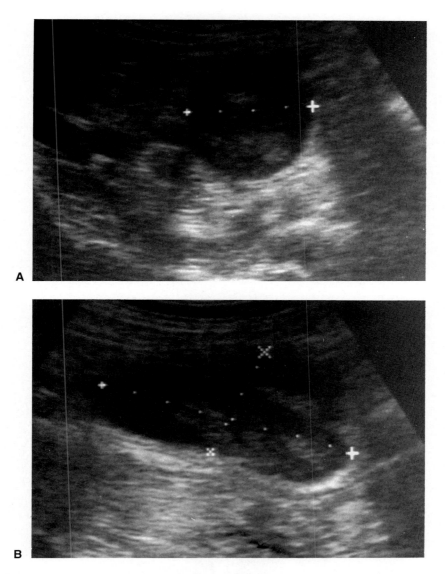

Figure 6-6. Mucocele of the appendix. Transverse (A) and longitudinal (B) sonograms of the mucocele show an ovoid thin-walled cystic mass with marked through transmission and internal echoes related to mucin. (C) A CT scan shows the mass (m), with attenuation slightly lower than muscle, near the cecal tip.

viewed in cross-section and a "pseudokidney" or "sandwich" appearance when viewed in longitudinal section. These descriptive terms refer to a thick outer hypoechoic rim surrounding an echogenic central mass (Figure 6-8). Another appearance that has been reported is a concentric-ring

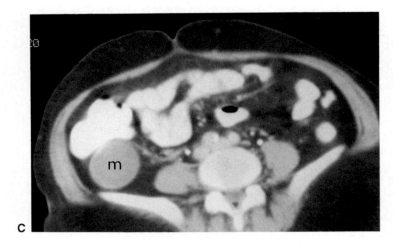

Figure 6-6 (Continued)

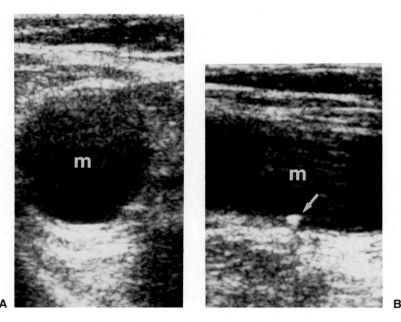

Figure 6-7. Mucocele with wall calcification. Transverse (A) and longitudinal (B) sonograms show the mucocele as a tubular cystic mass (m) containing a nonmobile wall calcification (arrow in panel B), identified as a punctate echogenic focus producing an acoustic shadow. The mass contains low-amplitude echoes related to mucin as well as near-field reverberations.

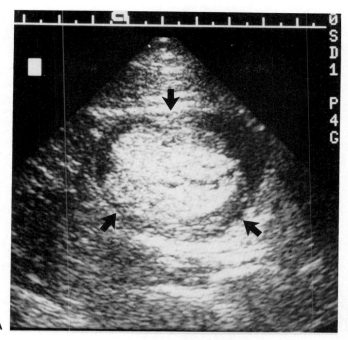

A

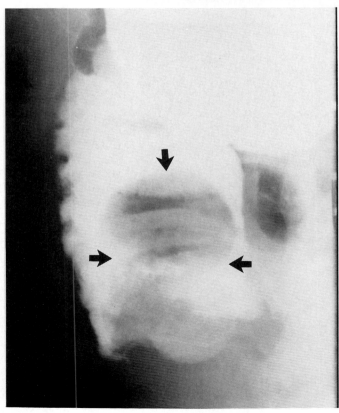

B

Figure 6-8.
Ileocolic intus-
susception.
(A) A transverse
sonogram
shows the clas-
sic target sign
(between ar-
rows), with a
large central
echogenic area
surrounded by a
thick hypo-
echoic rim.
(B) A film from a
barium enema
shows barium
outlining the in-
tussusceptum
(between ar-
rows). The lead
point was a cecal
polyp that con-
tained *in situ*
carcinoma.
(Case courtesy of
Paul Radecki,
M.D., Thomas
Jefferson Uni-
versity Hospi-
tal, Philadel-
phia, Pa.)

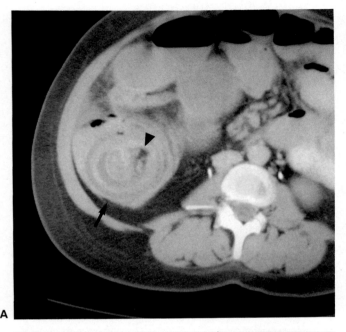

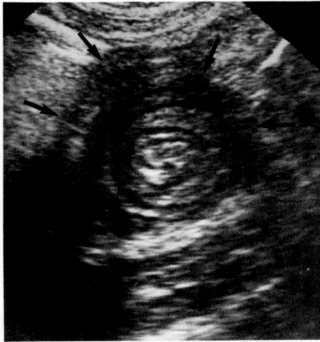

Figure 6-9. Intussusception with concentric-ring appearance. (A) A CT scan shows ileocolic intussusception as a mass with concentric rings (arrow) and containing mesenteric fat (arrowhead). (B) A sonogram from a different patient shows similar findings (arrows). (Panel B is reprinted with permission from Wilson [70].)

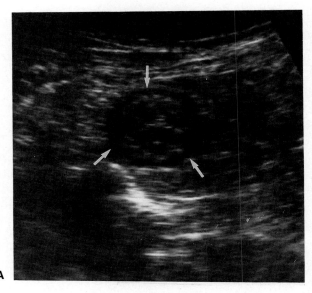

A

Figure 6-10. Crohn's disease of the small intestine. (A) A transverse sonogram shows a target sign (outlined by arrows), consisting of alternating hypoechoic and hyperechoic layers. The central echogenic lumen is narrowed.

pattern corresponding to the interfaces between the walls of the involved bowel loops, their mesenteries, and their respective lumens (Figure 6-9). At first glance, the concentric-ring appearance of the mass in the test images might suggest intussusception. However, only one loop of bowel is evident; there is no intussusceptum but rather a lumen containing fluid (Figure 6-2). In patients with intussusception, the lumen is filled with the intussusceptum (Figure 6-8) and is generally not visible in the manner observed in the test images. Other factors making intussusception unlikely are the patient's age (intussusception is relatively uncommon in adults) and the presence of gas in the bowel wall.

Crohn's disease (Option (E)) is a transmural granulomatous inflammatory disorder of the gastrointestinal tract. Involvement can occur anywhere in the gut from mouth to anus, but the terminal ileum and colon are most often affected. The usual sonographic findings in patients with Crohn's disease are segmental areas of circumferential bowel wall thickening and luminal narrowing (Figure 6-10). Dilated bowel loops can also be seen proximal to areas of stricture. Other reported findings include free fluid, abscess, matted bowel loops that can be difficult to distinguish from abscess, fat accumulation around the bowel, mesenteric lymph node enlargement, and linear bands of echoes caused by fistulas.

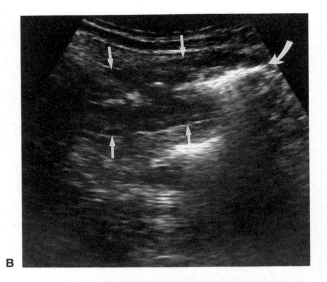

B

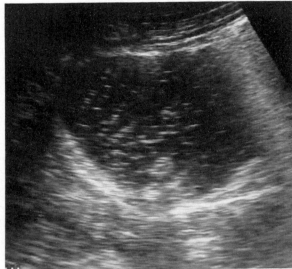

C

Figure 6-10 (Continued). Crohn's disease of the small intestine. (B) A longitudinal sonogram of the same bowel loop (between the straight arrows) shows the sandwich sign (curved arrow points to gas in the narrowed lumen). (C) A sonogram shows a dilated small bowel loop proximal to the narrowed bowel loop. Internal echoes are related to bowel contents. (D) A CT scan obtained on the same day shows the thick-walled small bowel loops (arrowheads) with dilated proximal small bowel (d). The arrow indicates the ascending colon.

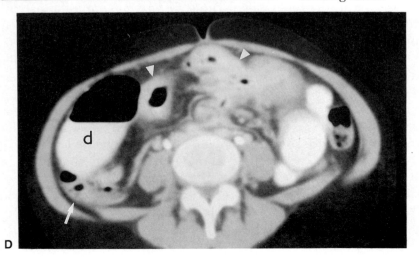

D

The normal bowel wall thickness, when distended, is 3 mm or less. Thickening up to 5 mm can be observed in normal bowel loops when not distended or during peristalsis. A persistent thickness of more than 5 mm should be considered pathologic. Normal bowel loops are usually compressible and show evidence of peristalsis, whereas thickened bowel loops are noncompressible and usually aperistaltic. Thick bowel loops have a target or pseudokidney appearance similar to that described for intussusception (Figures 6-11 and 6-12). However, in patients with bowel wall thickening, the thick hypoechoic outer rim corresponds to tumor or edematous bowel wall and the echogenic center corresponds to the lumen. Edema generally results in symmetric wall thickening, whereas asymmetric thickening suggests the diagnosis of tumor. The echogenic center is generally smaller in patients with bowel wall thickening than in those with intussusception because the compressed lumen is generally smaller than the intussusceptum (compare Figures 6-10 through 6-12 with Figure 6-8).

The finding of a thick-walled ascending colon in the test patient could be secondary to Crohn's disease. In fact, bowel wall thickening is a nonspecific finding that has a number of causes, including other colitides, tumor, diverticulitis, and neutropenic typhlitis. The gas in the bowel wall could even represent an intramural fistula, a potential feature of Crohn's disease but one that is infrequently demonstrated sonographically. However, Crohn's disease is less likely than ischemic colitis to produce these findings, particularly in an elderly man. There is a small incidence peak in the elderly, but Crohn's disease usually occurs in younger patients, most typically in the third decade of life. In addition, the lumen in patients with Crohn's disease is generally more narrowed than is observed in the test images. Therefore, Crohn's disease is not the most likely diagnosis.

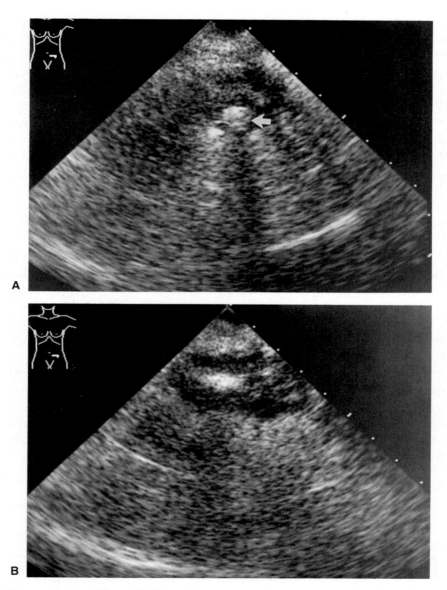

Figure 6-11. Diverticulitis. Transverse (A) and longitudinal (B) sonograms of thickened sigmoid colon were obtained by transvaginal sonography. The transverse view shows the target appearance, and the longitudinal view shows the pseudokidney appearance. Gas or stool is seen within a diverticulum (arrow in panel A).

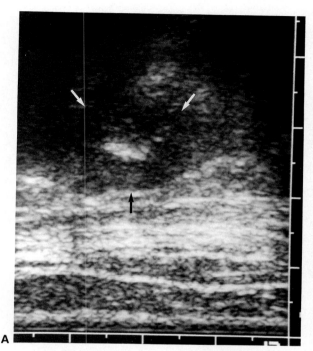

A

Figure 6-12. Other causes of bowel wall thickening. (A) A sonogram shows the target appearance caused by adenocarcinoma (arrows). (B) A sonogram shows thick-walled small bowel secondary to intramural hemorrhage in a patient with Henoch-Schönlein purpura. (C) A sonogram shows thick-walled cecum caused by neutropenic typhlitis lying in the iliac fossa.

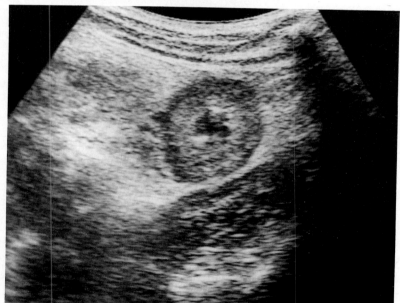

B

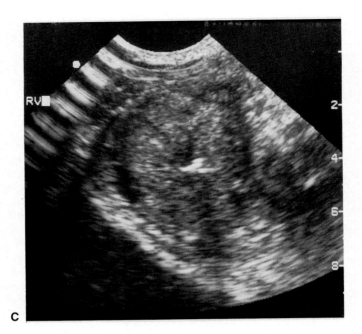

C

Question 27

Concerning appendicitis,

(A) the risk of appendiceal perforation is greatest in very young and very old patients
(B) the highest rate of negative laparotomy for suspected appendicitis occurs in children
(C) the normal upper limit for appendiceal diameter is 6 mm
(D) the criteria for normal appendiceal wall thickness in children are the same as those for adults
(E) free fluid around the cecum is a reliable sonographic sign of perforation

Acute appendicitis is the most common indication for emergency abdominal surgery and accounts for approximately 1% of all operations performed in the United States. Between 7 and 12% of people develop appendicitis at some time during their life. The incidence peaks during the second and third decades of life, but the disease can occur at any age.

Appendicitis results from luminal obstruction followed by infection. Hyperplastic lymphoid follicles account for the obstruction in up to 60% of cases, and fecaliths or viscid fecal masses are responsible for approximately 35% of cases. Rare causes include foreign bodies, strictures, and tumors. Following obstruction of the lumen, mucus accumulates and becomes infected (simple appendicitis). At this stage, the disease is still localized to the appendix and the visceral pain is referred to the epigastrium or periumbilical region. With progressive accumulation of pus within the lumen, there is sufficient pressure to disrupt venous outflow from the wall of the appendix, resulting in focal or extensive necrosis (gangrenous appendicitis) and eventually perforation (perforated appendicitis). At these later stages, pain shifts to the right lower quadrant as a result of peritoneal irritation. Decreased nerve sensitivity as a result of gangrene can result in temporary improvement of the patient's discomfort (the "treacherous calm of Dieulafoy"). The risk of perforation and abscess formation increases with the duration of appendicitis. In adults the likelihood of perforation rises rapidly after 24 hours, whereas in children an increased risk of perforation occurs as soon as 6 to 12 hours after onset of the process.

The overall rate of perforation in appendicitis is reported to be 10 to 30%. Although appendicitis occurs most commonly during the second and third decades of life, the risk of perforation is greatest in young children and elderly patients **(Option (A) is true).** This is because the diagnosis is usually delayed in these populations. The presentation of appendicitis can clinically simulate gastroenteritis or intussusception, both of which are common in children. Young children are also unable to give an accurate history. As a result, appendicitis is often not suspected until perforation has occurred. The frequency of perforation in children younger than 1 year of age approaches 100% and is as high as 50% at 5 years of age. Elderly patients frequently seek medical attention late, and once they do, the diagnosis is often delayed because the classic symptoms of appendicitis are less pronounced in this group. This results in a perforation rate exceeding 30%.

The diagnosis of appendicitis by experienced surgeons is straightforward in up to 80% of patients. Such patients usually do not require radiologic evaluation and are taken straight to surgery. However, an atypical presentation occurs in about 20% of patients. To avoid the complications of delayed diagnosis, surgeons have traditionally accepted a false-positive clinical diagnosis rate (and resulting negative laparotomy rate) of 15 to 20%. This number varies depending on the patient population at risk. The highest rate of negative laparotomy occurs in women of reproductive age **(Option (B) is false).** Rates as high as 45% have been reported for this group and result from the overlapping presentations of acute appendicitis and common gynecologic diseases. Imaging in general, and ultrasonography in particular, has proven to be of greatest benefit in these patients and in patients presenting with atypical symptoms.

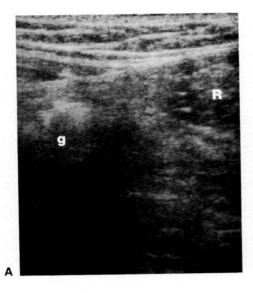

Figure 6-13. Value of graded-compression sonography. Transverse sonograms of the right lower abdomen before (A) and during (B) compression show that the rectus abdominus muscle (R) is compressed against the psoas major muscle (Ps). Intervening gas (g) is pushed away, allowing visualization of the external iliac artery (a) and vein (v).

The abdominal radiograph is abnormal in less than 50% of patients with appendicitis. Signs of appendicitis on abdominal radiographs include localized adynamic ileus, appendicolith, and right lower quadrant mass. Appendicoliths are present in 30 to 35% of patients with appendicitis but are apparent radiographically in only about 14%.

Barium enema has a reported accuracy of 50 to 84% for the diagnosis of appendicitis. The most reliable sign of appendicitis is mass effect on the cecal tip. Lack of filling of the appendix with barium has poor sensitivity and specificity by itself. Lack of appendiceal filling occurs in many individuals without appendicitis, and partial filling of the appendix does not exclude the diagnosis since appendicitis can be confined to the tip of the appendix.

CT can show the primary and secondary findings of appendicitis with far greater accuracy than does either abdominal radiography or barium enema. Primary findings of appendicitis include thickening and enhancement of the wall of the appendix, appendiceal enlargement or distension, and the presence of an appendicolith. Secondary findings include soft tissue attenuation in the periappendiceal fat, periappendiceal fluid, and periappendiceal abscess.

Puylaert was the first to describe the use of graded-compression sonography to diagnose appendicitis. The value of this technique has been confirmed by numerous investigators. By using gentle gradual pressure, the muscles of the anterior abdominal wall are compressed against those of the posterior abdominal wall. This results in displacement of

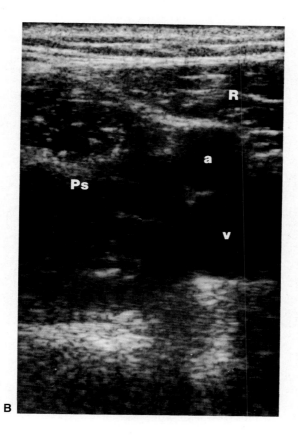

intervening gas-containing bowel loops and permits visualization of the deep abdominopelvic structures (Figure 6-13). The reduction in distance from the transducer allows the use of higher frequencies (usually 5 or 7.5 MHz), resulting in improved anatomic resolution. Linear-array or convex linear-array transducers are most effective because of their ability to apply pressure over a larger area. However, good results can be achieved with other transducers. The gentle gradual pressure applied can be tolerated by most patients, even those with abdominal pain. Obesity, ascites, severe ileus, or severe pain can result in an unsatisfactory examination, but this occurs in only a few patients.

In patients with localized pain, the appendix is often identified at the site of maximum discomfort. If this is not successful in identifying the appendix, a systematic approach is necessary. The transducer is placed transversely in the right upper abdomen and, by scanning inferiorly, the ascending colon should be identified as the largest tubular structure extending from the inferior liver margin to the right iliac fossa. The as-

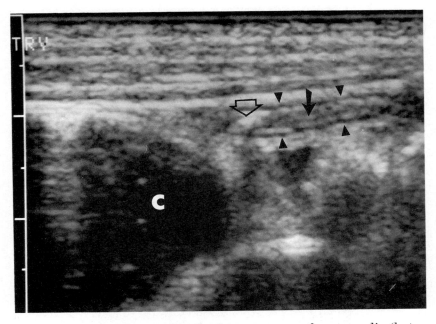

Figure 6-14. Normal appendix. In this sonogram the appendix (between arrowheads) is seen medial to the fluid-filled cecum (C) and just deep to the muscles of the abdominal wall. The central hyperechoic linear echo represents the lumen (solid arrow), which contains gas proximally; the gas is seen as an echogenic focus (open arrow). The diameter of the appendix is 3 mm, and the wall thickness is 1.5 mm. Note the characteristic gut signature.

cending colon often contains anechoic fluid, gas with shadowing, or echogenic fecal material (Figure 6-14). The absence of peristalsis is helpful in distinguishing the colon from small bowel, which usually shows active peristalsis. An attempt is made to identify the terminal ileum and the cecal tip, where the appendix should be located. The appendix is identified as a tubular blind-ending structure arising from the cecum (Figure 6-14). It is important to attempt to identify the entire length of the appendix since appendicitis can be confined to the distal portion of the appendix (Figure 6-15). Other valuable landmarks to identify because of their usual proximity to the appendix include the iliac fossa, psoas muscle, and external iliac vessels. Longitudinal scanning can be used as needed to supplement the search for the appendix. Rioux has reported that scanning with the bladder initially full and then empty and scanning in the left lateral decubitus position can be of value in identifying the appendix in some cases.

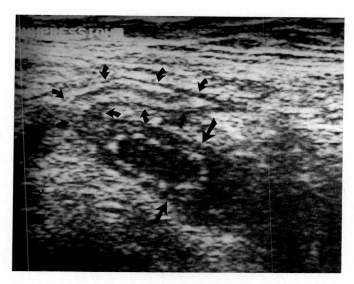

Figure 6-15. Simple appendicitis involving only the distal portion of the appendix. In this sonogram, the appendix has a normal diameter and wall thickness proximally (between small arrows) but appears distended and enlarged distally (between large arrows). The configuration of the appendix did not change with compression.

When the graded-compression technique was first reported by Puylaert, any visualization of the appendix was regarded as a sign of appendicitis. The identification of a normal appendix has subsequently been reported by several investigators, with visualization rates of 5 to 82% in patients without appendicitis. Therefore, criteria for distinguishing the normal from the abnormal appendix have been established. The abnormal appendix is noncompressible (i.e., its configuration and size do not change with compression). Distinct wall layers corresponding to the different histologic layers can be observed in both normal and abnormal appendices (Figures 6-4, 6-14, and 6-15; see also Figures 6-18 and 6-19). In general, as the wall edema becomes more severe, the wall architecture becomes more disorganized and indistinct (Figures 6-16 through 6-18). Body habitus, age, and sonographic resolution also play a role in the ability to identify distinct wall layers; therefore, this feature alone cannot be relied on to distinguish normal from abnormal appendices. Other criteria for appendicitis include an appendiceal diameter greater than 6 mm **(Option (C) is true)** and a wall thickness greater than 2 to 3 mm (Figure 6-19). These criteria are the same for adults and children **(Option (D) is true).** If the lumen of a normal appendix contains fluid or stool, the diameter can exceed 6 mm but the appendiceal lumen should be com-

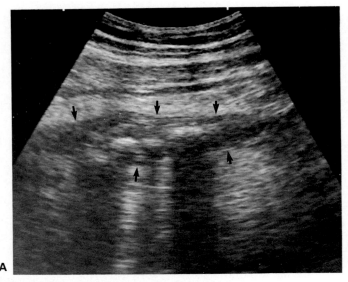

A

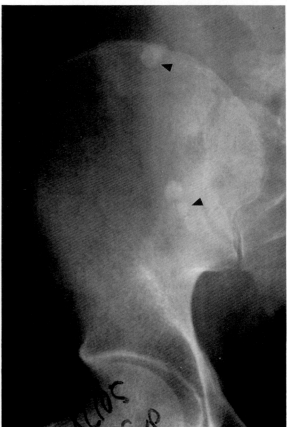

B

Figure 6-16. Gangrenous appendicitis with multiple appendicoliths. (A) A longitudinal sonogram shows that the appendix (arrows) contains multiple appendicoliths. The wall is thickened to various degrees without visualization of distinct layers. (B) An abdominal radiograph shows the appendicoliths (arrowheads).

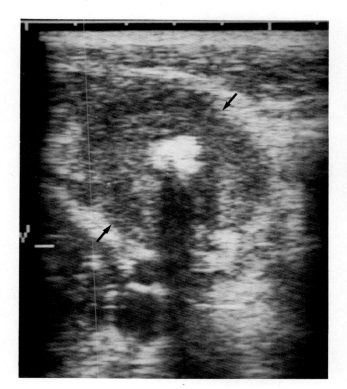

Figure 6-17 (left). Gangrenous appendicitis. In this sonogram, the appendix (arrows) is markedly enlarged. The wall is very thick, and the distinct histologic layers are absent. An appendicolith with distal shadowing is present in the lumen.

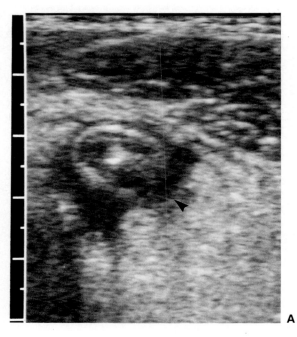

Figure 6-18 (right and on the following page). Perforated appendicitis. (A) A transverse sonogram of the appendix shows an appendicolith, asymmetric wall thickening, and discontinuity of the echogenic submucosal layer (arrowhead).

A

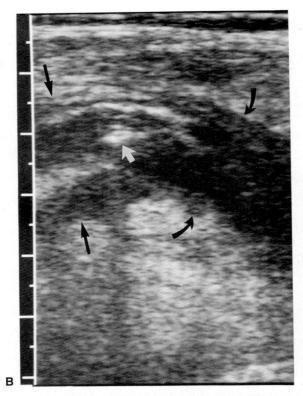

B

Figure 6-18 (Continued).
Perforated appendicitis.
(B) A longitudinal sono-
gram of the appendix
shows loss of the bowel
wall layers distally
(curved arrows) compared
with proximally (straight
black arrows). The white
arrow indicates an appen-
dicolith. (C) A CT scan
shows the enlarged,
thickened appendix (ar-
rowhead) and adjacent in-
flammatory process (ar-
row).

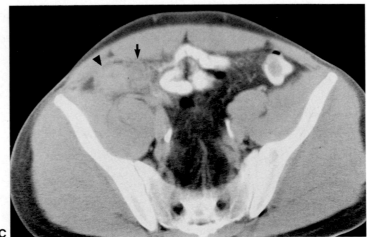

C

pressible. One or more appendicoliths may also be identified (Figures
6-4, 6-16, and 6-17).

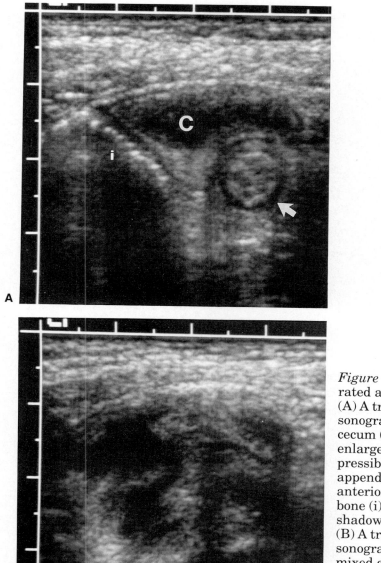

Figure 6-19. Perforated appendicitis. (A) A transverse sonogram shows the cecum (C) and an enlarged noncompressible retrocecal appendix (arrow) anterior to the iliac bone (i) and the shadow it produces. (B) A transverse sonogram shows mixed cystic and solid areas, representing a complex periappendiceal abscess.

As mentioned above, simple appendicitis progresses to gangrenous and then perforated appendicitis. Sonographic observation during the gangrenous phase often reveals progressive fluid distension of the appendiceal lumen, increasing diameter, and progression of wall thickening

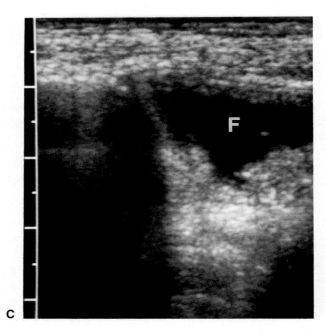

C

Figure 6-19 (Continued). Perforated appendicitis. (C) A sonogram shows that free fluid (F) is also present.

(Figure 6-17). There is loss of the distinct submucosal layer, resulting in a more uniform hypoechoic wall (Figures 6-16 and 6-17). Sonographic findings associated with perforation include (1) lack of tenderness during compression despite abnormal sonographic findings; (2) ileus or thickening of adjacent bowel loops (Figure 6-5); (3) interloop fluid pockets; (4) free fluid with or without debris (Figure 6-19); (5) asymmetric thickening of the appendiceal wall (Figure 6-18); (6) loss of the echogenic submucosal layer (Figure 6-18); (7) prominent pericecal fat (Figure 6-5); and (8) periappendiceal mass or abscess (Figures 6-20 through 6-22). However, the sensitivity of sonography for detection of perforation is lower than it is for detection of appendicitis. This is probably related to inadequate compression of the appendix because of localized peritonitis, poor visualization caused by localized adynamic ileus, and extensive necrosis or disintegration of the appendix rendering its visualization difficult. Of the findings listed above, Borushok et al. found only loculated pericecal fluid, prominent pericecal fat (>10 mm thick), and circumferential loss of the echogenic submucosal layer to be statistically associated with appendiceal perforation. However, none of these findings had a sensitivity for perforation greater than 59%. The presence of free fluid alone is nonspecific and can be seen in patients with many diseases associated with abdominal pain **(Option (E) is false).** Once perforation occurs, it is

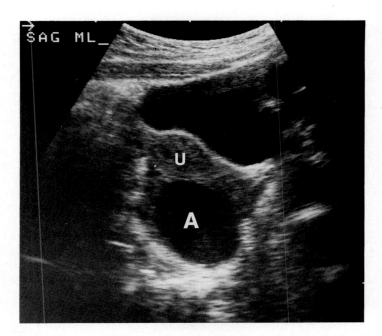

Figure 6-20. Periappendiceal abscess. In this sonogram, a large abscess (A) is seen in the cul-de-sac posterior to the uterus (U). The appendix is not visible.

often walled off by adjacent omental or mesenteric fat (Figure 6-5), or a phlegmon or one or more abscesses can form (Figures 6-5 and 6-19 through 6-22). As mentioned above, the appendix is often difficult to visualize at this stage. The abscess can appear cystic (Figures 6-5 and 6-20), complex (Figure 6-19), or solid (Figure 6-21). The presence of gas within the abscess can make visualization difficult or can result in its being mistaken for bowel (Figure 6-22).

There have been many published studies about the use of graded-compression sonography to diagnose appendicitis. Several investigators have suggested that the rate of negative laparotomy can be significantly reduced by the use of sonography. Sensitivities of 75 to 94%, specificities of 86 to 96%, positive predictive values of 89 to 93%, negative predictive values of 89 to 98%, and overall accuracies of 90 to 96% have been reported. In addition, Gaensler et al. have reported that sonography can result in a different diagnosis in 70% of patients presenting with symptoms suggestive of appendicitis in whom another diagnosis is ultimately established. Gynecologic, hepatobiliary, and genitourinary disorders are among the entities that enter into the clinical differential diagnosis and for which sonography has value in arriving at an alternative diagnosis.

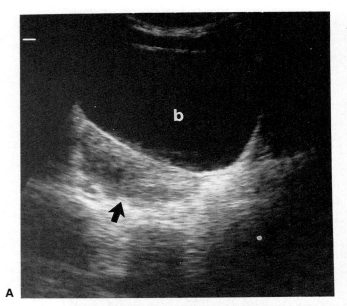

Figure 6-21. Echogenic solid-appearing periappendiceal abscess. (A) An abscess (arrow) with an echogenic sonographic appearance is seen posterior to the bladder (b). The appendix is not visible. (B) CT scan shows the same abscess (arrow) to have fluid attenuation. Sigmoid colon is interposed between the abscess and bladder.

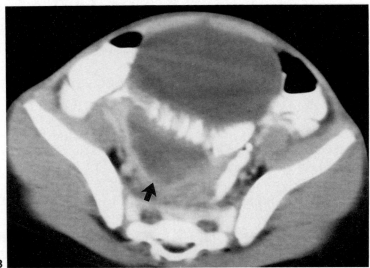

Sonography can also distinguish appendicitis from other gastrointestinal disorders that have a similar clinical picture. Included among these are mesenteric adenitis with acute terminal ileitis and Crohn's disease. Mesenteric adenitis with acute terminal ileitis is an infectious disease usually caused by *Yersinia enterocolitica*. A similar syndrome can be caused by *Campylobacter jejuni* or can follow upper respiratory infec-

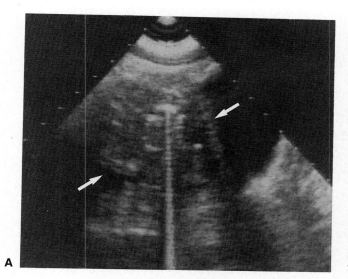

Figure 6-22. Periappendiceal abscess containing gas. (A) A sagittal sonogram of the right hemipelvis shows an abscess (arrows) containing numerous echogenic foci, some producing ringdown artifact. The appendix is not visible. (B) A CT scan shows a large abscess (arrow) containing gas.

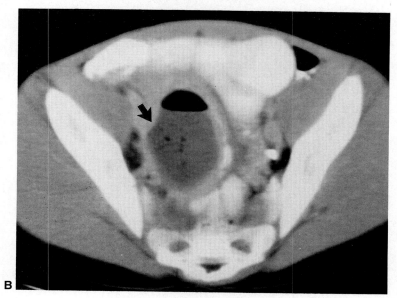

tions. The sonographic findings include thickening of the terminal ileum and an increased number of enlarged adjacent mesenteric lymph nodes (defined as greater than 4 mm in anteroposterior diameter) (Figure 6-23). Crohn's disease commonly involves the ileocecal region and can involve the appendix as well. Rarely, isolated involvement of the appendix occurs, with "appendicitis" being the initial manifestation of the dis-

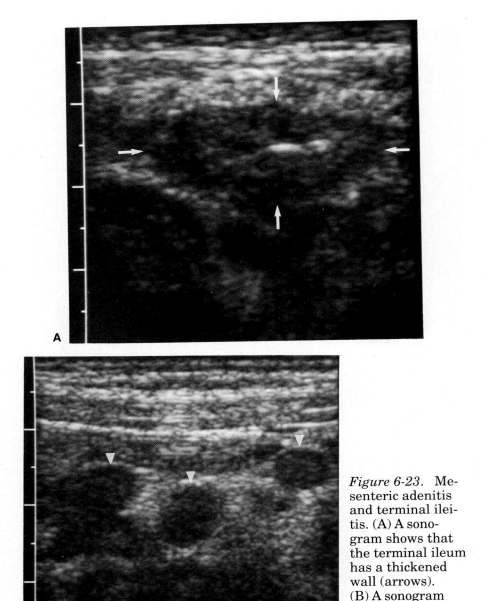

Figure 6-23. Mesenteric adenitis and terminal ileitis. (A) A sonogram shows that the terminal ileum has a thickened wall (arrows). (B) A sonogram shows that enlarged mesenteric lymph nodes (arrowheads) are also present nearby.

ease. In 1988, Puylaert et al. reported that thickening of the ileum and cecum is severe in patients with Crohn's disease, whereas the infiltrative changes around the inflamed appendix are minimal. In contrast, appendiceal findings usually predominate in patients with appendicitis, and thickening of the ileum and cecum is mild.

Question 28

Concerning mucocele of the appendix,

(A) it occurs most commonly in middle-aged to elderly women
(B) it is due to a benign lesion in approximately 90% of cases
(C) it generally appears as an anechoic mass in the right lower quadrant
(D) the presence of wall calcification in a right-lower-quadrant mass should suggest the diagnosis
(E) pseudomyxoma peritonei is a frequent complication

Mucocele of the appendix is a descriptive term that refers to an abnormal accumulation of mucin within the appendix. It has a reported prevalence of 0.2 to 0.3% in appendectomy specimens. There is a female to male predominance of 4:1 and a mean age at presentation of 55 years **(Option (A) is true)**. A right lower quadrant mass is palpated in about 50% of cases. Approximately two-thirds of patients report some right lower quadrant pain, but nearly one-quarter of patients are asymptomatic.

Mucoceles were once thought to arise most often from appendiceal obstruction caused by postinflammatory stricture or fecalith. This still occurs in some cases, resulting essentially in retention cysts filled with mucin and having normal mucosa. In such cases, appendicitis apparently does not result because there is no secondary bacterial infection. However, more recent evidence suggests that mucoceles result from a primary abnormality of the appendiceal mucosa. Higa et al. have classified these lesions into three groups: (1) focal or diffuse mucosal hyperplasia analogous to a colonic hyperplastic polyp, (2) mucinous cystadenoma with neoplastic epithelium similar to colonic villous adenoma and adenomatous polyp, and (3) mucinous cystadenocarcinoma with neoplastic epithelium analogous to mucin-producing adenocarcinoma of the colon. The reported association of mucocele with neoplasms elsewhere in the colon supports this theory. Wolff and Ahmed reported a concomitant neoplasm in the colon in 21% of patients with mucocele, and one-third of these patients had more than one colonic neoplasm. Even with this system of classification, nearly 90% of these lesions are benign and are due to either mucosal hyperplasia or mucinous cystadenoma **(Option (B) is true)**.

The imaging feature of a mucocele is a mass in the expected region of the appendix. Imaging cannot distinguish benign from malignant causes of mucocele. Masses up to 10 cm in diameter have been reported, but 4 to 6 cm is the most common size at presentation. The appendix can be retrocecal, and so the mass can develop posterior to the cecum. Conventional abdominal radiographs can show mass effect on adjacent bowel or bladder. Barium enema shows mass effect on the cecum, terminal ileum, or sigmoid colon. The typical appearance on CT is a smooth-walled, well-encapsulated, low-attenuation mass near the cecal tip (Figure 6-6). The attenuation of the mass is usually that of fluid, but masses approaching soft tissue attenuation have been reported. The attenuation depends on the amount and nature of mucin within the mass; the consistency of the mucin can vary from liquefied to gelatinous. These differences in the mucin also account for the variable sonographic appearance. Typically, sonography shows a well-defined ovoid cystic mass containing internal echoes and exhibiting excellent through transmission (Figure 6-6). The inner wall can be irregular secondary to mucin or epithelial hyperplasia. Anechoic mucoceles have been reported but are not typical **(Option (C) is false).** Mucoceles often contain punctate or curvilinear wall calcifications (Figure 6-7), which are most easily demonstrated by CT but can also be seen on conventional radiographs and sonography. The sonographic appearance of a wall calcification is that of a highly echogenic focus; shadowing is produced if the calcification is large enough in relation to the width of the ultrasound beam and if it is close to the focal zone of the transducer. The wall calcification results from chronic inflammation incited by the mucin in the appendiceal wall. Another rare form of calcification that can be seen in association with mucocele is myxoglobulosis, which is seen in 0.35 to 8% of patients. This entity represents opaque globules composed of necrotic tissue floating in mucus. When these calcify, they can be seen on imaging studies.

The differential diagnosis of mucocele includes other cystic masses in the right lower quadrant. Periappendiceal abscess (Figures 6-5 and 6-19 through 6-22) and ovarian cystic lesions are the most common. The former can usually be distinguished from mucocele by the clinical presentation. In addition, periappendiceal abscess is often associated with a thick-walled, noncompressible appendix (Figure 6-19). Less common entities that might be confused with mucocele include duplication, mesenteric, or omental cysts; mesenteric hematoma or tumor; lymphoma (Figure 6-24); and retroperitoneal masses (in patients with retrocecal mucocele). The presence of curvilinear or punctate wall calcification should strongly suggest the diagnosis of mucocele **(Option (D) is true).**

Complications of mucocele are rare and include torsion, hemorrhage, intussusception, and pseudomyxoma peritonei **(Option (E) is false).** Pseudomyxoma peritonei results from rupture of the mucocele and is characterized by accumulation of mucus within the peritoneal cavity and

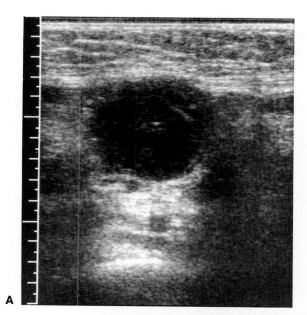

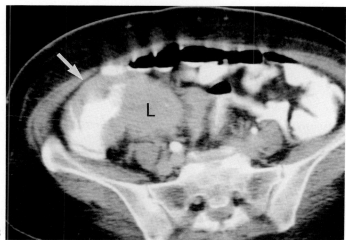

Figure 6-24. Lymphoma mimicking periappendiceal abscess or mucocele. (A) A right pelvic sonogram shows a hypoechoic mass with enhanced through transmission, giving the impression of a cystic mass. (B) A CT scan shows a solid mass (L) and adjacent cecal wall thickening (arrow).

implants of mucinous epithelial cells on the peritoneal surfaces. Controversy exists concerning whether pseudomyxoma peritonei is a complication of benign as well as malignant mucocele. This controversy results partly because of inconsistencies in the definition of pseudomyxoma peritonei. Benign and malignant mucoceles can cause mucus accumulation in the peritoneal cavity. However, only malignant mucoceles result in implants of mucinous epithelium. The prognosis for benign "pseudomyxoma" is excellent, whereas the prognosis for malignant pseudomyxoma is very poor (5-year survival of approximately 25%). Adhesions and bowel obstruction are frequent complications.

CT and sonography can show the changes of pseudomyxoma peritonei. Both show ascites with mass effect on adjacent structures. Implants near the liver, for example, cause scalloping of the liver margin. Sonography shows ascites that can contain internal echoes. These intraperitoneal collections of mucin can also calcify, often in a rimlike fashion.

Question 29

Concerning intussusception,

- (A) it is the most common cause of bowel obstruction in patients between 2 months and 5 years of age
- (B) the spontaneous perforation rate is about 5%
- (C) a malignant tumor acts as the lead point in about 75% of adult patients
- (D) it is characterized by a "coiled-spring" appearance on sonograms
- (E) free fluid contraindicates enema reduction

Intussusception represents the invagination or "telescoping" of one bowel loop (the intussusceptum) into another (the intussuscipiens). In the vast majority of cases, the intussusceptum represents a segment of intestine that is proximal to the intussuscipiens. This disease has different clinicopathologic implications in the pediatric and adult populations.

Intussusception is relatively common in children, with a reported frequency of 2 to 4 per 1,000, and represents the most common cause of bowel obstruction in children between the ages of 2 months and 5 years **(Option (A) is true).** The average age at presentation is 6 to 7 months, with most intussusceptions occurring between 4 and 10 months of age; 65% of patients are younger than 1 year of age, and approximately 80% are younger than 2 years of age. A male-to-female predominance has consistently been reported and ranges from 1.5:1 to 3:1.

Approximately 90 to 95% of cases of intussusception in children are idiopathic, meaning that there is no mass acting as a lead point for the intussusception. Most intussusceptions in children are ileocolic or ileoileocolic. Areas of swollen intramural intestinal lymph tissue in the terminal ileum (Peyer's patches) have been implicated as the cause in this population. This hypothesis is supported by the common association with antecedent viral infections, such as upper respiratory infections, measles, and gastroenteritis syndromes. A pathologic lead mass can be seen at any age; however, a particular effort to identify such a mass should be made in patients falling outside of the typical age range for idiopathic intussusception, i.e., neonates and patients over 3 years of age.

The clinical presentation in children is often classic. A previously healthy child usually presents with abdominal pain, which spontaneously abates but recurs with increasing frequency in ensuing hours. This progresses to vomiting and rectal bleeding. The stool appears dark red and gelatinous, giving rise to the descriptive term, "currant jelly" stool. In many cases, the presentation is not typical and gastroenteritis is initially suspected. Physical examination often reveals a sausage-shaped abdominal mass in the right upper quadrant and absence of bowel in the right lower quadrant (Dance's sign). Abdominal distension occurs as small bowel obstruction develops. Signs of peritonitis can develop, although the spontaneous perforation rate is low (reported to be 1 in 300 cases) **(Option (B) is false).**

Intussusception is uncommon in adults, accounting for only about 5% of intestinal obstructions in this population. Idiopathic intussusception is uncommon in adults; 75 to 85% of adult intussusceptions are associated with a pathologic lead point. Most small bowel lead points are benign, whereas up to 50% of colon lead points have been reported to be malignant. Therefore, although there is a significant rate of malignancy, particularly in patients with colonic intussusceptions, fewer than half of the lesions overall are malignant **(Option (C) is false).** Examples of pathologic lead points in adults or children include lipomas, polyps, benign and malignant tumors, abnormal appendices, appendiceal stumps, ectopic mucosa, Meckel's diverticula, gastrointestinal duplications, and suture lines. Intussusception can also occur without lead points in patients with sprue, cystic fibrosis, or Henoch-Schönlein purpura.

The clinical presentation in adults is less characteristic than in children. Patients tend to complain of chronic abdominal pain that is minimal or mild. Vomiting and/or diarrhea can also occur, but rectal bleeding is uncommon. An abdominal mass is palpated in only about 25% of patients.

Conventional abdominal radiographs are usually the first radiographic studies performed. They may show a mass, usually in the right abdomen, that corresponds to the intussusception. Various degrees of small bowel distension are observed, depending on the severity of the obstruction caused by the intussusception. Signs of perforation are rare.

The barium enema has been the traditional next step in the radiographic evaluation of suspected intussusception, both for diagnosis and for reduction in patients in whom intussusception is found. The appearance on barium enema depends on the degree of obstruction to the retrograde flow of barium. Complete obstruction results in abrupt termina-

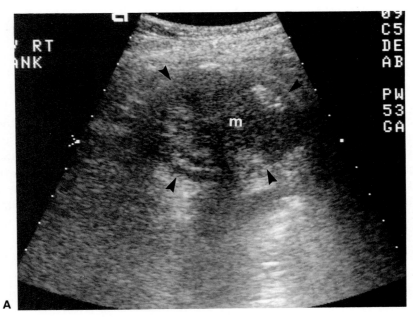

A

Figure 6-25. Intussusception seen as a complex mass, secondary to a cecal mass. (A) A peripheral hypoechoic wall (arrowheads) surrounds a central mass (m) containing areas of various echogenicities. (B) The mesenteric arteries could be traced into the mass on color Doppler sonography. The Doppler waveform tracing shows the typical high-impedance flow pattern in the fasting state expected with a mesenteric artery. (C) A CT scan obtained on the same day shows the intussusception as a mass (m) surrounded by contrast.

tion of the barium column, or barium may outline a small portion of the lead point (see Figure 6-8). If barium is able to flow between the inner wall of the intussuscipiens and the outer wall of the intussusceptum, the classic "coiled-spring" appearance results. Successful reduction depends on the age of the patient, the presence or absence of a pathologic lead point, and the duration of the intussusception. In general, enema reduction is successful less often in patients with long-standing intussusception and in those with a pathologic lead point. Success rates of 45 to 75% have been reported. Recently, the use of air alone for reduction of intussusception has been advocated by some investigators, and success rates comparable to those of barium reduction have been reported.

On CT, intussusception appears as either an abrupt termination of the intraluminal contrast column or an intraluminal mass surrounded by contrast (Figure 6-25). Fat can be observed within the mass, corresponding to mesenteric fat drawn into the intussusception, and concen-

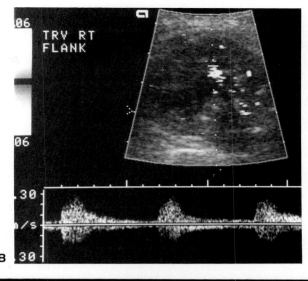

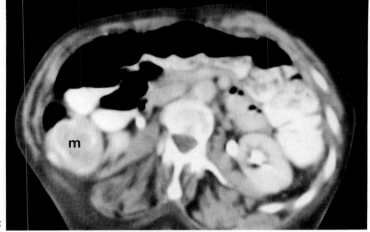

tric rings of alternating high and low attenuation can also be observed (Figure 6-9A).

On sonography, the intussusception is usually observed as a mass with a diameter of 3 to 5 cm. Three sonographic patterns have been described. The first is the target or doughnut appearance, in which the intussusception, viewed in cross-section, appears as a hypoechoic halo surrounding an echogenic central mass (Figure 6-8). The corresponding longitudinal appearance has been described as the pseudokidney or sandwich sign. The thick outer hypoechoic wall and the inner echogenic

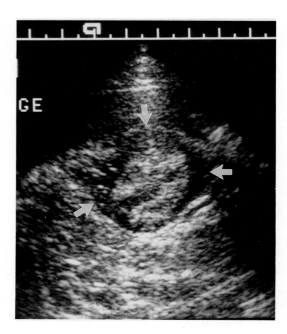

Figure 6-26. Villous adenoma of the cecum. A large villous adenoma of the cecum mimics the classic target appearance of intussusception (between arrows). In this case, the villous adenoma is the large central echogenic mass and is surrounded by the hypoechoic cecal wall. (Case courtesy of Paul Radecki, M.D.)

mass were originally attributed to the thickened wall of the intussuscipiens and to the compressed layers of the intussusceptum, respectively. More recently, Montali et al. and Swischuk and Stansberry have suggested that the hypoechoic portion represents the entering and returning edematous walls of the intussusceptum. The second sonographic pattern is the "concentric-ring" appearance (Figure 6-9B). This corresponds to the multiple interfaced layers between the walls of the intussusceptum and intussuscipiens and their respective lumens. This finding can be observed with improving sonographic resolution or with lesser degrees of bowel wall edema. The third and least common pattern that has been described is that of a complex mass (Figure 6-25). In some cases, the lead mass can be identified. A "coiled-spring" appearance has not been reported as a sonographic finding in patients with intussusception **(Option (D) is false).**

The concentric-ring appearance is pathognomonic for intussusception. The sonographic demonstration of a target sign, while suggestive of intussusception, is not pathognomonic (Figure 6-26). Any cause of bowel wall thickening can theoretically lead to this appearance (see Figures 6-10 through 6-12). As mentioned above, the central echogenic component is generally larger in patients with intussusception than in patients with bowel wall thickening not related to intussusception. In most patients, the presentation aids in suggesting the correct diagnosis; in fact, sonography has been shown by a number of investigators to be highly accurate for diagnosing or excluding intussusception. In Europe and Asia, it has become the first diagnostic imaging modality used in suspected cases of intussusception. There is growing use in North America, and some authors are now advocating its use as an initial diagnostic examination in this clinical setting.

Sonography has also been used with excellent results to monitor hydrostatic saline reduction in patients with intussusception. Some authors have suggested that the thickness of the outer hypoechoic wall can be used as an indicator of reducibility by enema. Pracros et al. found that when the wall was more than 8 to 10 mm thick, hydrostatic reduction was often difficult or impossible. Lee et al. found that no cases associated with a wall thickness ≥16 mm could be successfully reduced. However, Verschelden et al. found no correlation between wall thickness and reduction rate. Free fluid has been found by several investigators in uncomplicated cases of intussusception and is not by itself a contraindication to attempted enema reduction **(Option (E) is false).** Contraindications to enema reduction are clinical findings of peritonitis, shock, signs of perforation on abdominal radiographs or sonography, and signs of high-grade bowel obstruction.

Gary M. Kellman, M.D.
Paul L. Goldberg, M.D.

SUGGESTED READINGS

ISCHEMIC COLITIS

1. Alpern MB, Glazer GM, Francis IR. Ischemic or infarcted bowel: CT findings. Radiology 1988; 166:149–152
2. Dickstein G, Boley SJ. Colonic ischemia. In: Zuidema GD (ed), Shackelford's surgery of the alimentary tract, 3rd ed. Philadelphia: WB Saunders; 1991:84–94
3. Goldberg SM, Nivatvongs S, Rothenberger DA. Colon, rectum, and anus. In: Schwartz (ed), Principles of surgery, 5th ed. New York: McGraw-Hill; 1989:1249–1250
4. Ouellet JY, Duprat G Jr, Laperrière J, Grégoire A, Fontaine A. Pyocolon: an unusual manifestation of colon ischemia. Can Assoc Radiol J 1988; 39:235–237
5. Reeders JW, Rosenbusch G, Tytgat GN. Radiological aspects of ischemic colitis. A review. Diagn Imaging 1981; 50:4–16
6. Thoeni RF, Margulis AR. Inflammatory diseases. In: Margulis AR, Burhenne HJ (eds), Alimentary tract radiology, 4th ed. St Louis: CV Mosby; 1989:992–995

APPENDICITIS

7. Abu-Yousef MM, Bleicher JJ, Maher JW, Urdaneta LF, Franken EA Jr, Metcalf AM. High-resolution sonography of acute appendicitis. AJR 1987; 149:53–58

8. Balthazar EJ, Megibow EJ, Siegel SE, Birnbaum BA. Appendicitis: prospective evaluation with high-resolution CT. Radiology 1991; 180:21–24

9. Blane CE, White SJ, Wesley JR, Coran AG. Sonography of ruptured appendicitis. Gastrointest Radiol 1986; 11:357–360

10. Borushok KF, Jeffrey RB Jr, Laing FC, Townsend RR. Sonographic diagnosis of perforation in patients with acute appendicitis. AJR 1990; 154:275–278

11. Brown JJ. Acute appendicitis: the radiologist's role (editorial). Radiology 1991; 180:13–14

12. Gaensler EH, Jeffrey RB Jr, Laing FC, Townsend RR. Sonography in patients with suspected acute appendicitis: value in establishing alternative diagnoses. AJR 1989; 152:49–51

13. Hayden CK Jr, Kuchelmeister J, Lipscomb TS. Sonography of acute appendicitis in childhood: perforation versus nonperforation. J Ultrasound Med 1992; 11:209–216

14. Jeffrey RB Jr, Jain KA, Nghiem HV. Pictorial essay. Sonographic diagnosis of acute of appendicitis: interpretive pitfalls. AJR 1994; 162:55–59

15. Jeffrey RB Jr, Laing FC, Lewis FR. Acute appendicitis: high-resolution real-time US findings. Radiology 1987; 163:11–14

16. Jeffrey RB Jr, Laing FC, Townsend RR. Acute appendicitis: sonographic criteria based on 250 cases. Radiology 1988; 167:327–329

17. Larson JM, Peirce JC, Ellinger DM, et al. 1989 ARRS President's Award. The validity and utility of sonography in the diagnosis of appendicitis in the community setting. AJR 1989; 153:687–691

18. Lewis FR, Holcroft JW, Boey J, Dunphy E. Appendicitis: a critical review of diagnosis and treatment in 1000 cases. Arch Surg 1975; 110:677–682

19. Mindelzun RE, McCort JJ. Acute abdomen. In: Margulis AR, Burhenne HJ (eds), Alimentary tract radiology, 4th ed. St Louis: CV Mosby; 1989:299–302

20. Nghiem HV, Jeffrey RB Jr. Acute appendicitis confined to the appendiceal tip: evaluation with graded compression sonography. J Ultrasound Med 1992; 11:205–207

21. Puylaert JB. Acute appendicitis: US evaluation using graded compression. Radiology 1986; 158:355–360

22. Puylaert JB, Rutgers PH, Lalisang RI, et al. A prospective study of ultrasonography in the diagnosis of appendicitis. N Engl J Med 1987; 317:666–669

23. Quillin SP, Siegel MJ. Appendicitis in children: color Doppler sonography. Radiology 1992; 184:745–747

24. Rioux M. Sonographic detection of the normal and abnormal appendix. AJR 1992; 158:773–778

25. Schrock TR. Acute appendicitis. In: Sleisenger MH, Fordtran JS (eds), Gastrointestinal disease: pathophysiology, diagnosis, management. Philadelphia: WB Saunders; 1989:1382–1388

26. Spear R, Kimmey MB, Wang KY, Sillery JK, Benjamin DR, Sawin RS. Appendiceal US scans: histologic correlation. Radiology 1992; 183:831–834

27. Telford GL, Condon RE. Appendix. In: Zuidema GD (ed), Shackelford's surgery of the alimentary tract, 3rd ed. Philadelphia: WB Saunders; 1991:133–141

28. Vignault F, Filiatrault D, Brandt ML, Garel L, Grignon A, Ouimet A. Acute appendicitis in children: evaluation with US. Radiology 1990; 176:501–504

MUCOCELE

29. Aho AJ, Heinonen R, Lauren P. Benign and malignant mucocele of the appendix. Histological types and prognosis. Acta Chir Scand 1973; 139:392–400

30. Athey PA, Hacken JB, Estrada R. Sonographic appearance of mucocele of the appendix. JCU 1984; 12:333–337

31. Dachman AH, Lichtenstein JE, Friedman AC. Mucocele of the appendix and pseudomyxoma peritonei. AJR 1985; 144:923–929

32. Higa E, Rosai J, Pizzimbono CA, Wise L. Mucosal hyperplasia, mucinous cystadenoma, and mucinous cystadenocarcinoma of the appendix. A re-evaluation of appendiceal "mucocele". Cancer 1973; 32:1525–1541

33. Horgan JG, Chow PP, Richter JO, Rosenfield AT, Taylor KJ. CT and sonography in the recognition of mucocele of the appendix. AJR 1984; 143:959–962

34. Madwed D, Mindelzun R, Jeffrey RB Jr. Mucocele of the appendix: imaging findings. AJR 1992; 159:69–72

35. Sandler MA, Pearlberg JL, Madrazo BL. Ultrasonic and computed tomographic features of mucocele of the appendix. J Ultrasound Med 1984; 3:97–100

36. Skaane P, Ruud TE, Haffner J. Ultrasonographic features of mucocele of the appendix. JCU 1988; 16:584–587

37. Wolff M, Ahmed N. Epithelial neoplasms of the vermiform appendix (exclusive of carcinoid). II. Cystadenomas, papillary adenomas, and adenomatous polyps of the appendix. Cancer 1976; 37:2511–2522

INTUSSUSCEPTION

38. Alzen G, Funke G, Truong S. Pitfalls in the diagnosis of intussusception. JCU 1989; 17:481–488

39. Bisset GS III, Kirks DR. Intussusception in infants and children: diagnosis and therapy. Radiology 1988; 168:141–145

40. Bowerman RA, Silver TM, Jaffe MH. Real-time ultrasound diagnosis of intussusception in children. Radiology 1982; 143:527–529

41. Ein SH, Stephens CA. Intussusception: 354 cases in 10 years. J Pediatr Surg 1971; 6:16–27

42. Holt S, Samuel E. Multiple concentric ring sign in the ultrasonographic diagnosis of intussusception. Gastrointest Radiol 1978; 3:307–309

43. Lee HC, Yeh HJ, Leu YJ. Intussusception: the sonographic diagnosis and its clinical value. J Pediatr Gastroenterol Nutr 1989; 8:343–347

44. Montali G, Croce F, De Pra L, Solbiati L. Intussusception of the bowel: a new sonographic pattern. Br J Radiol 1983; 56:621–623

45. Pracros JP, Tran-Minh VA, Morin de Finfe CH, Deffrenne-Pracros P, Louis D, Basset T. Acute intestinal intussusception in children. Contribution of ultrasonography (145 cases). Ann Radiol (Paris) 1987; 30:525–530

46. Swischuk LE, Hayden CK, Boulden T. Intussusception: indications for ultrasonography and an explanation of the doughnut and pseudokidney signs. Pediatr Radiol 1985; 15:388–391

47. Swischuk LE, Stansberry SD. Ultrasonographic detection of free peritoneal fluid in uncomplicated intussusception. Pediatr Radiol 1991; 21:350–351

48. Verschelden P, Filiatrault D, Garel L, et al. Intussusception in children: reliability of US in diagnosis—a prospective study. Radiology 1992; 184:741–744

49. Wang GD, Liu SJ. Enema reduction of intussusception by hydrostatic pressure under ultrasound guidance: a report of 377 cases. J Pediatr Surg 1988; 23:814–818

50. Weinberger E, Winters WD. Intussusception in children: the role of sonography. Radiology 1992; 184:601–602

51. Weissberg DL, Scheible W, Leopold GR. Ultrasonographic appearance of adult intussusception. Radiology 1977; 124:791–792

52. Wood SK, Kim JS, Suh SJ, Paik TW, Choi SO. Childhood intussusception: US-guided hydrostatic reduction. Radiology 1992; 182:77–80

CROHN'S DISEASE

53. Agha FP, Ghahremani GG, Panella JS, Kaufman MW. Appendicitis as the initial manifestation of Crohn's disease: radiologic features and prognosis. AJR 1987; 149:515–518

54. Dubbins PA. Ultrasound demonstration of bowel wall thickness in inflammatory bowel disease. Clin Radiol 1984; 35:227–231

55. Kaftori JK, Pery M, Kleinhaus U. Ultrasonography in Crohn's disease. Gastrointest Radiol 1984; 9:137–142

56. Khaw KT, Yeoman LJ, Saverymuttu SH, Cook MG, Joseph AE. Ultrasonic patterns in inflammatory bowel disease. Clin Radiol 1991; 43:171–175

57. Puylaert JB, van der Werf S, Ulrich C, Veldhuizen RW. Crohn disease of the ileocecal region: US visualization of the appendix. Radiology 1988; 166:741–743

58. Worlicek H, Lutz H, Heyder N, Matek W. Ultrasound findings in Crohn's disease and ulcerative colitis: a prospective study. JCU 1987; 15:153–163

59. Yeh HC, Rabinowitz JG. Granulomatous enterocolitis: findings by ultrasonography and computed tomography. Radiology 1983; 149:253–259

GASTROINTESTINAL TRACT—GENERAL AND MISCELLANEOUS

60. Downey DB, Wilson SR. Pseudomembranous colitis: sonographic features. Radiology 1991; 180:61–64

61. Fleischer AC, Muhletaler CA, James AE Jr. Sonographic assessment of the bowel wall. AJR 1981; 136:887–891

62. Goerg C, Schwerk WB, Goerg K. Gastrointestinal lymphoma: sonographic findings in 54 patients. AJR 1990; 155:795–798
63. Matsumoto T, Iida M, Sakai T, Kimura Y, Fujishima M. *Yersinia* terminal ileitis: sonographic findings in eight patients. AJR 1991; 156:965–967
64. McAlister WH. Gastrointestinal tract. In: Siegel MJ (ed), Pediatric sonography. New York: Raven Press; 1991:179–211
65. Mittelstaedt CA. The gastrointestinal tract. In: Mittelstaedt CA (ed), Abdominal ultrasound. New York: Churchill Livingstone; 1987:605–656
66. Puylaert JB. Mesenteric adenitis and acute terminal ileitis: US evaluation using graded compression. Radiology 1986; 161:691–695
67. Puylaert JB, Lalisang RI, van der Werf SD, Doornbos L. *Campylobacter* ileocolitis mimicking acute appendicitis: differentiation with graded-compression US. Radiology 1988; 166:737–740
68. Teefey SA, Montana MA, Goldfogel GA, Shuman WP. Sonographic diagnosis of neutropenic typhlitis. AJR 1987; 149:731–733
69. Wada M, Kikuchi Y, Doy M. Uncomplicated acute diverticulitis of the cecum and ascending colon: sonographic findings in 18 patients. AJR 1990; 155:283–287
70. Wilson SR. The gastrointestinal tract. In: Rumack CM, Wilson SR, Charboneau JW (ed), Diagnostic ultrasound. St. Louis: Mosby-Year Book; 1991:181–207
71. Wilson SR, Toi A. The value of sonography in the diagnosis of acute diverticulitis of the colon. AJR 1990; 154:1199–1202

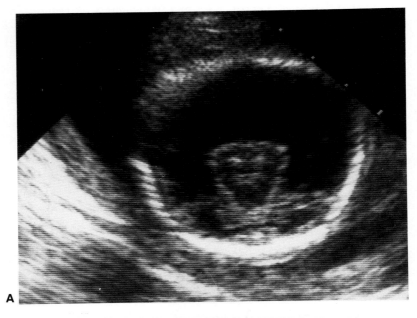

A

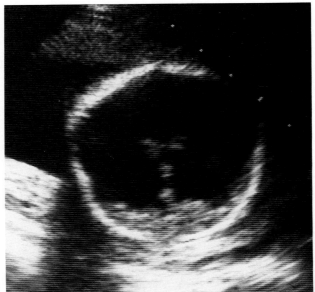

B

Figure 7-1. This 33-year-old woman had a maternal α-fetoprotein level in serum elevated three multiples of the mean at 16 weeks gestation. You are shown four images of the fetal head obtained during a fetal sonographic examination performed at 18 weeks gestation.

Case 7: Holoprosencephaly

Question 30

Which *one* of the following is the MOST likely diagnosis?

- (A) Hydranencephaly
- (B) Porencephaly
- (C) Hydrocephalus
- (D) Semilobar holoprosencephaly
- (E) Agenesis of the corpus callosum

Figure 7-1A is a coronal sonogram of the fetal head with fused thalami (see Figure 7-2) projecting into a crescent-shaped monoventricle. There is no evidence of the formation of distinct lateral ventricles. Figures 7-1B and C are transaxial sonograms of the fetal head and demonstrate an incomplete falx and an irregular mantle of cerebral cortical tissue. In Figure 7-1D, also a transaxial image, cursors have been placed to measure the biocular (+) and intraocular (x) distances. The intraocular distance is short, indicating hypotelorism. These findings are most consistent with a diagnosis of semilobar holoprosencephaly **(Option (D) is correct).**

Hydranencephaly (Option (A)) is characterized by complete or near-complete absence of the cerebral hemispheres, which are replaced with cerebrospinal fluid (CSF) contained within the intact meninges and skull. Occasionally, a minute amount of cerebral cortex within the orbital surfaces of the frontal lobes and the innermost aspects of the temporo-occipital lobes is preserved. This small amount of cortical tissue, however, is usually not detectable by sonography. In hydranencephalic fetuses, sonography of the fetal head demonstrates no cortical mantle. The finding of an irregular cortical mantle in the fetus in the test case eliminates hydranencephaly as a diagnostic possibility.

Porencephaly (Option (B)) is a term used to describe a CSF-filled cyst or cavity within the brain, which may communicate with the ventricular system. This disorder is generally divided into two types. The first type occurs because of abnormal migration of neuronal cells destined to form

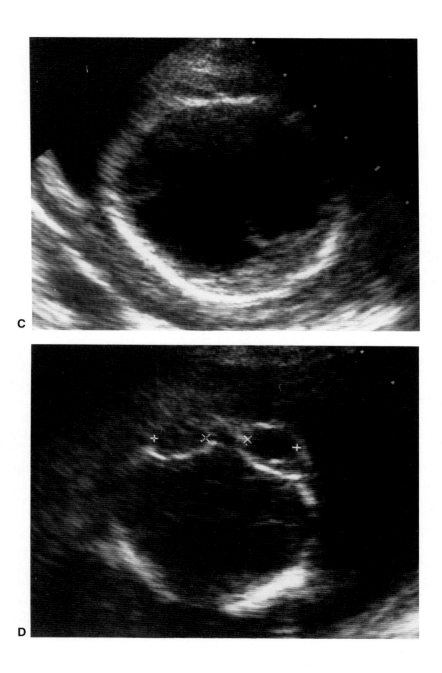

C

D

the cerebral cortex, a disorder called schizencephaly or "cleft brain." The
result is an intraparenchymal defect of both gray and white matter,
which becomes filled with CSF. The defect is often bilateral and tends to
occur in the parenchyma within the vascular distribution of the middle

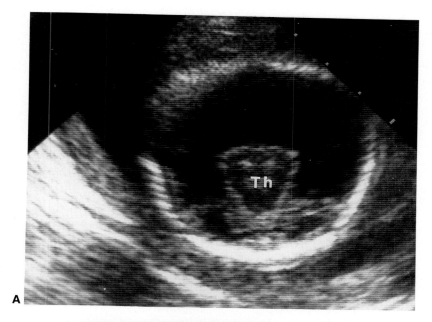

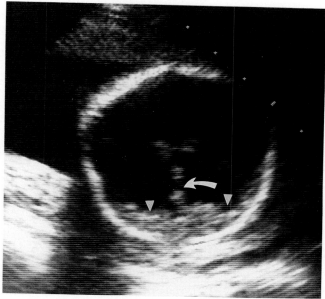

Figure 7-2 (Same as Figure 7-1). Holoprosencephaly. (A) A coronal sonogram of the fetal head at 18 weeks gestation demonstrates a horseshoe-shaped single ventricle surrounding fused thalami (Th). (B) A transaxial sonogram shows an incomplete falx (arrow) and a thin mantle of cerebral cortex (arrowheads) pancaked anteriorly. (C) A transaxial sonogram at a slightly more cephalic level than panel A demonstrates the partial falx (arrow) and the small amount of cerebral cortical tissue (arrowheads). (D) A transaxial sonogram of the fetal face at the level of the orbits (O) shows hypotelorism; the distance between the inner aspects of the orbits (the intraocular distance) as measured by the x cursors is too short. The + cursors measure the biocular distance.

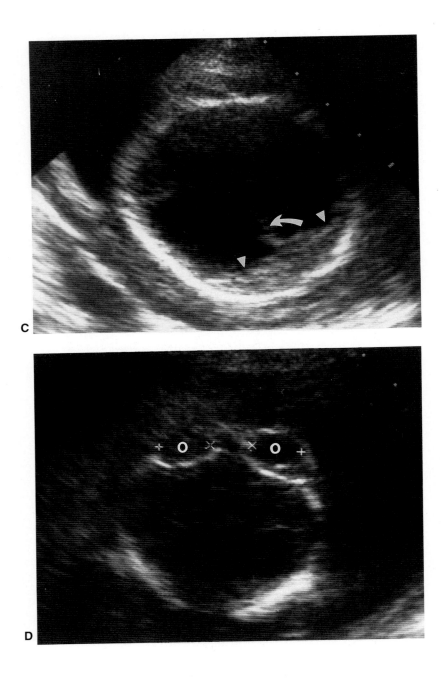

C

D

cerebral artery (Figure 7-3). In the second type, the cystic space is thought to be the consequence of a vascular, traumatic, or infectious destructive process that focally damages the parenchyma. This type is almost always unilateral. Several authors consider porencephaly to be

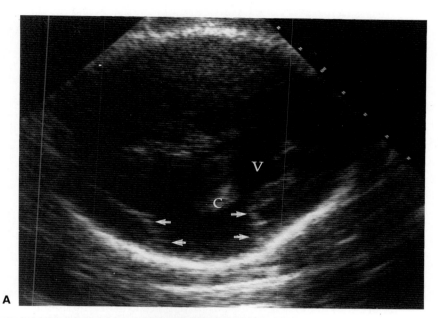

A

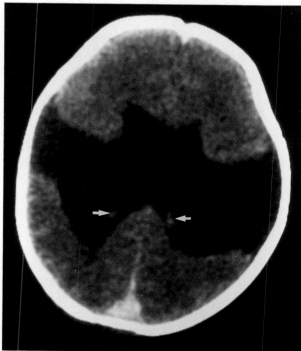

B

Figure 7-3. Schizencephaly. (A) A transaxial fetal sonogram at 32 weeks gestation demonstrates a cleft of the cortical mantle allowing the ventricle (V) to communicate with the subarachnoid space. The edges of the cerebral tissue are marked by arrows. C = choroid plexus. (B) A CT scan after birth confirms the finding of a wide cleft of the brain mantle and demonstrates the abnormality to be present bilaterally. Arrows mark the choroid plexus.

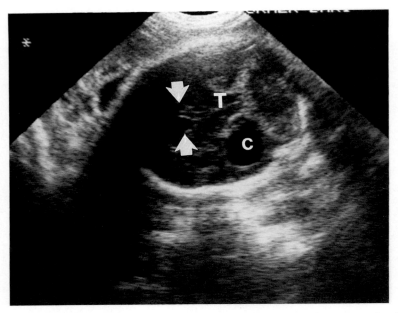

Figure 7-4. Porencephalic cyst. A slightly off-axis sonogram at the level of the thalami (T) demonstrates a porencephalic cyst (C) of the occipital parenchyma. There is mild dilatation of the frontal horns of the lateral ventricles (arrows).

part of a continuum of destructive central nervous system (CNS) processes, with hydranencephaly being the most severe type. The prenatal sonographic findings of porencephaly include a cystic space in the expected location of the normal brain parenchyma and a normally formed ventricular system; also, although hydrocephalus is occasionally present (Figure 7-4), the infratentorial structures and face are typically normal. Porencephaly is a less likely diagnosis in the test case because of the abnormal facies and ventricular system shown in the test images.

The term hydrocephalus (Option (C)) describes a heterogeneous group of disorders in which there is dilatation of the ventricular system. The cerebral cortex is present but can be markedly thinned in fetuses with very severe hydrocephalus. The falx and other midline structures are normal. Additionally, clear definition or separation of the frontal horns of the lateral ventricles is always present but can be difficult to detect in fetuses with massive hydrocephalus. The thalami are normally formed and, in fact, may be splayed by dilatation of the third ventricle rather than fused, as seen in fetuses with holoprosencephaly. The absence of distinct lateral ventricles and the apparent fusion of the thalami make hydrocephalus an unlikely diagnosis.

Agenesis of the corpus callosum (Option (E)) can be complete or partial depending on the gestational age at which callosal development is arrested. Complete agenesis is thought to be a primary process, occurring before 12 menstrual weeks. The absence of the normal corpus callosum produces characteristic changes within the cerebral hemispheres and the ventricular system. Superior displacement and dilatation of the third ventricle, often referred to as an interhemispheric "cyst," are the most characteristic findings but are often the most variable. The lateral ventricles are abnormally shaped and pointed. More-subtle findings include disproportionate enlargement of the occipital horns, a more parallel course of the ventricle wall than is normally seen, and demonstration of both the medial and lateral walls of the lateral ventricle at a level where demonstration of a single periventricular line is normal (Figure 7-5). The superiorly displaced third ventricle can become rather large and can superficially mimic the monoventricle of holoprosencephaly; however, careful examination of the fetus will reveal morphologically abnormal yet distinct and separate lateral ventricles. Another differential feature is the falx, which is always present in fetuses with callosal agenesis and is often unusually deep. Patients with agenesis of the corpus callosum are likely to have hypertelorism rather than hypotelorism, which is more typical of holoprosencephaly. Agenesis of the corpus callosum is part of the spectrum of cranial abnormalities associated with holoprosencephaly; however, the crescent-shaped monoventricle, fused thalami, and hypotelorism in the test images indicate that this is not the most likely diagnosis.

Holoprosencephaly is a CNS malformation that describes a spectrum of cerebral and facial malformations resulting from incomplete differentiation and cleavage of the prosencephalon (forebrain). Early in the organogenesis of the fetal brain, there is formation of three vesicles: the prosencephalon, the mesencephalon, and the rhombencephalon. As the prosencephalon grows, the various germinal matrices that will make the cerebral hemispheres and deep cortical nuclei begin to develop. The normal prosencephalon then undergoes extensive diverticulation and cleavage. Cleavage in the transverse plane results in the separation of the telencephalon (the cerebral hemispheres, lateral ventricles, caudate nucleus, and putamen) from the diencephalon (thalamus, hypothalamus, and globus pallidus). Sagittal division along the mesodermal folds forms the rudimentary cerebral hemispheres and lateral ventricles, which are separated in the midline by the early falx. In fetuses with holoprosencephaly, there is both abnormal sagittal and transverse division.

Pathologically, holoprosencephaly represents a continuum of anomalous development; however, it is convenient to characterize the malformation into three categories (alobar, semilobar, and lobar) depending on

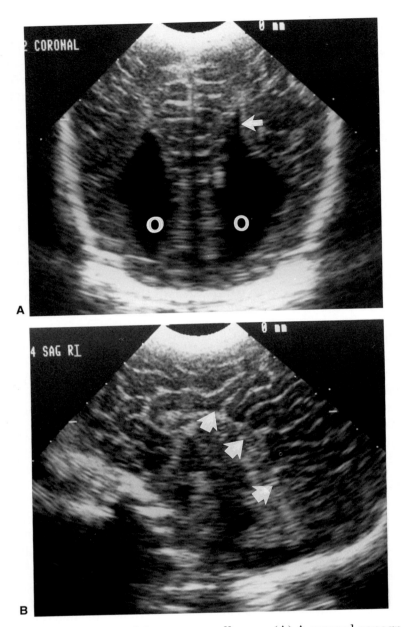

Figure 7-5. Agenesis of the corpus callosum. (A) A coronal sonogram of the head of a baby born with agenesis of the corpus callosum demonstrates disproportionate dilatation of the occipital horns (O) and lateral pointing of the frontal horns (arrow). The ventricles are actually displaced laterally. (B) A sagittal sonogram demonstrates the characteristic radial array of medial cerebral gyri (arrows) toward the midline and the absence of the corpus callosum.

the degree of forebrain cleavage. The most severe form is alobar holoprosencephaly, in which no cleavage of the prosencephalon has occurred.
The brain is small and lacks a normal ventricular system. Instead of distinct lateral ventricles, a monoventricular cavity is present. Absence of
the third ventricle results in thalamic fusion. If the cleavage abnormality
is less severe, an intermediate form of holoprosencephaly, termed semilobar holoprosencephaly, results. A monoventricular cavity with rudimentary occipital horns is present, and the thalamus and basal ganglia are
totally or partially fused. The test case is an example of semilobar holoprosencephaly. The test images demonstrate an irregular cortical mantle, a crescent-shaped monoventricle, and thalamic fusion, findings that
are diagnostic of this malformation. In the least severe type, lobar holoprosencephaly, the two hemispheres and lateral ventricles are better separated; although the frontal horns are hypoplastic, the remainder of the
ventricular system develops nearly normally. The basal ganglia and thalami may be fused but are usually separated. The changes in lobar holoprosencephaly are very subtle and are usually not detectable on prenatal
sonography.

Question 31

Concerning hydranencephaly,

(A) associated anomalies are common
(B) the prognosis is uniformly poor
(C) macrocephaly is nearly always present *in utero*
(D) the presence of a partial falx distinguishes it from holoprosencephaly
(E) the absence of infratentorial structures distinguishes it from holoprosen-
cephaly

Hydranencephaly is a condition in which there is complete or near-
complete destruction of the cerebral hemispheres. The supratentorial
structures begin to develop normally but suffer an insult that destroys
the parenchyma. The most commonly accepted etiology for this disorder
is *in utero* occlusion of the supraclinoid carotid arteries. Greene et al.
have described a case in which massive intracranial hemorrhage was
shown to evolve into hydranencephaly over serial fetal ultrasound examinations. Toxoplasmosis and cytomegalovirus infection have also been
documented to play a role in some cases.

The term hydranencephaly is derived from a combination of the
terms hydrocephalus and anencephaly. However, hydranencephaly is
dissimilar to both these entities. Unlike anencephaly, in which there is a
defect of the cranial vault accompanying the absence of cerebral hemi-

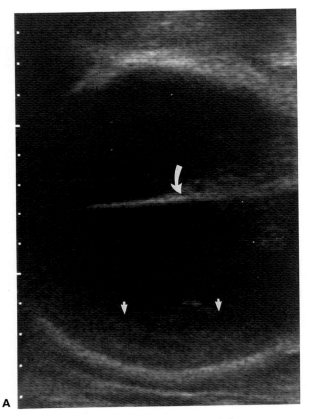

A

Figure 7-6. Hydranencephaly. (A) A transaxial sonogram of a fetus at 34 weeks gestation with hydranencephaly demonstrates an enlarged calvarium without recognizable cerebral cortex. The falx cerebri is intact (curved arrow). A side-lobe artifact causes echoes to be present adjacent to the calvarium in the far field (straight arrows), which may be confused with cerebral tissue. This artifact is not present in the near field. (B) A transaxial view demonstrates normal choroid plexi (straight arrows) and dural attachments (curved arrow). (C) At a slightly more caudal level than panel B, a transaxial view demonstrates distinct paired thalami (T), a finding that distinguishes hydranencephaly from the fused thalami of holoprosencephaly (see Figure 7-2A).

spheres, the cranium, dura, and leptomeninges are completely intact in hydranencephaly. In contrast to hydrocephalus, in which the cerebral hemispheres are present but thinned, the cerebral cortex is nearly completely absent in fetuses affected with hydranencephaly.

The diagnosis of hydranencephaly should be suspected when there is no discernible cortical tissue detected during ultrasonic evaluation of the fetal head. The sonographic features of hydranencephaly include an intact cranium filled with fluid, which may be anechoic or contain inter-

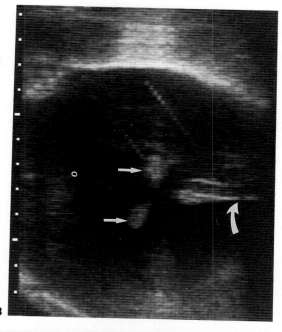

B

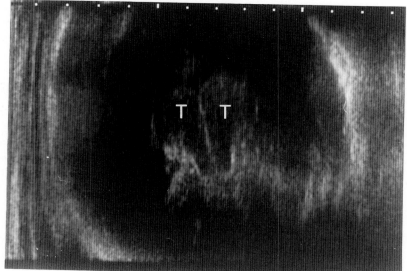

C

nal echoes related to prior intracranial hemorrhage. The midbrain, basal ganglion, and posterior fossa are generally normal, presumably since their blood supply is not principally derived from the supraclinoid carotid arteries **(Option (E) is false).** The falx, tentorium, and dural attachments are usually preserved and are typically easily identifiable because they are surrounded by large amounts of fluid (Figure 7-6).

Although the falx is usually intact in fetuses with hydranencephaly, it has been reported to be partially deficient or absent similar to the appearance of the falx in fetuses with semilobar holoprosencephaly. The finding of a partial falx is therefore not a distinguishing feature between these two conditions **(Option (D) is false).**

Hydranencephaly needs to be distinguished from severe hydrocephalus and alobar holoprosencephaly, two conditions that may appear as large bilateral "fluid" collections within the cranium. In severe hydrocephalus, the cortical tissue is present but may be markedly thinned and compressed against the inner table of the skull by the enlarged ventricles. The detection of the thin rind of cortex was more difficult with older ultrasound equipment. However, with current technology the presence of the intact cortical mantle should be readily detected.

In some cases of alobar holoprosencephaly, the cerebral mantle may be present in scant amounts anteriorly within the cranium and be largely deficient overlying the superior and posterior areas of the brain. Alobar holoprosencephaly can be distinguished by the detection of the fused thalami and the commonly associated facial and extra-CNS anomalies associated with this disorder. Hydranencephaly is considered to be a random, destructive event that occurs sporadically. Therefore, facial and other anomalies are generally not associated with this disorder **(Option (A) is false).** Also, unlike many other cerebral malformations, there is no increased risk of chromosomal abnormalities or occurrence in subsequent pregnancies.

The head circumference of fetuses with hydranencephaly is usually normal or slightly increased at birth **(Option (C) is false).** Macrocephaly, however, rapidly develops in infants who survive the first few weeks of life. The prognosis is uniformly poor, with the most severely affected neonates dying within the first few days of life; few infants survive beyond 3 months **(Option (B) is true).**

Question 32

Findings frequently associated with semilobar holoprosencephaly include:

- (A) absence of the septum pellucidum
- (B) large dorsal cyst
- (C) renal dysplasia
- (D) agenesis of the corpus callosum
- (E) macrocephaly

In addition to the characteristic abnormalities of the ventricular system that occur with holoprosencephaly, there is maldevelopment of the

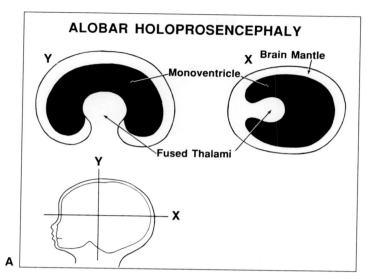

ALOBAR HOLOPROSENCEPHALY

Figure 7-7. Diagrams of holoprosencephaly. (A) Alobar holoprosencephaly. Note the presence of the monoventricle and the fused midline thalami, as well as the absence of falx. (B) Semilobar holoprosencephaly with dorsal sac. Note the absence of falx, the partial fusion of thalami, and the partially separated ventricles The dorsal sac widely communicates with the ventricle. (C) Three morphologic types of alobar (and semilobar) holoprosencephaly in sagittal view. (1) "Pancake type." The residual brain mantle is flattened at the base of the brain. The dorsal sac is correspondingly large. (2) "Cup type." More brain mantle is present, but it does not cover the monoventricle. The dorsal sac communicates widely with the monoventricle. (3) "Ball type." The brain mantle completely covers the monoventricle, and a dorsal sac may be present. (Reprinted with permission from Nyberg DA, Mahony BS, Pretorius DH. Diagnostic ultrasound of fetal anomalies: text and atlas. St. Louis: Mosby-Yearbook; 1990:101–102.)

midline intracranial structures (Figure 7-7). In fetuses with alobar holoprosencephaly, the corpus callosum, falx, and interhemispheric fissure are typically completely absent. In fetuses with the semilobar form, the interhemispheric fissure and the falx are usually partially formed posteriorly but deficient anteriorly. In fetuses with the lobar form, a more complete interhemispheric fissure and falx are present extending into the frontal area of the brain. The corpus callosum is usually absent in fetuses with semilobar holoprosencephaly, although the presence of a splenium-like structure has been noted in some fetuses **(Option (D) is true).** However, the septum pellucidum is absent in all forms of holoprosencephaly **(Option (A) is true).**

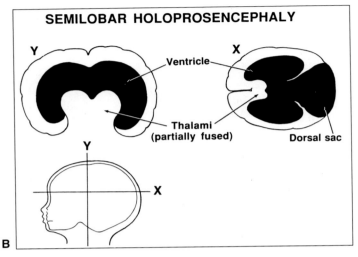

SEMILOBAR HOLOPROSENCEPHALY

Y   X

Ventricle

Thalami
(partially fused)

Dorsal sac

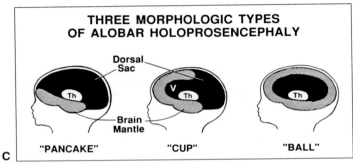

THREE MORPHOLOGIC TYPES
OF ALOBAR HOLOPROSENCEPHALY

Dorsal
Sac

Brain
Mantle

"PANCAKE"   "CUP"   "BALL"

The appearance of the brain in alobar and semilobar holoprosencephaly has been further characterized as "pancake," "cup," and "ball" types,
terms that describe the morphologic appearance of the cortical mantle
when viewed by the pathologist (Figure 7-7). The different configurations
reflect the degree to which the monoventricular cavity is covered by the
cortical tissue. In the pancake type, the residual cortex is flattened anteriorly and inferiorly at the base of the calvarium. In the cup type, more
cortical tissue is present partially covering the monoventricle anteriorly
and superiorly. In the ball type, the brain mantle nearly completely covers the monoventricle. When the cortex fails to cover the ventricle, the
membranous roof of the ventricle expands outward to form a "dorsal
cyst" or "dorsal sac" (Figure 7-8) **(Option (B) is true).** It is important to
identify this structure correctly as a dorsal cyst and not mistake it for
other cystic masses including Dandy-Walker cyst, arachnoid cyst, "interhemispheric cyst" of agenesis of the corpus callosum, or a vein of Galen

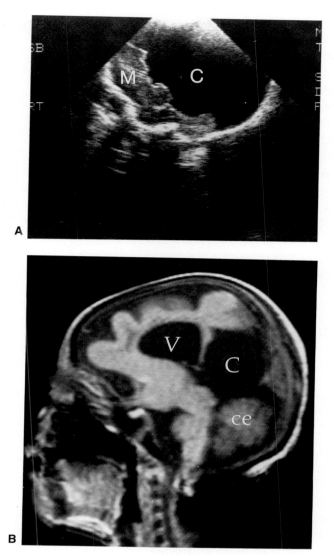

Figure 7-8. Dorsal cyst of holoprosencephaly. (A) Pancake type. A sagittal sonogram performed on a newborn with holoprosencephaly demonstrates the pancake type of cerebral cortex. The cortical tissue is present as a flat mantle (M) anteriorly. The membranous roof of the ventricle expands outward to form a dorsal cyst (C) or sac between the residual cerebral cortex and the calvarium. (B) Cup type. A sagittal T1-weighted MR image of a newborn with semilobar holoprosencephaly. More cortical tissue is present, but it does not completely cover the monoventricle. The dorsal cyst (C) lies superior to the cerebellum (ce) and communicates with the ventricle (V).

aneurysm. The dorsal cyst of holoprosencephaly lies superior to the cerebellum and often has a characteristic crescentic or boomerang shape. The other characteristic intracranial findings of holoprosencephaly (lack of defined lateral ventricles, fused thalami, and absence of midline structures) will also help to differentiate these anomalies.

A variety of extracranial malformations have been noted in up to 50% of fetuses with semilobar and alobar holoprosencephaly, often in association with a chromosomal abnormality. Cardiac defects and renal dysplasia are the most common anomalies **(Option (C) is true).** Polydactyly, omphalocele, and meningomyelocele have also been reported.

The head circumference in fetuses with holoprosencephaly may be normal, decreased, or increased. In fetuses with an enlarged ventricle, presumably due to obstruction of CSF flow, the fetal head becomes macrocephalic **(Option (E) is true).** However, ventriculomegaly is not always present in holoprosencephaly. Microcephaly may be present if cerebral hypoplasia is severe and the ventricular cavity is at the upper limit of normal size to mildly enlarged.

Question 33

Concerning holoprosencephaly,

    (A) the detection of cyclopia or ethmocephaly is diagnostic
    (B) the absence of facial anomalies excludes the diagnosis of the alobar form
    (C) trisomy 13 is the most commonly associated chromosomal abnormality
    (D) it is prognostically important to distinguish the alobar form from the semilobar form
    (E) most cases are sporadic and clinically unsuspected

In addition to the distinctive intracranial malformations noted in fetuses affected with holoprosencephaly, there are specific facial anomalies that also occur. Early in fetal life, as the prosencephalon is undergoing cleavage, the central facial structures (the optic disks, the olfactory placodes, and the premaxillary segment of the face) are also migrating and differentiating. It is believed that the same embryologic maldevelopment that results in failure of cleavage and differentiation of the prosencephalon also causes maldevelopment of the eyes, nose, and premaxillary segment in fetuses with holoprosencephaly. The most severe facial anomalies are most often seen in fetuses with alobar holoprosencephaly but also occur in the other forms. These anomalies are characterized as cyclopia (a single midline orbit, fleshy proboscis above the orbit, and absent nose), ethmocephaly (a median proboscis between hypoteloric orbits), and cebocephaly (a singular nostril with ocular hypotelorism) (Figure

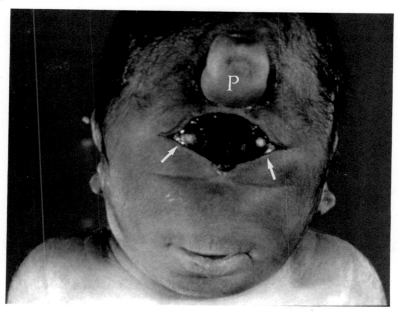

A

Figure 7-9. Facial anomalies associated with holoprosencephaly. (A) Cyclopia. A gross-specimen photograph of a fetus with alobar holoprosencephaly demonstrates a single midline orbit. Two globes (arrows) are present, but they have failed to migrate laterally. A midline proboscis (P) is present above the orbit, and the nasal structures are absent. (B) Ethmocephaly. A fetal sonogram demonstrates a proboscis (arrow) projecting as a beaklike structure between hypoteloric orbits. (C) Ethmocephaly. A gross pathologic specimen of the aborted fetus shown in panel B demonstrates the proboscis, hypotelorism, and the absence of the nasal structures and premaxilla. (D) Premaxillary agenesis (also termed arhinencephaly with cleft lip). This condition is sometimes found in fetuses with less-severe forms of holoprosencephaly. Note the small flat nose (straight arrow), hypotelorism, and absent intermaxillary segment of the face (curved arrow). On pathologic review, the fetus in the test case demonstrated premaxillary agenesis.

7-9). Other fetuses may have less severe facial anomalies such as mild hypotelorism, flat nose, and premaxillary agenesis (midline facial cleft). Examination of the fetal face is, therefore, extremely important when a cerebral malformation is detected. Identification of a proboscis, single orbit, single nostril, or severe hypotelorism confirms the diagnosis of holoprosencephaly **(Option (A) is true).**

Although severe midline facial anomalies are specific to the diagnosis of holoprosencephaly, their absence does not exclude the diagnosis. A normal face can be present in up to 29% of infants born with alobar and

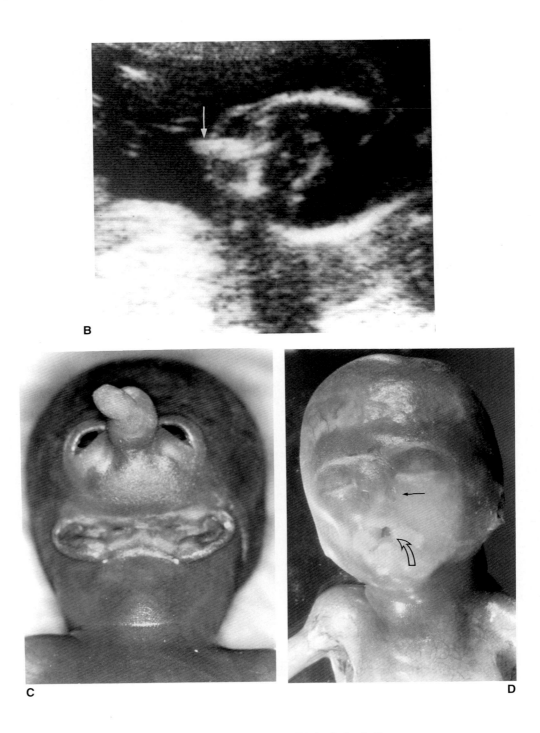

B

C

D

semilobar holoprosencephaly **(Option (B) is false).** In some cases, prenatal ultrasonography may not detect facial anomalies; the less severe

anomalies may not be recognized, or anomalies may be overlooked despite the severity. McGahan et al. noted facial anomalies to be present at birth or autopsy in 24 of 27 (89%) fetuses with alobar or semilobar holoprosencephaly; however, prenatal ultrasonography detected only 14 (58%) of the 24 abnormalities. In this series, midline facial cleft, the most common anomaly, was present in eight fetuses but diagnosed sonographically in only four cases. This series also included eight fetuses (five fetuses with cyclopia and three with ethmocephaly) with a proboscis, two of which were not detected with prenatal ultrasonography.

The incidence of holoprosencephaly has been estimated to be 1 in 16,000 live births; however, the actual incidence may be higher with some affected fetuses escaping detection because of spontaneous abortion. Holoprosencephaly is usually a sporadic occurrence detected on routine prenatal ultrasonography **(Option (E) is true).** The etiology of this malformation is heterogeneous and unknown in the majority of cases. Some series have reported a chromosomal abnormality to be present in up to 50% of affected fetuses. When a chromosomal aberration is noted, trisomy 13 occurs most frequently **(Option (C) is true).** Trisomy 18, triploidy, 13q-, and 18p- have also been noted. The recessively inherited Meckel syndrome is the most well know monogenetic cause of holoprosencephaly. Familial occurrence has also been documented. Autosomal recessive inheritance with variable expression has been suggested in some families, and autosomal dominant inheritance with incomplete penetrance has been suggested in others.

The diagnosis of holoprosencephaly signals the need for chromosomal determination to guide the management of future pregnancies. In the absence of a chromosomal abnormality, an empiric recurrence risk of 6% has been calculated. A chromosomal anomaly may predict a relatively low recurrence risk (less than 1%) if a trisomy is detected or a much higher risk if the aneuploidy is secondary to a translocation and one of the parents is a carrier of the translocation chromosome. In the familial cases, the risk may be 25% if associated with autosomal recessive inheritance or higher if autosomal dominant inheritance with variable penetrance is suspected.

The prognosis of fetuses with holoprosencephaly depends on the severity of the malformation. Most children with alobar holoprosencephaly die shortly after birth. The prognosis of fetuses with the semilobar form is generally very poor as well, with those surviving having profound mental retardation. Therefore, it is not important to differentiate the alobar from the semilobar form, as both have poor prognoses **(Option (D) is false).** Infants with the more severe facial anomalies (cyclopia and ethmocephaly) generally die in the immediate neonatal period. The prognosis of the lobar form is variable. Patients often survive childhood and may in fact have a normal lifespan. Mental retardation can range from mild to severe. Visual and olfactory disturbances are common. It is possible that some individuals with very subtle forms of lobar holoprosencephaly may have only very limited neurologic abnormalities.

Question 34

Concerning sonography of the fetal brain,

    (A) the ratio of the lateral ventricular width to the hemispheric width is relatively constant throughout gestation

    (B) the width of the lateral ventricle measured at the level of the atrium is relatively constant throughout gestation

    (C) a lateral ventricular atrial width greater than 10 mm is considered abnormal

    (D) the choroid plexus normally fills the entire ventricular width

    (E) ventriculomegaly is usually an isolated fetal abnormality

Fetal hydrocephalus is a heterogeneous group of disorders, with more than 86% of the affected fetuses having other associated malformations **(Option (E) is false).** Detection of the concurrent abnormalities is important for determining the appropriate treatment, mode of delivery, and patient counseling. Most fetuses have one or more CNS malformations, most commonly myelomeningocele. For these reasons, assessment of ventricular size has become an important part of routine prenatal sonography.

Siedler and Filly have demonstrated that the telencephalon is relatively small in early gestation, and so the choroid plexus and lateral ventricles constitute a major component of the intracranial volume. The ventricles, however, demonstrate little if any increase in diameter; therefore, later in gestation, as the brain grows, the ventricles occupy a smaller proportion of the cranial width. This is reflected in the ratio of lateral ventricle width to hemispheric width, which progressively decreases throughout gestation **(Option (A) is false).** Normal values for this ratio have been published by several investigators. The ratio, which is normally high during early pregnancy (approximately 71% at 15 weeks), progressively decreases to approximately 33% at 24 weeks and remains at this level until term. Therefore, the ratio has proved to be most useful after 24 weeks, when, as a rule, any measurement greater than 50% is considered abnormal. However, the wide variation of normal values in early pregnancy limits this measurement. In contrast, the ventricular atrium maintains a relatively stable size throughout gestation and can therefore provide an age-independent measurement to assess ventriculomegaly **(Option (B) is true).** Cardoza et al. defined the mean atrial

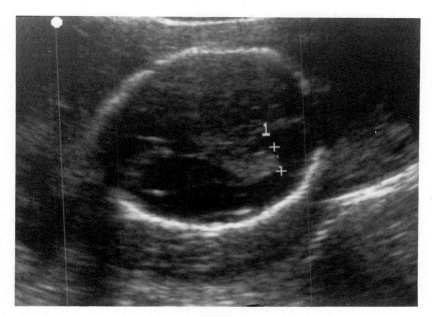

Figure 7-10. Measurement of the lateral ventricle. A transaxial sonogram of a 16-week-old fetus shows that the normal choroid plexus fills the lateral ventricle. The ventricle is measured from the medial to lateral echogenic lines that surround the ventricle, as demonstrated by the cursors.

diameter as 7.6 ± 0.6 mm with a range of 6 to 9 mm. Therefore, fetuses with atrial measurements greater than 10 mm are considered to have ventriculomegaly and warrant a careful examination for associated anomalies **(Option (C) is true).**

The atrium was chosen as the preferential site for measurement for several reasons. Its walls are perpendicular to the ultrasound beam in the axial plane and can be identified in nearly all normal fetuses. The choroid plexus is largest at the level of the atrium, where it fills the lateral ventricle and therefore provides a conspicuous landmark **(Option (D) is true).** Additionally, dilatation of the atrium and occipital horns may be the earliest finding in fetuses with mild hydrocephalus (Figure 7-10). An associated finding in hydrocephalus has been described as the "dangling choroid" sign. In fetuses with hydrocephalus, the choroid plexus in the far ventricle separates from the medial wall of the lateral ventricle and lies in a dependent position. It gives the appearance of dangling in the enlarged ventricle (Figure 7-11). The documentation of normal-sized lateral ventricles, however, does not exclude significant CNS

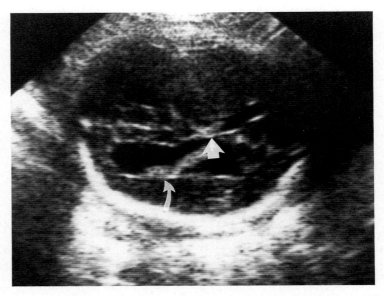

Figure 7-11. Dangling choroid sign. A transaxial sonogram of a fetus with myelomeningocele and mild hydrocephalus shows that the choroid plexus in the far ventricle is heavier that the surrounding CSF; it falls away from the medial ventricular wall and lies dependently against the lateral wall (curved arrow). The choroid plexus in the near ventricle is also dangling (straight arrow).

abnormalities. A few fetuses with myelomeningocele and encephaloceles may demonstrate no evidence of ventricular dilatation. It is also important, therefore, to assess the cisterna magna for effacement, which may be a subtle sign of myelomeningocele.

Jill E. Langer, M.D.
Beverly G. Coleman, M.D.

SUGGESTED READINGS

HOLOPROSENCEPHALY

1. Chervenak FA, Issacson G, Hobbins JC, Chitkara U, Tortora M, Berkowitz RL. Diagnosis and management of fetal holoprosencephaly. Obstet Gynecol 1985; 66:322–326
2. Cohen MM. An update on the holoprosencephalic disorders. J Pediatrics 1982; 101:865–869

3. DeMyer W, Zeman W, Palmer CG. The face predicts the brain: diagnostic significance of median facial anomalies for holoprosencephaly (arhinencephaly). Pediatrics 1964; 34:256–263

4. Filly RA, Chinn DH, Callen PH. Alobar holoprosencephaly: ultrasonic prenatal diagnosis. Radiology 1984; 151:455–459

5. Fitz CR. Holoprosencephaly and related entities. Neuroradiology 1983; 25:225–238

6. Jeanty P, Dramaix-Wilmet M, Van Gansbeke D, Van Regemorter N, Rodesch F. Fetal ocular biometry by ultrasound. Radiology 1982; 143:513–516

7. McGahan JP, Nyberg DA, Mack LA. Sonography of facial features of alobar and semilobar holoprosencephaly. AJR 1990; 154:143–148

8. Nyberg DA, Mack LA, Bronstein A, Hirsch J, Pagon RA. Holoprosencephaly: prenatal sonographic diagnosis. AJR 1987; 149:1051–1058

HYDRANENCEPHALY

9. Dublin AB, French BN. Diagnostic image evaluation of hydranencephaly and pictorially similar entities, with emphasis on computed tomography. Radiology 1980; 137:81–91

10. Greene MF, Benacerraf B, Crawford JM. Hydranencephaly: US appearance during *in utero* evaluation. Radiology 1985; 156:779–780

PORENCEPHALY

11. Raybaud C. Destructive lesions of the brain. Neuroradiology 1983; 25:265–291

HYDROCEPHALUS

12. Cardoza JD, Filly RA, Podrasky AE. The dangling choroid plexus: a sonographic observation of value in excluding ventriculomegaly. AJR 1988; 151:767–770

13. Cardoza JD, Goldstein RB, Filly RA. Exclusion of fetal ventriculomegaly with a single measurement: the width of the lateral ventricular atrium. Radiology 1988; 169:711–714

14. Filly RA, Cardoza JD, Goldstein RB, Barkovich AJ. Detection of fetal central nervous system anomalies: a practical level of effort for a routine sonogram. Radiology 1989; 172:403–408

15. Filly RA, Goldstein RB, Callen PW. Fetal ventricle: importance of routine obstetric sonography. Radiology 1991; 181:1–7

16. Hertzberg BS, Bowie JD, Burger PC, Marshburn PB, Djang WT. The three lines: origin of sonographic landmarks in the fetal head. AJR 1987; 149:1009–1012

17. Nyberg DA, Mack LA, Hirsch J, Pagon RO, Shepard TH. Fetal hydrocephalus: sonographic detection and clinical significance of associated anomalies. Radiology 1987; 163:187–191

18. Siedler DE, Filly RA. Relative growth of higher fetal brain structures. J Ultrasound Med 1987; 6:573–576

AGENESIS OF THE CORPUS CALLOSUM

19. Babcock DS. The normal, absent, and abnormal corpus callosum: sonographic findings. Radiology 1984; 151:449–453
20. Bertino RE, Nyberg DA, Cyr DR, Mack LA. Prenatal diagnosis of agenesis of the corpus callosum. J Ultrasound Med 1988; 7:251–260

FETAL CRANIAL SONOGRAPHY—GENERAL

21. Carrasco CR, Stierman ED, Harnsberger HR, Lee TG. An algorithm for prenatal ultrasound diagnosis of congenital CNS abnormalities. J Ultrasound Med 1985; 4:163–168
22. McGahan JP, Ellis W, Lindfors KK, Lee BC, Arnold JP. Congenital cerebrospinal fluid-containing intracranial abnormalities: a sonographic classification. JCU 1988; 16:531–544

Notes

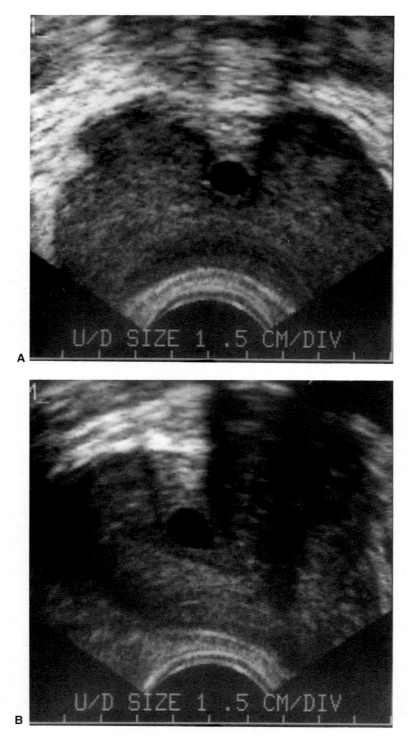

Figure 8-1. This 60-year-old man was referred for transrectal sonography of the prostate gland because of urinary frequency and postvoid dribbling. You are shown transverse (A) and midline sagittal (B) images.

Case 8: Prostatic Utricle Cyst

Question 35

Which *one* of the following is the MOST likely diagnosis?

(A) Cystic carcinoma
(B) Ejaculatory duct cyst
(C) Prostatic utricle cyst
(D) Seminal vesicle cyst
(E) Retention cyst

Figure 8-1A is a transverse sonogram through the base of the prostate. In the midline there is a 5-mm round, anechoic cystic structure (Figure 8-2A). The hypoechoic smooth muscle of the ejaculatory ducts is seen on either side of the cystic mass. The sagittal image (Figure 8-1B) shows that this cyst is 8 mm in length, nearly surrounded by prostatic tissue, and teardrop shaped (Figure 8-2B). The clinical history of postvoid dribbling is useful since, of the options listed, only the prostatic utricle normally communicates with the urethra. The appearance is not completely specific, but the small, midline cyst and the course of the ejaculatory duct around the mass, combined with the clinical history of postvoid dribbling, are most consistent with a prostatic utricle cyst **(Option (C) is correct).**

The sonographic appearance of prostate cancer (Option (A)) is varied, although the lesions are usually solid and in the peripheral area of the gland (Figure 8-3). Only a few cases of cystic cancer have been reported. Unlike the appearance in the test images, these cancers have had large, irregularly shaped cystic spaces associated with wall nodularity. The anechoic areas are secondary to necrosis, and the solid wall components represent the tumor. The small, smooth, simple cystic appearance of the mass in the test patient should not suggest cystic carcinoma.

Ejaculatory duct cysts (Option (B)) do not typically present with obstructive or dribbling symptoms. They have a near-midline location at the level of the verumontanum, and toward the base of the prostate they lie in the expected course of the ejaculatory duct within the central zone

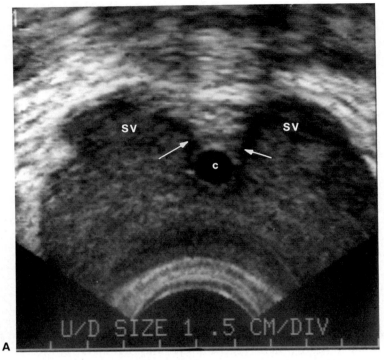

A

Figure 8-2 (Same as Figure 8-1).   Utricle cyst. (A) A transverse sonogram through the base of the prostate shows a 5-mm anechoic midline cyst (c). A portion of the seminal vesicle (SV) can be identified on each side. The hypoechoic smooth muscle of the ejaculatory ducts (arrows) is also identified coursing around the cyst on each side. (B) A sagittal image of the prostate shows the cyst (c) to be teardrop shaped and nearly surrounded by prostatic tissue. The cyst lies anterior to and separate from the ejaculatory duct (arrow). U = area of urethra.

(Figures 8-4 and 8-5). The ejaculatory duct can be identified lateral and posterior to the cyst in the test patient (Figure 8-2). Ejaculatory duct cyst should be considered in the differential diagnosis of the test patient; however, given the sonographic appearance and presenting symptoms, it is not the best diagnosis.

Seminal vesicle cysts (Option (D)) are not midline lesions and are extraprostatic. Sonographically they are identified cephalic to the base of the prostate (Figure 8-6). They should not be surrounded by prostatic tissue, as is the lesion in the test patient.

Retention cysts (Option (E)) are generally not midline lesions and are frequently discovered incidentally (Figure 8-7). They are only infrequently symptomatic and do not communicate with the urethra. Rarely,

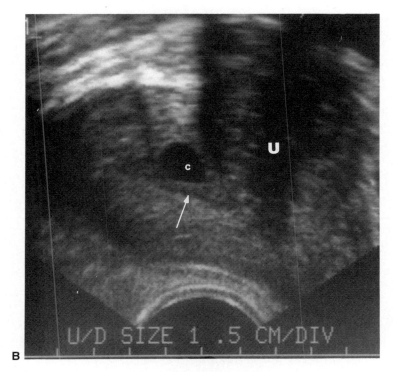

U/D SIZE 1 .5 CM/DIV

B

Figure 8-2 (Continued)

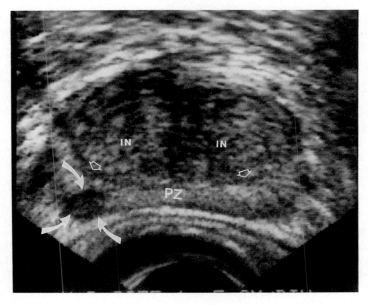

Figure 8-3. Hypoechoic carcinoma. A transverse image of the prostate at a level between the midgland and the apex shows a discrete, hypoechoic 6-mm nodule in the right peripheral zone (curved arrows). The normal hyperechoic outer gland peripheral zone (PZ) is separated from the inner gland (IN) by the hypoechoic surgical capsule (open arrows). Mild changes of BPH are present in the inner gland. At surgery this was a stage B cancer, with a Gleason score of 5.

231

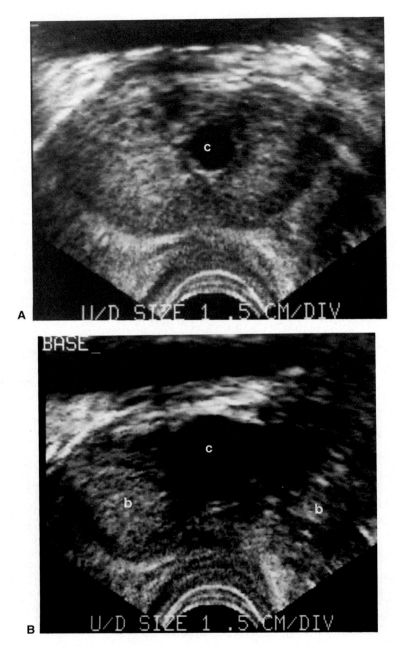

Figure 8-4. Ejaculatory duct cyst. (A) A transverse sonogram through the midgland shows an 8-mm cystic mass (c) slightly to the left of the midline. (B) A more cephalic transverse image through the prostate base (b) shows that the cyst (c) projects to the left and is 17 mm in the transverse dimension. The more lateral position of the cyst in the base of the gland is consistent with the expected course of the ejaculatory duct. (C) A transverse scan at the level of the seminal vesicles (sv) shows the cyst (c) to lie between these two structures. (D) A sagittal image shows the cyst (c) to project beyond the prostate base (arrows) and to course through the central zone (cz), which is slightly more echogenic than the peripheral zone (PZ).

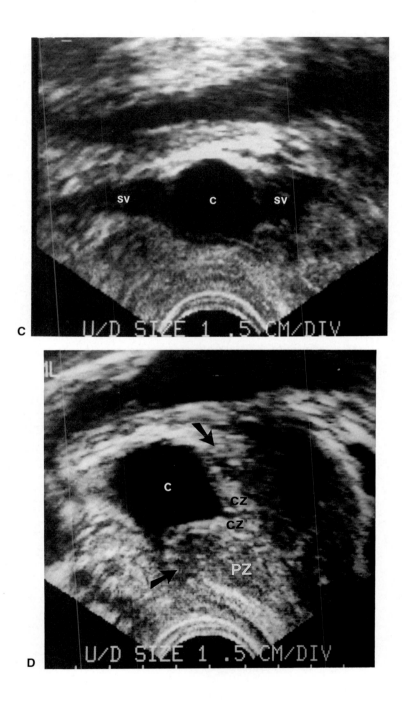

they attain sufficient size to cause obstructive symptoms if they are located near the urethra. Therefore, postvoid dribbling symptoms would not be expected and retention cyst is not the best diagnosis.

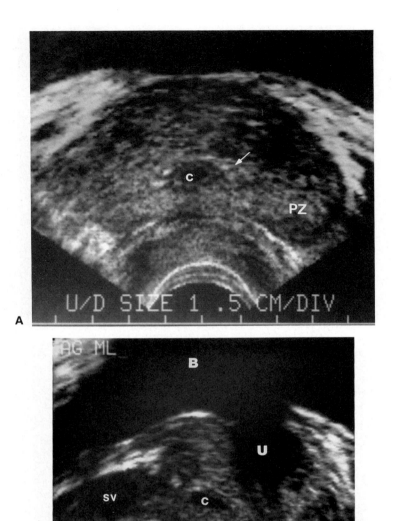

Figure 8-5. Small ejaculatory duct cyst. (A) A transverse sonogram through the midgland shows a small, ovoid 4-mm cyst (c) projecting slightly to the right of the midline. The cyst is in the central zone (arrow), which is slightly more echogenic than the peripheral zone (PZ). (B) A sagittal image shows the cyst (C) to be oblong, 8 mm long, and in the course of the ejaculatory duct. The seminal vesicle (SV) is cephalic to the gland. B = bladder; U = urethra.

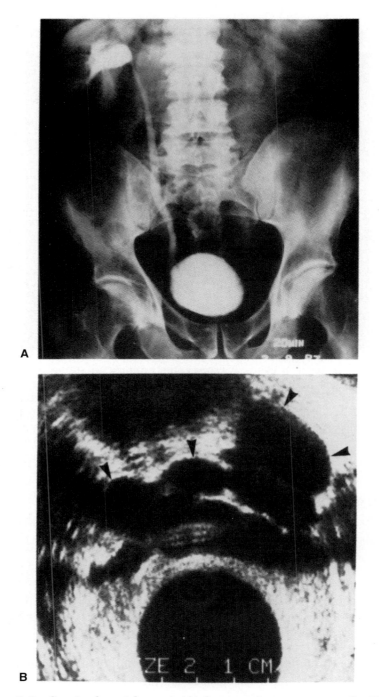

Figure 8-6. Seminal vesicle cyst. (A) An excretory urogram of a 53-year-old man with a history of chronic prostatitis shows a solitary right kidney. Cystoscopy revealed a maldeveloped left hemitrigone. (B) A transverse endorectal sonogram reveals a septated cystic mass of the left seminal vesicle (arrowheads). At surgery, a multiloculated cyst of the left seminal vesicle was found. (Reprinted with permission from King et al. [4].)

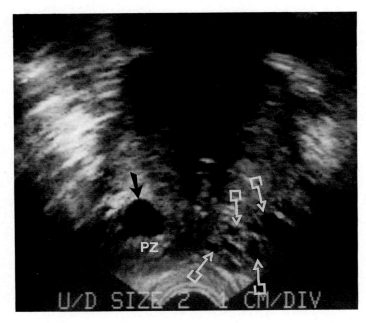

Figure 8-7. Retention cysts. A transverse endorectal sonogram shows a large cyst (black arrow) in the right midgland peripheral zone (PZ) and numerous smaller cysts (white arrows) in the left peripheral zone. None of the cysts are midline in location. The cysts were an incidental finding and are consistent with the diagnosis of retention cysts.

Question 36

Concerning carcinoma of the prostate,

   (A) most cases arise within the transition zone of the gland
   (B) it usually appears hypoechoic on sonography
   (C) it frequently contains cystic areas caused by tumor necrosis
   (D) the sensitivity of transrectal sonography for its detection is greater than 90%
   (E) it is accurately staged by transrectal sonography

Prostatic carcinoma is the most common malignant neoplasm in the world, the most frequently diagnosed cancer in American men, and the second most lethal cancer in American men. There appears to be no correlation of prostatic carcinoma with diet, venereal disease, sexual habits, smoking, or occupational exposure. Higher testosterone levels have been proposed as a major determinant of risk. It is more common among blacks and much less common among Asians than among whites. It is variously estimated that 10 to 50% of men in the sixth decade have microscopic foci of well-differentiated adenocarcinoma. Every decade of aging nearly doubles the frequency of such tumors, so that by the ninth decade up to 80% of men will develop prostatic cancer and nearly all men over 90 years of age will have detectable cancer. Fortunately, 90% of these cancers are latent and remain undetected and clinically unimportant for decades. This prevalence of latent tumors appears to be unique to the prostate gland. There is a 6 to 10% chance of developing clinically overt disease, with 75% of cases affecting men 60 to 79 years of age.

Before the location, appearance, and spread of prostatic carcinoma can be discussed, the anatomy of the gland must be reviewed. Conventional lobar anatomy, in which the prostate is divided into five distinct major lobes, has been replaced by the zonal approach. In current practice the anatomic description of the prostate is divided according to histologic zonal anatomy, not positional differences. The prostate gland is divided into three major areas: the anterior aspect, the inner gland, and the outer gland (Figure 8-8). The anterior fibromuscular stroma occupies the anterior aspect of the gland and is devoid of prostatic acinar tissue. It is composed of fibrous and muscular tissue; it is thick anteriorly and thins as it surrounds the prostate gland laterally and posteriorly to form the prostate capsule.

The inner or central gland is composed of the smooth muscle of the internal urethral sphincter and the urethra, a thin lining of proximal prostatic urethra called the periurethral glandular tissue, and the transition zone. The bilobed transition zone, found on each side of the internal urethral sphincter just cephalic to the verumontanum, is acinar tissue and initially accounts for 5% of glandular tissue volume. The transition zone is the only part of the prostate that is acinar tissue and not part of the outer gland.

The outer or peripheral gland is composed of central and peripheral zones, both of which are acinar tissue. Not all authors agree on the inclusion of the central zone within the outer gland. Both Lee et al. (1989) and Rifkin et al. (1989) consider the central zone and peripheral zone to be outer gland tissues; sonographic and anatomic similarities between the two zones seem to make this a logical classification. The sonographic appearance of the two zones is similar, and both are separated from the inner gland by the surgical capsule. The central zone is situated posterior to, and is distinctly separate from, the central gland. It extends from the base to the level of the verumontanum and surrounds the paired ejaculatory ducts. The peripheral zone comprises the posterior, apical (inferior), lateral, posterolateral, and anterolateral portions of the prostate. It is the largest portion of the prostate, accounting for approximately 75% of the volume of the normal postpubescent gland.

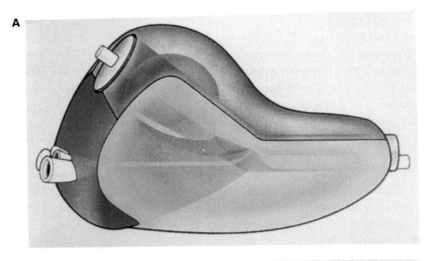

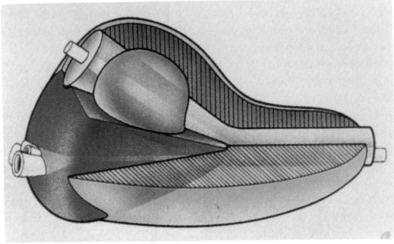

Figure 8-8. Zonal anatomy of the prostate gland. (A) Illustration of zonal anatomy with the entire prostate viewed from the side. Yellow = peripheral zone; orange = central zone; blue = transition zone; green = anterior fibromuscular stroma. The anterior gray tubular structure is the urethra. Tubular structures projecting from the base are ejaculatory ducts. (B) Illustration with a portion of the peripheral zone cut away. In both panels A and B, anterior is toward the top of the page, posterior toward the bottom, cranial to the left, and caudal to the right. (Reprinted with permission from Lee et al. [20].)

The sonographic echotextures of the different areas of the prostate vary, with the outer gland being hyperechoic compared with the inner gland (Figure 8-3). In addition, within the outer gland the central zone is sometimes minimally hyperechoic to the peripheral zone (Figures 8-4D

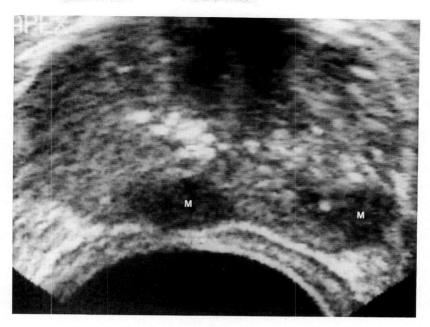

Figure 8-12. Granulomatous prostatitis. A transverse sonogram through the prostate toward the apex of the gland shows two focal hypoechoic masses (M). They are both in the peripheral zone, and the one to the right slightly bulges the contour of the gland. The sonographic appearance is nonspecific but suspicious for carcinoma. Biopsy revealed granulomatous prostatitis.

score. Components with a score of 4 or greater are associated with a worse prognosis. DNA ploidy may also be promising as a predictor of biologic behavior. Patients whose tumors have normal diploid DNA content have a more favorable prognosis and are more sensitive to surgical, hormonal, or radiation therapy than are patients with DNA-nondiploid (aneuploid) tumors. Aneuploid tumors tend to grow more rapidly and metastasize early, and they are less responsive to current treatments.

Prostatic carcinoma is generally designated stage A, B, C, or D. Stages A and B disease are confined to the prostate. Stage A cancer is defined as nonpalpable cancer detected in a specimen obtained by transurethral prostatectomy. Stage B disease is a palpable lesion confined to one or both sides of the prostate. Stage C disease extends through the prostatic capsule into the periprostatic fat, neurovascular bundle, or seminal vesicles. Stage D disease includes lymphatic spread to lymph nodes in the obturator, iliac, or periaortic locations or hematogenous spread to bones or, less often, lung and liver. Patients with tumors confined to the gland are usually considered candidates for radical surgery, whereas those with more advanced disease are usually treated by radiation therapy or chemotherapy.

Lee et al. showed in 1991 that inner gland and outer gland cancers tend to escape from the prostate at different locations. Outer gland tumors most frequently extend to and escape from the gland at the prostatic capsule (38%), at either the apex or the base. The seminal vesicle (18%) and invaginated extraprostatic space (36%) (along the ejaculatory duct insertion into the central zone, which is devoid of capsule) are also frequent sites of extension. Routes for extension of inner gland tumors are more limited, with the anterior fibromuscular stroma and surgical capsule acting as highly resistant barriers to tumor extension. It has been suggested that a transurethral resection of the prostate disrupts these natural barriers, thereby explaining the spread of some inner gland tumors. Inner gland tumors most frequently invade the anterior fibromuscular stroma (61%), but only 9% exhibit extraprostatic extension. When the escape occurs, it is most often at the junction of prostatic capsule and anterior fibromuscular stroma at the apex of the gland. Overall, in the series of Lee et al., 22 and 48% of inner gland and outer gland tumors, respectively, had escaped the gland.

Ideally, a cross-sectional imaging study should accurately stage carcinoma and reliably differentiate stage B and C disease. Numerous studies have been undertaken to determine whether sonography is sufficiently sensitive for this purpose. Capsular invasion was studied by Hamper et al., with criteria for invasion defined as discontinuity of capsular echoes (i.e., irregularity or clear disruption of bright periprostatic fat) and the presence of local contour deformity or bulge that was created by the tumor (Figures 8-9 and 8-10). The sensitivity of sonographic detection of capsular penetration was 68%, with a specificity of 91% and a positive predictive value of 80%. The detection rate was more accurate with increasing penetration. Hamper et al. also evaluated the ability of sonography to detect invasion of the neurovascular bundle. Involvement of the neurovascular bundle is important in deciding whether sexual function can be preserved in patients undergoing radical prostatectomy. Invasion of the neurovascular bundle was diagnosed when the tumor was close to the posterolateral aspect of the gland, causing a bulge or irregularity of the posterolateral tumor outline and echogenic periprostatic fat. Sonography could identify both neurovascular bundles in only 50% of cases and could not identify either bundle in 19% of cases. The sensitivity for predicting invasion was 66%, the specificity was 78%, and the positive predictive value was 51%, with the accuracy again increasing with increasing depths of penetration. It is important to detect seminal vesicle invasion since it carries an extremely poor prognosis when treated with radical prostatectomy, even in the absence of lymph node spread. Middleton et al. showed that the 5-year outcome of patients with microscopic tumor extension into the capsule of a radical prostatectomy specimen was virtually as good as for that for patients with tumor confined histologically to the capsule. In this study, 91% of patients with confined disease and 87% of patients with microscopic invasion of the prostate capsule were free of disease at 5 years. In contrast, only 50% of patients with microscopic invasion of the seminal vesicles were free of disease at 5 years. Unfortunately, the sonographic accuracy for detection of seminal vesicle invasion is quite varied from study to study. According to Terris et al., sonographic findings of invasion include relative hyperechogenicity plus a combination of two or more of the following: asymmetry, enlargement (i.e., seminal vesicle size of 1 cm or more in anteroposterior dimension on transverse scan), and anterior displacement greater than 1 cm from the midline rectal wall on transverse scan. The sensitivity of hyperechogenicity and a combination of two or more abnormalities was 71%, with a specificity of 94%. However, a multi-institutional study showed the sensitivity for seminal vesicle invasion to be only 22%.

The multi-institutional cooperative study was undertaken to compare sonography with MRI in staging early prostate cancer. The overall staging accuracy of sonography was 58%. Sonography was unable to reliably differentiate microscopic local disease from advanced disease in patients presenting with clinically localized disease. Sonography accurately staged confined disease and advanced disease in only 49 and 63% of patients, respectively **(Option (E) is false).** Unfortunately, the same study showed that MRI was only slightly better than sonography, with an overall accuracy of 69%. At this time, neither technique has the ability to identify microscopic spread of disease. MRI with rectal coils may improve results, but this remains to be studied.

Question 37

Factors of value in distinguishing cancer of the prostate from benign prostatic hyperplasia include:

(A) location of the lesion
(B) presence of urinary retention
(C) echogenicity of the lesion
(D) prostate gland volume
(E) level of prostate-specific antigen in serum

Benign prostatic hyperplasia (BPH) is generally defined as a well-demarcated, well-differentiated enlargement of the inner gland. The prostate usually maintains a normal size and weight until age 40. After age 50, 50% of men have some degree of BPH. The prostate may double in size from its normal 15 to 20 g to an average of 33 g as determined at autopsy. Up to 80% of men develop BPH, but only 10% require surgical intervention. Unlike prostatic carcinoma, which affects the inner gland transition zone in only 20 to 25% of patients, BPH affects the transition zone in 95% of patients and the periurethral glandular tissue in the remaining 5%. The location of carcinoma, which is predominantly an outer gland disease, with respect to that of BPH, which is an inner gland process, is a significant distinguishing feature **(Option (A) is true)**. BPH can present as a single, relatively well demarcated focus or as multiple benign hyperplastic nodules (adenomas). The surgical capsule separates the hyperplastic tissue from the compressed peripheral zone. The surgical capsule can be demarcated by a well-defined change in echogenicity (Figure 8-3), a hypoechoic rim (halo), or calcifications and corpora amylacea.

The clinical presentation of BPH depends on the site and size of the prostatic nodules. Even small nodules projecting into the prostatic urethra can cause stream reduction and bladder outlet obstruction, whereas large nodules arising laterally can be asymptomatic for a long period. The initial symptom is most commonly a reduction in the force of the urine stream. Nocturia is common, as is difficulty in initiating urination. Urinary retention can have a gradual or sudden onset. Sudden acute urinary retention is an indication for surgery, but 50% of patients are relieved by catheter drainage and may pass urine relatively well before requiring surgery. The presence of urinary retention is suggestive of BPH, but it does not exclude the possibility of an associated carcinoma or a carcinoma positioned so that it could cause bladder outlet obstruction **(Option (B) is false)**. In fact, most men with prostatic carcinoma probably also have BPH. Approximately 10% of specimens obtained during transurethral resection of the prostate contain carcinoma.

The primary types of BPH have been described and correlated with the sonographic appearance. Homogeneous stromal (or fibromuscular) hyperplasia is hypoechoic in appearance. Glandular hyperplasia is hypoechoic (Figure 8-3) or hyperechoic depending on the size of the gland and the variability of cystic structures. The third type, an admixture of stromal and glandular hyperplasia, is the most common and has mixed echogenicity (Figure 8-13). The frequent presence of hypoechoic foci in patients with BPH means that the cancer yield on biopsy within the transition zone is lower than from areas of similar echogenicity in the peripheral zones. In a 1989 study by Lee et al., biopsy of a hypoechoic lesion at least 1 cm in size in the transition zone had a positive yield of carcinoma of 13%. For lesions of comparable size in the peripheral zone,

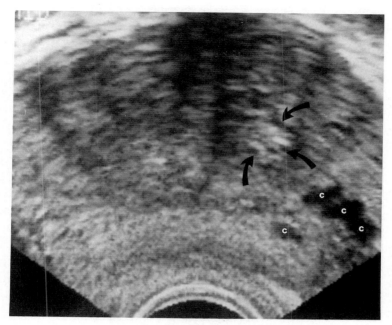

Figure 8-13. Benign prostatic hyperplasia. A transverse sonogram through the midgland shows a heterogeneous central gland in the left transition zone (arrows). Small left peripheral zone cysts (c) are consistent with retention cysts.

the positive yield was 41%. The most suspicious finding for carcinoma of the transition zone was localized asymmetry with a hypoechoic lesion. Echogenicity alone was not a reliable distinguishing feature of carcinoma versus BPH **(Option (C) is false).**

There is continued controversy about the value of screening for prostatic carcinoma. There is concern about whether screening will detect the latent cancers for which the morbidity and mortality of treatment may exceed those of the disease itself. Three screening methods are now generally available: digital rectal examination, prostate-specific antigen (PSA), and transrectal ultrasonography of the prostate. For many years, digital rectal examination was the only established means of diagnosing prostatic carcinoma. However, it is estimated that 50% of cancers arise anterior to the verumontanum and are nonpalpable. Sonography is not an ideal screening modality since it is expensive and lacks sufficient sensitivity, as discussed earlier.

The need for a screening tool that is objective, quantitative, well tolerated, and independent of the skill of the operator seems desirable. PSA appears to fulfill these objectives. It is a glycoprotein secreted exclusively by epithelial cells in the prostate and is produced in the cytoplasm of both benign and malignant prostate cells. Elevation in the level of PSA is common in patients with nonmalignant prostatic disease. From 30 to 50% of patients with BPH have elevated PSA concentrations in serum, depending on the size of the gland and the degree of obstruction. Elevated PSA levels can also result from prostatitis, recent prostate biopsy, and even recent digital rectal examination. The PSA concentrations are increased in 25 to 92% of patients with cancer of the prostate, depending on tumor volume. Littrup et al. have shown that when PSA levels are adjusted for the volume of the gland, the PSA levels in patients with cancer are more likely to exceed the volume-adjusted 95th percentile than are those in patients with a negative biopsy. Patients whose PSA level is greater than the volume-adjusted 95th percentile have a risk for cancer up to nine times that of the general screening population. Prostate volume alone cannot reliably differentiate carcinoma from BPH **(Option (D) is false),** but prostate volume correlated with PSA levels appears to be an important objective variable for screening programs. Gram for gram, the average prostatic cancer produces at least 10 times more PSA than is produced by normal prostatic tissue.

The upper limit of normal PSA levels is open to question, but a PSA level greater than 10 ng/mL is most unlikely to be due to BPH alone, and urologic evaluation is indicated. Up to 67% of these patients have carcinoma, whereas only 2% of patients with BPH have such an elevated PSA level **(Option (E) is true).** When the PSA level is greater than 10 ng/mL, the incidence of cancer is so high that some advocate the use of random biopsy when a lesion is not seen by transrectal sonography. When the PSA level is 4 to 10 ng/mL, there is considerable overlap of BPH with carcinoma. Current practice suggests that sonography be performed in these cases. If a discrete lesion is identified, biopsy is performed. If no discrete lesion is seen, the patient is monitored. A PSA level lower than 4 ng/mL is considered normal, although up to 21% of patients with localized carcinomas have normal PSA levels. It is therefore agreed that the PSA level should not displace a digital rectal examination in the early detection of prostate cancer.

It now appears that the most reasonable screening approach is to combine the three different methods: digital rectal examination, determination of the serum PSA level, and transrectal ultrasonography of the prostate. A study by Catalona et al. compared the various screening methods alone and in combination. In that study a PSA level greater than 4 ng/mL was considered abnormal. When all three screening methods were abnormal, a diagnosis of carcinoma was made in 56% of cases. When PSA plus sonography or digital rectal examination were abnormal, carcinoma was detected in 28% of cases. When the PSA level alone was abnormal, carcinoma was present in approximately 20% of cases. Current practice suggests that measurement of the PSA level in serum and rectal examination, combined with sonography in patients with abnormal findings, will provide a better method of detection of prostatic carcinoma than rectal examination alone.

Question 38

Concerning cysts seen on transrectal sonography,

    (A) seminal vesicle cysts are associated with autosomal dominant polycystic disease
    (B) ejaculatory duct cysts are associated with renal agenesis
    (C) ejaculatory duct cysts are associated with hematospermia
    (D) prostatic utricle cysts are associated with cryptorchidism
    (E) prostatic utricle cysts usually contain spermatozoa
    (F) retention cysts are usually associated with ejaculatory pain

Prostatic cysts are occasionally detected incidentally during evaluation for possible carcinoma. They can be associated with various clinical conditions or symptoms including prostatism, inflammatory conditions, pain, hematospermia, and infertility. Sonography is increasingly used in the workup of these conditions. The differential diagnosis of cystic lesions of the prostate can be difficult, but it is useful to categorize the lesion in question as either near or away from the midline. Association with other diseases or genitourinary anomalies, as well as needle aspiration, will help to narrow the diagnostic possibilities further (Table 8-1).

To understand the etiology of many of the cystic diseases, it is necessary to review the embryologic development of the prostate and adjacent structures. The prostate gland is formed from the urogenital sinus, an endodermal derivative, during the third month of fetal life. The other important precursors to development of the genitourinary system are the paired mesonephric (Wolffian) and paramesonephric (Müllerian) ducts (Figure 8-14A). These are both mesodermal derivatives and originate from the common urogenital fold. The Wolffian ducts develop into the epididymides, vasa deferentia, seminal vesicles, and ejaculatory ducts (Figure 8-14B). The Müllerian ducts fuse in the midline caudally, with the fused tip projecting into the posterior wall of the urogenital sinus as a small swelling, the Müllerian tubercle. The Müllerian tubercle gives rise to the prostatic utricle. There is controversy about whether the Müllerian tubercle is of mesodermal origin or whether it originates from the urogenital sinus (endoderm) and is induced to form as a result of the contact of the fused caudal Müllerian ducts with the urogenital sinus. By

Table 8-1: Cystic lesions of the prostate

Cyst type	Location	Association with other anomalies	Aspiration
Prostatic utricle	Midline	Yes—unilateral renal agenesis, hypospadias, incomplete testicular descent	Rare sperm
Müllerian duct	Midline	No	No sperm
Ejaculatory duct	Near midline	No	Sperm
Seminal vesicle	Near midline extra-prostatic	Yes—renal agenesis, ectopic ureter, vas deferens agenesis, autosomal dominant polycystic disease	Sperm
Benign prostatic hy-perplasia	Lateral in transition zone	No	Usually not necessary
Retention	Lateral in three glandular zones	No	Clear fluid, no sperm
Abscess	Lateral	No	Pus

the third fetal month, most of the Müllerian ductal system has regressed, with the only persistent derivative in the adult male being the appendix testis (Figure 8-14B).

Congenital seminal vesicle cysts have been found in association with abnormalities involving the kidneys and male urogenital tract. A presumed embryologic abnormality of the lower mesonephric duct leads to ipsilateral renal agenesis or dysgenesis, ectopic ureteral insertions, and vas deferens agenesis (Figure 8-6). Only recently described is the association of seminal vesicle cysts with autosomal dominant polycystic disease **(Option (A) is true).** The cysts in these patients are most probably acquired and due to a basement membrane defect, which allows cyst formation in multiple organs, including the seminal vesicles. Because of the association of seminal vesicle cysts with ipsilateral urogenital anomalies, and because only 60% of patients with autosomal dominant polycystic disease have a relevant family history, it has been suggested that patients with cross-sectional imaging evidence of seminal vesicle cysts should undergo renal sonography. Seminal vesicle dilatation can also be acquired as a result of processes that obstruct the seminal vesicle or ejac-

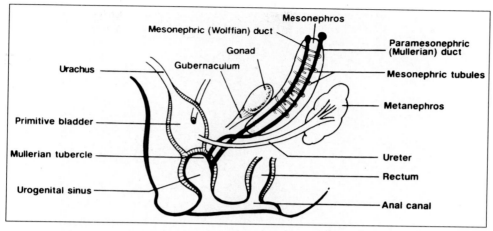

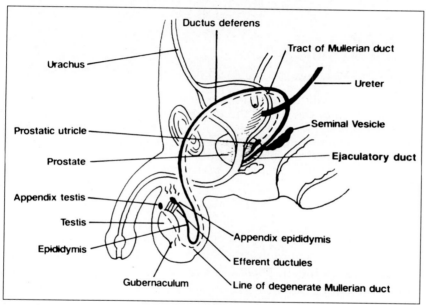

Figure 8-14. Genitourinary system embryology. (A) Sagittal diagram of the genitourinary system in a male fetus prior to sexual differentiation. Only one side of the paired structures is illustrated. (B) Sagittal diagram of the derivatives of the urogenital sinus, Wolffian duct, and Müllerian duct. A dotted line shows the course of the regressed Müllerian duct. See text for discussion. (Reprinted with permission from Nghiem et al. [6].)

ulatory duct (Figure 8-15), or it can be due to either BPH or prior prostatic surgery.

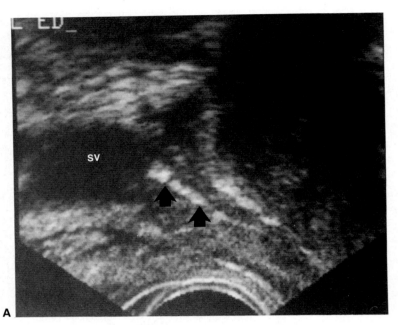

A

Figure 8-15. Ejaculatory duct stones and seminal vesicle dilatation. (A) A sagittal image to the left of the midline shows a line of echogenic foci (arrows) within the ejaculatory duct. The seminal vesicle (SV) appears enlarged and hypoechoic. (B) A transverse image through the left seminal vesicle (outlined by arrows) confirms the enlargement and shows numerous anechoic areas consistent with cystic dilatation.

Unlike seminal vesicle cysts, ejaculatory duct cysts are not associated with other congenital genitourinary anomalies such as renal agenesis **(Option (B) is false).** These cysts can be either congenital or secondary to inflammation, resulting in an obstruction of the ejaculatory duct. Small cysts are usually not associated with symptoms and are detected incidentally (Figure 8-5). Prior to the widespread practice of prostatic sonography, they would have gone undetected. The cysts are classically identified in the central zone along the expected course of the ejaculatory duct.

Large ejaculatory duct cysts can be associated with perineal pain, dysuria, hematospermia **(Option (C) is true),** and ejaculatory pain. Occasionally, large cysts extend cephalad to the prostate (Figure 8-4). These large cysts can contain calculi and debris (Figure 8-16). They can appear midline in location and simulate the appearance of the other midline cystic lesions, primarily prostatic utricle and Müllerian duct cysts.

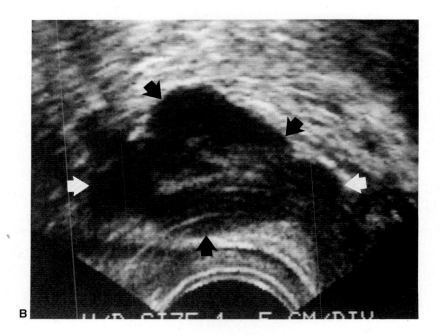

B

Prostatic utricle cysts and Müllerian duct cysts are both midline lesions (Figure 8-17) that are usually indistinguishable by imaging. Utricle cysts (Figure 8-2) are usually smaller than Müllerian duct cysts and are generally intraprostatic. The utricle communicates with the urethra, and so patients may present with the classic symptom of postvoid dribbling; also, fluid is sometimes expressed from the cyst at the time of a rectal examination. Prostatic utricle cysts are associated with a variety of genitourinary abnormalities. These include hypospadias, incomplete testicular descent **(Option (D) is true),** and unilateral renal agenesis. In contrast, Müllerian duct cysts do not communicate with the urethra and are not associated with other genitourinary anomalies. For this reason, it is believed that the utricle cysts have a different embryologic origin than the Müllerian duct cysts.

Müllerian duct cysts arise from the region of the verumontanum. They can become quite large and extend cephalad to the prostate. The cephalic portion of the Müllerian duct develops lateral to the midline, so that cysts developing from these remnants of the Müllerian duct theoretically can extend slightly lateral to the midline or can occur anywhere along the path of Müllerian duct regression, from the scrotum to the utricle. They usually occur in the third and fourth decades of life but have been found in children and older men.

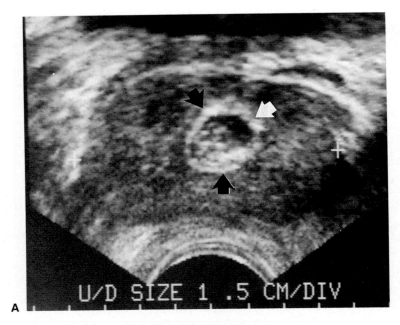

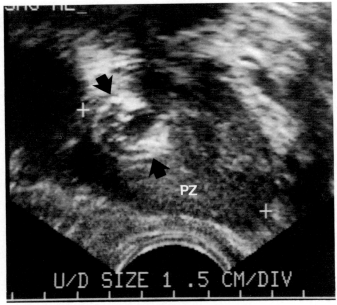

Figure 8-16. Ejaculatory duct cyst with debris. Two images from a prostate sonogram of a 34-year-old man with hematospermia are shown. (A) A transverse image reveals a 1-cm round mass (arrows) with echogenic margins. Internal echogenic debris is identified within the anechoic center of the mass. (B) A sagittal image again shows the mass (arrows) in the base of the gland, anterior to the peripheral zone (PZ). The location of the mass, in combination with the history, is most consistent with the diagnosis of complicated ejaculatory duct cyst.

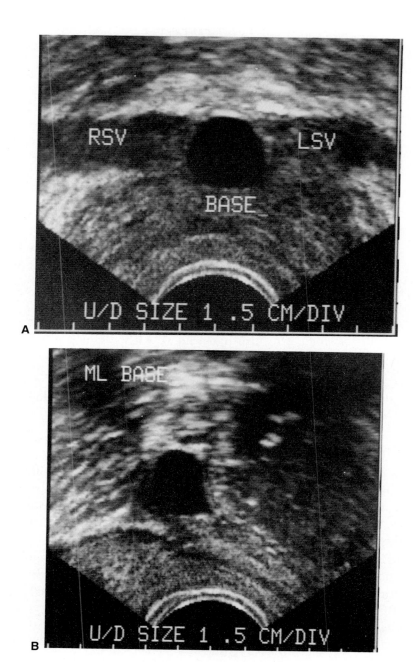

Figure 8-17. Midline cyst. (A) A transverse sonogram through the prostate base shows a discrete, round midline cyst between the right (RSV) and left (LSV) seminal vesicles. (B) A sagittal midline image again shows the cyst at the base of the gland. This could represent either a Müllerian duct cyst or utricle cyst.

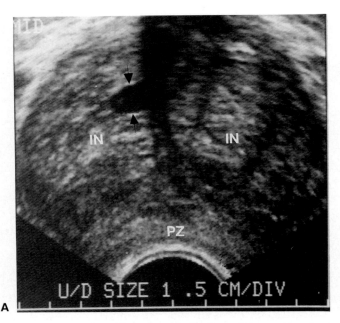

Figure 8-18. Benign prostatic hyperplasia with cystic change. (A) A transverse sonogram through the mid-prostate gland shows an enlarged heterogeneous inner gland (IN) with a cyst (arrows) on the right. PZ = peripheral zone. (B) A transverse sonogram through the apex of the same gland shows several areas of cystic change (arrows) in the left inner gland (IN). PZ = peripheral zone.

Aspiration can help differentiate among the various midline and near-midline cysts. Assuming normal testicular function, aspiration of an ejaculatory duct cyst will yield spermatozoa. In contrast, Müllerian duct cysts never, and prostatic utricle cysts rarely, contain spermatozoa **(Option (E) is false).**

The prostatic cysts discussed above have been located in a midline or near-midline location. There is a group of cystic diseases that are intraprostatic and usually nonmidline in location. These are cysts associated with BPH, retention cysts, and abscesses. Most retention cysts and abscesses are located away from the midline, simply because they are processes of glandular tissue, most of which is located away from the midline. The extraprostatic location of seminal vesicle cysts is also not midline.

The cysts associated with BPH are the most commonly observed cystic lesions (Figure 8-18). They are located in the hyperplastic transition zone, often in association with hyperplastic nodules. They are typically small and do not cause symptoms. They may contain corpora amylacea,

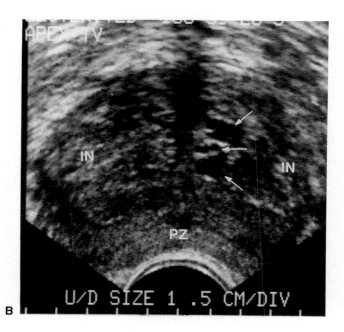

calculi, or hemorrhagic fluid as a result of infarction and necrosis of hyperplastic nodules.

Infectious processes of the prostate can result in cystic change. Cavitary prostatitis results in a "Swiss cheese" appearance to the gland, with cysts of various size distributed throughout the glandular portions of the prostate (Figure 8-19). Usually there is a history of long-standing genitourinary infection. Prostatic abscesses can involve any portion of the gland. Often there is a clinical history of diabetes. The abscess appears as a focal hypoechoic or anechoic mass with thickened or irregular walls, septations, or internal echoes (Figure 8-20). These abscesses are usually not midline. The appearance can be quite similar to that of reported cases of cystic carcinoma.

Retention cysts result from obstruction of prostatic glandular ductules, causing dilatation of the glandular acini (Figures 8-7 and 8-13). They are true acquired cysts; aspiration yields clear or occasionally viscid fluid but never spermatozoa. Retention cysts do not usually cause symptoms (they occasionally do so if located close to the bladder neck), but they can cause obstruction. They are not associated with ejaculatory pain **(Option (F) is false).**

Retention cysts are smooth-walled, unilocular, and less than 2 cm in diameter on sonography. They can be found in any of the three glandular zones of the prostate. Typically they occur in the fifth and sixth decades

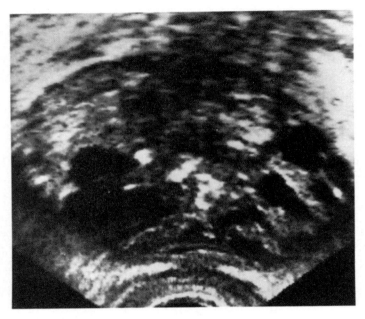

Figure 8-19. Cavitary prostatitis. A transverse scan of a patient with long-standing symptoms of prostatitis shows disorganized prostate tissue with numerous cysts of varying sizes throughout the glandular zones of the prostate. (Reprinted with permission from Nghiem et al. [6].)

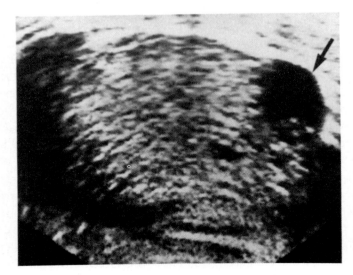

Figure 8-20. Prostatic abscess. A sagittal scan shows an irregular anechoic mass containing solid debris (arrow) in the anterior apical region. Aspiration yielded purulent fluid, which grew *E. coli.* (Reprinted with permission from Nghiem et al. [6]).

of life. If they are located within the transition zone, they can be indistinguishable from cystic change due to BPH. However, neither of these is usually symptomatic, so the distinction is not important.

Karen J. Stuck, M.D.
Gary M. Kellman, M.D.

SUGGESTED READINGS

CYSTIC DISEASES OF THE PROSTATE

1. Alpern MB, Dorfman RE, Gross BH, Gottlieb CA, Sandler MA. Seminal vesicle cysts: association with adult polycystic kidney disease. Radiology 1991; 180:79–80
2. Hamper UM, Epstein JI, Sheth S, Walsh PC, Sanders RC. Cystic lesions of the prostate gland: a sonographic-pathologic correlation. J Ultrasound Med 1990; 9:395–402
3. King BF, Hattery RR, Lieber MM, Berquist TH, Williamson B Jr, Hartman GW. Congenital cystic disease of the seminal vesicle. Radiology 1991; 178:207–211
4. King BF, Hattery RR, Lieber MM, Williamson B Jr, Hartman GW, Berquist TH. Seminal vesicle imaging. RadioGraphics 1989; 9:653–676
5. Littrup PJ, Lee F, McLeary RD, Wu D, Lee A, Kumasaka GH. Transrectal US of the seminal vesicles and ejaculatory ducts: clinical correlation. Radiology 1988; 168:625–628
6. Nghiem HT, Kellman GM, Sandberg SA, Craig BM. Cystic lesions of the prostate. RadioGraphics 1990; 10:635–650

PROSTATE CARCINOMA AND BENIGN PROSTATIC HYPERPLASIA

7. Baran GW, Golin AL, Bergsma CJ, et al. Biologic aggressiveness of palpable and nonpalpable prostate cancer: assessment with endosonography. Radiology 1991; 178:201–206
8. Bude R, Bree RL, Adler RS, Jafri SZ. Transrectal ultrasound appearance of granulomatous prostatitis. J Ultrasound Med 1990; 9:677–680
9. Catalona WJ, Smith DS, Ratliff TL, et al. Measurement of prostate-specific antigen in serum as a screening test for prostate cancer. N Engl J Med 1991; 324:1156–1161
10. Chantelois AE, Parker SH, Sims JE, Horne DW. Malacoplakia of the prostate sonographically mimicking carcinoma. Radiology 1990; 177:193–195
11. Dyke CH, Toi A, Sweet JM. Value of random US-guided transrectal prostate biopsy. Radiology 1990; 176:345–349
12. Gittes RF. Carcinoma of the prostate. N Engl J Med 1991; 324:236–245
13. Hamper UM, Sheth S, Walsh PC, Epstein JI. Bright echogenic foci in early prostatic carcinoma: sonographic and pathologic correlation. Radiology 1990; 176:339–343

14. Hamper UM, Sheth S, Walsh PC, Holtz PM, Epstein JI. Carcinoma of the prostate: value of transrectal sonography in detecting extension into the neurovascular bundle. AJR 1990; 155:1015–1019

15. Hamper UM, Sheth S, Walsh PC, Holtz PM, Epstein JI. Capsular transgression of prostatic carcinoma: evaluation with transrectal US with pathologic correlation. Radiology 1991; 178:791–795

16. Hamper UM, Sheth S, Walsh PC, Holtz PM, Epstein JI. Stage B adenocarcinoma of the prostate: transrectal US and pathologic correlation of nonmalignant hypoechoic peripheral zone lesions. Radiology 1991; 180:101–104

17. Lee F, Littrup PF, Torp-Pedersen ST, et al. Prostate cancer: comparison of transrectal US and digital rectal examination for screening. Radiology 1988; 168:389–394

18. Lee F, Siders DB, Torp-Pedersen ST, Kirscht JL, McHugh TA, Mitchell AE. Prostate cancer: transrectal ultrasound and pathology comparison. A preliminary study of outer gland (peripheral and central zones) and inner gland (transition zone) cancer. Cancer 1991; 67:1132–1142

19. Lee F, Torp-Pedersen S, Littrup PJ, et al. Hypoechoic lesions of the prostate: clinical relevance of tumor size, digital rectal examination, and prostate-specific antigen. Radiology 1989; 170:29–32

20. Lee F, Torp-Pedersen ST, Siders DB, Littrup PJ, McLeary RD. Transrectal ultrasound in the diagnosis and staging of prostatic carcinoma. Radiology 1989; 170:609–615

21. Lee F Jr, Bronson JP, Lee F, et al. Nonpalpable cancer of the prostate: assessment with transrectal US. Radiology 1991; 178:197–199

22. Lile R, Thickman D, Miller GJ, Crawford ED. Prostatic comedocarcinoma: correlation of sonograms with pathologic specimens in three cases. AJR 1990; 155:303–306

23. Littrup PJ, Kane RA, Williams CR, et al. Determination of prostate volume with transrectal US for cancer screening. Part I. Comparison with prostate-specific antigen assays. Radiology 1991; 178:537–542

24. Littrup PJ, Williams CR, Egglin TK, Kane RA. Determination of prostate volume with transrectal US for cancer screening. Part II. Accuracy of *in vitro* and *in vivo* techniques. Radiology 1991; 179:49–53

25. Llewellyn CH, Holthaus LH. Cystic carcinoma in the prostate: findings on transrectal sonography. AJR 1991; 157:785–786

26. McClennan BL. Transrectal US of the prostate: is the technology leading the science? Radiology 1988; 168:571–575

27. Middleton RG, Smith JA Jr, Melzer RB, Hamilton PE. Patient survival and local recurrence rate following radical prostatectomy for prostatic carcinoma. J Urol 1986; 136:422–424

28. Rifkin MD, Dahnert W, Kurtz AB. State of the art: endorectal sonography of the prostate gland. AJR 1990; 154:691–700

29. Rifkin MD, McGlynn ET, Choi H. Echogenicity of prostate cancer correlated with histologic grade and stromal fibrosis: endorectal US studies. Radiology 1989; 170:549–552

30. Rifkin MD, Zerhouni EA, Gatsonis CA, et al. Comparison of magnetic resonance imaging and ultrasonography in staging early prostate cancer. Results of a multi-institutional cooperative trial. N Engl J Med 1990; 323:621–626

31. Sheth S, Hamper UM, Walsh PC, Holtz PM, Epstein JI. Stage A adenocarcinoma of the prostate: transrectal US and sonographic-pathologic correlation. Radiology 1991; 179:35–39

32. Steinfeld AD. Questions regarding the treatment of localized prostate cancer. Radiology 1992; 184:593–598

33. Terris MK, McNeal JE, Stamey TA. Invasion of the seminal vesicles by prostatic cancer: detection with transrectal sonography. AJR 1990; 155:811–815

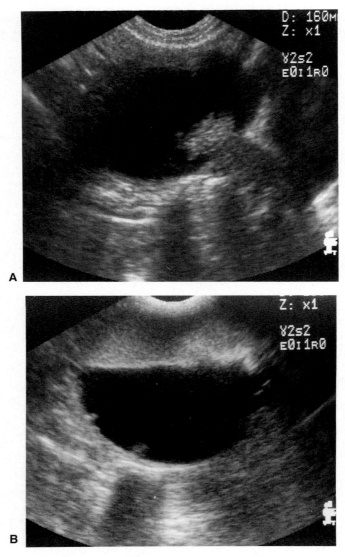

Figure 9-1. This 40-year-old woman complained of vague lower abdominal discomfort. A mass was palpable on pelvic examination. You are shown longitudinal (A) and transverse (B) sonograms of the right pelvis.

Case 9:   Cystic Teratoma

Question 39

Which *one* of the following is the MOST likely diagnosis?

(A) Chronic ectopic pregnancy
(B) Cystic teratoma
(C) Endometrioma
(D) Ovarian cystadenocarcinoma
(E) Appendiceal abscess

Palpable adnexal masses in patients with vague symptoms pose difficulties for the examining gynecologist. Ultrasonography is clearly the procedure of choice for the initial evaluation of such masses. Figure 9-1A is a sagittal transabdominal sonogram of the left adnexa. It displays a large, complex mass that is predominantly cystic, with acoustic shadowing beyond a focal echogenic nodule (Figure 9-2A). Figure 9-1B is a transverse midline sonogram that demonstrates an echogenic fat-fluid level with several additional nodules in the inferior cystic component (Figure 9-2B). There is no identifiable free fluid in the pelvis.

Cystic teratoma is the most likely diagnosis on the basis of the clinical history and the sonographic characteristics of this mass **(Option (B) is correct)**. MRI (Figure 9-3) confirmed the presence of fat, fluid, and soft tissue components within this mass.

The echogenic mural focus with associated acoustic shadowing represents the dermoid plug, a finding that is virtually pathognomonic of a cystic teratoma. The acoustic shadowing caused by the dermoid plug reflects its composition as a mixture of hair and sebum as well as fragments of bone or teeth (Figure 9-4).

Chronic ectopic pregnancy (Option (A)) is an insidious form of tubal pregnancy that is characterized by slow or repeated episodes of hemorrhage and a nonviable embryo. The growth of trophoblastic tissue in the fallopian tube results in a hematosalpinx, which progresses to gradual disintegration of the tubal wall. The episodic hemorrhage incites a local inflammatory response in the peritoneal cavity, which becomes mani-

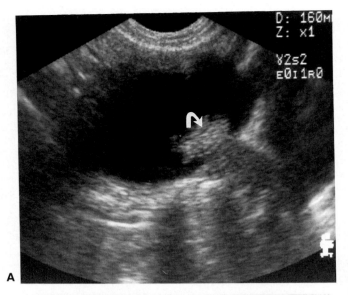

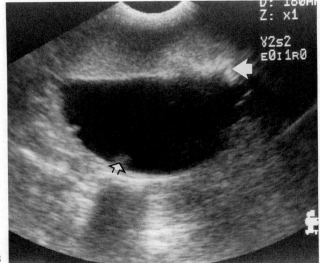

Figure 9-2 (Same as Figure 9-1). Cystic teratoma. (A) A sagittal sonogram of the left adnexa displays a predominantly cystic mass with a focal nodule (arrow) that produces distal acoustic shadowing. (B) A transverse midline scan shows an echogenic fat-fluid level (solid arrow) and small nodular excrescences (open arrow) in the inferior cystic component. These features are virtually pathognomonic for cystic teratoma.

fested as a complex adnexal mass. Adhesions often develop between the mass, adjacent bowel loops, and uterus. The age and vague symptoms of the test patient could support the diagnosis of chronic ectopic pregnancy. However, the sonographic findings of a fat-fluid level and a focal nodule with acoustic shadowing make chronic ectopic pregnancy an unlikely diagnosis.

Chronic ectopic pregnancy has a nonspecific sonographic pattern of a complex adnexal mass, which must be differentiated from endometriosis

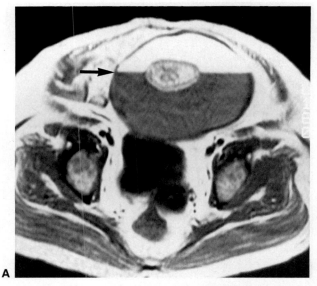

A

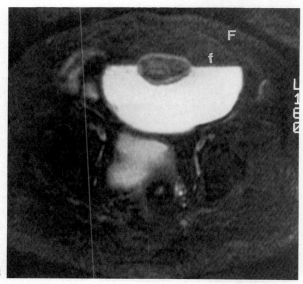

B

Figure 9-3. Same patient as in Figures 9-1 and 9-2. Cystic teratoma. (A) An axial T1-weighted MR image shows the mixed-intensity nodule at the fat-fluid interface (arrow). Fat has a high signal intensity on T1-weighted images, and fluid is dark. (B) An axial T2-weighted MR image confirms that the fat (f) within the dermoid is similar in intensity to the subcutaneous fat (F). Fluid has a high signal intensity on T2-weighted images. (C) A sagittal MR image shows the location of the large teratoma anterior to the uterine fundus (u).

and pelvic inflammatory disease (PID). The mass tends not to be discrete and often involves both the adnexa and the cul-de-sac, and sonography cannot distinguish the posterior aspect of the uterus from the pelvic hematocele. Most of the masses described in a series of 22 cases by Bedi et al. were predominantly solid with scattered cystic components. This appearance was thought to be related to variable amounts of fresh hemorrhage, organized hematoma, degenerating products of conception, and

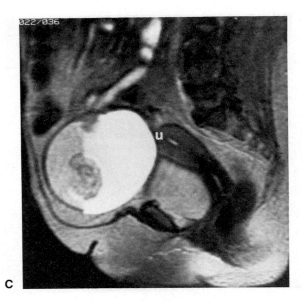

C

Figure 9-3 (Continued)

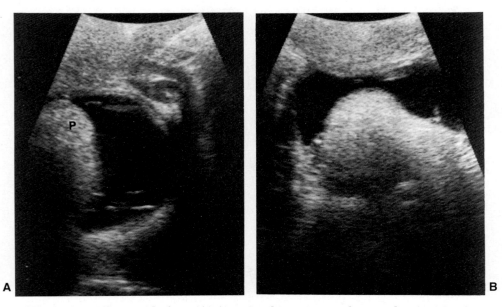

A

B

Figure 9-4. Dermoid plug. (A) A sagittal sonogram shows a benign cystic teratoma with acoustic shadowing from the dermoid plug (P). (B) A coronal sonogram shows the dermoid plug protruding into the cystic component of the teratoma.

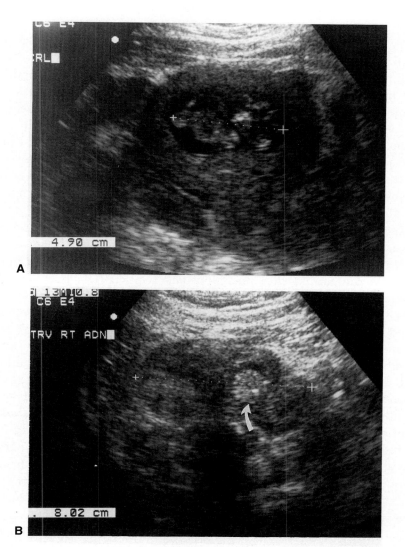

Figure 9-5. Chronic ectopic pregnancy. This 29-year-old woman presented with abdominal cramping for 1 week. She had been amenorrheic
for 11 weeks. (A) Sagittal midline sonogram of the first-trimester intrauterine pregnancy with cursors outlining the embryonic length. (B) A
transverse sonogram shows the complex right-adnexal mass (cursors),
which, at surgery, represented a right ectopic pregnancy with attached
blood clot (arrow) and degenerating products of conception located in the
muscular wall of the fallopian tube.

surrounding extensive adhesions (Figure 9-5). There is no specific time-
table that helps in the differentiation of acute from chronic ectopic preg-

nancy. Usually patients with chronic ectopic pregnancy have an 8-week history of amenorrhea and symptoms of vaginal bleeding and pelvic pain of 2 to 3 weeks duration. This is a relatively long period compared with the duration of symptoms associated with acute ectopic pregnancy. The lower abdominal pain and vaginal bleeding experienced by patients with chronic ectopic pregnancy are often less severe than the excruciating pain, profuse bleeding, and, sometimes, shock in patients with acute ectopic pregnancy. Free peritoneal blood in the cul-de-sac is noted to be less frequent in chronic than in acute ectopic pregnancy. In addition, only half the patients with chronic ectopic pregnancy have a positive serum test for the beta subunit of human chorionic gonadotropin, compared with all patients with acute ectopic pregnancy.

Endometriosis is characterized by the presence of ectopic endometrial tissue with a secondary chronic inflammatory reaction. It most commonly affects women of childbearing age. The clinical history of the test patient is compatible with endometrioma (Option (C)), but the sonographic features are atypical. Endometriomas, or "chocolate cysts," are focal collections of blood that can be anechoic or complex with evenly disbursed echoes, nodules due to clots, or fluid-debris levels (Figure 9-6). The vast majority have thin walls; however, walls of variable thickness and diffusely thickened walls have been described. Septations and loculated areas within the mass can occur but are unusual. Athey and Diment noted septations in 40% (16 of 40) of cases: single in seven endometriomas and multiple in nine. However, in four previous studies, septations were mentioned in only a few lesions. As in patients with PID, the inflammatory reaction sometimes obscures pelvic tissue planes. Associated adhesions and scar tissue can block the fallopian tubes. In severe cases, multiple collections can be seen with hemorrhage in various stages. The dermoid plug and fat-fluid level seen in the test images make endometrioma a very unlikely diagnosis.

Both the clinical history of the test patient and the sonographic features in the test images preclude the diagnosis of ovarian cystadenocarcinoma (Option (D)). Ovarian tumors are common throughout adult life, but malignancies occur most frequently in postmenopausal women. The incidence of ovarian carcinoma increases with age, peaking in the sixth and seventh decades of life. Most tumors that are diagnosed early are discovered serendipitously in asymptomatic patients. Cystadenocarcinomas tend to be quite large, averaging 15 to 30 cm in diameter at the time of presentation. The lack of initial symptoms means that more than two-thirds of patients have advanced disease at presentation, resulting in a poor 5-year survival rate. Depending on their size and mobility, these tumors can be located in the adnexa, superior to the uterine fundus, or low in the cul-de-sac either in the rectovaginal pouch of Douglas or

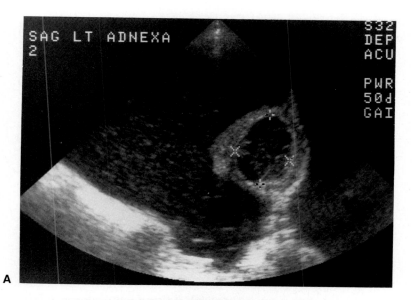

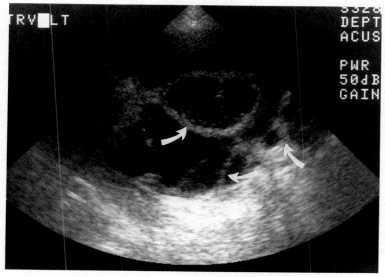

Figure 9-6. Endometrioma. This 43-year-old woman has had prior exploratory laparotomies for endometriosis involving both ovaries. (A) Sagittal sonogram of the left adnexal mass with a thick-walled nodule (cursors) and fine low-level internal echoes. (B) A transverse sonogram through the nodule shows multiple loculations (arrows) within this mass. The appearance is likely due to numerous episodes of hemorrhage over a long period of time. (C) A transverse sonogram through another portion demonstrates a fluid-debris level (arrow) within another loculated component. There is good sound transmission through the entire mass, indicating its cystic nature. This constellation of findings without constitutional signs or symptoms is most suggestive of endometrioma.

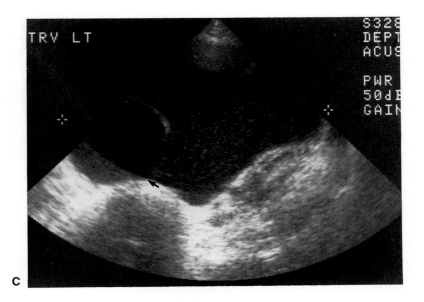

C

between the bladder and uterus. The main histologic cell types are serous and mucinous tumors. These tumors are primarily multiloculated
masses, often containing abundant papillary projections (Figure 9-7),
which is in contrast to the fat-fluid level in the test image. Turbid or
bloody fluid is usually found on pathologic examination. The solid nodules within these tumors do not contain fat, hair, bone, or teeth and are
therefore not hyperechogenic with acoustic shadowing.

Appendiceal abscess (Option (E)) is a complication of acute appendicitis, a disease that can occur at any age but is most prevalent in adolescence. Abscesses are estimated to form in approximately 2 to 7% of
patients with appendicitis. The frequency of perforation in acute appendicitis is approximately 15%; however, only in one-third of cases with
perforation does the process evolve to frank abscess formation. Patients
with both complicated and uncomplicated appendicitis typically have
some systemic symptoms, including fever, leukocytosis, and an elevated
erythrocyte sedimentation rate. Sonographic signs of appendiceal perforation include localized right lower quadrant fluid collections, occasionally with demonstration of the appendiceal lumen as a fingerlike, hyperechoic projection; free intraperitoneal fluid; and a complex paracecal
mass or lower pelvic mass with increased through sound transmission.
The inflammatory mass of an appendiceal abscess appears anechoic or
hypoechoic with thickened walls and ill-defined borders. It can contain
variable amounts of internal debris. However, the fat-fluid level and
acoustic shadowing seen in the test image should not be confused with a

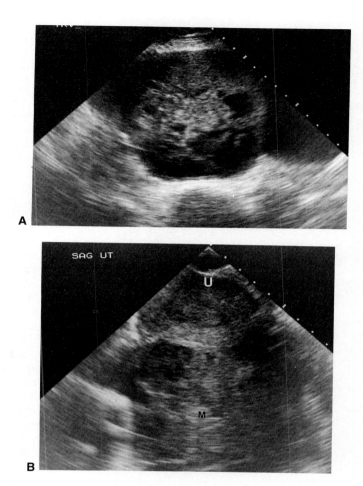

Figure 9-7. Left ovarian cystadenocarcinoma. (A) A transverse sonogram demonstrates a complex mass with solid and cystic components.
(B) A sagittal transvaginal sonogram demonstrates the uterus (U), which
is separate from the mass (M). At surgery, a large endometrioid carcinoma containing bloody fluid and focal solid areas of grade III carcinoma
intermixed with grade I and II carcinoma was found.

gas-containing abscess or an appendicolith. Reflection of the ultrasound
beam at a soft tissue-gas interface generally produces acoustic shadowing with reverberation/ring-down artifacts from air in the nondependent
portion of the abscess cavity. If the transducer is angled so that the fluid
portion of an abscess is initially encountered, a dense echogenic line can
be produced at the fluid-gas interface as a result of almost total reflection
of the ultrasound beam. In some cases, a gas-containing abscess appears
as a very densely echogenic mass with acoustic shadowing or as a more

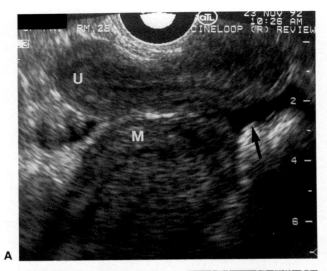

A

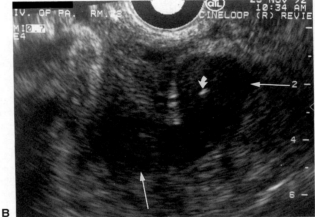

B

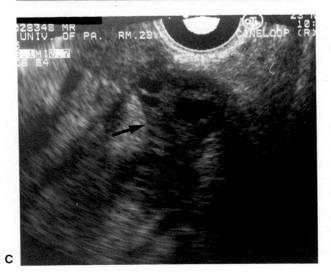

C

Figure 9-8. Appendicitis with abscess. This 20-year-old woman presented with right lower quadrant pain and fever. Sonograms were taken to rule out pelvic inflammatory disease. (A) A midline sagittal transvaginal scan shows cul-de-sac fluid (arrow) and a moderately echogenic mass (M) with echotexture similar to that of the uterus (U). (B) A sagittal transvaginal sonogram of the right adnexa shows a tubular hypoechoic mass (straight arrows) with a shadowing echogenic focus representing an appendicolith (curved arrow). (C) A sagittal transvaginal sonogram of the right adnexa shows small follicles in a normal-appearing right ovary (arrow). At surgery a large mass was removed; it contained a tubular structure filled with hemorrhage and was surrounded by a fibrous tissue reaction. The final histopathologic diagnosis was suppurative appendicitis and serositis.

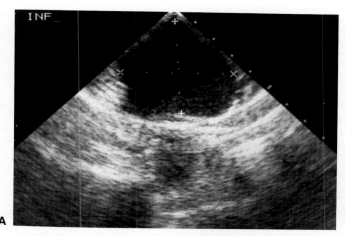

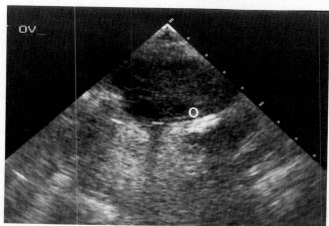

Figure 9-9. Appendiceal rupture with abscess formation. (A) A sagittal transvaginal sonogram shows a pelvic fluid collection (cursors) in a 22-year-old woman with pain, noncontributing clinical history, and limited pelvic examination. (B) A coronal transvaginal sonogram shows the separate edematous right ovary (O) with numerous follicles.

complex mass with several regions of shadowing due to numerous gas pockets. An appendicolith appears as a small, punctate, echodense focus with distal acoustic shadowing (Figure 9-8). The pelvis is a frequent site of intraperitoneal spread of infection; therefore, inflammatory disease of the appendix can be difficult to differentiate from tubo-ovarian processes. Ultrasonography is occasionally of value in clarifying the nature of a palpable right lower quadrant mass in a female patient by demonstrating the mass as separate from the normal ovaries (Figure 9-9).

Question 40

Concerning cystic teratoma,

    (A) it is the most common germ cell tumor
    (B) the purely cystic form is uncommon
    (C) it often simulates bowel on sonography
    (D) the "tip of the iceberg" sign refers to acoustic shadowing from teeth
    (E) there is a 10% risk of malignant transformation

The three major functional and anatomic components that may give rise to ovarian tumors are the germinal cells, the stroma composed of sex cord and mesenchymal cells, and the surface epithelium. Of the germ cell tumors, only cystic teratoma (dermoid cyst) is benign. It is by far the most common type in this group, accounting for approximately 15% of all primary ovarian tumors **(Option (A) is true).**

Generally, germ cell tumors of the ovary occur in much younger patients than do tumors originating from the epithelium. There is a very wide age distribution for cystic teratomas (prepubertal to postmenopausal); however, the vast majority occur during the reproductive years. Malignant transformation of a benign cystic teratoma is rare; the estimated risk is approximately 2 to 4% **(Option (E) is false).** It has been well documented that this occurs mainly in the dermoid plug in postmenopausal patients, with squamous cell carcinoma being the most common malignant lesion.

Cystic teratomas arise from all three germ layers and therefore display different sonographic appearances depending on the variable proportions of internal elements such as fat, hair, teeth, and skin. The overall heterogeneity of these lesions is reflected in their variable gross and microscopic appearances. Pure sebum consists of complex lipids derived from keratinizing epidermis and sebaceous glands. It mimics simple fluid on sonography because of its homogeneity (Figure 9-10). The sebum in these tumors is frequently mixed with hair, and therefore a classic, purely cystic appearance on ultrasonography is uncommon **(Option (B) is true).**

Teratomas that contain only fluid have been shown on histologic inspection to be lined by neuroectoderm. Sheth et al. compared the ultrasonographic and CT features of 23 teratomas and noted that only 2 (8.7%) were entirely anechoic. Most of the dermoid cysts appeared as complex lesions containing both hyperechoic and hypoechoic components. The poorly echogenic regions on sonography corresponded to fluid on CT in 5 cases and to very low-attenuation fat in 12 cases.

Benign cystic teratomas can vary from 0.5 to 40 cm in diameter, but most measure less than 10 cm in maximum dimension. They are usually

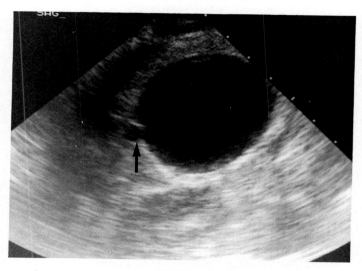

Figure 9-10. Cystic teratoma mimicking simple cyst. A sagittal trans-vaginal sonogram of the right adnexa demonstrates a predominantly cystic mass with a nodular area (arrow) in the wall. This mass did not resolve after several menstrual cycles, and therefore surgery was performed. Hair was noted to be growing from a 1-cm protuberance on the inner lining of the cyst, which contained clear translucent fluid and thick cheesy material.

unilocular but can be divided by a few thin septa into two or more compartments. The wall is 2 to 5 mm thick and is typically regular. The cystic teratoma in the test patient has distinctive ultrasonographic characteristics that help differentiate it from other adnexal masses. The fat-fluid level, which is due to the fat-fluid or hair-fluid interface, is a relatively infrequent finding but is a unique feature of dermoid cysts. In such cases, large quantities of hair or fat actually float on the aqueous fluid. This often has a different appearance from the fluid-debris levels that are seen more often in hemorrhagic ovarian cysts or endometriomas (Figure 9-11). The proteinaceous debris from prior hemorrhage lies in a dependent position with serous fluid on top. Posterior acoustic shadowing beyond the dermoid cyst has varied appearances and can be produced by hair, fat, teeth, or bone fragments. A mixture of sebum and hair is highly echogenic, with acoustic shadowing that can totally obscure the back wall of a very large mass. In such cases, the near wall of the teratoma is usually recognized, hence the term "tip of the iceberg" sign (Figure 9-12). Of all the echogenic components, calcium from bone or teeth is less common than fat or hair, and acoustic shadowing from such small calcific foci is generally very discrete **(Option (D) is false).**

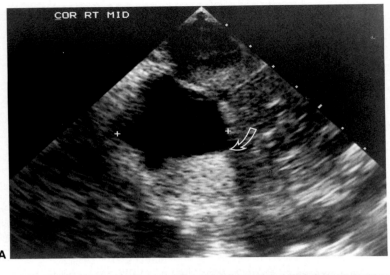

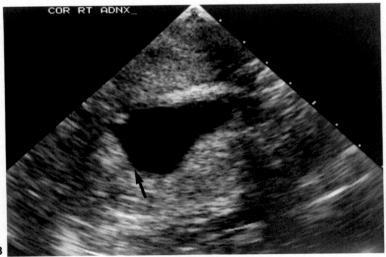

Figure 9-11. Cystic teratoma. This 41-year-old woman presented to the emergency room with abdominal pain. (A) A coronal transvaginal sonogram of the right adnexa demonstrates a complex mass (cursors) with a fluid-debris level (arrow). (B) The level (arrow) shifted on repositioning the patient. At surgery, this cyst was found to contain sebaceous material, hair, and calcification.

Some ovarian teratomas can mimic gas- or feces-filled bowel loops within the pelvis because of their heterogeneous internal architecture and distal acoustic shadowing **(Option (C) is true)** (Figure 9-13). In

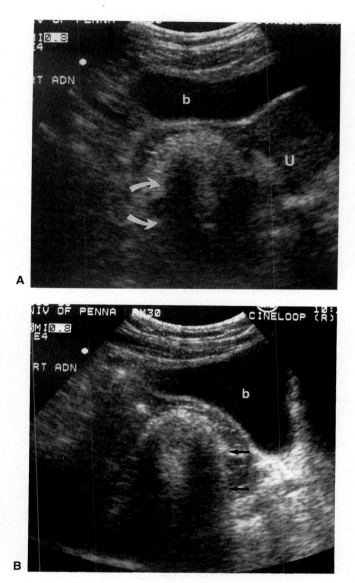

Figure 9-12. "Tip of the iceberg" sign. Transverse (A) and sagittal (B) sonograms demonstrate extensive acoustic shadowing (arrows) beyond a highly echogenic teratoma. b = bladder; U = uterus.

addition, they can be pedunculated and located superior to the uterine fundus; this is also a possible explanation for previously reported failures to diagnose these tumors by transabdominal ultrasonography. In an early series by Laing et al. of 51 surgically proven cases of teratoma, approximately 24% were missed by sonography. Continued technological

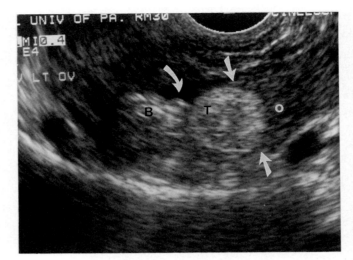

Figure 9-13 (left). Cystic teratoma. A coronal transvaginal sonogram shows bowel (B) with echogenicity similar to that of an adjacent small teratoma (T). There are "beaks" of normal ovarian tissue (straight arrows) surrounding the more sharply marginated tumor. The curved arrow represents fluid. o = ovary.

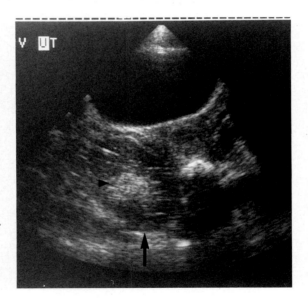

Figure 9-14 (right). Bowel simulating cystic teratoma. This 22-year-old woman presented with a history of constipation and possible pelvic mass. A sonogram of the right adnexa shows an ill-defined heterogeneous mass (arrow) with an echogenic center (arrowhead), which changed little after administration of a water enema. Radiographs (not shown) revealed only bowel without evidence of fat or calcium.

improvements, including transvaginal sonography and color Doppler imaging, coupled with techniques such as the water enema, have been very helpful in visualizing the peristaltic activity in echogenic areas containing bowel (Figure 9-14). The test case demonstrates another classic sign of cystic teratoma. The Rokitansky nodule or dermoid plug is an echogenic focus that protrudes from the inner wall of a predominantly cystic mass. These nodules often demonstrate acoustic shadowing as a result of a large variety of tumorous tissues (Figure 9-4). Buy et al. noted an 80% frequency of dermoid plugs in a series of 43 tumors. These dermoid plugs ranged in diameter from 1 to 6.5 cm and were frequently round or oval with a regular border. They tended to make an acute angle with the cyst wall. In view of the above-described features, careful scanning with state-of-the-art ultrasonography equipment should yield higher sensitivity and specificity rates for the diagnosis of cystic teratoma.

Question 41

Concerning endometrioma,

- (A) it is the most common form of endometriosis
- (B) age is helpful in distinguishing it from cystadenocarcinoma
- (C) the most common sonographic appearance is a simple cystic mass
- (D) the ovary is the most common site
- (E) acoustic shadowing differentiates it from cystic teratoma

The exact pathogenesis of endometriosis remains controversial. Probably the most widely accepted theory is that of transtubal retrograde implantation of endometrial tissue during menstruation. Other explanations include hematogenous or lymphatic dissemination and müllerian metaplasia of peritoneal mesothelium into functional endometrium. This disease afflicts premenopausal women, with a mean age range reported in several series as 28 to 35 years. Cystic ovarian neoplasms occur most frequently in postmenopausal women. In a large series of 170 epithelial ovarian tumors, Buy et al. found the mean patient age for various lesions as follows: benign, 50 years; borderline, 52 years; and malignant, 57 years. Thus, age is helpful in distinguishing endometrioma from cystadenoma or cystadenocarcinoma **(Option (B) is true).**

Endometriosis is an enigmatic disorder characterized by the growth of functioning endometrial tissue within the peritoneal cavity yet outside the uterus, usually on the surface of abdominal and pelvic organs. It has two distinct clinical and sonographic presentations: diffuse and focal (Figure 9-15). In the diffuse form, which is the more common **(Option (A) is false),** endometrial tissue implants on the serosal surfaces of the peritoneum and bowel and on the uterosacral ligaments.

These very tiny nodules, usually less than a few millimeters in size, can be extremely difficult to depict by any imaging modality. The ectopic endometrial tissue responds to hormonal changes and bleeds during menses; therefore, a variable size and appearance may be noted during different phases of a patient's cycle or with the onset of reactive fibrosis.

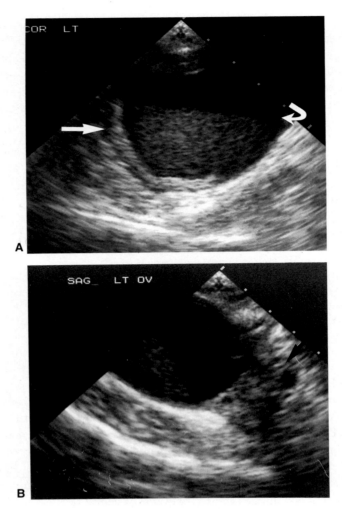

Figure 9-15. Diffuse and focal endometriosis. This 38-year-old woman presented with a history of a questionable pelvic mass. (A) A coronal transvaginal sonogram of the left adnexus demonstrates a thick-walled mass (straight arrow) with a fluid-debris level (curved arrow). (B) A sagittal transvaginal sonogram shows the mass projecting off the left ovary (arrow). At surgery there were diffuse endometrial implants involving the peritoneal cavity and both fallopian tubes, as well as a focal left endometrioma.

These deposits may be more evident when free peritoneal fluid is present. Transvaginal and transrectal sonograms may offer some help in localizing small implants involving the bladder and rectosigmoid colon. CT and MRI generally have the same difficulty as sonography in diagnosing the diffuse form of endometriosis. An isolated CT case report by

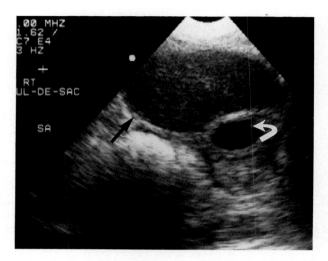

Figure 9-16. Endometrioma. This 48-year-old woman presented with a history of menorrhagia, dysmenorrhea, and persistent mass behind an enlarged, irregular uterus. A sagittal sonogram of the right cul-de-sac demonstrates a thin-walled mass (straight arrow) filled with fine, evenly disbursed echoes. An adjacent small follicle (curved arrow) was also noted. At surgery, there was a cystic structure with direct communication to the distal right fallopian tube. The cyst had a smooth, inner mucosal surface and contained old blood; there was also an adjacent, very small cyst containing brown fluid.

Nardi et al. described peritoneal seeding and endometrial involvement of the greater omentum and mesentery, which mimicked a case of peritoneal carcinomatosis. At present, however, no imaging procedure is either sensitive or specific enough to evaluate diffuse endometriosis, and a definitive diagnosis still requires operative intervention.

On the other hand, the sonographic, CT, and MR features of the localized form of endometriosis (endometrioma) have been extensively studied. When implants become greater than 1 to 2 cm in size, they can usually be identified readily by ultrasonography. The masses tend to be round or ovoid, but lobulated and bilobed masses have been reported. Athey and Diment described posterior acoustic enhancement in almost 90% of cases. This is believed to be due to the fluid nature of the blood products of variable age within the masses. Endometriomas range in size from 3 to 20 cm. Their internal architecture frequently exhibits a pattern of diffuse, fine, evenly disbursed echoes without septations (Figure 9-16). The presence of these echoes excludes the diagnosis of a simple cyst **(Option (C) is false).** The overall appearance of endometriomas can closely simulate that of hemorrhagic ovarian cysts, however. Clumps of

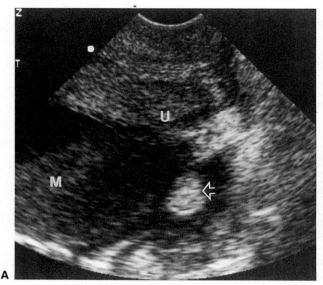

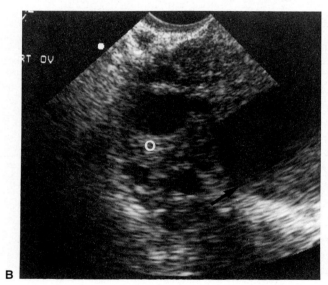

Figure 9-17. Endometriosis mimicking cystic teratoma. This 48-year-old woman presented for sonography to rule out ovarian cyst. (A) A sagittal transvaginal sonogram shows a complex mass (M) in the cul-de-sac posterior to the uterus (U). Note the very echogenic solid nodule (arrow), which lacked acoustic shadowing. (B) A coronal transvaginal sonogram shows a normal right ovary (O) with numerous small follicles adjacent to this predominantly cystic mass with a fluid-debris level (arrow), which appears different from the fat-fluid level in the test case.

high-intensity echoes secondary to clots occasionally occur within endometriomas (Figure 9-17). However, acoustic shadowing, which is often seen beyond various tissues in a cystic teratoma, is not a feature of endometriomas **(Option (E) is true).** Endometriosis has been found in the heart, lungs, pleura, lower extremities, and subarachnoid space, but most cases involve the pelvis. The diffuse form typically occurs in numerous sites including the cul-de-sac, rectovaginal septum, and fallopian tubes. Endometriomas are most often located within the ovary **(Option (D) is true)**. Schiller et al. described a series of 23 endometriomas, of which 15 could not be distinguished sonographically from the ipsilateral ovary, 7 appeared intraovarian, and 1 was clearly extraovarian.

Question 42

Concerning cystadenocarcinomas,

  (A) they arise from the ovarian stroma
  (B) septations and papillary excrescences are typical of both mucinous and serous tumors
  (C) they are the most common cause of simple unilocular ovarian cysts in postmenopausal patients
  (D) they are the most common cause of pseudomyxoma peritonei
  (E) Doppler sonography usually shows abnormally high diastolic flow

Cystadenocarcinomas are classified as epithelial ovarian tumors, which collectively arise from the surface epithelium that covers the ovary **(Option (A) is false)** and are the most common ovarian tumors, accounting for 70 to 75% of cases. Germ cell tumors constitute 15 to 20%, sex cord stromal tumors account for 10%, and metastatic tumors to the ovary account for 5%. Bilateral involvement is frequent with ovarian carcinoma, occurring in 20 to 60% of carcinomas of various histologic types (Figure 9-18).

Ovarian tumors often contain several different cell types, and generally the tumor is named for the predominant type. Epithelial tumors are believed to arise from mesothelial inclusion cysts that result from invagination of the mesothelium after the rupture of ovarian follicles. The exact etiology of the neoplastic transformation is unknown. Intraperitoneal spread is the primary mode of dissemination of the most common epithelial tumors. Lymphatic spread and local invasion of contiguous structures are also common (Figure 9-18). Hematogenous metastases tend to occur late in the disease. Peritoneal seeding results when the ovarian capsule has been penetrated (Figures 9-18 through 9-20). This is often evident initially as abdominal and pelvic ascites. Tumor invasion of lymphatic channels has been postulated as the cause of the ascitic fluid. Organs with the largest peritoneal surfaces such as the liver, bowel, and omentum are commonly involved in cases of extensive disease (Figure 9-20). Pseudomyxoma peritonei refers to the gross appearance of the abdomen when filled with a gelatinous material resembling the contents of the primary tumor. This is most often due to mucinous cystadenocarcinomas; only 2 to 5% are due to mucinous cystadenomas **(Option (D) is**

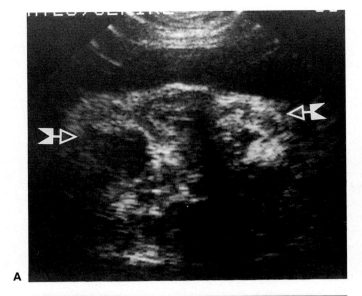

A

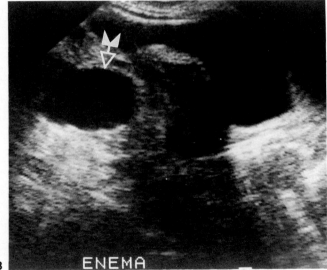

B

Figure 9-18. Bilateral serous papillary cystadenocarcinoma. This 61-year-old woman presented with an 18-month history of abdominal discomfort, weight loss, and decreased stool caliber. (A) A transverse sonogram shows ill-defined bilateral adnexal masses (arrows). (B) A sagittal sonogram taken after a water enema shows a large right cystic component (arrow). Water was noted to enter and leave portions of the mass, suggesting bowel involvement by tumor.

true). Rarely, pseudomyxoma peritonei is appendiceal in origin secondary to a mucinous adenocarcinoma or a type of foreign-body peritonitis.

Cystadenocarcinomas are papillary tumors lined with cells that secrete either a mucous or a serous substance. The serous variety is the most common ovarian epithelial tumor, constituting 30% of all ovarian tumors and 40% of all ovarian cancers. Serous tumors are benign (60%), borderline (15%), or malignant (25%). The mucinous variety is the sec-

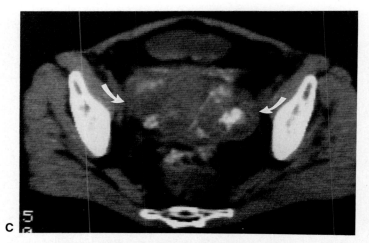

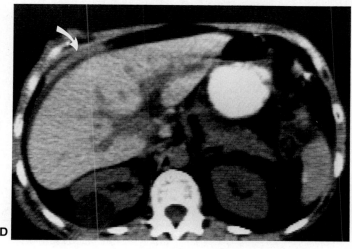

Figure 9-18 (Continued). Bilateral serous papillary cystadenocarcinoma. (C) A CT scan of the pelvis shows bilateral calcified masses (arrows). (D) A CT scan of the abdomen shows peritoneal studding (arrow). A right renal cyst is noted incidentally. At surgery, hysterectomy was not possible because of bulky disease involving the parietal peritoneum, mesentery, bowel, uterus, and liver. Numerous psammoma bodies were noted.

ond most common type of ovarian epithelial tumor, accounting for 20 to 25% of all ovarian tumors and 10% of all ovarian cancers. About 80% are benign, 10 to 15% are borderline, and 5% are malignant. Sonographically, both the serous and mucinous tumors are predominantly fluid-filled masses with multiple septations and nodular vegetations (Figure 9-21) **(Option (B) is true).** These solid areas are more common in malignant masses than in benign ones (Figure 9-22). The more solid and irregular the internal morphology of an epithelial tumor on ultrasonography, the more likely it is to be malignant. Mucinous tumors tend to contain more septa and echogenic debris than do serous ones (Figure 9-23). Benign serous tumors can appear unilocular with a smooth internal surface or only a solitary septum or few papillary projections. Some con-

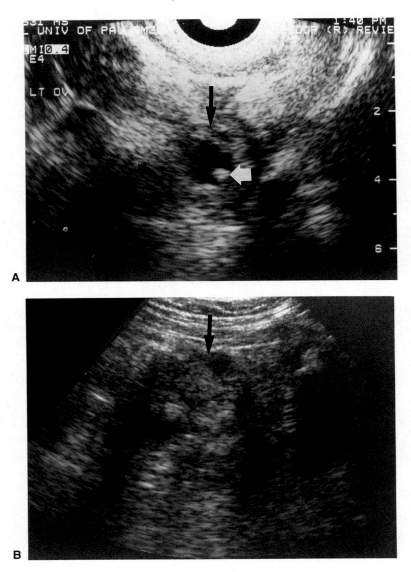

Figure 9-19. Metastatic serous cystadenocarcinoma. This 28-year-old woman had a right salpingo-oophorectomy 3 years earlier for "border-line" malignancy. (A) A coronal transvaginal sonogram shows a small, thick-walled left ovarian mass (black arrow) with echogenic focus (white arrow) protruding into the cystic central cavity. (B) Persistence of a solid, ill-defined mass (arrow) after water enema confirmed the validity of the observation and excluded a loop of bowel. (C) A CT scan confirmed the presence of a serous tumor (arrow).

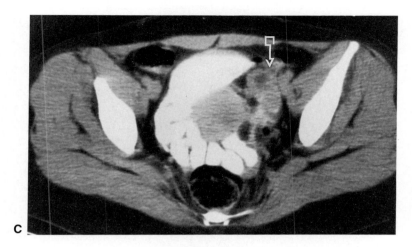

Figure 9-19 (Continued)

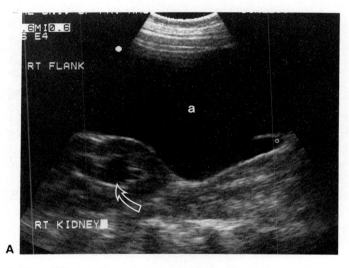

Figure 9-20. Bilateral serous cystadenocarcinoma. This 33-year-old woman at 17 weeks gestation complained of rapidly increasing abdominal girth. (A) A sagittal sonogram of the right flank shows a large amount of ascites (a) and hydronephrosis (arrow). (B and C) Transverse sonograms of a complex mass involving both ovaries. Panel C shows a large, solid mass (M) superior to the uterus.

fusion can occur during attempts to differentiate these serous tumors from other cystic pelvic abnormalities (Figure 9-24). Unilocular cystic masses have a very low risk of malignancy irrespective of the patient's

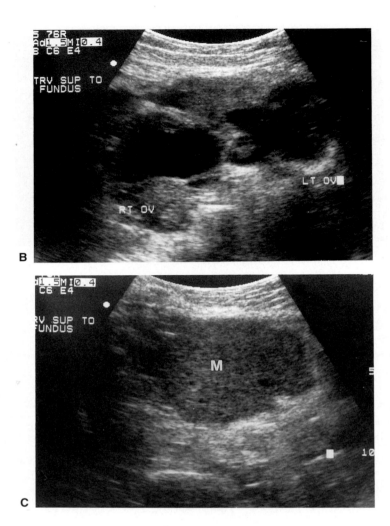

age. The most common cause of such lesions in postmenopausal patients is a benign cyst **(Option (C) is false).** The prevalence of unilateral cysts in postmenopausal women is 10 to 20%. The exact stimulus for post-menopausal cyst formation is unknown. Wolf et al. showed that there is no significant difference in cyst prevalence between patients being given various hormone regimens and those not taking hormones. It is possible, however, that sequential hormone treatment stimulates the postmeno-pausal ovary to form cysts. It is not known whether ovaries actively pro-ducing cysts have a higher potential for malignancy.

Transvaginal sonography has significantly improved our ability to characterize the internal morphology of cystic ovarian masses. The addi-

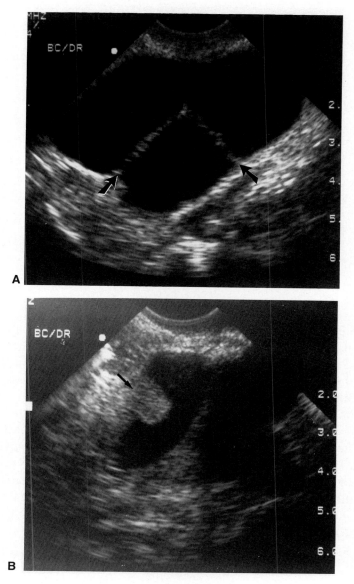

Figure 9-21. Serous cystadenoma. This 71-year-old woman had a palpable right adnexal mass and a history of total abdominal hysterectomy, left salpingo-oophorectomy, and appendectomy more than 25 years earlier. (A through C) Coronal transvaginal sonograms demonstrate numerous thick septa (arrows in panel A) within a predominantly cystic mass. There are solid nodular excrescences (arrow in panel B) extruding into a lateral component of the mass. There is a fluid-debris level within one loculated compartment (arrow in panel C).

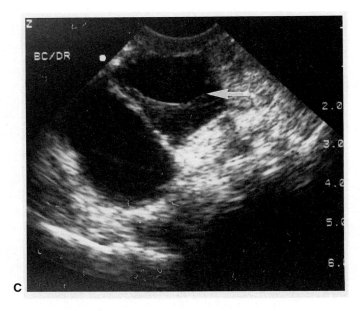

C

tion of duplex and color Doppler sonography to vaginal probes may further increase our ability to differentiate benign from malignant ovarian masses. Preliminary investigative reports indicate that color Doppler sonography can detect blood flow in small, low-resistance vessels that form in tumors. Pulsed Doppler can then be used to quantify and characterize flow patterns in areas of tumor neovascularity. Malignancies show increased diastolic flow, presumably secondary to deficient muscle in the walls of neovessels and possibly to arteriovenous shunting **(Option (E) is true)**. In our sonography laboratory, when we interrogate vessels in and around an ovarian mass, we are currently using a pulsatility index of <1.0 and a resistive index of <0.4 as indicators worrisome for malignancy. Unfortunately, even at this level there is significant overlap between benign and malignant disorders.

Beverly G. Coleman, M.D.

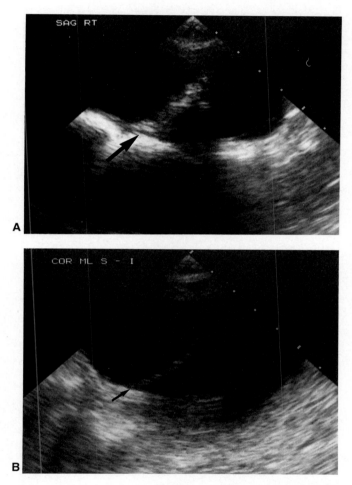

Figure 9-22. Serous cystadenofibroma. This 67-year-old woman presented with a history of mass on intravenous urogram. (A) A sagittal
transvaginal sonogram shows a predominantly cystic mass anterior and
superior to the uterus, with a very thickened, irregular septum (arrow).
(B) A coronal transvaginal sonogram shows a thin septum (arrow) in
another portion of this mass. The ovaries were not visualized.

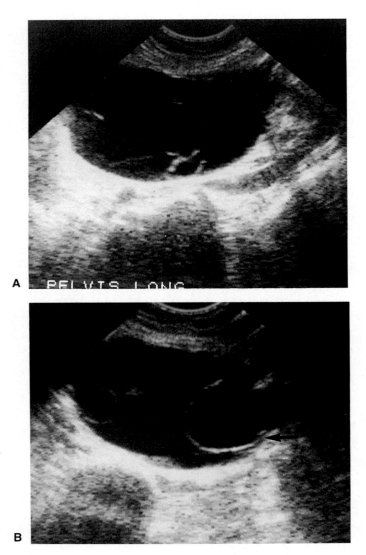

Figure 9-23. Mucinous cystadenoma. (A) A sagittal sonogram shows a multiloculated, cystic pelvic mass in an asymptomatic 50-year-old woman. (B) A transverse sonogram shows a polypoid vegetation (arrow) arising from the wall of the cystic mass. A mucin-filled cyst was found at surgery.

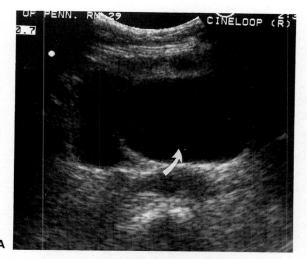

A

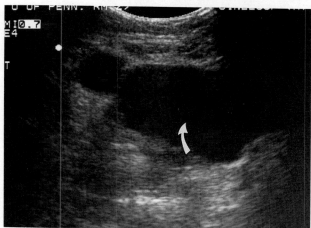

B

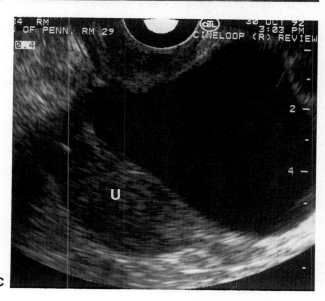

C

Figure 9-24. Serous cystadenoma simulating bladder diverticulum. This 53-year-old patient presented with vaginal bleeding and a history of polycystic ovary disease. Transverse (A) and sagittal (B) sonograms of the pelvis demonstrate a cystic mass (arrow), which appeared larger on postvoid scans. (C) A transvaginal sonogram shows the cystic mass impressing the anterior aspect of the uterus (U). The question of bladder diverticulum was raised, and MRI was performed. Axial T1-weighted (D) and T2-weighted (E) MR scans confirm the presence of a large cystic mass (M) deforming the bladder (B).

293

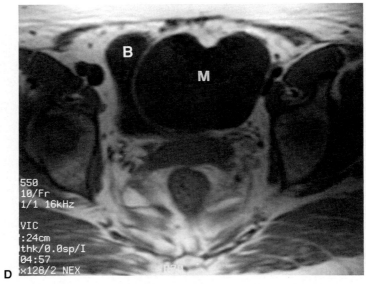

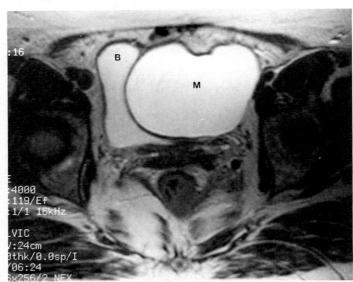

SUGGESTED READINGS

CYSTIC TERATOMA

1. Buy J-N, Ghossain MA, Moss AA, et al. Cystic teratoma of the ovary: CT detection. Radiology 1989; 171:697–701
2. Guttman PH Jr. In search of the elusive benign cystic ovarian teratoma: application of the ultrasound "tip of the iceberg" sign. JCU 1977; 5:403–406

3. Laing FC, Van Dalsem VF, Marks WM, Barton JL, Martinez DA. Dermoid cysts of the ovary: their ultrasonographic appearances. Obstet Gynecol 1981; 57:99–104

4. Quinn SF, Erickson F, Black WC. Cystic ovarian teratomas: the sonographic appearance of the dermoid plug. Radiology 1985; 155:477–478

5. Sheth S, Fishman EK, Buck JL, Hamper UM, Sanders RC. The variable sonographic appearances of ovarian teratomas: correlation with CT. AJR 1988; 151:331–334

6. Sisler CL, Siegel MJ. Ovarian teratomas: a comparison of the sonographic appearance in prepubertal and postpubertal girls. AJR 1990; 154:139–141

7. Skaane P, Klott KJ. Fat-fluid level in a cystic ovarian teratoma. J Comput Assist Tomogr 1981; 5:577–579

CHRONIC ECTOPIC PREGNANCY

8. Bedi DG, Fagan CJ, Nocera RM. Chronic ectopic pregnancy. J Ultrasound Med 1984; 3:347–352

9. Bedi DG, Moeller D, Fagan CJ, Winsett MZ. Chronic ectopic pregnancy. A comparison with acute ectopic pregnancy. Eur J Radiol 1987; 7:46–48

10. Cole T, Corlett RC Jr. Chronic ectopic pregnancy. Obstet Gynecol 1982; 59:63–68

ENDOMETRIOMA

11. Athey PA, Diment DD. The spectrum of sonographic findings in endometriomas. J Ultrasound Med 1989; 8:487–491

12. Baltarowich OH, Kurtz AB, Pasto ME, Rifkin MD, Needleman L, Goldberg BB. The spectrum of sonographic findings in hemorrhagic ovarian cysts. AJR 1987; 148:901–905

13. Birnholz JC. Endometriosis and inflammatory disease. Semin US CT MR 1983; 4:184–192

14. Friedman H, Vogelzang RL, Mendelson EB, Neiman HL, Cohen M. Endometriosis detection by US with laparoscopic correlation. Radiology 1985; 157:217–220

15. Lande IM, Hill MC, Cosco FE, Kator NN. Adnexal and cul-de-sac abnormalities: transvaginal sonography. Radiology 1988; 166:325–332

16. Nardi PM, Ruchman RB. CT appearance of diffuse peritoneal endometriosis. J Comput Assist Tomogr 1989; 13:1075–1077

CYSTADENOCARCINOMA

17. Brammer HM III, Buck JL, Hayes WS, Sheth S, Tavassoli FA. From the archives of the AFIP. Malignant germ cell tumors of the ovary: radiologic-pathologic correlation. RadioGraphics 1990; 10:715–724

18. Buy J-N, Ghossain MA, Sciot C, et al. Epithelial tumors of the ovary: CT findings and correlation with US. Radiology 1991; 178:811–818

19. Dachman AH, Lichtenstein JE, Friedman AC. Mucocele of the appendix and pseudomyxoma peritonei. AJR 1985; 144:923–929

20. Fleischer AC, Rogers WH, Rao BK, Kepple DM, Jones HW. Transvaginal color Doppler sonography of ovarian masses with pathological correlation. Ultrasound Obstet Gynecol 1991; 1:275–278

21. Granberg S, Norström A, Wikland M. Comparison of endovaginal ultrasound and cystological evaluation of cystic ovarian tumors. J Ultrasound Med 1991; 10:9–14

22. Kurjak A, Zalud I, Alfirevic Z. Evaluation of adnexal masses with transvaginal color ultrasound. J Ultrasound Med 1991; 10:295–297

23. Levine DL, Gosink BB, Wolf SI, Feldesman MR, Pretorius DH. Simple adnexal cysts: the natural history in postmenopausal women. Radiology 1992; 184:653–659

24. Williams AG, Mettler FA, Wicks JD. Cystic and solid ovarian neoplasms. Semin US CT MR 1983; 4:166–183

25. Wolf SI, Gosink BB, Feldesman MR, et al. Prevalence of simple adnexal cysts in postmenopausal women. Radiology 1991; 180:65–71

APPENDICEAL ABSCESS

26. Abu-Yousef MM, Franken EA Jr. An overview of graded compression sonography in the diagnosis of acute appendicitis. Semin US CT MR 1989; 10:352–363

27. Machan L, Pon MS, Wood BJ, Wong AD. The "coffee bean" sign in periappendiceal and peridiverticular abscess. J Ultrasound Med 1987; 6:373–375

28. Ngo C, Wong L, Yaghmai I. Unusual sonographic appearance of a perforated appendiceal abscess. Pediatr Radiol 1989; 19:335–336

29. Nunez D Jr, Yrizarry JM, Casillas VJ, Becerra J, Russell E. Percutaneous management of appendiceal abscesses. Semin US CT MR 1989; 10:348–351

30. Sutton CL, McKinney CD, Jones JE, Gay SB. Ovarian masses revisited: radiologic and pathologic correlation. RadioGraphics 1992; 12:853–877

31. Terry J, Forrest T. Sonographic demonstration of salpingitis. Potential confusion with appendicits. J Ultrasound Med 1989; 8:39–41

Notes

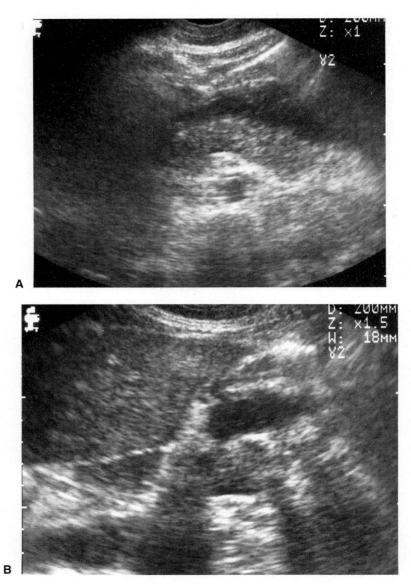

Figure 10-1. This 33-year-old woman has upper abdominal pain. You are shown selected axial (A) and sagittal (B) upper abdominal sonograms and a coronal sonogram through the left flank (C).

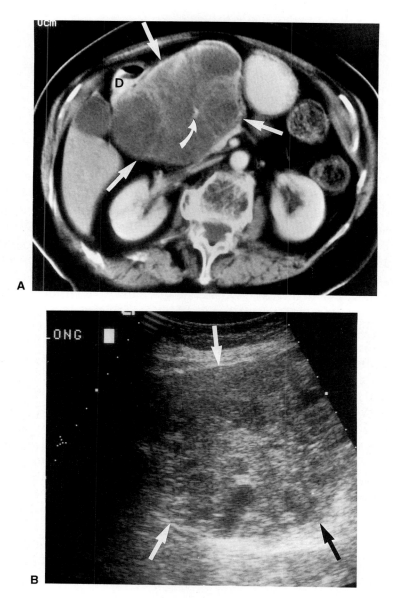

Figure 10-10. Microcystic adenoma. (A) A postcontrast CT scan demonstrates a 12-cm low-attenuation mass (straight arrows) in the head of the pancreas. There is a small central calcification (curved arrow). D = duodenum. (B) A transverse sonogram through the mass (arrows) demonstrates that the mass is very echogenic as a result of innumerable tiny cysts. Several of the larger cysts are visualized. The pancreatic origin of the mass was more clearly defined on the CT study.

Question 44

Concerning chronic pancreatitis,

    (A) the sonographic finding of pancreatic ductal calcification is diagnostic
    (B) it is associated with characteristic changes in pancreatic parenchymal echogenicity
    (C) it is rarely focal
    (D) it is a progressive disease
    (E) it is rarely caused by gallstones

Intraductal pancreatic calcifications are virtually pathognomonic of chronic pancreatitis and can be identified by sonography, CT, and radiography **(Option (A) is true).** In the United States, intraductal pancreatic calcifications are most often associated with alcohol-induced chronic pancreatitis but may develop in patients with chronic pancreatitis of other etiologies. Among patients with chronic pancreatitis and calcification demonstrable on radiography, chronic alcoholism is present in 75 to 90%. The frequency of pancreatic calculi in patients with alcohol-induced chronic pancreatitis is 20 to 40%; it is 2% or less in patients with pancreatitis related to biliary tract disease. Other uncommon causes of pancreatic calculi include hereditary pancreatitis, hyperparathyroidism with pancreatitis, kwashiorkor (protein-calorie malnutrition), cystic fibrosis, and idiopathic causes (nonspecific ductal obstruction).

Calcification can occasionally be seen within the pancreatic parenchyma or within pancreatic masses. Calcification of the parenchyma can occur after trauma or infarction when there has been intraparenchymal hemorrhage. Although they are uncommon pancreatic neoplasms, up to 20 to 30% of islet cell tumors and 10 to 20% of cystic pancreatic neoplasms contain calcification. Pancreatic pseudocysts occasionally have a rim of calcification. Calcification within pancreatic adenocarcinoma is extremely rare; however, a carcinoma can develop in a patient with chronic calcific pancreatitis.

The pathogenesis of pancreatic ductal calculi is poorly understood. Several factors may be responsible, including physicochemical properties of pancreatic fluid and hydrodynamic forces. The calcifications are almost always true stones lying free in the pancreatic ductal system rather than in the parenchyma. They contain a protein matrix and varying amounts of calcium carbonate.

Sonographically, pancreatic calcifications are seen as small, highly reflective particles that sometimes give the gland a stippled appearance (Figures 10-6 through 10-8). Acoustic shadowing behind the calcifications can be present (Figure 10-6). When they are located in a dilated main pancreatic duct, they are often surrounded by fluid and their intraductal location is confirmed sonographically (Figure 10-8). Calculi located in side branches of the main duct can appear parenchymal at sonography since dilatation of side branches is usually not demonstrated.

Chronic pancreatitis is an inflammatory process of the pancreas characterized by progressive sclerosis with destruction of parenchyma. Infiltration with inflammatory cells can be present to varying degrees, as can edema and focal necrosis. Small retention cysts and pseudocysts can be present. Both sonography and CT are useful procedures for evaluating patients with known or suspected chronic pancreatitis. Sonography can provide valuable information about the size and texture of the gland, the presence of pancreatic fluid collections or calcifications, biliary duct dilatation, and the presence of gallstones. The entire pancreas is visualized in most patients high-resolution real-time scanners with an average technical failure rate of 15%. With CT, the pancreas is imaged satisfactorily in essentially 100% of patients. Extrapancreatic pseudocysts can be more easily seen and their relationship to adjacent structures more accurately ascertained by CT than by sonography.

Both sonography and CT are sensitive in identifying an abnormal pancreas, but the accuracy for a specific diagnosis of chronic pancreatitis is relatively low. In one series, the accuracy of CT for a specific diagnosis in 50 patients with chronic pancreatitis was 56%. In another series, the specific detection rate for chronic pancreatitis with sonography was 48%.

Sonographic pancreatic morphology in patients with chronic pancreatitis is variable. Typically, in patients with severe chronic pancreatitis the main pancreatic duct is dilated and measures greater than 3 mm in diameter. The duct can be irregular, with increased echogenicity of the walls. Intraductal filling defects, calculi, and ductal narrowing can be seen. The pancreatic parenchymal echotexture is typically heterogeneous. In one series of 42 cases of chronic pancreatitis evaluated with sonography, pancreatic echogenicity was characterized as normal in 2%, generally increased in 31%, generally decreased in 2%, heterogeneous in 62%, and focally decreased in 2%. Although heterogeneous echogenicity was the most common pattern seen in chronic pancreatitis, it was also identified in 29% of patients with recurrent acute pancreatitis, 14% of patients with cancer, and 1% of normal patients in this series. Thus, there are no characteristic sonographic changes in parenchymal echogenicity in patients with chronic pancreatitis **(Option (B) is false).**

The pancreas can be normal in size, be diffusely enlarged or atrophic, or contain focal areas of enlargement. Diffuse enlargement is most often correlated with a more acute process, whereas focal areas of enlargement with irregular contours or diffuse atrophy are correlated with greater chronicity of symptoms. In one series, focal enlargement was reported in

Table 10-1: Causes of pancreatitis

Acute	Chronic
Alcohol ingestion	Alcohol ingestion
Biliary tract disease (gallstones)	Biliary tract disease
Trauma	Trauma
Metabolic (hyperlipidemia, hyperparathyroidism, renal failure)	Metabolic (primary hyperparathyroidism)
Hereditary	Hereditary
Infection (mumps, viral hepatitis, other viral infections, mycoplasma, ascariasis)	Idiopathic
	Cystic fibrosis
Drugs	Severe protein-calorie malnutrition
Vasculitis-associated connective tissue disorders	
Penetrating duodenal ulcer	
Obstruction of ampulla of Vater	

12% of 42 patients with chronic pancreatitis evaluated by ultrasonography and in 30% of 56 patients evaluated with CT **(Option (C) is false).**

Morphologic changes within the pancreas depicted at sonography do not accurately predict the severity of clinical findings or the functional impairment of the gland. The calculi seen in chronic alcohol-induced pancreatitis usually develop after 5 to 10 years of episodic abdominal pain. Ductal obstruction due to intraductal protein precipitates results in atrophy of acinar cells and fibrosis. A continuing inflammatory process results characterized by irreversible morphologic change and progressive loss of exocrine and endocrine function **(Option (D) is true).** Acute exacerbations can occur, but the condition may be painless. Steatorrhea, diabetes mellitus, and vitamin B_{12} malabsorption are manifestations of functional impairment of the gland but cannot be predicted based on sonographic findings.

Chronic and acute pancreatitis can be due to alcohol ingestion, biliary disease, trauma, metabolic abnormalities, hereditary factors, and various infections and drugs (Table 10-1). The pancreatitis associated with gallstones, however, is predominantly acute and rarely chronic **(Option (E) is true).** A cholecystectomy, typically performed in patients after the first or second attack of gallstone-induced acute pancreatitis, cures this form of pancreatitis.

Question 45

Concerning cystic pancreatic neoplasms,

(A) microcystic adenoma (serous cystadenoma) has virtually no malignant potential
(B) a specific diagnosis can often be made on the basis of imaging features alone
(C) mucinous cystic tumors commonly demonstrate multiple tiny cysts on sonography
(D) amorphous calcifications are commonly present within the center of a microcystic adenoma
(E) the glycogen-rich cytoplasm of the cells lining the cyst of a microcystic adenoma is a diagnostic feature

Most pancreatic cysts are pseudocysts or retention cysts related to pancreatitis or trauma. Cystic pancreatic neoplasms are uncommon and account for only 5 to 15% of all pancreatic cystic lesions and for less than 1% of pancreatic malignancies. These tumors are pathologically classified into microcystic (serous) adenomas and mucinous cystic neoplasms. Mucinous cystic neoplasms are further subdivided into mucinous (macrocystic) cystadenoma and mucinous (macrocystic) cystadenocarcinoma. This classification is important clinically because microcystic adenomas are believed to have virtually no malignant potential **(Option (A) is true)**. Recently, however, a case report described a primary tumor of the pancreas that was histologically indistinguishable from microcystic adenoma but which behaved in a malignant fashion with associated metastases. All previously documented cases of microcystic (serous) adenomas have been benign. On the other hand, mucinous cystic neoplasms either are frankly malignant or have malignant potential.

The clinical presentation of patients with cystic pancreatic neoplasms is nonspecific. The most common presenting symptom is either abdominal pain or vague abdominal discomfort. Other symptoms include weight loss, vomiting, and jaundice. A case of microcystic adenoma presenting with acute hemoperitoneum due to rupture into the lesser peritoneal sac has been reported. When asymptomatic, the mass can be discovered by the patient or physician or incidentally during imaging procedures performed for unrelated reasons. These tumors are more common in women than men and tend to present in the sixth to eighth decade of life.

A specific diagnosis of microcystic adenoma or mucinous cystic neoplasm can often he made on the basis of imaging features alone **(Option (B) is true)**. In a blinded review of 16 cases of microcystic adenoma and 29 cases of mucinous cystic neoplasm, CT features allowed a correct diagnosis in 93% of microcystic adenomas and 95% of mucinous cystic

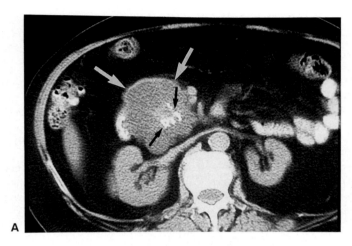

A

Figure 10-11. Microcystic adenoma. (A) A noncontrast CT scan shows an 8-cm low-attenuation mass (white arrows) in the head of the pancreas. There is calcification (black arrows) of a central scar. (B) A postcontrast CT scan demonstrates enhancement of fine septa within the mass (white arrows) and again shows the calcified scar (black arrows). (Case courtesy of David H. Stephens, M.D., Mayo Clinic, Rochester, Minn.)

neoplasms. Sonography accurately diagnosed 78% of microcystic adenomas and 93% of mucinous cystic neoplasms.

Microcystic adenomas have been reported to range in size from 1 to 25 cm, with a mean of 10.8 cm. At sonography, they are ovoid masses that may lack a demonstrable wall (Figure 10-9). They can appear totally echogenic when the cysts are very small. Frequently, however, multiple larger (but typically less than 2 cm) cysts are identified within the echogenic mass (Figure 10-10). Occasionally, a central scar, which can be calcified, is seen (Figures 10-10 through 10-12). On CT scans obtained without intravenous contrast enhancement, the attenuation of the tumor is generally low and may be within the range of attenuation values for water. Enhancement of all or part of the tumor is seen in most cases after contrast agent administration (Figures 10-9 through 10-12). Septa within the tumor become visible, and a honeycomb appearance is seen. Often, CT does not reveal the full extent of fine septa and other solid elements seen by sonography (Figure 10-10). The central scar is well demonstrated by CT, especially when calcified. These tumors can be located in any part of the pancreas, but most (approximately two-thirds) occur in the body and tail.

Mucinous cystic neoplasms have been reported to range in size from 2 to 19 cm, with a mean of 10.5 cm. They are most commonly located in

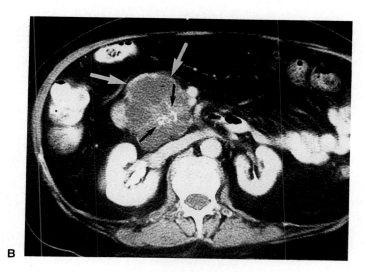

Figure 10-11 (Continued)

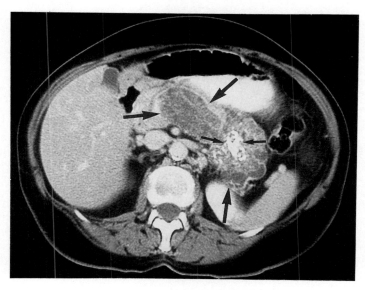

Figure 10-12. Microcystic adenoma. A postcontrast CT scan demonstrates a large tumor (large arrows) with multiple small cysts. Central calcification (small arrows) is present in the tail of the pancreas. (Case courtesy of David H. Stephens, M.D.)

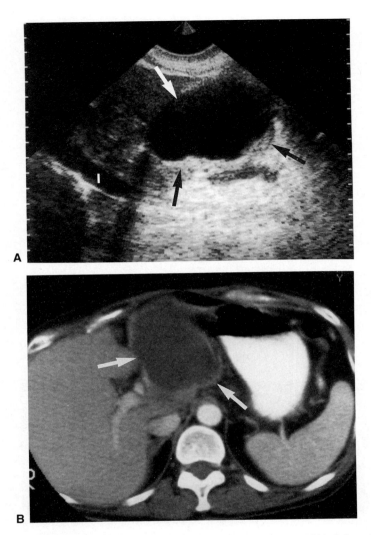

Figure 10-13. Mucinous cystic tumor of the pancreas. (A) A longitudinal sonogram demonstrates a large cystic pancreatic mass (arrows). The fluid within the mass is primarily echo-free, similar to a simple cyst, but there is nodularity and focal thickening of the posterior wall. I = inferior vena cava. (B) A postcontrast CT scan demonstrates the large cystic mass in the pancreas (arrows). Several regions of the wall of the mass are minimally thickened, and they enhanced with the contrast agent.

the body or tail of the pancreas. On sonography, they can be unilocular or multilocular cystic lesions (Figure 10-13). The individual cysts are less numerous and larger than in microcystic adenomas. They are generally greater than 2 cm in diameter and are often much larger **(Option (C) is**

false). Obvious cystic and near-water-density regions are demonstrated on CT (Figure 10-13). Both sonography and CT reveal the thick wall common in these neoplasms. Sonography tends to show the thick septa and papillary excrescences more clearly, whereas the pancreatic origin of the mass is often better depicted on CT. Differentiation of mucinous cystadenoma from cystadenocarcinoma is not possible unless there is evidence of local invasion or distant metastasis.

Calcification within cystic pancreatic neoplasms is not uncommon. It is found less frequently in mucinous cystic tumors than in microcystic adenomas. Imaging can demonstrate amorphous, random calcifications in the wall or peripherally within the mass in mucinous cystic tumors. When calcification is present within the central scar of a microcystic adenoma, a sunburst pattern is characteristic **(Option (D) is false).**

Microcystic adenomas and mucinous cystic tumors have very distinct microscopic features. Epithelial cells line the cysts of microcystic adenomas evenly and contain a glycogen-rich cytoplasm that is a diagnostic feature **(Option (E) is true).** Mucin is not demonstrated within the cells. The large cystic spaces in mucinous cystic tumors are lined by mucin-producing cells arranged in a varying architectural pattern, ranging from single rows to cellular stratification to invasive adenocarcinoma. Benign and malignant epithelia can be juxtaposed within a cyst. Stains for mucin demonstrate both intracellular and extracellular mucin. Glycogen is not identified. Appropriate staining techniques should be requested from the pathologist when imaging-directed fine-needle aspiration biopsies are performed for suspected cystic pancreatic neoplasms.

Mucinous cystic tumors should be surgically resected, because they are either malignant or potentially malignant neoplasms. Surgical resection remains the treatment of choice in many cases of microcystic adenoma because these tumors have the potential to enlarge slowly and compress adjacent structures, sometimes leading to gastrointestinal hemorrhage, common bile duct obstruction, and pancreatic duct obstruction. In patients who are poor surgical candidates or in certain asymptomatic patients, observation alone may be considered. Fine-needle aspiration biopsy can be used to increase the confidence in the diagnosis.

Question 46

Concerning carcinoma of the pancreas,

- (A) dilatation of the pancreatic duct is common
- (B) the presence of a pseudocyst effectively excludes the diagnosis
- (C) it most often appears as a focal, relatively hypoechoic pancreatic mass
- (D) on contrast-enhanced dynamic CT, significant enhancement of the tumor mass is common
- (E) at the time of diagnosis, it is rarely confined to the pancreas

Either sonography or CT can be used to evaluate patients with suspected pancreatic carcinoma. Sonography is often used for initial evaluation of patients presenting with suspected obstructive jaundice. It is highly accurate in determining whether the jaundice is surgical (obstructive) or medical (nonobstructive). It can also be valuable in evaluating the etiology of biliary obstruction. Therefore, sonography is an excellent initial imaging modality for patients with carcinoma of the head of the pancreas who present with obstructive jaundice (Figure 10-14). It is less accurate than CT in evaluating tumors in the body and tail of the pancreas.

The primary sonographic or CT findings of pancreatic carcinoma are a tumor mass with associated pancreatic and/or bile duct dilatation and evidence of metastatic disease. Dilatation of the pancreatic duct upstream from a focal pancreatic tumor is common (Figure 10-15) and has been reported in up to 67% of patients on CT **(Option (A) is true).** Chronic obstruction of the pancreatic duct causes atrophy of the surrounding parenchyma. Obstruction of the main pancreatic duct can also cause rupture of a side branch duct, resulting in formation of a postobstructive pseudocyst. The presence of a pseudocyst does not exclude the diagnosis of pancreatic cancer and has been found in up to 11% of patients **(Option (B) is false).**

Pancreatic carcinoma can be identified sonographically as a focal change in echotexture, but most often it presents sonographically as a focal, contour-deforming, relatively hypoechoic pancreatic mass (Figure 10-16) compared with the remainder of the parenchyma **(Option (C) is true).** These lesions are usually 2 cm or more in diameter. Smaller tumors are occasionally identified on the basis of a change in echotexture alone, without relying on distortion of the size or shape of the pancreas for diagnosis.

On CT, a pancreatic carcinoma most often presents as a focal mass (Figure 10-17). A diffuse mass, encompassing most of the gland, is uncommon. The tumor mass typically enhances less than the surrounding parenchyma on contrast-enhanced dynamic CT **(Option (D) is**

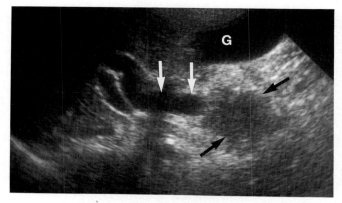

Figure 10-14. Adenocarcinoma of the pancreas. A longitudinal sonogram demonstrates a hypoechoic mass (black arrows) in the head of the pancreas. The common bile duct (white arrows) is dilated down to the level of the mass, where it is obstructed. G = gallbladder.

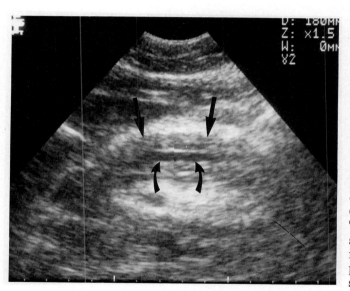

Figure 10-15. Pancreatic duct dilatation as a result of pancreatic adenocarcinoma. A transverse sonogram through the body of the pancreas (straight arrows) demonstrates dilation of the pancreatic duct (curved arrows). The small obstructing tumor in the head of the pancreas is not visualized.

false). A central zone of diminished attenuation within the mass is believed to represent the hypovascular, scirrhous tumor, whereas the remainder of the mass represents normal parenchyma or inflammatory tissue caused by obstructive pancreatitis.

Endoscopic sonography is a new diagnostic modality that was initially developed to visualize the wall of the gastrointestinal tract. With an ultrasound transducer positioned at the tip of an endoscope in the

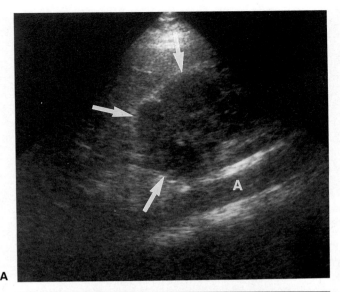

A

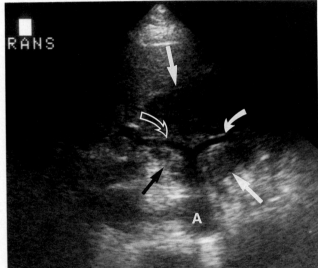

B

Figure 10-16.
Adenocarcinoma of
the pancreas. Lon-
gitudinal (A) and
transverse (B)
sonograms demon-
strate a large
hypoechoic tumor
(straight arrows)
extending cephalad
from the body of
the pancreas and
encasing the celiac
artery and its
branches. The
curved open arrow
represents the he-
patic artery, and
the curved solid ar-
row represents the
splenic artery. A =
aorta.

stomach or duodenum, the pancreatic parenchyma and duct can be evaluated in great detail. This requires skill in endoscopic techniques and
knowledge of regional anatomy to identify landmarks. This modality is
highly sensitive in visualizing pancreatic tumors, especially when they
are small. Local metastatic involvement of the portal venous system, portions of the celiac axis, and adjacent lymph nodes can be assessed. Liver
and other distant metastases cannot be evaluated because of the small
field of view and limited depth penetration of the transducers.

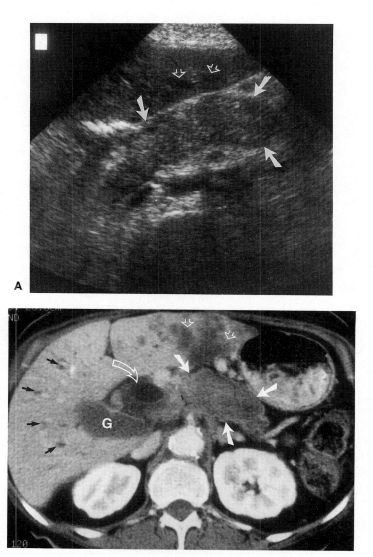

Figure 10-17. Pancreatic carcinoma with liver metastases. (A) A transverse sonogram demonstrates a mass in the body of the pancreas (solid arrows). Several small hypoechoic lesions (open arrows) in the left lobe of the liver suggest the presence of liver metastases. (B) A postontrast CT scan confirms the presence of liver metastases (straight open arrows) and a relatively nonenhancing tumor mass in the body of the pancreas (solid white arrows). The common bile duct (curved open arrow) is obstructed by the tumor. Black arrows represent dilated intrahepatic bile ducts. G = gallbladder.

A focal pancreatic mass with ductal dilatation is not specific for pancreatic carcinoma. Other primary pancreatic neoplasms, metastatic disease, and pancreatitis can result in similar findings. Ancillary sonographic and CT findings of pancreatic carcinoma include hepatic or lymph node metastasis, vascular involvement (encasement, invasion, and occlusion), local tumor extension, contiguous organ involvement, and ascites (Figures 10-16 and 10-17). Identification of these findings may allow a more specific diagnosis to be made and is used to assess tumor resectability.

Pancreatic carcinoma remains a lethal disease. In 99% of patients, it has already metastasized by the time symptoms appear or a diagnosis is made **(Option (E) is true).** Surgical excision continues to provide the only possibility of cure, but the overall resectability rate is low (5 to 10%) and the median survival time after curative resection is 17 to 20 months. Patients presenting with small cancers (2 to 3 cm) in the head of the pancreas have the best chance for curative resection. Tumors greater than 4 cm in diameter are unlikely to be resectable, and body and tail lesions are hardly ever curable by surgical resection. The sonographic and CT criteria of a resectable pancreatic carcinoma are an intrapancreatic neoplasm, usually less than 2 to 3 cm in diameter, surrounded by normal parenchyma and with no evidence of local or extracapsular extension, vascular invasion, or metastases.

Mary C. Olson, M.D.
Thomas L. Lawson, M.D.

SUGGESTED READING

ACUTE PANCREATITIS

1. Freeny PC, Lawson TL. Radiology of the pancreas. New York: Springer-Verlag; 1982:169–222
2. Gonzales AC, Bradley EL, Clements JL Jr. Pseudocyst formation in acute pancreatitis: ultrasonographic evaluation of 99 cases. AJR 1976; 127:315–317
3. Hashimoto BE, Laing FC, Jeffrey RB Jr, Federle MP. Hemorrhagic pancreatic fluid collections examined by ultrasound. Radiology 1984; 150:803–808
4. Jeffrey RB Jr. Sonography in acute pancreatitis. Radiol Clin North Am 1989; 27:5–17
5. Jeffrey RB Jr, Laing FC, Wing VW. Extrapancreatic spread of acute pancreatitis: new observations with real-time US. Radiology 1986; 159:707–711
6. Lawson TL. Acute pancreatitis and its complications. Computed tomography and sonography. Radiol Clin North Am 1983; 21:495–513

CHRONIC PANCREATITIS

7. Ammann RW, Muench R, Otto R, Buehler H, Freiburghaus AU, Siegenthaler W. Evolution and regression of pancreatic calcification in chronic pancreatitis. A prospective long-term study of 107 patients. Gastroenterology 1988; 95:1018–1028
8. Cotton PB, Lees WR, Vallon AG, Cottone M, Croker JR, Chapman M. Grayscale ultrasonography and endoscopic pancreatography in pancreatic diagnosis. Radiology 1980; 134:453–459
9. Ferrucci JT, Wittenberg J, Black EB, Kirkpatrick RH, Hall DA. Computed body tomography in chronic pancreatitis. Radiology 1979; 130:175–182
10. Freeny PC. Classification of pancreatitis. Radiol Clin North Am 1989; 27:1–3
11. Freeny PC, Lawson TL. Radiology of the pancreas. New York: Springer-Verlag; 1982:223–305
12. Jones SN, Lees WR, Frost RA. Diagnosis and grading of chronic pancreatitis by morphological criteria derived by ultrasound and pancreatography. Clin Radiol 1988; 39:43–48
13. Luetmer PH, Stephens DH, Ward EM. Chronic pancreatitis: reassessment with current CT. Radiology 1989; 171:353–357
14. Minagi H, Margolin FR. Pancreatic calcifications. Am J Gastroenterol 1972; 57:139–145
15. Ring EJ, Eaton SB Jr, Ferrucci JT Jr, Short WF. Differential diagnosis of pancreatic calcification. AJR 1973; 117:446–452
16. Weinstein BJ, Weinstein DP, Brodmerkal GJ Jr. Ultrasonography of pancreatic lithiasis. Radiology 1980; 134:185–189

CYSTIC PANCREATIC NEOPLASMS

17. Alpert LC, Truong LD, Bossart MI, Spjut HJ. Microcystic adenoma (serous cystadenoma) of the pancreas. A study of 14 cases with immunohistochemical and electron-microscopic correlation. Am J Surg Pathol 1988; 12:251–263
18. Buck JL, Hayes WS. From the archives of the AFIP. Microcystic adenoma of the pancreas. RadioGraphics 1990; 10:313–322
19. Compagno J, Oertel JE. Microcystic adenomas of the pancreas (glycogen-rich cystadenomas) a clinicopathologic study of 34 cases. Am J Clin Pathol 1978; 69:289–298
20. Compagno J, Oertel JE. Mucinous cystic neoplasms of the pancreas with overt and latent malignancy (cystadenocarcinoma and cystadenoma). A clinicopathologic study of 41 cases. Am J Clin Pathol 1978; 69:573–580
21. Freeny PC, Weinstein CJ, Taft DA, Allen FH. Cystic neoplasms of the pancreas: new angiographic and ultrasonographic findings. AJR 1978; 131:795–802
22. Friedman AC, Lichtenstein JE, Dachman AH. Cystic neoplasms of the pancreas. Radiological-pathological correlation. Radiology 1983; 149:45–50
23. George DH, Murphy F, Michalski R, Ulmer BG. Serous cystadenocarcinoma of the pancreas: a new entity? Am J Surg Pathol 1989; 13:61–66
24. Johnson CD, Stephens DH, Charboneau JW, Carpenter HA, Welch TJ. Cystic pancreatic tumors: CT and sonographic assessment. AJR 1988; 151:1133–1138

25. Kamei K, Funabiki T, Ochiai M, Amano H, Kasahara M, Sakamoto T. Multifocal pancreatic serous cystadenoma with atypical cells and focal perineural invasion. Int J Pancreatol 1991; 10:161–172

26. Rubin GD, Jeffrey RB Jr, Walter JF. Pancreatic microcystic adenoma presenting with acute hemoperitoneum: CT diagnosis. AJR 1991; 156:749–750

27. Warshaw AL, Compton CC, Lewandrowski K, Cardenosa G, Mueller PR. Cystic tumors of the pancreas. New clinical, radiologic, and pathologic observations in 67 patients. Ann Surg 1990; 212:432–445

28. Wolfman NT, Ramquist NA, Karstaedt N, Hopkins MB. Cystic neoplasms of the pancreas: CT and sonography. AJR 1992; 138:37–41

PANCREATIC CARCINOMA

29. Campbell JP, Wilson SR. Pancreatic neoplasms: how useful is evaluation with US? Radiology 1988; 167:341–344

30. Freeny PC. Radiologic diagnosis and staging of pancreatic ductal adenocarcinoma. Radiol Clin North Am 1989; 27:121–128

31. Ormson MJ, Charboneau JW, Stephens DH. Sonography in patients with a possible pancreatic mass shown on CT. AJR 1987; 148:551–555

32. Rosch T, Braig C, Gain T, et al. Staging of pancreatic and ampullary carcinoma by endoscopic ultrasonography. Comparison with conventional sonography, computed tomography, and angiography. Gastroenterology 1992; 102:188–199

33. Rosch T, Lorenz R, Braig C, et al. Endoscopic ultrasound in pancreatic tumor diagnosis. Gastrointest Endosc 1991; 37:347–352

34. Warshaw AL, Swanson RS. Pancreatic cancer in 1988. Possibilities and probabilities. Ann Surg 1988; 208:541–553

Notes

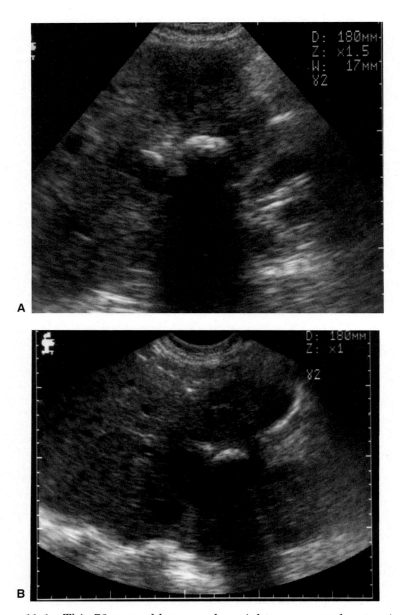

Figure 11-1. This 72-year-old woman has right upper quadrant pain and jaundice. You are shown transverse (A) and longitudinal (B) right upper quadrant sonograms.

Case 11: Carcinoma of the Gallbladder

Question 47

Which *one* of the following is the MOST likely diagnosis?

(A) Carcinoma of the gallbladder
(B) Hepatocellular carcinoma
(C) Hepatic abscess
(D) Acute cholecystitis
(E) Carcinoma of the hepatic flexure of the colon

Transverse and longitudinal right upper quadrant sonograms (Figure 11-1) demonstrate a relatively hypoechoic, poorly defined mass involving the porta hepatis and both lobes of the liver (Figure 11-2). In the center of this mass, there is an echogenic focus with acoustic shadowing. This should suggest a large gallstone, although the gallbladder is not identified. The gallbladder is engulfed by the mass, which is also invading the liver. This represents an advanced carcinoma of the gallbladder **(Option (A) is correct).** CT (Figure 11-3) confirms that the porta hepatis contains a mass that has replaced the gallbladder and has invaded the liver. The gallstone is better demonstrated by sonography than by CT.

Gallbladder carcinoma can have one of three sonographic patterns closely corresponding to gross pathologic morphology. It can present as: (1) a subhepatic mass that fills or replaces the gallbladder; (2) focal or diffuse gallbladder wall thickening; or (3) a discrete intraluminal polypoid mass.

A subhepatic mass that fills or replaces the gallbladder is the most common form of gallbladder carcinoma, accounting for 40 to 65% of gallbladder carcinomas at diagnosis, and is the type demonstrated in the test images. This form can be difficult to distinguish from other masses of the porta hepatis, including primary hepatic masses, metastatic disease, and inflammatory conditions of the gallbladder or right upper quadrant. Ancillary findings of embedded calculi, nonvisualization of a

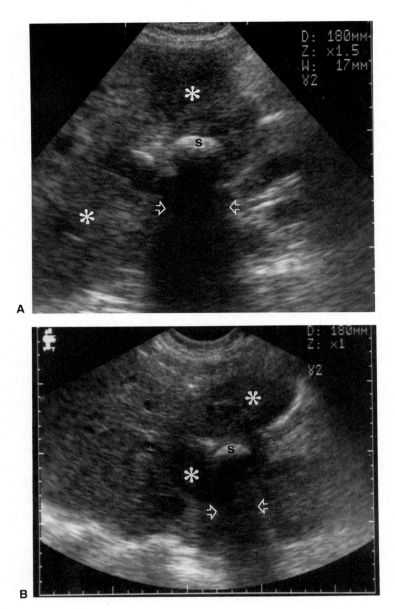

Figure 11-2 (Same as Figure 11-1). Gallbladder carcinoma with hepatic invasion. Transverse (A) and longitudinal (B) sonograms of the right upper quadrant demonstrate a large gallstone (s) with acoustic shadowing (open arrows). The gallbladder is replaced by a hypoechoic mass (✳), which is also invading the right and left lobes of the liver.

normal gallbladder, hepatic invasion, and a typical subhepatic location are very helpful in making the diagnosis of gallbladder carcinoma.

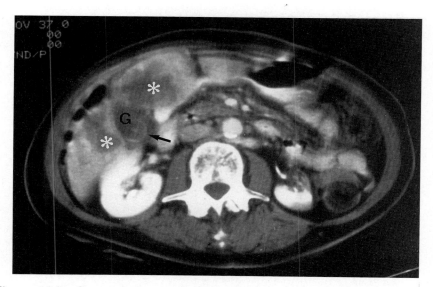

Figure 11-3. Same patient as in Figures 11-1 and 11-2. Gallbladder carcinoma with hepatic invasion. A CT scan confirms the presence of a mass (✳) that involves the gallbladder (G) and both lobes of the liver. The gallstone (arrow) is poorly visualized by CT.

Focal or diffuse gallbladder wall thickening is the next most common form of gallbladder carcinoma, making up 20 to 30% of tumors. Sonographic detection of focal wall thickening can be difficult (Figure 11-4). Acoustic shadowing from gallstones can obscure focal areas of thickening (Figure 11-5). This form of gallbladder carcinoma can be simulated by adenomyomatosis or adherent biliary sludge (Figure 11-6). Diffuse wall thickening by carcinoma can simulate acute or chronic cholecystitis, although the wall thickening associated with carcinoma is often more asymmetric or irregular (Figure 11-7).

The least common form of gallbladder carcinoma is an intraluminal polypoid mass, representing 15 to 25% of tumors (Figure 11-8). Polypoid tumors grow into the lumen of the gallbladder before invading the wall, and so the prognosis is better. Even when the primary tumor is large, hepatic invasion and metastatic spread are less common. These lesions often occur along the dependent wall of the gallbladder and can be simulated by tumefactive sludge (Figure 11-9), acute cholecystitis with desquamation of the mucosa (Figure 11-10), cholesterol polyps, blood clots, adenomas, and papillomas. Tumefactive sludge and blood clots are excluded when motion of these structures, relative to the gallbladder, is demonstrated as the patient changes position. Other nonmobile polyps

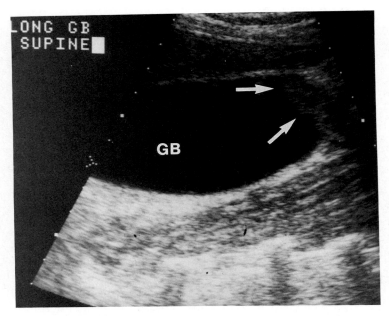

Figure 11-4. Gallbladder carcinoma. A longitudinal sonogram of the gallbladder (GB) reveals focal wall thickening (arrows) in the fundus. (Case
courtesy of Kika Dudiak, M.D., Mayo Clinic, Rochester, Minn.)

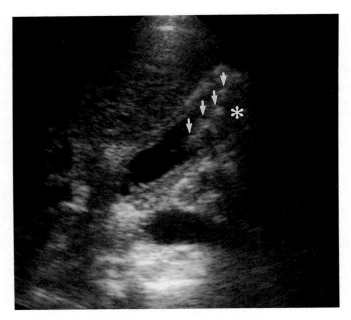

Figure 11-5. Gallbladder carcinoma. A longitudinal sonogram reveals a
fundal mass (✱) partially obscured by acoustic shadowing from gallstones (arrows). The presence of gallstones displaced from the dependent
gallbladder wall may be a sign of gallbladder carcinoma. (Case courtesy
of Robert S. Perret, M.D., Medical College of Wisconsin, Milwaukee,
Wis.)

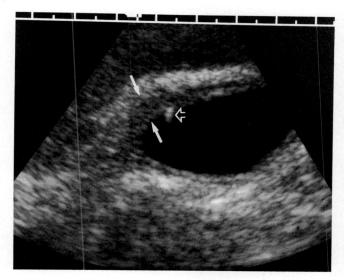

Figure 11-6. Adenomyomatosis of the gallbladder simulating gallbladder carcinoma. A longitudinal sonogram shows focal wall thickening (solid arrows). The echogenic reverberation artifact (open arrow) along the nondependent gallbladder wall represents a cholesterol crystal embedded in a Rokitansky-Aschoff sinus.

should be monitored if small, and some authors advocate cholecystectomy for polypoid masses greater than 1 cm in size.

Hepatocellular carcinoma (Option (B)), also known as hepatoma, is the most common primary malignant tumor of the liver. Its incidence, risk factors, and morphology vary in different parts of the world. In Asia and sub-Saharan Africa, hepatocellular carcinoma is the most common hepatic neoplasm, whereas in the United States metastatic disease is 20 times more frequent. Risk factors include chronic liver disease and cirrhosis; viral hepatitis, particularly that due to hepatitis B virus; alcoholic liver disease; and carcinogens such as aflatoxin. Hepatocellular carcinoma is also associated with hemochromatosis, alpha 1-antitrypsin deficiency, anabolic steroids, and long-term oral contraceptive use. Hepatitis B-related liver disease is the most common risk factor in Asia, and alcoholic liver disease is the most common risk factor in the United States. The morphologic forms of hepatocellular carcinoma include unifocal and multifocal masses and diffusely infiltrating tumor. Unifocal and multifocal masses are more common than diffusely infiltrating tumor in both the United States and Asia. However, tumor encapsulation, fatty metamorphosis, and arterioportal shunting are much more common in Asian populations.

In view of the association of hepatocellular carcinoma with chronic liver disease, screening by ultrasonography and by measurement of serum α-fetoprotein levels has been advocated and has been effective in Japan. Patients with alcoholic cirrhosis and fatty liver, in whom sono-

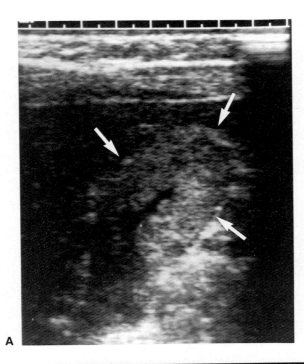

A

Figure 11-7. Gallbladder
carcinoma. A sonogram
(A) and a CT scan (B) re-
veal diffuse irregular
thickening of the gall-
bladder wall (arrows).
(Case courtesy of Kika
Dudiak, M.D.)

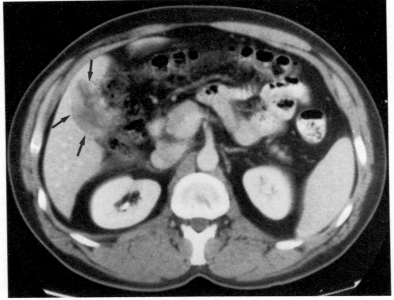

B

graphic examination may be limited, can be further evaluated with MRI
or CT.

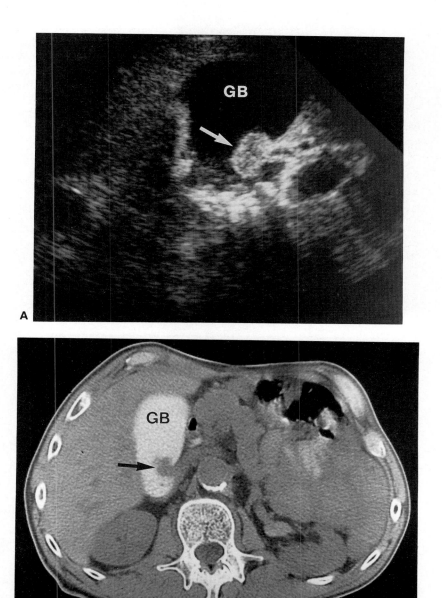

Figure 11-8. Gallbladder carcinoma. A sonogram (A) and a CT scan (B) demonstrate a polypoid mass (arrow) protruding into the gallbladder lumen (GB). The intraluminal contrast material is from recent endo-scopic retrograde cholangiopancreatography.

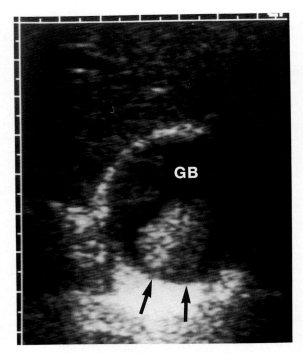

Figure 11-9 (left). Tumefactive sludge simulating gallbladder carcinoma. A transverse sonogram demonstrates a solid intraluminal mass (arrows) that simulates a polypoid carcinoma of the gallbladder (GB). This mass moved when the patient changed position.

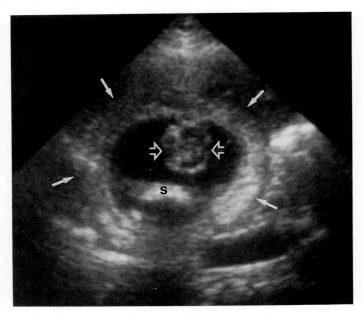

Figure 11-10. Acute cholecystitis simulating gallbladder carcinoma. A transverse gallbladder sonogram demonstrates a gallstone (s), diffuse wall thickening (solid arrows), and a polypoid mass (open arrows) arising from the nondependent gallbladder wall. Pathologic examination revealed acute cholecystitis with transmural inflammation of the wall of the gallbladder and mucosal sloughing. However, there was no malignancy.

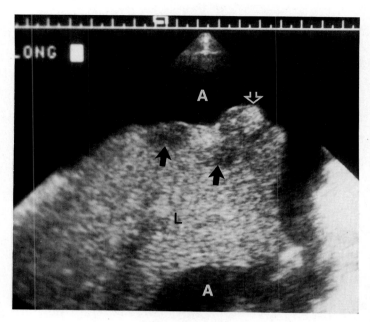

Figure 11-11. Multifocal hepatocellular carcinoma in a cirrhotic liver. The smaller nodules (solid arrows) are hypoechoic, whereas the largest nodule (open arrow) contains an area of increased echogenicity. The cirrhotic liver (L) is nodular in contour and is surrounded by ascitic fluid (A).

The sonographic appearance and echogenicity of hepatocellular carcinomas are variable. Small tumors are usually hypoechoic, being composed of solid sheets of tumor cells without necrosis (Figure 11-11). Larger tumors tend to be more echogenic as a result of areas of nonliquefactive necrosis, hemorrhage, fibrosis, sinusoidal dilation, and fatty change (Figure 11-12). The mass in the test images is uniformly hypoechoic, which would be unusual for a hepatocellular carcinoma of this size. Vascular invasion is a characteristic feature of hepatocellular carcinoma. The portal vein is invaded most commonly, although the inferior vena cava and hepatic veins can also be involved by tumor. Local extension occurs and can involve the liver capsule, diaphragm, abdominal wall, and pancreatic bed. Dissemination to regional lymph nodes is common. Calcification is relatively rare in hepatoma. It is a common feature of fibrolamellar hepatocellular carcinoma, a variant of hepatocellular carcinoma, but this is a rare disease that usually occurs in young patients. The sonographic features in the test images do not suggest hepatocellular carcinoma.

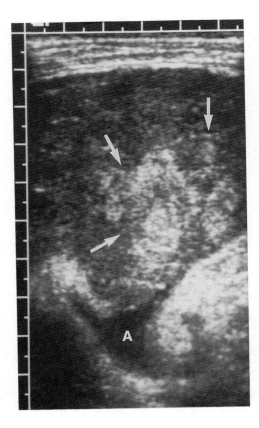

Figure 11-12. Infiltrating hepatocellular carcinoma. A transverse sonogram of the liver reveals ill-defined areas of increased echogenicity (arrows) invading the liver. A = ascites.

Hepatic abscesses (Option (C)) are variable in sonographic appearance. They can be hypoechoic or hyperechoic. The wall ranges from poorly defined to well defined. An abscess containing gas can be sonographically hyperechoic and can demonstrate ill-defined acoustic shadowing. Some features of the test images mimic an abscess, but the appearance is not typical for an abscess. In addition, the centrally located echogenic focus in the test case demonstrates very sharp acoustic shadowing, which is much more typical for calcification than for gas.

Patients with acute cholecystitis (Option (D)) usually present with distension of the gallbladder, thickening of the gallbladder wall, gallstones, and pericholecystic fluid. If the acute cholecystitis is uncomplicated, the gallbladder itself is invariably identified, unlike in the test images. Occasionally, if the acute cholecystitis is complicated by gallbladder necrosis and abscess formation or by emphysematous cholecystitis, the gallbladder itself is not well visualized (Figure 11-13). However, these features are not present in the test images.

Carcinoma of the hepatic flexure of the colon (Option (E)) can present with a right upper quadrant mass. If metastases are present, focal liver

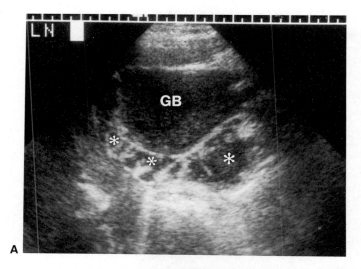

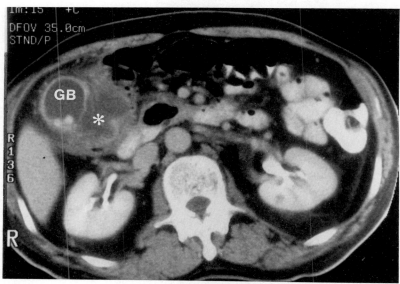

Figure 11-13. Acute cholecystitis with perforation. (A) A transverse sonogram of the gallbladder (GB) demonstrates intraluminal sludge and inflammatory debris, as well as pericholecystic fluid collections (∗) compatible with perforation. (B) A CT scan confirms the presence of an inflammatory fluid collection (∗) surrounding the gallbladder (GB), which contains several gallstones.

lesions can also be seen. The mass of a colon carcinoma is usually separate and distinct from the edge of the liver (Figure 11-14). A central echogenic lumen that contains gas can be seen; it should be linear on at

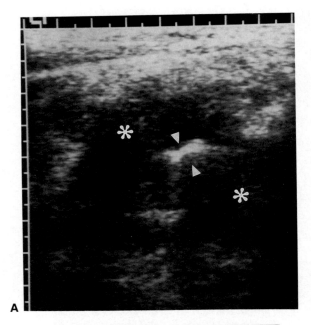

A

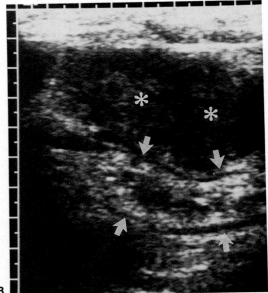

B

Figure 11-14. Colon carcinoma. (A) A transverse sonogram of the right lower quadrant demonstrates a hypoechoic mass (∗) with an echogenic central lumen (arrowheads). (B) A longitudinal sonogram lateral to the colonic lumen confirms the presence of a mass (∗) adjacent to a normal loop of ileum (arrows). (C) A CT scan shows abnormal annular thickening of the right colon (arrows) representing colon carcinoma. (Case courtesy of Bruce Silver, M.D., Rush Presbyterian-St. Luke's Medical Center, Chicago, Ill..)

least one scan plane. In the test images, the central echogenic focus is round on two scan planes. In addition, the mass is inseparable from the liver. Therefore, carcinoma of the hepatic flexure of the colon is not the correct diagnosis.

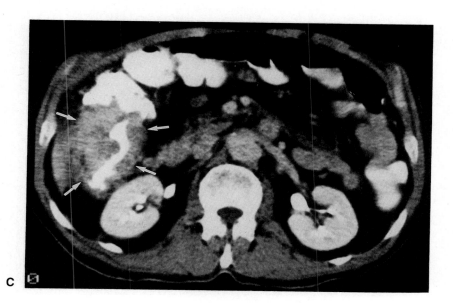

C

Question 48

Concerning gallbladder carcinoma,

(A) it is more common in women than in men
(B) it is commonly associated with gallstones
(C) there is an increased incidence in patients with porcelain gallbladder
(D) it frequently obstructs the common bile duct
(E) regional metastases are frequently present at the time of diagnosis

Gallbladder carcinoma is the most common malignancy of the biliary system, although it represents only 1 to 2% of all gastrointestinal tract malignancies. Gallbladder carcinoma is primarily a disease of the elderly, with a mean age at diagnosis of 72 years. Women are affected more commonly than men, with a ratio of 3:1 **(Option (A) is true).** Gallbladder carcinoma is associated with gallstones in 75 to 98% of affected individuals **(Option (B) is true).** There is also an increased incidence of carcinoma in patients with porcelain gallbladder **(Option (C) is true).** Gallbladder carcinoma is an incidental surgical finding in 1% of cholecystectomies but occurs in 22% of cases with calcification of the gallbladder wall (Figures 11-15 and 11-16). The strong association of gallbladder carcinoma with both cholelithiasis and porcelain gallbladder suggests the presence of an etiologic link. It is proposed that long-term inflammation

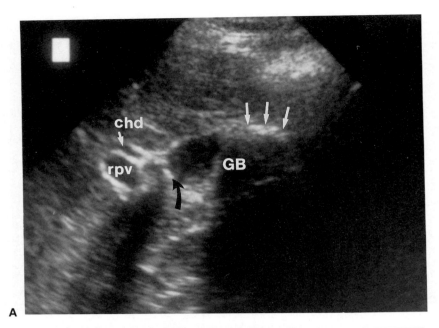

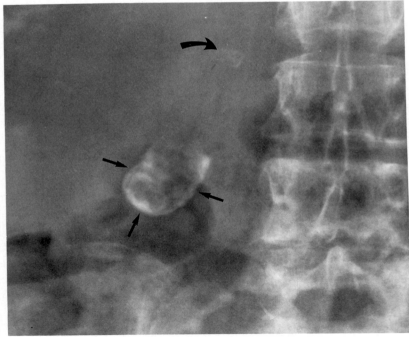

Figure 11-15. Porcelain gallbladder. (A) A longitudinal sonogram reveals the lower half of the gallbladder (GB) to be obscured by shadowing from a rim of calcium in the wall (straight arrows). A stone (curved arrow) is embedded in the gallbladder neck. chd = common hepatic duct; rpv = right portal vein. (B) A radiograph of the abdomen confirms calcification of the gallbladder fundus (straight arrows) and a stone in the gallbladder neck (curved arrow).

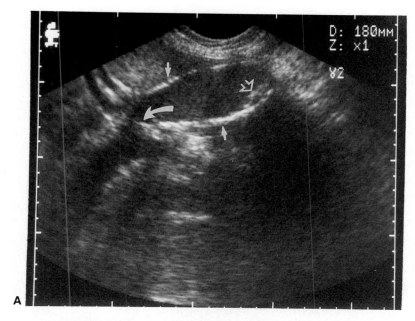

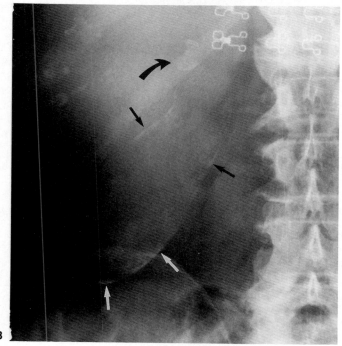

Figure 11-16. Gallbladder carcinoma in a patient with porcelain gallbladder. (A) A longitudinal sonogram demonstrates calcification of the
gallbladder wall (solid straight arrows), a stone (curved arrow) in the
neck of the gallbladder, and a fundal gallbladder carcinoma (open arrow).
(B) A radiograph of the abdomen shows calcification of the gallbladder
wall (straight arrows) and a stone (curved arrow) in the neck of the gallbladder.

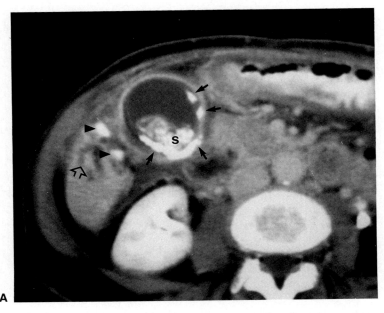

Figure 11-17. Locally invasive gallbladder carcinoma. (A) A CT scan at the level of the gallbladder fundus demonstrates calcification of the gallbladder wall (solid arrows), gallstones (s), and dilated right hepatic ducts (open arrow). A portion of a biliary drainage catheter is visible (arrowheads). (B) A CT scan at a slightly more cephalic level demonstrates a mass (✻) in the liver compatible with local hepatic invasion by gallbladder carcinoma. The right and left biliary ducts are dilated (open arrows). A drainage catheter is seen entering the right lobe of the liver (arrowheads).

of the gallbladder associated with cholelithiasis predisposes to dystrophic mural calcification as well as carcinoma.

The primary histologic type of gallbladder carcinoma is adenocarcinoma, which accounts for 90% of cases. Adenocarcinoma of the gallbladder can be either infiltrating, which is the most common form, or polypoid. Fibrosis, acute and chronic inflammatory cells, and extensive desmoplasia are often present. Squamous cell carcinoma makes up 5 to 10% of gallbladder carcinoma. The prognosis is poor for all types of gallbladder carcinoma. At the time of diagnosis, most carcinomas, other than those diagnosed incidentally during cholecystectomy, are in an advanced stage.

Gallbladder carcinoma spreads by several pathways. These include direct extension through the gallbladder wall and into adjacent structures, lymphatic invasion, hematogenous dissemination, and intraperito-

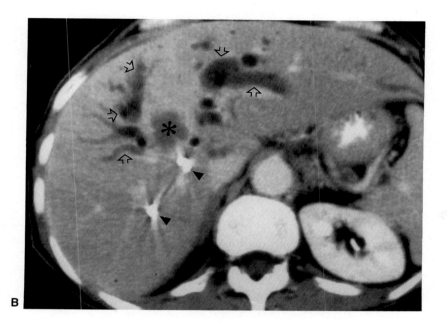

B

neal seeding. Direct invasion occurs readily because of the absence of a submucosal layer and the presence of a single instead of a double muscular layer in the gallbladder wall. At presentation, invasion of the liver is present in 50 to 80% of cases (Figure 11-17). Direct involvement of the stomach, duodenum, and colon can also occur, occasionally complicated by cholecystoenteric fistulas.

Biliary obstruction is present in 35 to 70% of cases, most often resulting from encasement of the common hepatic duct and common bile duct by tumor at the porta hepatis **(Option (D) is true).** Tumor can also directly invade the cystic duct and common bile duct, leading to obstruction and jaundice. This occurs in 4 to 25% of cases.

Regional lymph node metastasis is present in 50% of patients at presentation **(Option (E) is true)** (Figures 11-18 and 11-19). Tumor invades the rich lymphatic plexus of the gallbladder wall and disseminates to regional lymph nodes. The cystic duct node and common bile duct nodes are involved initially, and their subsequent neoplastic enlargement provides an additional mechanism for biliary obstruction. Further lymphatic dissemination extends to the peripancreatic and para-aortic nodes. Bulky peripancreatic nodes with associated biliary obstruction can simulate pancreatic carcinoma. Hematogenous metastases to the liver are present in 10 to 40% of patients (Figure 11-19). Pulmonary and

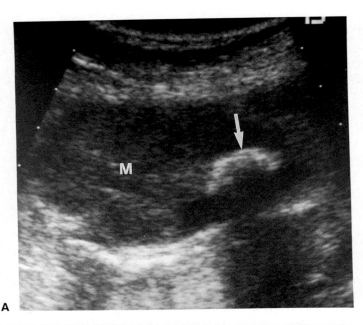

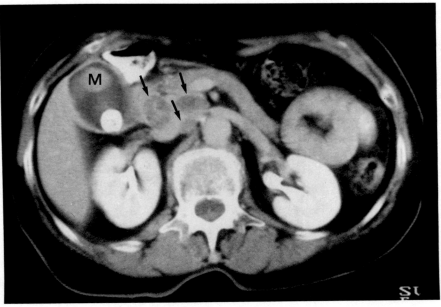

Figure 11-18. Gallbladder carcinoma with lymphadenopathy. (A) A longitudinal sonogram reveals a gallstone (arrow) in the fundus and a mass (M) filling most of the gallbladder lumen. (B) A CT scan demonstrates a portion of the intraluminal polypoid mass (M) of the gallbladder and peripancreatic adenopathy (arrows). (Case courtesy of Kika Dudiak, M.D.)

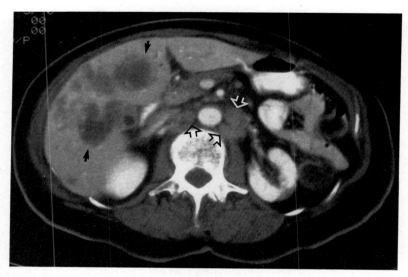

Figure 11-19. Metastatic gallbladder carcinoma. A CT scan through the liver reveals multiple low-attenuation hepatic metastases (solid arrows) and retroperitoneal adenopathy (open arrows).

osseous metastases can also occur. Ascites, which indicates seeding of the peritoneum, is an uncommon finding.

Question 49

Concerning hepatic abscess,

- (A) it most commonly appears as an anechoic mass
- (B) its appearance on contrast-enhanced CT is generally diagnostic
- (C) hepatic candidiasis commonly presents as multiple microabscesses
- (D) it is a complication of amebic colitis in about 50% of patients

Factors that predispose to the development of intrahepatic abscesses include biliary diseases such as suppurative cholangitis, cholecystitis and obstruction, abdominal surgery, trauma, diverticulitis, neoplasm, and immunocompromised status. Infectious agents reach the liver by extension through the biliary system, portal venous system, or hepatic artery, and, rarely, by direct extension (e.g., in trauma). The most frequent infectious agents are pyogenic bacteria, particularly *Escherichia coli*, although anaerobic bacteria, fungi, and parasites can also be responsible.

The sensitivity of sonography in the detection of hepatic abscesses is approximately 70 to 80%. The sonographic appearance of pyogenic he-

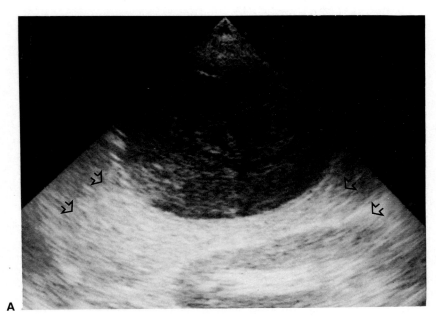

A

Figure 11-20. Hepatic abscess. (A) A longitudinal sonogram demonstrates a large hypoechoic abscess with internal echoes secondary to debris. There is acoustic enhancement (arrows), indicating the fluid nature of the mass. (B) A CT scan reveals a unilocular low-attenuation fluid collection (arrow).

patic abscesses is variable. Echogenicity varies from hypoechoic to markedly hyperechoic. Purely anechoic abscesses are rare **(Option (A) is false).** Early-stage hepatic abscesses, which contain cellular necrosis and neutrophils without frank liquefaction, can appear sonographically as solid lesions. Later stage abscesses often appear more cystic, although internal echoes in the form of septations, fluid-fluid interfaces, or debris are usually demonstrated (Figures 11-20 and 11-21). Intensely echogenic abscesses usually contain gas (Figure 11-22). Gas-containing abscesses can demonstrate acoustic shadowing or ring-down artifact. Occasionally the gas takes the form of microbubbles, which cannot be demonstrated by radiographs. The walls of hepatic abscesses are irregular in most patients but are occasionally well defined. The walls can be thick or thin. Acoustic enhancement is common, occurring in at least half of all patients (Figures 11-20 and 11-21). The size of pyogenic abscesses varies from very large to less than 1 cm. Abscesses are solitary in most patients, although multiple abscesses can occur. The right lobe is involved more often than the left.

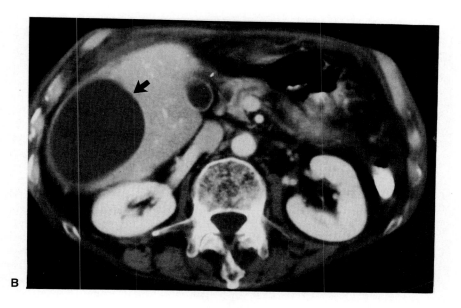

B

There are no sonographic features of hepatic abscesses that reliably differentiate them from benign cystic masses or necrotic neoplasms (Figure 11-23). Hepatic abscesses are also nonspecific in their appearance on plain and contrast-enhanced CT images **(Option (B) is false).** They are usually less dense than adjacent liver, although their attenuation values can range from that of serous fluid to significantly higher than serous fluid, depending on their composition. Abscesses are generally detected more easily following intravenous iodinated contrast administration, because the lesions are more conspicuous by comparison with the enhanced hepatic parenchyma (Figure 11-24). Rim enhancement is infrequent. The presence of gas bubbles or air-fluid levels strongly suggests abscess but is seen in fewer than 20% of patients. Gas bubbles are also a rare feature of some necrotic or superinfected neoplasms. CT readily identifies patients with multiple abscesses and demonstrates both unilocular and multilocular abscesses (Figures 11-24 and 11-25).

Percutaneous drainage of hepatic abscesses in concert with antibiotic therapy is the preferred therapeutic option in most cases, with a success rate of 70 to 90%. Drainage procedures can be performed with sonography or CT guidance. Preliminary diagnostic images are important for determining whether a safe access route that avoids diaphragm, bowel, or major blood vessels exists. Deciding whether to use CT or sonography for imaging guidance depends on the patient, abscess location, and, most importantly, the preference of the radiologist. The advantages of sonog-

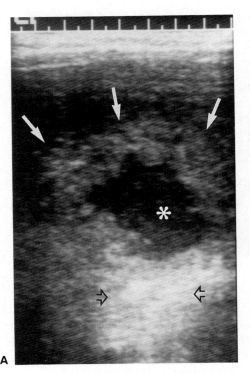

A

Figure 11-21. Hepatic abscess.
(A) A sonogram demonstrates a
central hypoechoic region (✳) that
contains debris, surrounded by a
rim of increased echogenicity
(solid arrows). Acoustic enhancement is present (open arrows). (B)
A contrast-enhanced CT demonstrates a multilocular mass (arrow) within the right lobe of the
liver. The appearance is nonspecific. (C) A radiograph taken after
injection of contrast into a percutaneous hepatic drainage catheter demonstrates the intercom-
munication of multiple peripheral
locules (arrows). This abscess was
successfully treated by percutaneous drainage. (Case courtesy
of F. Steven Davis, M.D., Hinsdale Hospital, Hinsdale, Ill.)

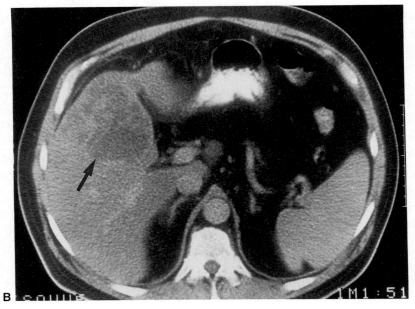

B

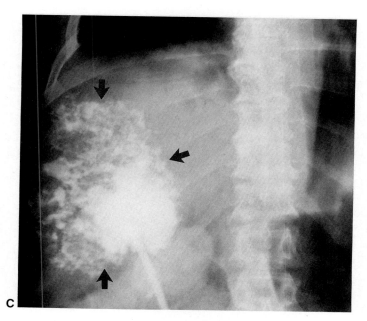

Figure 11-21 (Continued)

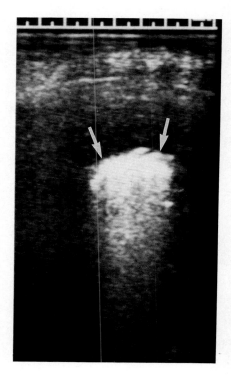

Figure 11-22. Gas-containing hepatic abscess. A sonogram demonstrates a densely echogenic focus within the liver (arrows) with ringdown artifact typical of gas.

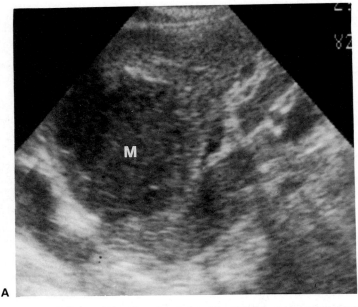

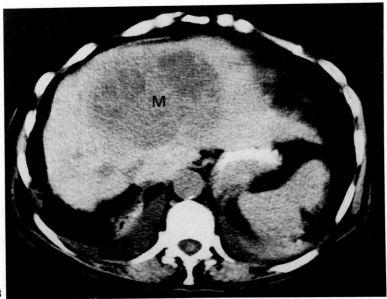

Figure 11-23. Hepatic abscess mimicking a solid hepatic lesion in a patient with adenocarcinoma of the colon. (A) A longitudinal sonogram demonstrates a relatively hypoechoic mass (M) in the left lobe of the liver. (B) A CT scan demonstrates a heterogeneous, poorly defined, low-attenuation mass (M) near the dome of the liver. Aspiration revealed purulent material.

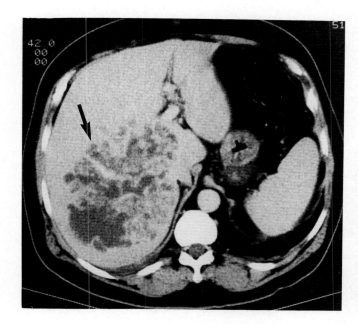

Figure 11-24 (left). Hepatic abscess. A post-contrast CT scan demonstrates a large multilocular abscess (arrow) within the right lobe of the liver. There is no rim enhancement.

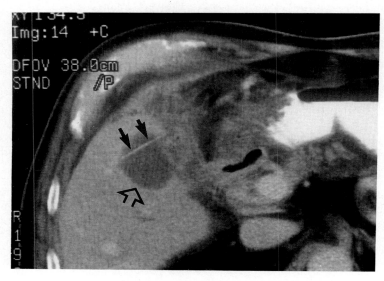

Figure 11-25. Unilocular hepatic abscess as a complication of surgery. A small sheared catheter fragment (solid arrows) inadvertently remains following laparoscopic cholecystectomy, and an abscess subsequently formed (open arrow). (Case courtesy of F. Steven Davis, M.D.)

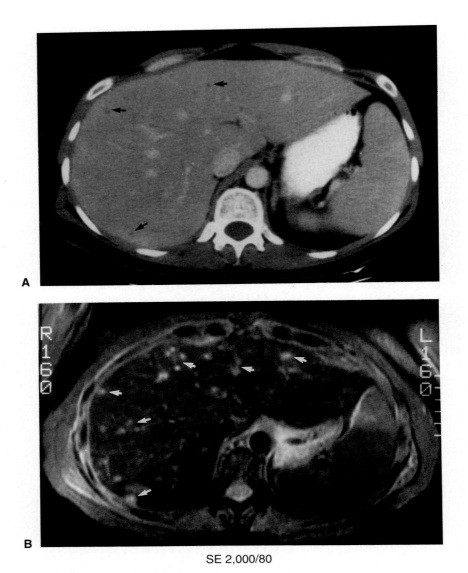

SE 2,000/80

Figure 11-26. *Candida* microabscesses in a patient with leukemia. (A) A postcontrast CT scan demonstrates multiple hepatic microabscesses (arrows). (B) A corresponding T2-weighted MR scan demonstrates a greater number of abnormal hyperintense foci (arrows) than did the CT scan.

raphy include the ability to image in multiple planes, real-time visualization of needle placement, and portability for unstable intensive care patients. CT is often preferred in complicated cases of extensive or multiple abscesses when several catheters may be required. Percutaneous abscess drainage is less successful in cases of multiple noncommunicating abscesses and in cases of superinfection of preexistent hepatic lesions such as hepatic tumors, cysts, or hematomas. Prolonged drainage may be necessary if there is an associated biliary fistula. In cases of associated biliary obstruction, simultaneous biliary drainage is required in order to achieve a cure.

Hepatic fungal microabscesses are most commonly due to *Candida albicans* and typically occur in immunocompromised hosts as opportunistic infections. They are usually hematogenously disseminated. Other mycoses that can be associated with microabscesses include cryptococosis, histoplasmosis, aspergillosis, and mucormycosis.

Hepatic candidiasis commonly presents as multiple microabscesses **(Option (C) is true)** (Figure 11-26). These exhibit several sonographic patterns depending on their stage of evolution (Figure 11-27). The earliest pattern consists of an echogenic focus containing a central hypoechoic nidus surrounded by a hypoechoic rim. This has been termed the "wheel within a wheel" sign. The central hypoechoic nidus consists of necrosis and can contain fungal elements. The surrounding echogenic zone represents inflammation, while the peripheral hypoechoic rim corresponds to fibrosis on histologic examination. The second pattern, also known as the "bull's-eye" or "target" lesion, consists of a central focus of increased echogenicity surrounded by a hypoechoic rim. The third pattern is the most common and consists of a uniformly hypoechoic lesion corresponding to fibrosis. The fourth pattern is an echogenic focus with acoustic shadowing secondary to calcification. These patterns are visible only when the neutrophil count is near normal and the host is able to mount an inflammatory response.

Hepatic amebic abscesses occur in 3 to 9% of patients with amebic colitis **(Option (D) is false).** *Entamoeba histolitica*, the causative organism is a parasite that burrows into the intestinal wall, usually the ascending colon and cecum, leading to inflammation with thickening and ulceration. Hepatic abscess, the most common extraintestinal complication, can result if amebic trophozoites are carried from the colon to the liver by the portal circulation. Most amebic abscesses occur in the right lobe of the liver. This can be explained by the preferential streaming of blood from the superior mesenteric vein, which drains the cecum and ascending colon, into the right portal vein; most splenic and inferior mesenteric venous flow enters the left portal vein. Amebic abscesses are usually round or oval, are hypoechoic relative to liver parenchyma, and commonly display homogeneous low-level echoes. Other features include a peripheral location, the presence of acoustic enhancement, and the lack of a discernable wall. However, there are no pathognomonic sonographic features that distinguish an amebic abscess from a pyogenic abscess. The

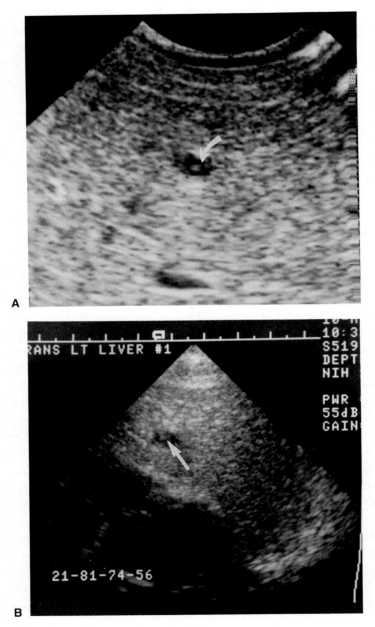

Figure 11-27. Sonographic patterns of hepatic candidiasis. (A) Pattern
I—"wheel within a wheel" sign. A central hypoechoic nidus (curved
arrow) of necrosis is surrounded by an echogenic ring of inflammation
and a peripheral hypoechoic halo of fibrosis. (B) Pattern II—"bull's-eye"
lesion. A central echogenic focus (arrow) is surrounded by a lucent halo.
(C) Pattern III. A uniformly hypoechoic lesion (open arrows) is demonstrated. (Cases courtesy of Thomas H. Shawker, M.D., Georgetown University Medical Center, Washington, D.C.)

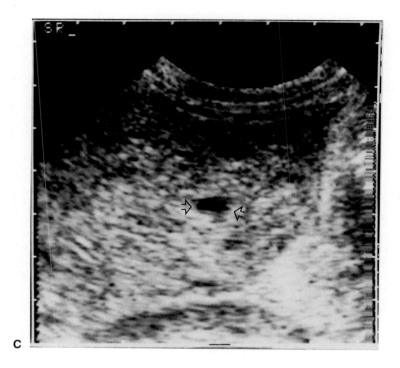

C

diagnosis is based on clinical history, laboratory data, and sonographic appearance. In some cases, percutaneous aspiration is helpful if the diagnosis is not confirmed. The appearance of the aspirated material is often described as similar to anchovy paste. Complications of amebic abscess include transdiaphragmatic spread into the pleural space, which is seen in approximately 15% of cases, and rupture into the pericardium, peritoneum, and retroperitoneum.

Medical treatment with metronidazole is usually successful. Following the institution of proper therapy, the time to healing is variable, ranging from 2 to 24 months. The wall becomes better defined, and the internal echogenicity can change. Enlarging anechoic areas are common, as are focal areas of increased echogenicity (Figure 11-28). The abscess usually resolves completely. In some cases, residual cysts, indistinguishable from simple cysts, remain. Percutaneous drainage is rarely required, although it has a role in the treatment of amebic abscesses with pyogenic superinfection and juxtacardiac abscesses that are at risk for rupture into the pericardium.

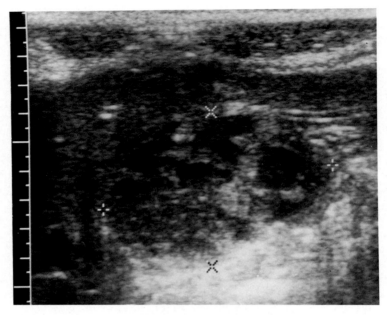

Figure 11-28. Partially treated amebic abscess. A complex mass in the left lobe of the liver contains anechoic regions as well as foci of increased echogenicity. Electronic caliper markers delineate the mass.

Question 50

Causes of gallbladder wall thickening include:

    (A) nephrotic syndrome
    (B) constrictive pericarditis
    (C) hepatic veno-occlusive disease
    (D) leukemia
    (E) Kawasaki's disease

The normal gallbladder wall is up to 3 mm thick. This measurement should be obtained perpendicular to the near wall to avoid pseudothickening, which occurs when the ultrasound beam is oblique relative to the gallbladder wall. Gallbladder contraction can also cause pseudothickening and should be suspected when the gallbladder measures less than 2 cm along the short axis.

Diffuse wall thickening is the most common abnormality of the gallbladder detected by sonography, although it is a nonspecific finding. Sonographically, the thickened gallbladder wall often appears as a hypo-

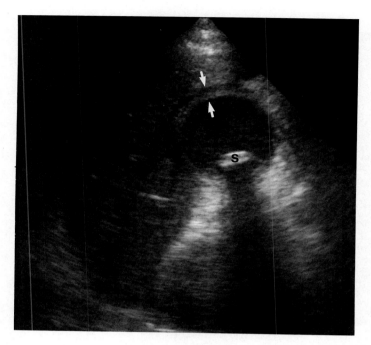

Figure 11-29. Acute cholecystitis. A transverse sonogram of the gall-bladder demonstrates diffuse thickening of the wall (arrows) of the gall-bladder and a gallstone (s).

echoic zone between two echogenic rings. An alternate sonographic appearance consists of "striated lucencies" alternating with echogenic bands in a thickened gallbladder wall. This form of wall thickening was initially believed specific for acute cholecystitis, but it is in fact seen in patients with many conditions. Biliary tract diseases causing gallbladder wall thickening include acute cholecystitis (particularly likely if the wall thickness exceeds 5 mm), chronic cholecystitis, and gallbladder carcinoma (Figures 11-29 and 11-30). There are numerous causes of wall thickening unrelated to biliary tract disease. Several pathophysiologic mechanisms are involved, and in some cases the mechanism is multifactorial.

Renal disease and the nephrotic syndrome can cause gallbladder wall thickening **(Option (A) is true).** The nephrotic syndrome is a manifestation of multiple different renal diseases, including those caused by immune or vascular mechanisms, metabolic abnormalities, and toxic insults. Heavy proteinuria secondary to glomerular damage is the hallmark of the disease. If the disease is severe enough, the plasma albumin level decreases and the plasma oncotic pressure falls. Intravascular fluid

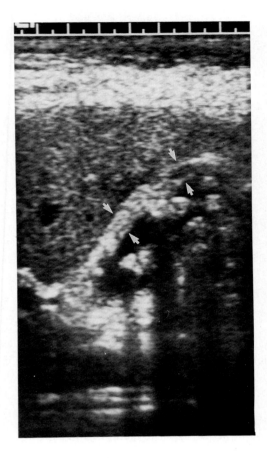

Figure 11-30. Acute cholecystitis. A longitudinal sonogram of the gallbladder reveals diffuse thickening of the wall (arrows) of the gallbladder with intramural striated lucencies. Multiple gallstones are present.

enters the interstitial tissues, resulting in generalized edema, including edema of the gallbladder wall. This leads to gallbladder wall thickening.

Constrictive pericarditis and other causes of right heart failure can also lead to diffuse gallbladder wall thickening **(Option (B) is true).** The fibrosis that encases the heart in patients with constrictive pericarditis impedes ventricular filling and leads to high atrial and systemic venous pressures. Congestive hepatomegaly develops. Increased portal venous pressure can contribute to gallbladder wall thickening. If congestive hepatomegaly is long-standing, hepatic function is impaired, leading to hypoalbuminemia, which also contributes to gallbladder wall thickening.

Several hepatic disorders can also lead to gallbladder wall thickening. Hepatic veno-occlusive disease is the progressive obliteration of small centrilobular veins. It is a common complication of bone marrow transplantation and is associated with gallbladder wall thickening

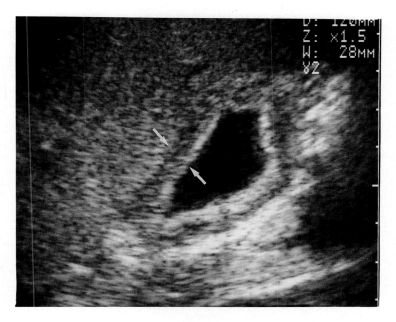

Figure 11-31. Hepatitis. A longitudinal sonogram of the gallbladder demonstrates diffuse gallbladder wall thickening (arrows).

(Option (C) is true). The obstruction of postsinusoidal blood flow, which results from obliteration of small centrilobular hepatic veins, leads to portal hypertension. Since the venous drainage of the gallbladder is to the right portal vein, referred portal hypertension leads to an increase in interstitial fluid and gallbladder wall edema. Cirrhosis can also cause gallbladder wall thickening as a result of both hypoalbuminemia and portal venous hypertension. Wall thickening secondary to viral hepatitis is felt to be the result of edema from a viral pericholecystitis that follows biliary excretion of virus (Figure 11-31). AIDS is also associated with wall thickening, most likely secondary to cytomegalovirus or cryptosporidiosis.

Pancreatitis and lymphoma with periportal adenopathy can cause obstruction of the lymphatic system of the gallbladder, with subsequent wall thickening. Leukemia rarely involves the gallbladder, but thickening has been reported as a result of transmural involvement of the wall by leukemic infiltrates **(Option (D) is true)** (Figure 11-32).

Acute hydrops of the gallbladder has been found in patients with Kawasaki's disease. The gallbladder is markedly distended, but the wall thickness is normal **(Option (E) is false)** (Figure 11-33). The pathophysiologic mechanism has not been completely elucidated, although

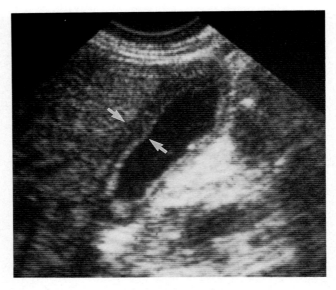

Figure 11-32. Leukemia. A longitudinal gallbladder sonogram demonstrates diffuse wall thickening (arrows).

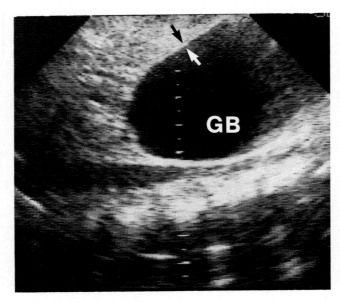

Figure 11-33. Kawasaki's disease with hydrops of the gallbladder. The gallbladder (GB) is distended, and the wall (arrows) is paper thin. (Case courtesy of Marilyn J. Siegel, M.D., Mallinckrodt Institute of Radiology, St. Louis, Mo.)

vasculitis is believed to play a role. Patients can have abnormal liver function studies and right upper quadrant pain, and the gallbladder can be palpable as a mass. This condition usually resolves without surgical intervention. Kawasaki's disease, also known as mucocutaneous lymph node syndrome, is a multisystem disorder of children. Common features include a high fever, lymphadenopathy, changes in the skin and mucous membranes, a fine macular rash, and scleral injection. Cardiovascular manifestations are less common and include myocarditis, pericarditis, and coronary artery aneurysms with resultant cardiomegaly, myocardial ischemia, and infarction.

Christine M. Dudiak, M.D.
Thomas L. Lawson, M.D.

SUGGESTED READINGS

GALLBLADDER CARCINOMA

1. Berk RN, Armbuster TG, Saltzstein SL. Carcinoma in the porcelain gallbladder. Radiology 1973; 106:29–31
2. Cooperberg PL, Gibney RG. Imaging of the gallbladder, 1987. Radiology 1987; 163:605–613
3. Franquet T, Montes M, Ruiz de Azua Y, Jimenez FJ, Cozcolluela R. Primary gallbladder carcinoma: imaging findings in 50 patients with pathologic correlation. Gastrointest Radiol 1991; 16:143–148
4. Kane RA, Jacobs R, Katz J, Costello P. Porcelain gallbladder: ultrasound and CT appearance. Radiology 1984; 152:137–141
5. Kumar A, Aggarwal S, Berry M, Sawhney S, Kapur ML, Bhargava S. Ultrasonography of carcinoma of the gallbladder: an analysis of 80 cases. JCU 1990; 18:715–720
6. Kuo YC, Liu JY, Sheen IS, Yang CY, Lin DY, ChangChein CS. Ultrasonographic difficulties and pitfalls in diagnosing primary carcinoma of the gallbladder. JCU 1990; 18:639–647
7. Lane J, Buck JL, Zeman RK. Primary carcinoma of the gallbladder: a pictorial essay. RadioGraphics 1989; 9:209–228
8. Polk HC. Carcinoma and the calcified gallbladder. Gastroenterology 1966; 50:582–585
9. Smathers RL, Lee JK, Heiken JP. Differentiation of complicated cholecystitis from gallbladder carcinoma by computed tomography. AJR 1984; 143:255–259
10. Soiva M, Aro K, Pamilo M, Päivänsalo M, Suramo I, Taavitsainen M. Ultrasonography in carcinoma of the gallbladder. Acta Radiol 1987; 28:711–714
11. Tsuchiya Y. Early carcinoma of the gallbladder: macroscopic features and US findings. Radiology 1991; 179:171–175
12. Weiner SN, Koenigsberg M, Morehouse H, Hoffman J. Sonography and computed tomography in the diagnosis of carcinoma of the gallbladder. AJR 1984; 142:735–739

HEPATOCELLULAR CARCINOMA

13. Choi BI, Kim CW, Han MC, et al. Sonographic characteristics of small hepatocellular carcinoma. Gastrointest Radiol 1989; 14:255–261

Case 11 / 359

14. Choi BI, Takayasu K, Han MC. Small hepatocellular carcinomas and associated nodular lesions of the liver: pathology, pathogenesis, and imaging findings. AJR 1993; 160:1177–1187
15. Dodd GD III, Miller WJ, Baron RL, Skolnick ML, Campbell WL. Detection of malignant tumors in end-stage cirrhotic livers: efficacy of sonography as a screening technique. AJR 1992; 159:727–733
16. Ezaki T. Screening methods for hepatocellular carcinoma. AJR 1991; 156:869
17. Freeny PC, Baron RL, Teefey SA. Hepatocellular carcinoma: reduced frequency of typical findings with dynamic contrast-enhanced CT in a non-Asian population. Radiology 1992; 182:143–148
18. Friedman AC, Lichtenstein JE, Goodman Z, Fishman EK, Siegelman SS, Dachman AH. Fibrolamellar hepatocellular carcinoma. Radiology 1985; 157:583–587
19. Kew MC, Popper H. Relationship between hepatocellular carcinoma and cirrhosis. Semin Liver Dis 1984; 4:136–146
20. LaBerge JM, Laing FC, Federle MP, Jeffrey RB Jr, Lim RC Jr. Hepatocellular carcinoma: assessment of resectability by computed tomography and ultrasound. Radiology 1984; 152:485–490
21. Miller WJ, Federle MP, Campbell WL. Diagnosis and staging of hepatocellular carcinoma: comparison of CT and sonography in 36 liver transplantation patients. AJR 1991; 157:303–306
22. Okuda K, Peters RL, Simson IW. Gross anatomic features of hepatocellular carcinoma from three disparate geographic areas. Proposal of new classification. Cancer 1984; 54:2165–2173
23. Sheu JC, Chen DS, Sung JL, et al. Hepatocellular carcinoma: US evolution in the early stage. Radiology 1985; 155:463–467
24. Tanaka S, Kitamura T, Imaoka S, Sasaki Y, Taniguchi H, Ishiguro S. Hepatocellular carcinoma: sonographic and histologic correlation. AJR 1983; 140:701–707
25. Teefey SA, Stephens DH, James EM, Charboneau W, Sheedy PF II. Computed tomography and ultrasonography of hepatoma. Clin Radiol 1986; 37:339–345

HEPATIC ABSCESS

26. Berry M, Bazaz R, Bhargava S. Amebic liver abscess: sonographic diagnosis and management. JCU 1986; 14:239–242
27. Callen PW, Filly RA, Marcus FS. Ultrasonography and computed tomography in the evaluation of hepatic microabscesses in the immunosuppressed patient. Radiology 1980; 136:433–434
28. Dewbury KC, Joseph AE, Millward Sadler GH, Birch SJ. Ultrasound in the diagnosis of the early liver abscess. Br J Radiol 1980; 53:1160–1165
29. Do H, Lambiase RE, Deyoe L, Cronan JJ, Dorfman GS. Percutaneous drainage of hepatic abscesses: comparison of results in abscesses with and without intrahepatic biliary communication. AJR 1991; 157:1209–1212
30. Dondelinger RF, Kurdziel JC, Gathy C. Percutaneous treatment of pyogenic liver abscess: a critical analysis of results. Cardiovasc Intervent Radiol 1990; 13:174–182

31. Halvorsen RA, Korobkin M, Foster WL, Silverman PM, Thompson WM. The variable CT appearance of hepatic abscesses. AJR 1984; 142:941–946

32. Ho B, Cooperberg PL, Li DK, Mack L, Naiman SC, Grossman L. Ultrasonography and computed tomography of hepatic candidiasis in immunosuppressed patients. J Ultrasound Med 1982; 1:157–159

33. Hochbergs P, Forsberg L, Hederström E, Andersson R. Diagnosis and percutaneous treatment of pyogenic hepatic abscesses. Acta Radiol 1990; 31:351–353

34. Hussain S, Dinshaw H. Ultrasonography in amebic colitis. J Ultrasound Med 1990; 9:385–388

35. Jaques P, Mauro M, Safrit H, Yankaskas B, Piggott B. CT features of intraabdominal abscesses: prediction of successful percutaneous drainage. AJR 1986; 146:1041–1045

36. Kressel HY, Filly RA. Ultrasonographic appearance of gas-containing abscesses in the abdomen. AJR 1978; 130:71–73

37. Kuligowska E, Connors SK, Shapiro JH. Liver abscess: sonography in diagnosis and treatment. AJR 1982; 138:253–257

38. Miller JH, Greenfield LD, Wald BR. Candidiasis of the liver and spleen in childhood. Radiology 1982; 142:375–380

39. Newlin N, Silver TM, Stuck KJ, Sandler MA. Ultrasonic features of pyogenic liver abscesses. Radiology 1981; 139:155–159

40. Pastakia B, Shawker TH, Thaler M, O'Leary T, Pizzo PA. Hepatosplenic candidiasis: wheels within wheels. Radiology 1988; 166:417–421

41. Powers TA, Jones TB, Karl JH. Echogenic hepatic abscess without radiographic evidence of gas. AJR 1981; 137:159–160

42. Ralls PW, Barnes PF, Johnson MB, De Cock KM, Radin DR, Halls J. Medical treatment of hepatic amebic abscess: rare need for percutaneous drainage. Radiology 1987; 165:805–807

43. Ralls PW, Barnes PF, Radin DR, Colletti P, Halls J. Sonographic features of amebic and pyogenic liver abscesses: a blinded comparison. AJR 1987; 149:499–501

44. Ralls PW, Colletti PM, Quinn MF, Halls J. Sonographic findings in hepatic amebic abscess. Radiology 1982; 145:123–126

45. Ralls PW, Quinn MF, Boswell WD, Colletti PM, Radin DR, Halls J. Patterns of resolution in successfully treated hepatic amebic abscess: sonographic evaluation. Radiology 1983; 149:541–543

46. Tandon N, Karak PK, Mukhopadhyay S, Kumar V. Amoebic liver abscess: rupture into retroperitoneum. Gastrointest Radiol 1991; 16:240–242

47. Terrier F, Becker CD, Triller JK. Morphologic aspects of hepatic abscesses at computed tomography and ultrasound. Acta Radiol [Diagn] (Stockh) 1983; 24:129–137

48. vanSonnenberg E, D'Agostino HB, Casola G, Halasz NA, Sanchez RB, Goodacre BW. Percutaneous abscess drainage: current concepts. Radiology 1991; 181:617–626

49. vanSonnenberg E, Mueller PR, Schiffman HR, et al. Intrahepatic amebic abscesses: indications for and results of percutaneous catheter drainage. Radiology 1985; 156:631–635

50. Wilson SR, Arenson AM. Sonographic evaluation of hepatic abscesses. J Can Assoc Radiol 1984; 35:174–177

51. Bradford BF, Reid BS, Weinstein BJ, Oh KS, Girdany BR. Ultrasonographic evaluation of the gallbladder in mucocutaneous lymph node syndrome. Radiology 1982; 142:381–384

52. Colli A, Cocciolo M, Buccino G, et al. Thickening of the gallbladder wall in ascites. JCU 1991; 19:357–359

53. Finlay DE, Mitchell SL, Letourneau JG, Longley DG. Leukemic infiltration of the gallbladder wall mimicking acute cholecystitis. AJR 1993; 160:63–64

54. Frick MP, Snover DC, Feinberg SB, Salomonowitz E, Crass JR, Ramsay NK. Sonography of the gallbladder in bone marrow transplant patients. Am J Gastroenterol 1984; 79:122–127

55. Herbetko J, Grigg AP, Buckley AR, Phillips GL. Venoocclusive liver disease after bone marrow transplantation: findings at duplex sonography. AJR 1992; 158:1001–1005

56. Hommeyer SC, Teefey SA, Jacobson AF, et al. Venocclusive disease of the liver: prospective study of US evaluation. Radiology 1992; 184:683–686

57. Marti-Bonmati L, Andres JC, Aguado C. Sonographic relationship between gallbladder wall thickness and the etiology of ascites. JCU 1989; 17:497–501

58. Nicolau C, Bru C, Carreras E, Bosch J, Bianchi L, Gilabert R, Vilana R. Sonographic diagnosis and hemodynamic correlation in veno-occlusive disease of the liver. J Ultrasound Med 1993; 12:437–440

59. Ralls PW, Quinn MF, Juttner HU, Halls JM, Boswell WD. Gallbladder wall thickening: patients without intrinsic gallbladder disease. AJR 1981; 137:65–68

60. Saverymuttu SH, Grammatopoulos A, Meanock CI, Maxwell JD, Joseph AE. Gallbladder wall thickening (congestive cholecystopathy) in chronic liver disease: a sign of portal hypertension. Br J Radiol 1990; 63:922–925

61. Shlaer WJ, Leopold GR, Scheible FW. Sonography of the thickened gallbladder wall: a nonspecific finding. AJR 1981; 136:337–339

62. Siegel MJ. Liver and biliary tract. In: Siegel MJ (ed), Pediatric sonography. New York: Raven Press; 1991:115–160

63. Teefey SA, Baron RL, Bigler SA. Sonography of the gallbladder: significance of striated (layered) thickening of the gallbladder wall. AJR 1991; 156:945–947

64. Wegener M, Börsch G, Schneider J, Wedmann B, Winter R, Zacharias J. Gallbladder wall thickening: a frequent finding in various nonbiliary disorders—a prospective ultrasonographic study. JCU 1987; 15:307–312

Notes

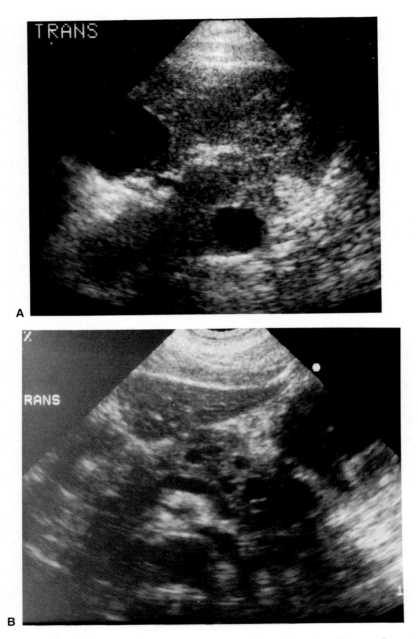

Figure 12-1. You are shown sonograms from two brothers. One is a transverse view of the lower pole of the left kidney in the 31-year-old brother (A), and one is a transverse view of the pancreatic body in the 27-year-old brother (B).

Case 12: von Hippel-Lindau Disease

Question 51

Which *one* of the following is the MOST likely diagnosis?

(A) Autosomal dominant polycystic disease
(B) Tuberous sclerosis
(C) Acquired cystic disease
(D) von Hippel-Lindau disease
(E) Cystic fibrosis

Figure 12-1A shows a hyperechoic mass (arrow, Figure 12-2A) and several cysts (C, Figure 12-2A) in the lower pole of the left kidney. Figure 12-1B shows multiple small cysts (arrows, Figure 12-2B) in the body of the pancreas. These findings in young-adult siblings suggest that they both suffer from an inherited disorder predisposing to visceral cyst formation. The solid hyperechoic mass in the kidney of one sibling suggests a predisposition to form solid renal tumors. Of the possibilities listed, von Hippel-Lindau disease is the most likely to produce all these abnormalities **(Option (D) is correct)**. In this case, the hyperechoic renal mass was surgically proven to be a small renal cell carcinoma.

Autosomal dominant polycystic disease (Option (A)) could explain the presence of renal and pancreatic cysts in a pair of siblings. However, the echogenic renal mass is harder to explain, since this disease is not associated with an increased risk of solid renal neoplasms. Cyst hemorrhage is common in patients with autosomal dominant polycystic disease and can result in a cyst with uniform low-level internal echoes, a fluid-debris level, or a complex cystic appearance (Figure 12-3). However, hemorrhagic cysts would not be expected to produce a homogeneous hyperechoic pattern, as seen in the test case. Therefore, autosomal dominant polycystic disease is not the most likely diagnosis.

Tuberous sclerosis (Option (B)) is another autosomal dominant genetic disorder. Renal angiomyolipomas, which typically appear homogeneous and hyperechoic, occur in 70 to 95% of patients with tuberous sclerosis and would certainly explain the solid mass in the kidney in one

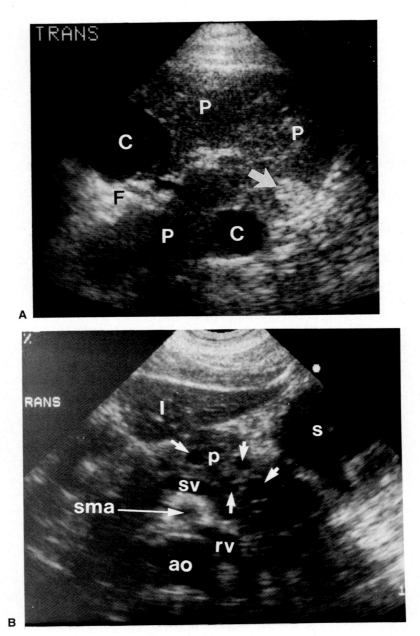

Figure 12-2 (Same as Figure 12-1). von Hippel-Lindau disease. (A) A transverse sonogram of the lower pole of the left kidney shows normal renal parenchyma (P) and normal renal sinus fat (F). Two cortical cysts (C) are also identified. A markedly hyperechoic solid mass (arrow) is seen in the lower-pole cortex. This solid mass was surgically proven to be a small renal cell carcinoma. (B) A transverse sonogram of the body of the pancreas demonstrates several normal anatomic structures including the left lobe of the liver (l), fluid in the stomach (s), splenic vein (sv), superior mesenteric artery (sma), aorta (ao), and left renal vein (rv). Multiple small cysts (arrows) are identified in the body of the pancreas (p).

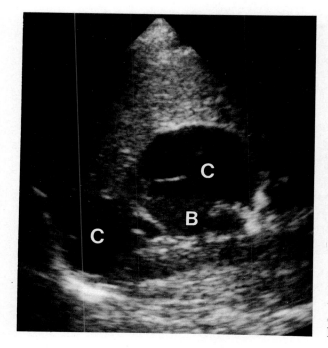

Figure 12-3. Autosomal dominant polycystic disease. A transverse sonogram through the upper pole of the right kidney shows different-sized partially septated cysts (C). The larger cyst contains layering blood products (B) in the dependent third due to hemorrhage.

of the siblings. Renal cysts also occur in patients with tuberous sclerosis and, rarely, can be the earliest manifestation of the disease. However, pancreatic cysts are not part of the spectrum of tuberous sclerosis; therefore, this is not the most likely diagnosis.

Acquired cystic disease (Option (C)) is seen in patients on chronic dialysis. Patients with acquired cystic disease are at increased risk of developing solid renal neoplasms. Therefore, the renal cysts and the solid renal mass in the test patients could be explained by acquired cystic disease. However, pancreatic cysts do not occur in patients with this disorder, and so acquired cystic disease is not the most likely diagnosis. In addition, acquired cystic disease would be expected to occur in siblings only if there were a familial cause of renal failure.

Cystic fibrosis (Option (E)) is a recessive disorder resulting in dysfunction of the exocrine secretory glands. In the pancreas, it causes inspissation and precipitation of pancreatic secretions. This leads to obstruction of the pancreatic ducts and can cause pancreatic cyst formation (Figure 12-4). Renal cysts and renal tumors are not part of the spectrum of cystic fibrosis, and therefore this is not the best diagnosis.

von Hippel-Lindau disease is an autosomal dominant disorder with variable penetrance that predisposes to the formation of a variety of vis-

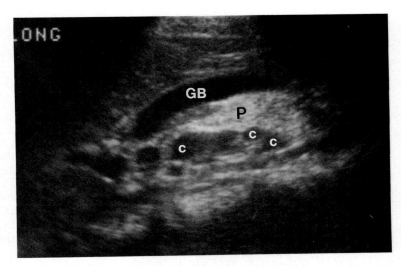

Figure 12-4. Cystic fibrosis. A longitudinal sonogram of the pancreatic head (P) using the gallbladder (GB) as a window shows several hypoechoic cystic structures (c) posteriorly.

ceral cysts and neoplasms. It is usually not recognized clinically until the third, fourth, or fifth decade of life. Patients most often present with signs or symptoms related to cerebellar or spinal cord disease or with visual changes, but occasionally abdominal cancers are diagnosed prior to the central nervous system (CNS) and orbital symptoms. The most common causes of morbidity and mortality are hemangioblastomas of the CNS, retinal angiomas, renal cell carcinoma, and pheochromocytoma.

The kidneys are involved in 30 to 70% of patients with von Hippel-Lindau disease. Renal cysts may be the first manifestation of the disease, and their detection can thus serve as the basis for genetic counseling. Although usually multiple, the renal cysts in patients with von Hippel-Lindau disease generally do not cause hypertension, renal insufficiency, or an overall enlargement in renal size as is seen in patients with autosomal dominant polycystic disease. Approximately 70% of renal cysts in patients with von Hippel-Lindau disease are stable over time. However, approximately 20% enlarge on follow-up studies and 10% become smaller or involute completely. The cysts can contain neoplastic elements in their walls and can evolve into renal cell carcinoma (Figure 12-5). Therefore, even benign-appearing cysts should be closely monitored.

Renal cell carcinoma occurs in 60 to 75% of patients with von Hippel-Lindau disease in whom the kidneys are involved. The tumors are bilateral in up to 75% and multifocal in 80 to 90% of these patients. They tend

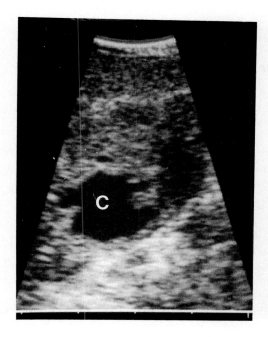

Figure 12-5. Renal cell carcinoma. An intraoperative sonogram of the kidney demonstrates a cystic mass (C) with a thick wall and marked mural nodularity. This was surgically proven to be a cystic renal cell carcinoma in a patient with von Hippel-Lindau disease.

to present at an earlier age than sporadic renal cell carcinoma, and the typical male predominance associated with sporadic renal cell carcinoma is not present in patients with von Hippel-Lindau disease.

Pheochromocytomas occur in up to 20% of patients with von Hippel-Lindau disease, but they are considerably more common in some families. They tend to be multiple, and they occur in extra-adrenal sites more commonly than do sporadic pheochromocytomas. On the other hand, they tend to produce clinical symptoms less often than do sporadic pheochromocytomas.

The most common pancreatic lesion in patients with von Hippel-Lindau disease is the simple cyst. Like pheochromocytomas, pancreatic cysts tend to be common in some families and infrequent in others. They are clinically asymptomatic in the vast majority of patients. Other pancreatic lesions reported in patients with von Hippel-Lindau disease include islet cell carcinoma, cystadenoma, and adenocarcinoma.

The dominant mode of inheritance means that half of the siblings and half of the children of affected individuals will develop the disease. All at-risk individuals should therefore have diagnostic tests directed at detecting the major manifestations of the disease when they are 18 to 20 years old. This will provide information useful for both therapeutic management and genetic counseling. Evaluation should include a careful

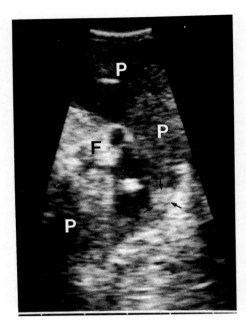

Figure 12-6. Renal cell carcinoma. An intraoperative sonogram of the kidney in a patient with von Hippel-Lindau disease demonstrates normal renal parenchyma (P) and renal sinus fat (F). A 5-mm solid echogenic mass (arrows) is seen along the periphery of the kidney. This mass could not be identified on preoperative CT or sonography and was not palpable at surgery. It was surgically proven to represent a small renal cell carcinoma.

physical examination of the neurologic system, an indirect ophthalmoscopic examination, and CT or MRI of the head and spine. The possible involvement of the kidneys, pancreas, and adrenal glands means that CT is probably the preferred means of screening the abdomen in at-risk individuals. In patients with known von Hippel-Lindau disease, CT is also the preferred means of surveillance. However, sonography is extremely valuable in evaluating indeterminate renal and pancreatic masses.

Once a solid or indeterminate renal mass is identified by CT or sonography, surgery should be performed to resect the mass and preserve as much normal renal parenchyma as possible. Intraoperative sonography is quite useful in localizing the suspicious lesion(s) so that resection can be minimized. It is also a valuable means of better characterizing indeterminate lesions and of identifying additional small lesions that require resection (Figure 12-6).

Question 52

Concerning acquired cystic disease of the kidney,

    (A) it occurs in patients undergoing either chronic hemodialysis or peritoneal dialysis

    (B) it occurs in patients with chronic renal disease who are not undergoing dialysis

    (C) it is usually sonographically apparent within the first year of dialysis

    (D) cyst hemorrhage is a common complication

    (E) sonography is more sensitive than CT in detecting solid renal lesions

Acquired cystic disease refers to the development of renal cysts in the failing kidney. It is a consequence of the progression of renal parenchymal diseases that cause chronic renal insufficiency. Occasionally, it may start before the time when dialysis becomes necessary **(Option (B) is true).** However, both peritoneal dialysis and hemodialysis allow patients to survive longer, and this allows acquired cystic disease to become more common and progressive **(Option (A) is true).** Acquired cystic disease generally does not become apparent on CT scans or sonograms until the patient has been on dialysis for more than 3 years **(Option (C) is false).** Approximately 90% of patients treated by dialysis for more than 10 years will develop identifiable acquired cystic disease.

The exact pathogenesis of the disease is unknown. One hypothesis is that dialysis fails to clear certain biologically active substances and that accumulation of these endogenous substances causes renal cysts to form. The facts that acquired cystic disease does not develop in uremic patients who undergo successful renal transplantation and subsequently enjoy prolonged periods of normal renal function and that renal transplantation may cause regression of acquired cystic disease both lend support to this theory.

Pathologically, the cysts in patients with acquired cystic disease are tubular in origin and generally range from microscopic to 2 to 3 cm in size (Figure 12-7). Most are smaller than 1 cm. They occur in both the cortex and medulla. The cysts can replace the entire kidney, but the kidneys usually remain small, a finding that helps to differentiate this condition from autosomal dominant polycystic disease. The kidneys do increase in volume with time and can eventually become larger than normal.

Renal tumors occur more commonly in patients with acquired cystic disease, with an estimated frequency of up to 7%. Generally, these tumors are small (<2 cm) and are usually detected incidentally. They can arise from cyst walls and project into the lumen of cysts, or they can be entirely solid (Figure 12-8). There is clear documentation that renal

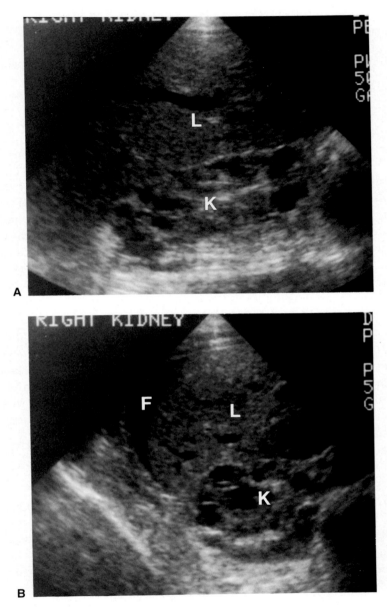

Figure 12-7. Acquired cystic disease. (A) A longitudinal sonogram of the right kidney (K) demonstrates multiple small cortical cysts. The kidney is small and slightly hyperechoic compared with the liver (L). (B) A transverse sonogram of the right kidney (K) again demonstrates multiple small cortical cysts. L = liver; F = peritoneal dialysis fluid.

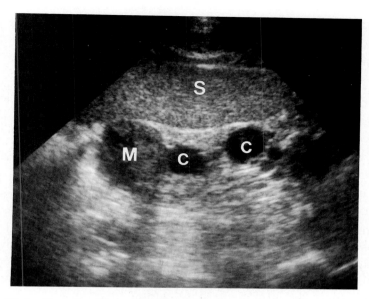

Figure 12-8. Renal cell carcinoma arising in a kidney in a patient with acquired cystic disease. An oblique sonogram of the left kidney demonstrates several small cysts (C) and a solid hypoechoic mass (M) that was surgically proven to be a renal cell carcinoma. Little normal renal parenchyma remains. S = spleen.

tumors are more common in the setting of acquired cystic disease, but the natural history of these tumors is not well understood. In fact, tumors that clearly exhibit malignant behavior may not be more common than in the general population. Therefore, the use of imaging studies to screen for renal cell carcinoma in dialysis patients is controversial. The combination of pre- and postcontrast CT is probably more sensitive than sonography in detecting solid masses in patients with acquired cystic disease **(Option (E) is false).** However, the expense of using CT screening to detect small solid lesions that will frequently have no clinical impact in this debilitated patient population is probably not justified. Sonography is less expensive and is capable of detecting most renal cell cancers before they metastasize, but the overall benefits of sonographic screening are also debatable. Currently, there are no generally agreed upon guidelines for screening dialysis patients for the development of renal tumors.

The most common complication of acquired cystic disease is renal hemorrhage. Bleeding disorders and heparinization during dialysis therapy may contribute to this complication. Approximately half the patients will develop hemorrhagic cysts **(Option (D) is true).** Approximately 10 to 20% of patients develop perinephric hematomas.

Question 53

Concerning tuberous sclerosis,

   (A) the classic clinical triad consists of mental retardation, seizures, and cutaneous lesions

   (B) it is associated with atrial myxomas

   (C) pulmonary involvement often results in spontaneous pneumothorax

   (D) associated angiomyolipomas are usually multiple and bilateral

   (E) associated angiomyolipomas occur in about 20% of patients

Tuberous sclerosis is a neurocutaneous syndrome that is characterized clinically by mental retardation, seizures, and cutaneous lesions **(Option (A) is true)**. It can be sporadic or inherited as an autosomal dominant trait. Multiple organs are usually involved. Cortical hamartomas (tubers), periventricular subependymal glial nodules, subependymal giant cell astrocytomas, and retinal hamartomas occur in the CNS. Approximately 30% of patients have cardiac involvement in the form of rhabdomyomas **(Option (B) is false)**. These lesions involve the ventricles more often than the atria and are usually multiple. Cardiac rhabdomyomas are usually asymptomatic, but they can protrude into the lumen and cause outflow obstruction. They can also affect contractility if they are extensive, and they can affect the cardiac conduction system. Pulmonary involvement is rare ($\leq$1%), usually occurs in females, and is identical to lymphangioleiomyomatosis. It causes honeycombing and subpleural blebs (Figure 12-9). Spontaneous perforation of the blebs produces pneumothorax in approximately 50% of affected individuals **(Option (C) is true)**. Unlike the situation for many of the other organ systems, pulmonary involvement almost always produces symptoms in patients with tuberous sclerosis. Skeletal lesions occur in approximately 50% of patients and are usually asymptomatic. Sclerotic patches can be seen in a variety of bones, and cystic lesions can be seen in the bones of the hands and feet. Periosteal reaction occurs particularly in the metatarsals. Hepatic hamartomas have been described but are unusual. They are similar to angiomyolipomas in that they contain large amounts of fat (Figure 12-10).

The kidneys are involved in up to 95% of patients with tuberous sclerosis who survive beyond childhood. The most common renal lesion associated with tuberous sclerosis is the angiomyolipoma, which occurs in 50 to 80% of patients **(Option (E) is false)**. As the name implies, angiomyolipomas are composed of variable amounts of fat, smooth muscle, and abnormal blood vessels. They are benign hamartomas that become symptomatic only when they bleed or compress adjacent structures. Angiomyolipomas associated with tuberous sclerosis are multiple and bilateral in

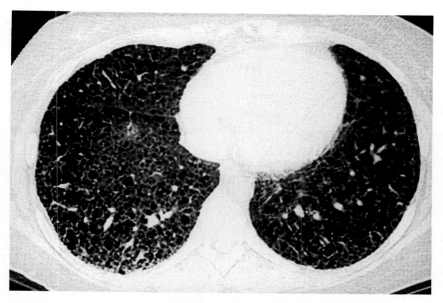

Figure 12-9. Lymphangioleiomyomatosis. A CT scan of the chest demonstrates marked honeycombing of the lungs with increased prominence of the interstitial tissues and parenchymal destruction with cystic air spaces, a pattern typical of lymphangioleiomyomatosis. (Case courtesy of David H. Stephens, M.D., Mayo Clinic, Rochester, Minn.)

approximately 90% of affected individuals **(Option (D) is true).** Rarely, they become so extensive that they cause renal insufficiency.

Sonographically, angiomyolipomas usually appear as homogeneous masses that are markedly hyperechoic compared with renal parenchyma. They are unencapsulated, but their margins are usually well demarcated from adjacent renal parenchyma. The angiomyolipomas associated with tuberous sclerosis are usually less than 1 cm in size (Figure 12-11), but they occasionally become considerably larger. In some patients with tuberous sclerosis, angiomyolipomas become so extensive that normal renal architecture is completely obscured and the kidneys become difficult to identify (Figure 12-12).

Benign renal cysts occur in 20 to 40% of patients with tuberous sclerosis. Cysts are more common in infants and children and may be the initial or occasionally the only manifestation of tuberous sclerosis in early childhood. Like angiomyolipomas, benign renal cysts are usually asymptomatic in this patient population, but they appear to be capable of producing hypertension and renal failure more often than angiomyolipomas do.

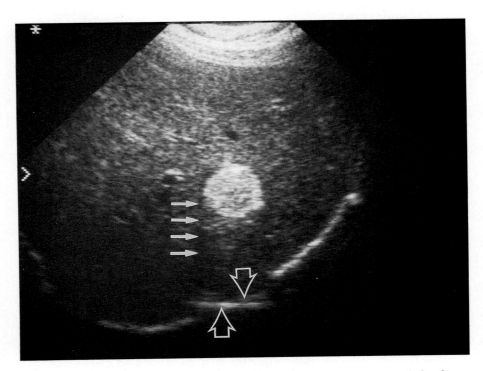

Figure 12-10. Hepatic hamartoma. A transverse sonogram of the liver demonstrates a markedly echogenic mass. This mass is composed predominantly of fat. Because the velocity of sound in fat is less than in the adjacent normal hepatic parenchyma, there are refractive effects at the edge of the lesion that result in redirection of the sound beam (solid arrows). This sound beam refraction causes misregistration of the diaphragmatic reflection (open arrows). This sonographic artifact distinguishes fat-containing tumors from other hyperechoic solid masses such as hemangiomas. (Case courtesy of David H. Stephens, M.D.)

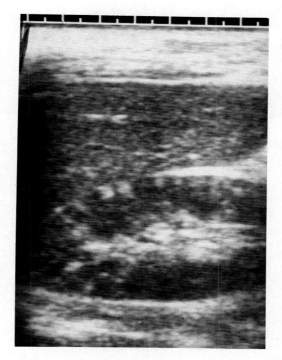

Figure 12-11. Tuberous sclerosis. A longitudinal sonogram of the right kidney shows multiple small angiomyolipomas as very echogenic masses in the renal cortex. (Case courtesy of David H. Stephens, M.D.)

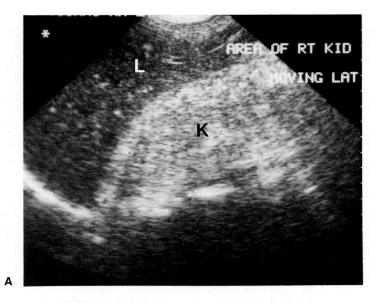

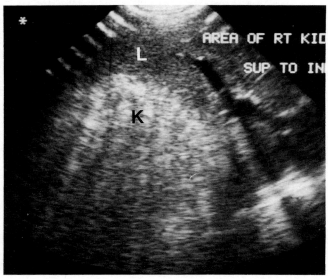

Figure 12-12. Tuberous sclerosis with complete replacement of the renal parenchyma by diffuse angiomyolipomas. Longitudinal (A) and transverse (B) sonograms of the right upper quadrant, obtained with the liver (L) as a window, show no normal renal parenchyma in the expected location of the right kidney (K). Attenuation of the sound beam by the angiomyolipomas is apparent as decreasing echogenicity in the deeper portions of the kidney. (C) A CT scan through the upper abdomen demonstrates marked enlargement of the kidneys bilaterally by multiple masses with attenuation values of fat. As on the sonograms, there is no normal renal parenchyma in the expected location of the kidneys (K). The enlarged kidneys in this patient have nearly filled the entire abdominal cavity. Bowel loops (B) are displaced centrally. (Case courtesy of Mary A. Middleton, M.D., Barnes-West County Hospital, St. Louis, Mo.)

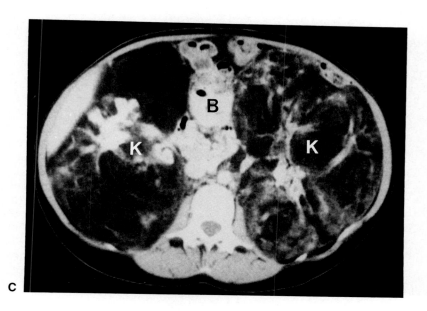

C

Question 54

Concerning sporadic renal angiomyolipoma,

    (A) it is a cause of spontaneous perinephric hematoma
    (B) sonography is diagnostic in most patients
    (C) it occurs more frequently in women than in men
    (D) calcification occurs in approximately 20% of patients
    (E) malignant degeneration occurs in about 5% of patients

Angiomyolipomas are benign hamartomas with no malignant potential **(Option (E) is false).** Except in patients with tuberous sclerosis, they are usually unilateral and solitary. They occur most often in middle age, and the female to male ratio is approximately 3:1 **(Option (C) is true).** They generally do not produce symptoms and are detected incidentally on imaging studies. However, the lack of normal elastic tissue in the walls of the tumor vessels means that they can bleed internally or into the renal parenchyma, collecting system, or retroperitoneum **(Option (A) is true).** Therefore, patients with angiomyolipomas can present with flank pain, hematuria, or life-threatening hemorrhage.

On sonography, 80% of angiomyolipomas are homogeneous and markedly hyperechoic compared with the renal cortex (Figure 12-13). However, hemorrhage, necrosis, and a predominance of nonfatty ele-

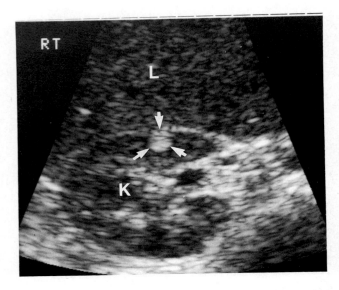

Figure 12-13. Typical angiomyolipoma. A transverse sonogram of the right kidney (K), obtained with the liver (L) as a window, demonstrates a markedly hyperechoic, homogeneous, well-defined mass (arrows) in the anterior cortex.

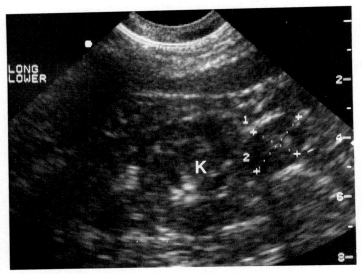

Figure 12-14. Atypical angiomyolipoma. An oblique sonogram of the right kidney (K) demonstrates an isoechoic exophytic mass (cursors) arising from the renal cortex. This mass had an attenuation value of –20 HU on CT, consistent with a fatty lesion.

ments can all result in atypical appearances (Figure 12-14). Therefore, approximately 12% of angiomyolipomas are hyperechoic but heterogeneous and 8% are either isoechoic or hypoechoic. Calcifications are extremely rare **(Option (D) is false).** A homogeneous renal mass that is as

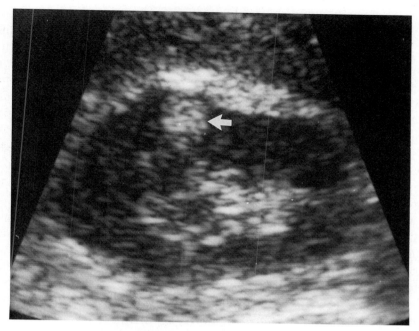

Figure 12-15. Hyperechoic renal cell carcinoma simulating an angiomyolipoma. A longitudinal sonogram through the lateral aspect of the left kidney demonstrates a markedly hyperechoic mass (arrow) that is similar in echogenicity to the renal sinus fat. This mass is sonographically identical to a typical angiomyolipoma, but it did not contain fat on CT and was surgically proven to be a renal cell carcinoma.

echogenic as renal sinus fat is very characteristic for angiomyolipoma, but this appearance is not diagnostic **(Option (B) is false).** In the early 1980s, Charboneau et al. and Hartman et al. documented that up to 5% of renal cell carcinomas have an appearance identical to that of angiomyolipoma. A more recent study by Forman et al. has demonstrated that small renal cell cancers (<3 cm) are even more likely to be hyperechoic (Figure 12-15). In their study, 32% of small renal cell cancers simulated angiomyolipomas whereas only 2% of larger renal cell cancers had this appearance. Smaller tumors are being detected more readily with current imaging modalities, and so these authors also documented an increasing frequency of detection of hyperechoic renal cell carcinomas, with 12% of all renal cancers appearing markedly hyperechoic.

Given the fact that a homogeneous, markedly hyperechoic renal mass is not pathognomonic for an angiomyolipoma, it is important that such masses be further evaluated in some fashion. If the mass is larger than 1 cm, CT should be performed to determine whether it contains fat.

Such CT scans should be performed without intravenous administration of contrast material, using thin sections (2 to 5 mm) to avoid volume-averaging artifacts. Detection of any fat within a renal mass is pathognomonic of angiomyolipoma. If fat is not detected in a renal mass larger than 1 cm in size, the mass should be considered a renal cell carcinoma and managed accordingly. CT documentation of fatty elements becomes progressively more difficult in angiomyolipomas less than 1 cm in size because of volume-averaging artifacts.

The clinical management of angiomyolipomas depends on both the symptoms and the certainty of the radiologic diagnosis. The first group of patients to consider are those in whom a hyperechoic mass is detected on sonography and subsequent CT confirms the presence of fatty elements, thus establishing an unequivocal diagnosis of angiomyolipoma. If patients in this group are asymptomatic, no further evaluation is required. Patients with mild symptoms such as flank pain or hematuria and angiomyolipomas smaller than 4 cm can be managed by angiographically directed embolization. If symptoms recur or if the initial lesion is larger than 4 cm, partial nephrectomy should be considered. Patients with CT-documented angiomyolipomas who present with severe, life-threatening hemorrhage require urgent surgery with preservation of as much renal parenchyma as possible. However, in some cases, total nephrectomy is unavoidable despite preoperative knowledge that the underlying renal mass is benign.

The other group of patients to consider are those in whom sonography demonstrates a markedly hyperechoic renal mass but CT demonstrates no detectable fatty elements. In this group of patients, if the mass is larger than 1 cm, it is very likely to represent a renal cell carcinoma and surgery should be considered if the patient's medical condition allows. Frozen sections should be obtained to determine whether the mass is malignant; if it is, a partial or radical nephrectomy should be performed. If malignancy cannot be confirmed by studying frozen sections, wedge resection or partial nephrectomy may be adequate. Patients with lesions that are less than 1 cm can either be monitored by serial sonograms or undergo surgical exploration as described above.

William D. Middleton, M.D.

SUGGESTED READINGS

VON HIPPEL-LINDAU DISEASE

1. Choyke PL, Glenn GM, Walther MM, et al. The natural history of renal lesions in von Hippel-Lindau disease: a serial CT study in 28 patients. AJR 1992; 159:1229–1234

2. Coulam CM, Brown LR, Reese DF. Hippel-Lindau syndrome. Semin Roentgenol 1976; 11:61–66
3. Fill WL, Lamiell JM, Polk NO. The radiographic manifestations of von Hippel-Lindau disease. Radiology 1979; 133:289–295
4. Horton WA, Wong V, Eldridge R. Von Hippel-Lindau disease: clinical and pathological manifestations in nine families with 50 affected members. Arch Intern Med 1976; 136:769–777
5. Levine E, Hartman DS, Smirniotopoulos JG. Renal cystic disease associated with renal neoplasms. In: Pollack HM (ed), Clinical urography. Philadelphia: WB Saunders; 1990:1126–1150

TUBEROUS SCLEROSIS

6. Bell DG, King BF, Hattery RR, Charboneau JW, Hoffman AD, Houser OW. Imaging characteristics of tuberous sclerosis. AJR 1991; 156:1081–1086
7. Bernstein J, Robbins TO. Renal involvement in tuberous sclerosis. Ann NY Acad Sci 1991; 615:36–49
8. Bernstein J, Robbins TO, Kissane JM. The renal lesions of tuberous sclerosis. Semin Diagn Pathol 1986; 3(2):97–105
9. Hoffman AD. Imaging of tuberous sclerosis lesions outside of the central nervous system. Ann NY Acad Sci 1991; 615:94–111
10. Lie JT. Cardiac, pulmonary, and vascular involvements in tuberous sclerosis. Ann NY Acad Sci 1991; 615:58–70
11. Narla LD, Slovis TL, Watts FB, Nigro M. The renal lesions of tuberosclerosis (cysts and angiomyolipoma)—screening with sonography and computerized tomography. Pediatr Radiol 1988; 18:205–209
12. Stapleton FB, Johnson D, Kaplan GW, Griswold W. The cystic renal lesion in tuberous sclerosis. J Pediatr 1980; 97:574–579
13. Stillwell TJ, Gomez MR, Kelalis PP. Renal lesions in tuberous sclerosis. J Urol 1987; 138:477–481
14. Wood BP, Lieberman E, Landing B, Marcus B. Tuberous sclerosis. AJR 1992; 158:750

ACQUIRED CYSTIC DISEASE

15. Jabour BA, Ralls PW, Tang WW, et al. Acquired cystic disease of the kidneys. Computed tomography and ultrasonography appraisal in patients on peritoneal and hemodialysis. Invest Radiol 1987; 22:728–732
16. Levine E, Slusher SL, Grantham JJ, Wetzel LH. Natural history of acquired renal cystic disease in dialysis patients: a prospective longitudinal CT study. AJR 1991; 156:501–506
17. Taylor AJ, Cohen EP, Erickson SJ, Olson DL, Foley WD. Renal imaging in long-term dialysis patients: a comparison of CT and sonography. AJR 1989; 153:765–767

ANGIOMYOLIPOMA

18. Andriole GL. Renal angiomyolipoma. In: Kursh ED, Resnick MI (eds), Current therapy in genitourinary surgery. St. Louis: Mosby-Year Book; 1992:46–50

19. Bosniak MA. The small (≤3.0 cm) renal parenchymal tumor: detection, diagnosis, and controversies. Radiology 1991; 179:307–317

20. Bosniak MA, Megibow AJ, Hulnick DH, Horii S, Raghavendra BN. CT diagnosis of renal angiomyolipoma: the importance of detecting small amounts of fat. AJR 1988; 151:497–501

21. Bret PM, Bretagnolle M, Gaillard D, et al. Small, asymptomatic angiomyolipomas of the kidney. Radiology 1985; 154:7–10

22. Charboneau JW, Hattery RR, Ernst EC III, James EM, Williamson B Jr, Hartman GW. Spectrum of sonographic findings in 125 renal masses other than benign simple cyst. AJR 1983; 140:87–94

23. Forman HP, Middleton WD, Melson GL, McClennan BL. Increasing frequency of detection of hyperechoic renal cell carcinomas. Radiology 1993; 188:431–434

24. Hartman DS, Goldman SM, Friedman AC, Davis CJ Jr, Madewell JE, Sherman JL. Angiomyolipoma: ultrasonic-pathologic correlation. Radiology 1981; 139:451–458

25. Päivänsalo M, Siniluoto T, Leinonen A, Kallioinen M. Sonographic findings in cases of benign renal tumours. J Med Imaging 1989; 3:164–170

26. Raghavendra BN, Bosniak MA, Megibow AJ. Small angiomyolipoma of the kidney: sonographic-CT evaluation. AJR 1983; 141:575–578

27. Yamashita Y, Takahashi M, Watanabe O, et al. Small renal cell carcinoma: pathologic and radiologic correlation. Radiology 1992; 184:493–498

Notes

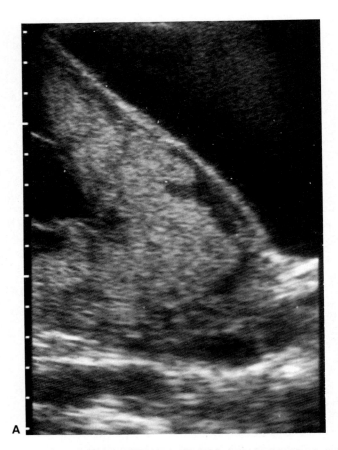

A

Figure 13-1. This 37-year-old gravida 3, para 1 woman underwent obstetric sonography at 23-weeks gestational age because of vaginal bleeding. You are shown longitudinal (A) and transverse (B) images through the lower uterus.

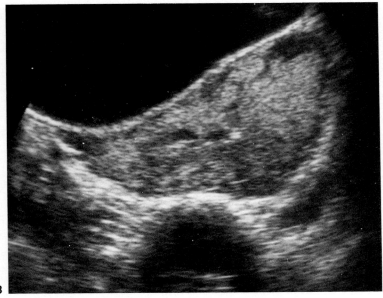

B

Case 13: Placenta Increta

Question 55

Which *one* of the following is the MOST likely diagnosis?

(A) Marginal placenta previa
(B) Placenta increta
(C) Subchorionic hemorrhage
(D) Gestational trophoblastic disease
(E) Abruptio placentae

The low midline sonogram through the uterus of the test patient (Figure 13-1A) shows a complete placenta previa, with the echogenic placenta covering the entire internal cervical os (Figure 13-2A). This is confirmed on the low transverse sonogram (Figure 13-1B), in which the placenta fills the lower uterine segment (Figure 13-2B). On both images the hypoechoic myometrium is of variable thickness secondary to invasion by the overlying placenta. The most likely diagnosis is therefore placenta increta **(Option (B) is correct).** During normal implantation, placental villi invade the decidual layer of the uterus, and during delivery the placenta is sheared off at that level. When there is a deficiency in the development of the decidual layer, the villous tissue invades deeper to implant into the myometrium, preventing complete placental detachment. The smallest degree of placental invasion into the myometrium is termed placenta accreta. Placenta increta refers to invasion extending to about 50% of the myometrial thickness, and placenta percreta is a full-thickness invasion with the potential for involvement of adjacent organs as well. Prior cesarean section increases the frequency of myometrial invasion by the placenta (accreta, increta, or percreta). Placenta accreta, increta, or percreta is also often associated with placenta previa, as in the test patient. The exact mechanism is unknown but is probably related to the relative inability of the lower uterine segment to respond during pregnancy to the normal hormonal influences for the creation of an adequate decidual layer. The antecedent formation of the placenta in the lower uterine segment, often culminating in placenta previa, also predisposes

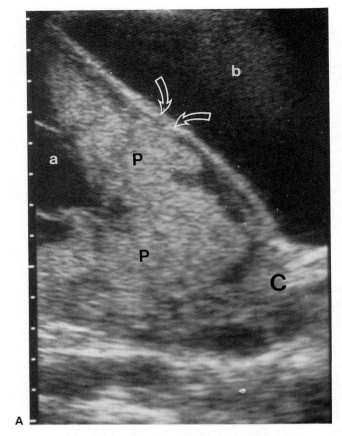

Figure 13-2 (Same as Figure 13-1). Placenta increta. (A) A longitudinal sonogram through the lower uterus shows echogenic complete placenta previa (P) over the cervix (C). a = amniotic fluid. The hypoechoic myometrium, which lies between the maternal bladder (b) and placenta, should be of uniform thickness, about 1 cm. The placenta is seen to be invading the myometrium (arrows). (B) A low transverse sonogram also shows the placenta invading the myometrium (arrows). b = maternal bladder.

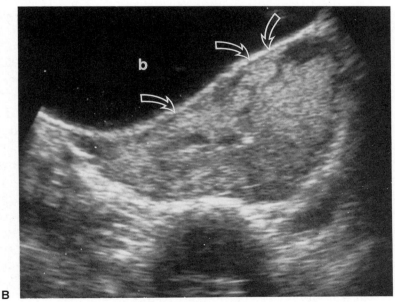

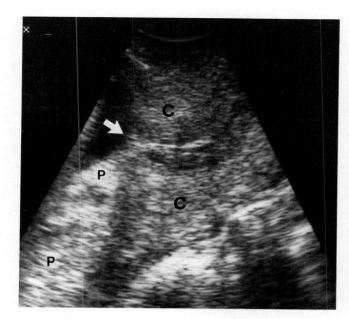

Figure 13-3. Marginal placenta previa. On a transvaginal scan, a midline sagittal image shows the cervix (C) with its echogenic lumen. The placenta (P) is posterior and stops at the edge of the cervix, short of the internal cervical os (arrow).

to the development of myometrial invasion. A placenta formed in the lower uterine segment is therefore more likely to extend over the cervix (placenta previa) and invade the myometrium (placenta accreta). Serious intra- or postpartum hemorrhage can result when the placenta is so involved. With extensive invasion or involvement of the larger uterine vessels, significant vaginal bleeding can occur and uterine rupture has been reported. Failure of placental separation at delivery can result in intractable bleeding, necessitating emergency hysterectomy.

On the basis of the location of the placenta relative to the internal cervical os, the following subsets of placenta previa have been described: (1) central/complete, in which the internal cervical os is totally covered by placental tissue, which clearly extends beyond the os in all directions; (2) partial, in which the internal cervical os is partially covered by placenta; (3) marginal, in which the edge of the placenta is at the margin of, but not frankly covering, the internal os; and (4) low lying, in which the placental edge is in close proximity to the cervix and lower uterine segment.

Functionally, the presence of placental tissue close to but not over the os can still require treatment as a frank placenta previa because of mechanical considerations. It has been suggested that a placenta within 2 cm of the internal os will often behave clinically as a placenta previa. However, by existing definitions, a marginal placenta previa does not extend over the cervical os (Figure 13-3). The test images clearly show a

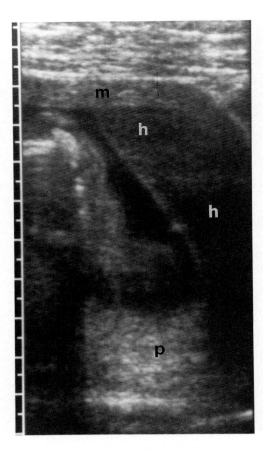

Figure 13-4. Subchorionic hemorrhage. A midline low sagittal sonogram shows a hypoechoic hematoma (h) between membranes and myometrium (m). The hematoma extends from the edge of the placenta (p).

complete placenta previa; therefore, marginal placenta previa (Option (A)) is not the correct diagnosis.

Subchorionic hemorrhage (Option (C)) is a common cause of vaginal bleeding during the late first or early second trimester. Sonographically it appears as an echogenic, isoechoic, or hypoechoic collection deep to the membranes, extending from the margin of the placenta for a variable distance (Figure 13-4). The edge of the placenta is often minimally elevated by the hemorrhage, since this represents a small marginal abruption. These features are not present in the test images.

Placental invasion of the myometrium occurs only with the malignant forms of gestational trophoblastic disease (Option (D)). Eighty percent of complete hydatidiform moles are benign, being confined to the intrauterine cavity. The classic sonographic appearance of a hydatidiform mole is that of an enlarged placenta containing multiple different-sized fluid-filled spaces corresponding to hydropic villi (Figure 13-5).

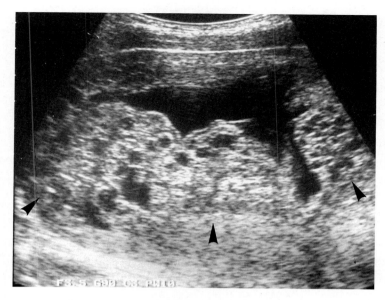

Figure 13-5. Complete hydatidiform mole. A transverse sonogram through the uterus shows an enlarged, bulky placenta (arrowheads) with multiple hypoechoic vesicles of different sizes.

These features are absent in the test images, in which the placenta is of normal echotexture and size.

Sonographic detection of abruptio placentae (Option (E)) is difficult, since findings are often nonspecific and are present in only a few instances. Described features, none of which are seen in the test images, include retroplacental fluid collection; fluid collection at the placental margin, elevating the adjacent membranes; basal intraplacental hypoechoic areas, suggesting infarction; and placental thickening beyond 6 cm or rounding of the placental edges, suggesting uterine contraction.

Question 56

Concerning placenta previa,

   (A) the presence of a succenturiate lobe can result in a false-positive diagnosis

   (B) transvaginal scanning is often necessary for diagnosis in the third trimester

   (C) myometrial contractions can cause a false-positive diagnosis in early pregnancy

   (D) placenta accreta is rarely associated with it

   (E) in most cases of central placenta previa diagnosed in early pregnancy, the placenta migrates to a nonobstructing position by the third trimester

Placenta previa refers to the presence of placental tissue over the cervix, secondary to low implantation. It is a leading cause of third-trimester vaginal bleeding, being found in 0.3 to 0.6% of third-trimester pregnancies. Its etiology is unknown. However, it is found most often in patients with a history of uterine surgery, including cesarean section and sharp curettage; in patients who have had previous abortions; and in women of advanced gestational age or multiparous status.

With growth and effacement of the lower uterus, a low placental implantation often results in vaginal bleeding. About 65% of patients with placenta previa have their first bleed after 30 weeks. A breech or transverse fetal lie in the third trimester should raise the suspicion of placenta previa.

A portion of the placenta separated from the main body of the placenta by a segment of membrane is termed an accessory or succenturiate lobe (Figure 13-6). The size of an accessory lobe can range from small to quite large, and the lobe can lie several centimeters from the primary placenta. In one-third of such placentas the umbilical cord inserts into the larger component; in the remaining two-thirds it is velamentous, or membranous, located between the two portions of placental tissues. A bilobed or bipartite placenta, occurring in about 1 in 350 pregnancies, has two roughly equal-sized lobes, usually with a central membranous cord insertion (Figure 13-7). Accessory or bipartite placentas are generally not clinically significant. However, failure to recognize a succenturiate lobe over the cervix while identifying a separate primary placenta remote to the cervix would result in a false-negative diagnosis of placenta previa **(Option (A) is false).** Vasa previa (the presence of placental vessels in the membranous components without overlying placental tissue) and retained placenta with postpartum hemorrhage are other potential complications that can elude diagnosis if not detected sonographically. The mechanism of formation of such placentas is not known, but it is possible that infarction or atrophy of a portion of a normal pla-

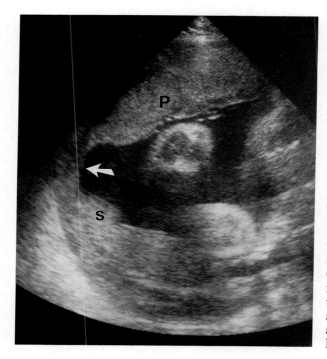

Figure 13-6. Succenturiate lobe. A longitudinal sonogram through the fundus shows separation (arrow) between the normal-appearing anterior placenta (P) and a small posterior accessory placental lobe (S).

centa occurred. This is supported by the cord insertion sites detected in these cases.

Imaging of the cervical region by transabdominal scanning can be difficult in the third trimester because of low fetal head position as well as general enlargement of the uterine and fetal structures (Figure 13-8A). Additionally, the inability of the maternal bladder to distend adequately can preclude visualization of this region. Exact relationships between the placenta and cervix may not be obvious, and transvaginal scanning is an important technique for defining these relationships (Figure 13-8B). With transvaginal scanning, proximity to the target organs allows use of higher-frequency probes with better resolution. It avoids problems with obesity, intervening fetal parts, and bladder filling. Careful transvaginal scanning has been proven safe under real-time visualization. With partial insertion of the probe, one can see the cervix and placenta and avoid blindly traumatizing the placenta, if placenta previa is present. Translabial scanning can also be used safely if active bleeding is present and the risk of transvaginal scanning is deemed too high. Transvaginal scanning is much less likely than transabdominal scanning to result in a false-positive diagnosis of placenta previa. The only false-positive diagnoses with transvaginal scanning have occurred with a mar-

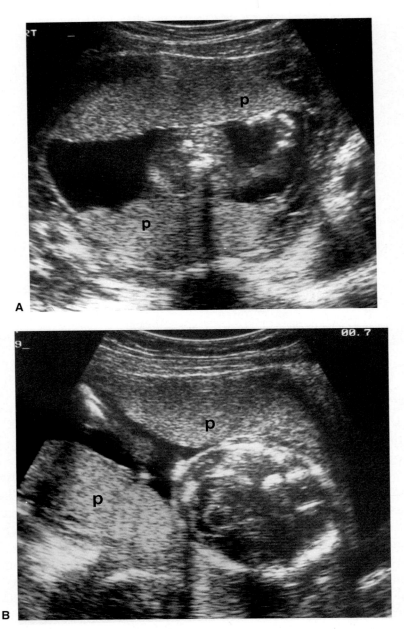

Figure 13-7. Bilobed placenta. Transverse (A) and longitudinal (B) images show equal-sized placental lobes (p) anteriorly and posteriorly in this singleton pregnancy.

ginal placenta previa imaged prior to 30 weeks. This probably results from differential lower uterine growth, with eventual enlargement of the

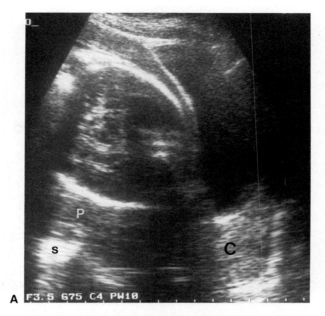

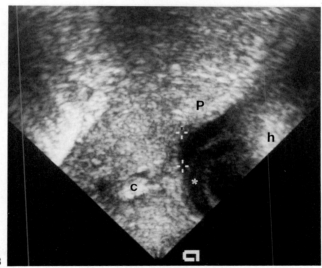

Figure 13-8. Marginal placenta previa. (A) A midline low transabdominal scan shows cephalic presentation, but the head is displaced anteriorly away from the sacrum (s) by a low posterior placenta (P). The exact relationship of the placenta to the cervix (C) could not be ascertained because of low head position; therefore, transvaginal scanning was performed. (B) A sagittal transvaginal scan shows the posterior placenta (P) not to be a frank placenta previa but rather to be a marginal placenta previa with the placental edge about 9 mm from the internal cervical os. c = cervical canal; h = fetal head. The asterisk indicates cord presentation between head and cervix, another potential complication best detected by transvaginal scanning.

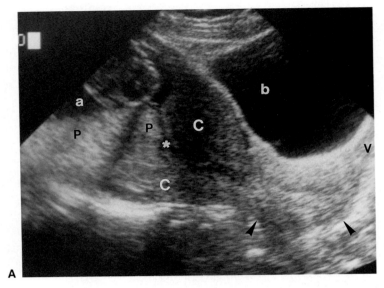

A

Figure 13-9. Uterine contraction causing appearance of placenta previa. (A) A midline low longitudinal image shows the cervix (arrowheads) and vagina (v) posterior to the bladder (b). Anterior and posterior contractions (C) of the lower uterus cause an apparent lengthening of the cervix. This results in an artificially high location of the internal cervical os (✳), which now appears to lie under the posterior placenta (P). (B) A midline low longitudinal image taken 13 minutes later, following relaxation of the contraction, again shows the cervix (arrowheads) and vagina (v) posterior to the bladder (B). The end of the placenta (P) is now clearly seen to stop well above the internal cervical os (✳). a = amniotic fluid.

distance between the cervix and the placenta. If a question of placenta previa exists, therefore, it is best to perform transvaginal scanning after 30 weeks because it is more reliable than transabdominal scanning in the third trimester **(Option (B) is true).**

The presence of myometrial contractions (Figure 13-9) or overdistension of the maternal bladder (Figure 13-10) can result in a false-positive diagnosis of placenta previa **(Option (C) is true).** In each instance there is a mass effect, which causes a coaptation of the anterior and posterior walls of the uterus superior to the cervix. This leads to a falsely elongated appearance of the cervix, which may abut placental tissue and hence be confused with placenta previa. Scanning over time to observe resolution of a contraction or serial scanning following partial voiding will often clarify these situations.

Invasion of the placenta into the myometrium, a pathologic condition termed placenta accreta, increta, or percreta with increasing depth of

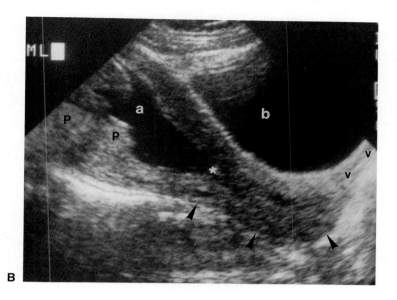

penetration, occurs primarily in areas of the uterus where the normal decidual response of pregnancy is subnormal. The two primary loci for this phenomenon are a site of prior cesarean section and the lower uterine segment, where placenta previa also occurs. Such placental invasion of the myometrium is found in up to 15% of patients with placenta previa (Figure 13-11) **(Option (D) is false).**

In the early second trimester it is often difficult to document the exact relationship between a "low-lying" placenta and the cervix. The appearance can simulate placenta previa if the location of the internal cervical os is misjudged. Up to 25% of placentas extend into the lower segment of the uterus in the early second trimester. In many of these cases, a diagnosis of placenta previa cannot be excluded; however, the actual frequency of placenta previa is only about 0.3 to 0.6% of third-trimester pregnancies. Rizos et al. found a 5.3% frequency of suspected placenta previa at midterm but only a 0.58% frequency at term. Overfilling of the bladder, uterine contractions, or a normal appearance prior to lower uterine growth can all result in a false-positive diagnosis of placenta previa. As the lower uterine segment grows and elongates during pregnancy, the separation between the cervix and the lower margin of the placenta becomes more apparent. Sometimes this apparent shift in placental position is referred to as placental "migration." True migration of the implanted placenta is not possible, but it is postulated that small infarctions at the edge of the placenta can result in focal atrophy and apparent movement of the placental edge to a position clearly separate

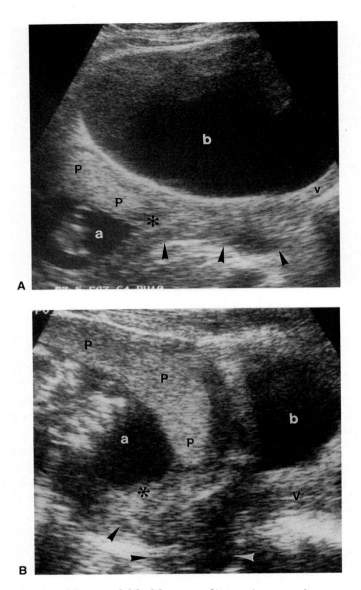

Figure 13-10. Maternal bladder overdistension causing appearance of placenta previa. (A) A midline low longitudinal image shows the cervix (arrowheads) and vagina (v) posterior to the bladder (b). The anterior placenta (P) appears to lie over the internal cervical os (*), due to over-distension of the maternal bladder with coaptation of the anterior and posterior walls of the lower uterus leading to an erroneously elongated cervical appearance. (B) Following near-complete bladder emptying, a midline low longitudinal image again shows the cervix (arrowheads) and vagina (v) posterior to the bladder (b). The inferior edge of the anterior placenta (P) stops above the internal cervical os (*). a = amniotic fluid.

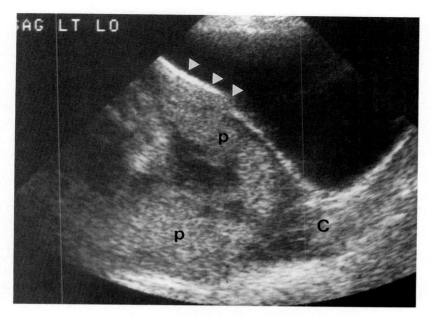

Figure 13-11. Placenta percreta. A midline low image shows complete placenta previa (p) over the cervix (C). The placenta has completely penetrated the myometrium and forms an external contour defect adjacent to the bladder wall (arrowheads).

from the cervix later in pregnancy. In patients in whom the placenta unequivocally covers the internal os early in pregnancy, the placenta should remain an obvious complete placenta previa throughout pregnancy (Figure 13-12). With a central placenta previa, as seen in the test patient, equal amounts of placental tissue extend in all directions from the os. Such a complete placenta previa does not change its position during pregnancy **(Option (E) is false).**

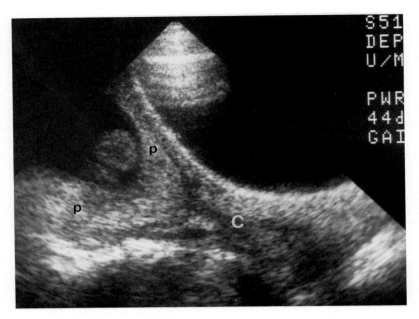

Figure 13-12. Placenta previa. A low midline scan at 16 weeks gestational age shows a predominantly posterior placenta (p) entirely covering the cervix (C) and extending onto the anterior uterine wall.

Question 57

Concerning pregnancy-related hemorrhage,

(A) about 50% of women with vaginal bleeding in the first 20 weeks of pregnancy have sonographic evidence of subchorionic hemorrhage
(B) subchorionic hemorrhage is identified sonographically by its predominantly retroplacental locus
(C) the sensitivity of sonography for detection of abruptio placentae is lower than 50%
(D) placenta accreta is a cause of persistent postpartum hemorrhage
(E) life-threatening hemorrhage is associated with velamentous cord insertion

Vaginal bleeding occurs in up to 30% of women in the first trimester of pregnancy and in 16 to 25% of women prior to the third trimester. Causes of first- and second-trimester bleeding include implantation bleeding, subchorionic hemorrhage (SCH), spontaneous abortion, threatened abortion, incomplete abortion, missed abortion, blighted ovum, ectopic pregnancy, molar pregnancy, and cervical diseases. In two large series of patients with vaginal bleeding, the frequency of SCH was 5 and

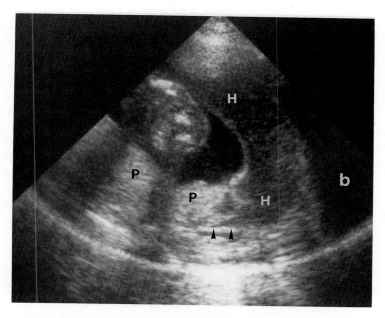

Figure 13-13. Subchorionic hemorrhage. A longitudinal sonogram shows a large contained hematoma (H), which has raised the placental margin (arrowheads) and extends away from the placenta (P). The hematoma is more echogenic than the amniotic fluid, which is separated from it by the membranes. b = maternal bladder.

18% **(Option (A) is false).** SCH is most often noted in the second trimester. It probably results from a marginal separation or abruption of the placental edge or marginal sinus. Only a small retroplacental collection is typically identified, with most of the blood dissecting away from the placenta deep to the membranes (Figure 13-13) **(Option (B) is false).** Retroplacental hemorrhage, termed abruption or abruptio placentae, is usually a third-trimester phenomena. Acute SCH can be echogenic, isoechoic, or even hypoechoic relative to the placenta. With time, most hemorrhages appear hypoechoic but are still more echogenic than the amniotic fluid. There are conflicting reports concerning the clinical significance of SCH. Some studies describe an increased fetal morbidity and mortality, particularly when a large bleed of more than 50 to 60 mL is identified. These results are not confirmed by all studies, however. Most reports indicate a relatively favorable outcome for these patients, particularly if the volume of the hematoma is less than 50 mL.

Placental abruption involves variable degrees of separation of the placenta from the underlying myometrium. Subsequent hemorrhage can

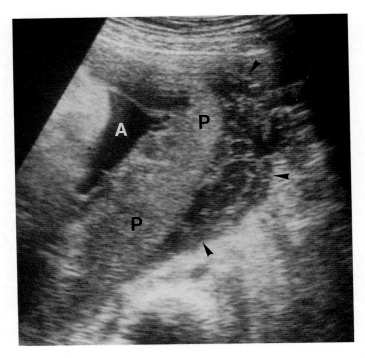

Figure 13-14. Retroplacental veins. A transverse sonogram shows a large, relatively anechoic area (arrowheads) deep to the placenta (P) Careful examination of the retroplacental area shows that it is composed of multiple tubular fluid collections, consistent with vessels. Flow can sometimes be visualized within such vessels on gray-scale imaging and is readily detected with color-flow Doppler sonography. A = amniotic cavity.

pass vaginally, accumulate retroplacentally, or do both. Uterine contractions occur in an effort to contain the hemorrhage. The variable degree, extent, and location of these processes lead to the sonographic features of abruption. A retroplacental fluid collection is pathognomonic, however infrequently imaged. Hypoechoic areas within the placenta, especially if basal, can suggest an infarction. Placental thickening and edge rounding can be seen with contractions. Unfortunately, several of these findings are not specific; when taken as a group, sonographic features suggesting abruption are seen in fewer than 50% of cases **(Option (C) is true).** Retroplacental hemorrhage is seen in 5% of placentas examined pathologically, although most of these hemorrhages are quite small. Approximately 30% of patients with a clinical abruption will have subsequent pathologic proof of a retroplacental hemorrhage. Sonography is not sensitive, however, for detecting most of these lesions. The differential diagnosis for retroplacental and intraplacental hypoechoic areas includes the normal basal veins (Figure 13-14), leiomyomas, contractions, nonpathologic placental fluid collections, and anechoic areas including venous lakes and old hematomas.

Pathologically, placenta accreta is an invasion of the underlying myometrium by the placental trophoblast. This relationship precludes clean separation of the placenta from the myometrium at delivery. If significant portions of the placenta are involved, this can result in continued postpartum hemorrhage since the uterus cannot adequately contract to halt bleeding at the placental implantation site or from the residual placenta **(Option (D) is true).** Life-threatening hemorrhage can occur, and a therapeutic hysterectomy might prove necessary.

Significant intrapartum hemorrhage is most often secondary to placenta previa or abruptio placenta. Placenta accreta, increta, or percreta can also result in life-threatening peripartum hemorrhage. A velamentous cord insertion, seen in about 1% of placentas, can also lead to life-threatening peripartum hemorrhage **(Option (E) is true).** When the umbilical cord inserts at or offset from the edge of the placenta, within the membranes, it is termed a velamentous cord. In this position the cord is more vulnerable to trauma, particularly if it is positioned over the internal cervical os (vasa previa). Massive hemorrhage can occur at delivery, either from direct fetal trauma or during rupture of the membranes. If rupture occurs, fetal mortality is 50 to 75%. Such cord insertions are more frequently seen in twin gestations and with a single umbilical artery. Velamentous cord insertion is rarely diagnosed with sonography *in utero*, as scanning is usually not directed specifically at the site of cord insertion into the placenta. Color-flow Doppler sonography could be useful, however, in making the diagnosis of velamentous cord insertion.

Question 58

Concerning gestational trophoblastic disease,

    (A) the typical vesicular appearance of a complete hydatidiform mole is usually not sonographically apparent until about 12 weeks

    (B) a normal placenta can be seen in association with a complete hydatidiform mole

    (C) a fetus seen in association with a partial hydatidiform mole usually has a triploid karyotype

    (D) about 50% of patients with a complete hydatidiform mole will develop persistent, invasive, or malignant trophoblastic disease

    (E) bilateral hemorrhagic corpus luteum cysts are seen in about 40% of patients with hydatidiform moles

Gestational trophoblastic disease can be subdivided into complete hydatidiform mole, partial hydatidiform mole, invasive mole, and choriocarcinoma.

A complete hydatidiform mole arises when an inactive oocyte is fertilized by a 23X sperm with subsequent chromosomal duplication, resulting in a 46XX conceptus, or simultaneously by both a 23X and a 23Y sperm, resulting in a 46XY conceptus. In either case, no embryo is formed and abnormal hyperplasia of the placental cytotrophoblast and syncytiotrophoblast results in the classic hydropic swelling of the placenta. On sonography the enlarged placenta appears as an echogenic masslike structure containing multiple fluid-filled vesicles of different sizes (Figures 13-15 and 13-16). This characteristic appearance is seen in the second trimester, because the evolving vesicles are generally too small to be resolved in the first trimester **(Option (A) is true)**. Some investigators have reported identification of typical vesicles in the first trimester, especially with transvaginal scanning, but the more common picture is one of a homogeneously solid mass or findings that suggest a missed abortion or blighted ovum.

The simultaneous presence of a complete hydatidiform mole and a fetus occurs in up to 2% of patients with a molar pregnancy, although the fetus is often dead **(Option (B) is true)**. Such an association does not occur with a singleton pregnancy, however, and is presumed to result from molar degeneration of one half of a dizygotic twin gestation. Typical sonographic features of a complete hydatidiform mole are noted along with an entirely normal fetus and placenta. Care should be taken to differentiate such a situation in which there is clear separation of normal and anomalous placental tissue, together with a normal fetus, from a partial hydatidiform mole, in which the abnormal placental tissue is more intermixed with the normal tissue and an associated fetus is anomalous.

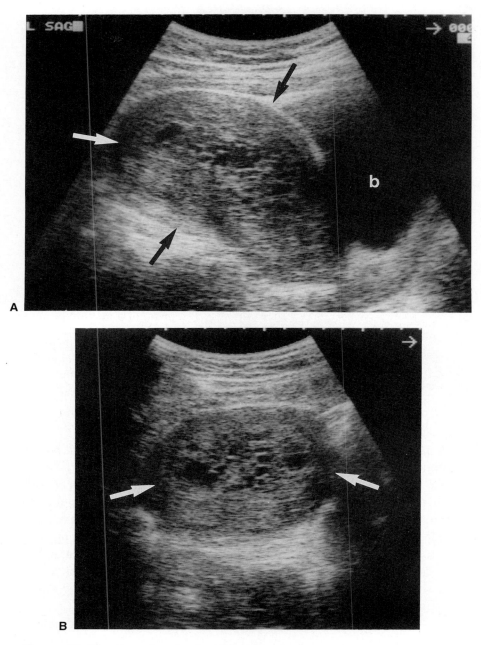

Figure 13-15. Complete hydatidiform mole. Longitudinal (A) and transverse (B) images show the enlarged uterus filled with heterogeneous echoes and multiple irregular fluid collections (arrows). b = bladder.

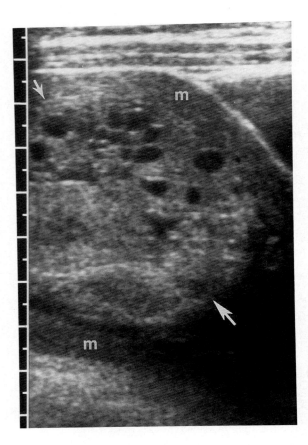

Figure 13-16. Complete hydatidiform mole. A high-resolution sonogram of a portion of an abnormal placenta (arrows) reveals multiple fluid-filled hypoechoic vesicles. m = myometrium.

A partial hydatidiform mole generally results when a normal oocyte is simultaneously fertilized by two sperm, resulting in a 69XXX or 69XXY karyotype. In contrast to a complete mole, which shows generalized hydropic edema of the villi throughout the placenta, a partial mole contains normal-appearing areas of placenta intermixed with regions of edematous villi. A fetus is often identified with a partial mole; however, the fetus tends to be markedly anomalous and severely growth retarded, and it is usually dead (Figure 13-17). When a fetus is present with a partial mole, it usually has a triploid karyotype, similar to the molar tissue **(Option (C) is true).**

The usual therapy for uncomplicated complete hydatidiform mole is dilation and curettage. When molar tissue invades the myometrium and cannot be removed by such surgical methods, persistent or invasive molar disease is present and metastatic disease is possible. There is a 12 to 25% potential for malignant transformation of benign complete hydatidiform mole **(Option (D) is false).** Partial mole has a significantly

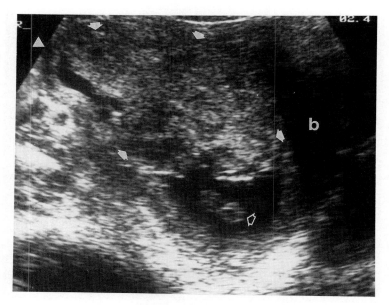

Figure 13-17. Partial hydatidiform mole. A sagittal image through the entire uterus (arrowhead indicates the fundus) shows an enlarged, heterogeneous placenta with several irregular fluid-filled areas (solid arrows). A nonliving embryo is noted (open arrow). b = bladder.

lower malignant potential, estimated at about 4%. Systemic methotrexate is the therapy of choice for invasive or metastatic disease. Gestational trophoblastic disease is associated with a marked elevation of the level of human chorionic gonadotropin (hCG), a protein secreted by the molar tissue; serial measurements of the hCG level are useful for monitoring the progress of therapy.

The increased quantities of hCG secreted by a complete hydatidiform mole stimulate the ovaries to form bilateral theca lutein cysts in 20 to 50% of patients (Figure 13-18). These cysts are derived from mesenchymal elements and are histologically distinct from functional cysts and other cysts derived from the ovary. A unilateral corpus luteum cyst is found in association with a normal early pregnancy and is not associated with elevated hCG levels. Elevated levels of hCG are not found with partial hydatidiform moles; therefore, theca lutein cysts are not associated with this entity **(Option (E) is false).**

Richard A. Bowerman, M.D.

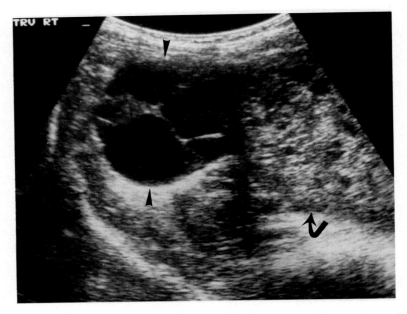

Figure 13-18. Theca lutein cysts. A transverse sonogram through the markedly enlarged right ovary (arrowheads) shows multiple large cysts. Similar findings were present on the left. Typical sonographic features of a hydatidiform mole are noted in the uterus (curved arrow).

SUGGESTED READINGS

PLACENTA ACCRETA, INCRETA, AND PERCRETA

1. Hoffman-Tretin JC, Koenigsberg M, Rabin A, Anyaegbunam A. Placenta accreta. Additional sonographic observations. J Ultrasound Med 1992; 11:29–34
2. Kerr de Mendonca L. Sonographic diagnosis of placenta accreta. Presentation of six cases. J Ultrasound Med 1988; 7:211–215
3. Pasto ME, Kurtz AB, Rifkin MD, Cole-Beuglet C, Wapner RJ, Goldberg BB. Ultrasonographic findings in placenta increta. J Ultrasound Med 1983; 2:155–159
4. Read JA, Cotton DB, Miller FC. Placenta accreta: changing clinical aspects and outcome. Obstet Gynecol 1980; 56:31–34
5. Tabsh KM, Brinkman CR III, King W. Ultrasound diagnosis of placenta increta. JCU 1982; 10:288–290

PLACENTA PREVIA

6. Artis AA III, Bowie JD, Rosenberg ER, Rauch RF. The fallacy of placental migration: effect of sonographic techniques. AJR 1985; 144:79–81

7. Farine D, Fox HE, Jakobson S, Timor-Tritsch IE. Vaginal ultrasound for diagnosis of placenta previa. Am J Obstet Gynecol 1988; 159:566–569

8. Gallagher P, Fagan CJ, Bedi DG, Winsett MZ, Reyes RN. Potential placenta previa: definition, frequency, and significance. AJR 1987; 149:1013–1015

9. Gianopoulos J, Carver T, Tomich PG, Karlman R, Gadwood K. Diagnosis of vasa previa with ultrasonography. Obstet Gynecol 1987; 69:488–491

10. Lim BH, Tan CE, Smith APM, Smith NC. Transvaginal ultrasonography for diagnosis of placenta previa. Lancet 1989; 1:444

11. Oppenheimer LW, Farine D, Ritchie JW, Lewinsky RM, Telford J, Fairbanks LA. What is a low-lying placenta? Am J Obstet Gynecol 1991; 165:1036–1038

12. Townsend RR, Laing FC, Nyberg DA, Jeffrey RB, Wing VW. Technical factors responsible for "placental migration": sonographic assessment. Radiology 1986; 160:105–108

INTRAPARTUM HEMORRHAGE

13. Jaffe MH, Schoen WC, Silver TM, Bowerman RA, Stuck KJ. Sonography of abruptio placentae. AJR 1981; 137:1049–1054

14. Jouppila P. Clinical consequences after ultrasonic diagnosis of intrauterine hematoma in threatened abortion. JCU 1985; 13:107–111

15. Nyberg DA, Cyr DR, Mack LA, Wilson DA, Shuman WP. Sonographic spectrum of placental abruption. AJR 1987; 148:161–164

16. Pedersen JF, Mantoni M. Prevalence and significance of subchorionic hemorrhage in threatened abortion: a sonographic study. AJR 1990; 154:535–537

17. Pedersen JF, Mantoni M. Large intrauterine haematomata in threatened miscarriage. Frequency and clinical consequences. Br J Obstet Gynecol 1990; 97:75–77

18. Rizos N, Doran TA, Miskin M, Benzie RJ, Ford JA. Natural history of placenta previa ascertained by diagnostic ultrasound. Am J Obstet Gynecol 1979; 133:287–291

19. Sauerbrei EE, Pham DH. Placental abruption and subchorionic hemorrhage in the first half of pregnancy: US appearance and clinical outcome. Radiology 1986; 160:109–112

20. Stabile I, Campbell S, Grudzinskas JG. Ultrasonic assessment of complications during first trimester of pregnancy. Lancet 1987; 2:1237–1240

21. Stabile I, Campbell S, Grudzinskas JG. Threatened miscarriage and intrauterine hematomas. Sonographic and biochemical studies. J Ultrasound Med 1989; 8:289–292

GESTATIONAL TROPHOBLASTIC DISEASE

22. Bagshawe KD. Risk and prognosis factors in trophoblastic neoplasia. Cancer 1976; 38:1373–1385

23. Hertzberg BS, Kurtz AB, Wapner RJ, et al. Gestational trophoblastic disease with coexistent normal fetus: evaluation by ultrasound-guided chorionic villus sampling. J Ultrasound Med 1986; 5:467–469

24. Rubenstein JB, Swayne LC, Dise CA, Gersen SL, Schwartz JR, Risk A. Placental changes in fetal triploidy syndrome. J Ultrasound Med 1986; 5:545–550

PLACENTA—GENERAL

25. Benirschke K, Kaufman P. Pathology of the human placenta. New York: Springer-Verlag; 1990

Notes

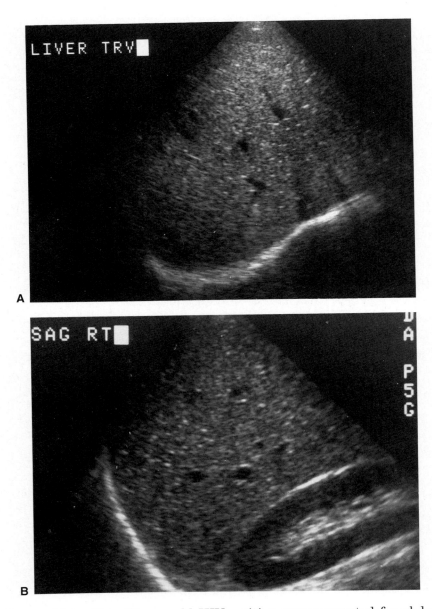

Figure 14-1. This 32-year-old HIV-positive man presented for abdominal sonography because of elevated liver enzyme levels. You are shown transverse (A), longitudinal (B), and magnified (C) views of the liver.

Case 14: *Pneumocystis carinii* Infection

Question 59

Which *one* of the following is the MOST likely diagnosis?

(A) Lymphoma
(B) Metastatic Kaposi's sarcoma
(C) *Pneumocystis carinii* infection
(D) Peliosis hepatis
(E) Viral hepatitis

Figure 14-1 shows innumerable tiny, highly reflective, nonshadowing foci distributed diffusely throughout the liver parenchyma. In a patient infected with human immunodeficiency virus (HIV), these findings are characteristic of a disseminated infectious process and have been reported most frequently with disseminated *Pneumocystis carinii* infection **(Option (C) is correct)**. Pathologically, the hyperechoic foci represent granulomas that are usually but not always calcified. There have been isolated case reports that disseminated *Mycobacterium avium-intracellulare* and cytomegalovirus (CMV) infection produce a similar sonographic appearance. However, even though disseminated infection is more common with *M. avium-intracellulare* than with *P. carinii*, these sonographic findings are more characteristic of the latter condition. Tuberculosis and fungal infections are common in patients with AIDS and can also result in calcified granulomas in the liver. Depending on geography, these infections can also be seen commonly in patients without AIDS. Typically, these granulomas are not as numerous, are larger, and often result in acoustical shadowing (Figure 14-2). The granulomas in patients with these diseases should not be confused with the innumerable tiny nonshadowing lesions seen in sonograms of patients with disseminated *Pneumocystis* infection.

Lymphoma (Option (A)) frequently has visceral involvement in patients with AIDS. It is seen as a hypoechoic mass or masses, sometimes with a central area that is isoechoic relative to normal liver parenchyma and with a hypoechoic halo (Figure 14-3). Lymphoma masses can

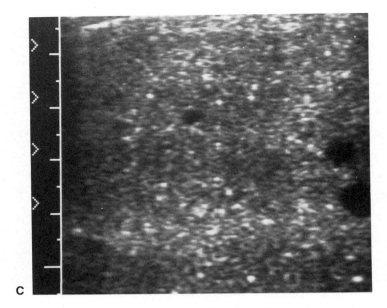

Figure 14-1 (Continued)

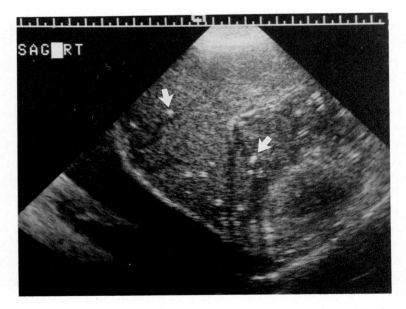

Figure 14-2. Hepatic granulomas in a patient without AIDS. Several punctate hyperechoic foci are seen in the liver, some producing acoustic shadowing (arrows). These are less numerous than the granulomas typically observed in patients with disseminated *P. carinii* infection.

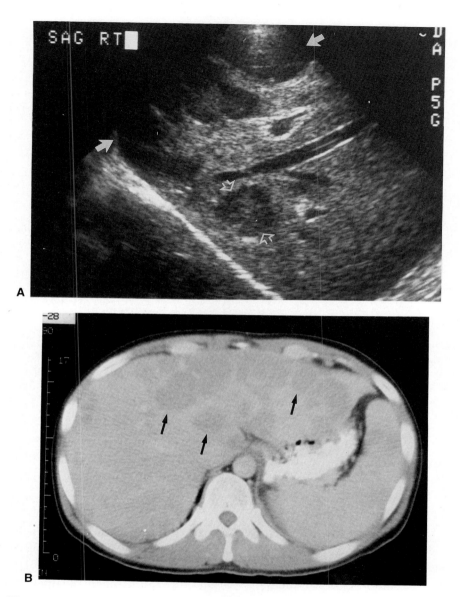

Figure 14-3. AIDS-related non-Hodgkin's lymphoma. (A) A sonogram shows that the liver contains multiple hypoechoic masses (between solid arrows). One mass has a central area that is isoechoic with normal hepatic parenchyma (open arrows). (B) A CT scan shows multiple low-attenuation masses corresponding to hepatic lymphoma (arrows).

be very hypoechoic with enhanced through transmission (Figure 14-4), features that can give the erroneous impression of a cystic mass such as

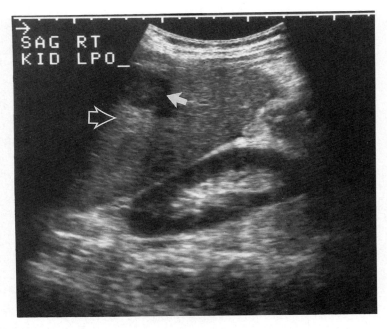

Figure 14-4. AIDS-related non-Hodgkin's lymphoma simulating a cystic mass. A sonogram shows that the liver contains a hypoechoic mass (solid arrow) with prominent enhanced through transmission (open arrow). This mass contains internal echoes; however, anechoic masses and even apparent septations have been reported in AIDS-related lymphoma.

a pyogenic abscess. Even apparent septations have been found within these masses. Lymphoma does not produce hyperechoic masses and has not been reported to produce tiny, highly reflective foci in the liver such as those in the test images.

Kaposi's sarcoma (KS) (Option (B)) is usually a multicentric disease in patients with AIDS and commonly involves the abdominal viscera. Aside from those with hepatomegaly, a very nonspecific finding in HIV-infected patients, the vast majority of patients with liver involvement do not have an abnormality detected by sonography. The few patients in whom sonographic evidence of hepatic involvement has been reported have shown disease in a periportal distribution, reflecting the perivascular manner in which this tumor typically spreads. The periportal tumor infiltration can appear hyperechoic or hypoechoic (Figure 14-5). From this perivascular location, the disease process spreads into the hepatic parenchyma. Discrete masses are rarely seen owing to the microscopic nature of the disease. In the few patients in whom discrete masses have been described, the masses have been small (5 to 12 mm) and hyperechoic. Tiny echogenic foci such as those seen in the test images have not been reported.

Peliosis hepatis (Option (D)) is an uncommon condition characterized by multiple blood-filled cystic spaces in the liver, ranging in size from less than 1 mm to several centimeters. These spaces may communicate with dilated hepatic sinusoids and may be lined by hepatocytes (parenchymal type) or endothelial cells (phlebectatic type). Peliosis most often involves the liver but can also affect the other reticuloendothelial organs (i.e., spleen, lymph nodes, and bone marrow). Involvement of the kidneys, lungs, pleura, and gastrointestinal tract has also been reported. Hepatic involvement is almost always present when other organs are involved. Presenting signs and symptoms most commonly include hepatomegaly, hepatocellular dysfunction, portal hypertension, and hemorrhage due to rupture of the involved organ, most often the liver or spleen. The diagnosis should be considered when these symptoms arise in a patient at risk for peliosis. HIV-infected patients are among those who are reported to be at increased risk for developing this disorder, possibly because of an effect of the virus on sinusoidal endothelial cells. It has also been suggested that inappropriate secretion of immunoregulatory factors can cause both peliosis and KS by acting on the vascular endothelium. Risk factors for peliosis other than HIV infection include chronic wasting disorders (e.g., tuberculosis, cancer, and hematologic diseases), exposure to hepatotoxic agents, and treatment with anabolic or other steroids. Resolution of the condition has been reported following cessation of steroid therapy.

In the past, peliosis has rarely been diagnosed prior to autopsy. When detected, the diagnosis has usually been made by blind core biopsy of the liver. Recently, a few case reports of the imaging findings in patients with peliosis have been published. When the cystic spaces are small, imaging findings are usually normal. As the cystic spaces enlarge, they can become visible on imaging studies. CT of patients with peliosis hepatis has shown small lesions ranging from 1 mm to 1 cm in diameter. These have a variable enhancement pattern, some remaining hypodense and others becoming isodense or hyperdense following intravenous administration of contrast material. On MRI, multiple hepatic foci that have increased signal intensity on T2-weighted images and variable signal intensity on T1-weighted and proton-density images are seen. The variable signal intensity reflects various stages of subacute hemorrhage, which also probably accounts for the variable enhancement pattern on CT. Few descriptions of the sonographic findings in patients with peliosis hepatis have been published. An MR case report by Maves et al. described "a coarsely echogenic liver with small, inhomogeneous areas of decreased echogenicity," but no images were shown. The pattern seen in

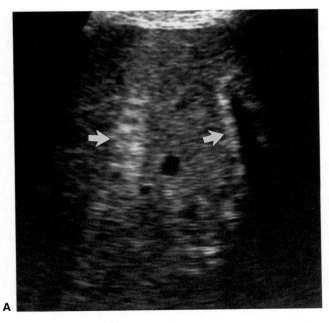

A

Figure 14-5. Hepatic AIDS-related Kaposi's sarcoma. (A) A sonogram shows hyperechoic periportal echoes (arrows) corresponding to tumor infiltration. (B) A sonogram shows small hyperechoic masses (arrows) in proximity to the portal veins. (C) A CT scan shows multiple central small masses (arrowheads) and periportal tumor infiltration that mimics the appearance of biliary dilation (arrows). Pathologic proof is lacking in this case, but the findings are characteristic of those that have been reported in the literature. The patient was known to have KS.

the test images has not been reported, nor would it be expected from the pathologic description of the lesion. Therefore, peliosis hepatis is not the best diagnosis. If the diagnosis of peliosis hepatis is suspected on the basis of imaging findings, confirmation generally requires core biopsy since fine-needle aspirates reveal only blood.

Viral hepatitis (Option (E)) can be acute or chronic. Acute hepatitis involves primarily the intralobular portion of the liver with sparing of the portal and periportal regions. Chronic hepatitis, which can be subdivided into chronic active hepatitis and chronic persistent hepatitis, involves primarily the perilobular, periportal, and portal regions of the liver. Fibrosis frequently accompanies chronic active hepatitis and can lead to cirrhosis.

As shown by Kurtz et al., the histopathologic distribution of these forms of hepatitis helps explain their different sonographic appearances.

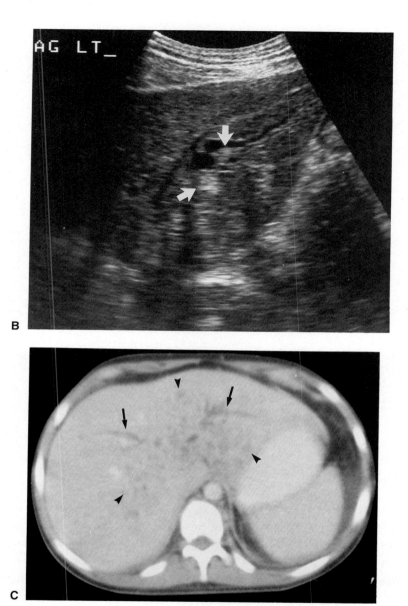

B

C

In patients with mild cases, the findings may be normal. Hepatomegaly is often present but is nonspecific. A distinctive pattern in patients with acute viral hepatitis results when the perilobular hepatic parenchyma appears very hypoechoic because of edema. This causes the portal triads to appear very echogenic in contrast to the hypoechoic parenchymal background and also results in the visualization of an increased number

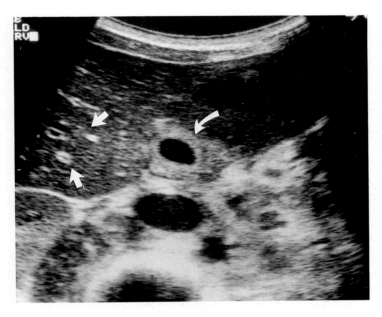

Figure 14-6. Acute viral hepatitis. A sonogram shows that the hepatic parenchyma is relatively hypoechoic, resulting in prominence and an increased number of visualized portal triads (straight arrows). There is associated thickening of the gallbladder wall (curved arrow).

of portal triads compared with the normal liver (Figure 14-6). This appearance has been referred to descriptively as the "starry sky" liver, a pattern that at least on superficial inspection could appear similar to that in the test images. However, the liver granulomas in patients with disseminated *P. carinii* infection are punctate and should be easily distinguished from the linear parallel nature of the portal triad echoes. In patients with chronic hepatitis, the portal triads usually become more difficult to identify because of the periportal distribution, and the liver appears hyperechoic with a coarsened echotexture secondary to fibrosis. Characteristic findings of cirrhosis can be seen in the late stages of this disease. However, in the AIDS population, increased hepatic echogenicity with loss of portal triad visualization is more often caused by granulomatous hepatitis (Figure 14-7) or fatty infiltration related to severe protein malnutrition (Figure 14-8). The presence of ultrasound attenuation by the liver favors the latter (Figure 14-8).

Viral hepatitis occurs with increased frequency in HIV-infected patients. Hepatitis B is transmitted through exposure to blood and blood products, during sexual contact, and from mothers to infants, primarily at the time of birth. These routes of transmission are the same as for

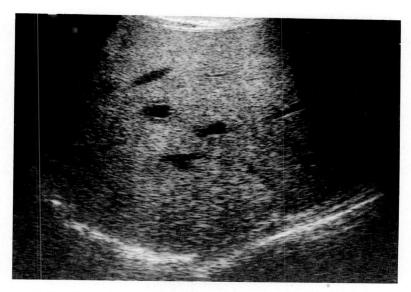

Figure 14-7. Granulomatous hepatitis caused by *M. avium-intracellulare*. A sonogram shows a diffuse increase in hepatic echogenicity with loss of the normal portal-triad echoes.

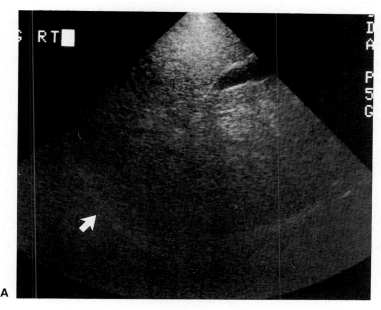

A

Figure 14-8. Fatty infiltration in a patient with AIDS. (A) A sonogram shows that the liver is diffusely hyperechoic with a coarse texture. There is marked attenuation of the ultrasound beam, resulting in poor visualization of the diaphragm (arrow). (B) A postcontrast CT scan shows a diffuse decrease in hepatic attenuation.

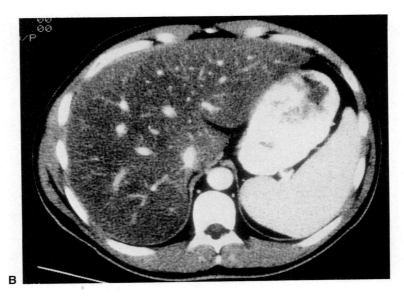

B

Figure 14-8 (Continued)

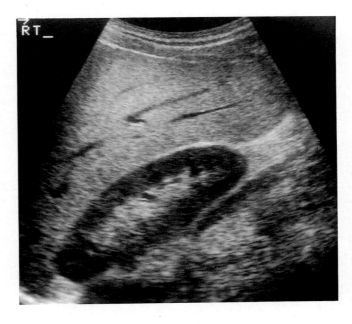

*Figure 14-9.
CMV hepatitis in
a patient with
AIDS. A sono-
gram shows that
the liver is dif-
fusely hyper-
echoic relative to
the kidney. There
is loss of the nor-
mal hyperechoic
portal triads.*

HIV, so it is not surprising that these infections have a predilection for
the same populations and can coexist. In addition, patients with AIDS,
because of impaired cellular immunity, are at risk for developing other,
more unusual forms of viral hepatitis. CMV infection is common in

identify other sites of involvement. This is successful most often in identifying lesions in the chest and gastrointestinal tract. Unfortunately, despite the high frequency of liver and spleen involvement at autopsy, imaging studies rarely demonstrate an abnormality in these organs **(Option (D) is false)**. Hepatic KS usually has a perivascular distribution at autopsy. It is an infiltrative neoplasm that tends to be localized to the subcapsular, hilar, and periportal areas of the liver, with invasion of the parenchyma from these sites. This process is generally microscopic or too subtle to identify on imaging studies. Histologically, the neoplasm is relatively hypocellular, consisting of periportal spindle cells and dense collagenous sheaths. Percutaneous needle biopsy of the liver rarely results in collection of affected tissue because of the hypocellular nature of the tumor and because focal lesions are rarely identified, resulting in biopsies that are blind. As a result, hepatic involvement has rarely been diagnosed prior to autopsy.

Several case reports showing hepatic involvement in patients with AIDS-related KS have been published in the imaging literature. Not surprisingly, the distribution of findings reflects the pathologic description above. Luburich et al. described the presence of hepatomegaly and multifocal hyperechoic nodules, ranging in size from 5 to 12 mm, both adjacent to the portal veins and diffusely infiltrating the liver parenchyma (Figure 14-5). One patient also had hyperechoic periportal tumor described as "bands" (Figure 14-5). On CT, both the nodules and the periportal bands had low attenuation values prior to and during the bolus intravenous administration of contrast material; they showed enhancement on delayed scans. Some lesions did not enhance or showed only peripheral enhancement, possibly because of intranodular thrombosis. Towers et al. also reported periportal tumor infiltration, but this appeared hypoechoic on sonography. They theorized that the difference between their case and those showing hyperechoic periportal tissue could be ascribed to a relative absence of fibrosis that was present in the previously reported cases and that this absence possibly represented an earlier manifestation of the disease. Hypoechoic nodules have not been reported as a finding in patients with hepatic KS **(Option (E) is false)**. The presence of hypoechoic nodules should suggest alternative diagnoses such as lymphoma or abscesses caused by pyogenic, mycobacterial, or fungal opportunistic infections. In addition to KS, the differential diagnosis for hyperechoic lesions in a patient with AIDS includes hemangiomas, metastases, fungal microabscesses, and an unusual manifestation of focal fatty infiltration (e.g., such as that described above for CMV hepatitis). In most cases, definitive diagnosis of hyperechoic or hypoechoic lesions requires needle biopsy or correlative imaging studies (Figure 14-14).

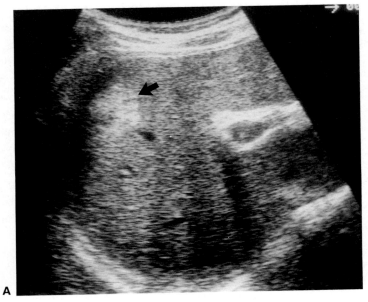

Anterior

Posterior

Figure 14-14. Hemangioma in a patient with AIDS-related Kaposi's sarcoma. (A) Sonography shows a hyperechoic mass (arrow) in the liver. The mass is larger than those reported in patients with KS, suggesting an alternative diagnosis. (B) A transaxial SPECT image with Tc-99m erythrocytes shows increased blood pool activity (arrow) within the lesion. This finding is characteristic of a hemangioma. The lesion was stable in appearance on serial sonographic examinations.

As mentioned above, lymph node involvement is very common in patients with AIDS-related KS. In most cases, an increased number of only slightly enlarged lymph nodes is demonstrated on imaging studies. The appearance most closely resembles PGL. Occasionally, in the lymphadenopathic subtype of KS, lymph node enlargement is massive. In each situation, the differential diagnosis includes lymphoma and opportunistic infections. Biopsy is required in most cases to establish a specific diagnosis. Biopsy is generally reserved for lymph nodes larger than 1.5 cm because of the common occurrence of small lymph nodes containing reactive hyperplasia and because of the technical difficulty of performing biopsy of these small lymph nodes.

Question 62

Concerning extrapulmonary *Pneumocystis carinii* infection,

    (A) it is uncommon

    (B) most patients with disseminated infection have a history of *P. carinii* pneumonia

    (C) it is characterized pathologically by granuloma formation

    (D) sonography is more sensitive than CT for detection of hepatic involvement

    (E) the sonographic patterns of hepatic and splenic involvement are different

P. carinii pneumonia represents the most common opportunistic infection in patients with AIDS, but extrapulmonary involvement has only rarely been reported. In recent years, extrapulmonary *P. carinii* infection has been seen with increased frequency, but it remains uncommon **(Option (A) is true).** The increased incidence can be related to a variety of factors, the most likely being the use of aerosolized pentamidine for treatment and prophylaxis of *P. carinii* pneumonia. Numerous reports of disseminated *P. carinii* infection appeared in the imaging literature shortly after early testing and subsequent Food and Drug Administration approval of this drug. It has been theorized that this therapy results in therapeutic levels of the drug in the lungs but not systemically, allowing the progression of infection in extrapulmonary sites. Other potential explanations for the increased reporting of this process include the growing number of patients with AIDS and their increased life span, a change in virulence factors of the *Pneumocystis* organism, and improved immune response secondary to treatment with antiviral drugs such as azidothymidine (AZT), resulting in radiographically demonstrable granuloma formation.

Clinical manifestations of disseminated infection are either absent or nonspecific. Patients can present with abdominal pain or abnormal labo-

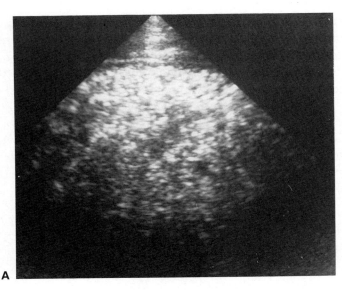

A

Figure 14-15. Disseminated *P. carinii* infection. (A and B) Sonograms show innumerable punctate hyperechoic foci in the liver (panel A) and spleen (panel B). These echogenic foci fall at the large end of the spectrum for this disease process but should not cause confusion with other granulomatous infections because they are so numerous. (C) A sonogram shows similar findings in the renal cortex, making the identification of renal margins difficult (arrows). The renal pyramids appear very hypoechoic by comparison.

ratory values such as elevation of alkaline phosphatase, hepatic transaminase, and creatinine levels. The vast majority of patients with extrapulmonary *P. carinii* infection also have pulmonary involvement either prior to or at the time of diagnosis **(Option (B) is true),** but exceptions have been reported. Therefore, the disease should still be considered when characteristic radiographic findings are present, even when there is no history of *P. carinii* pneumonia.

Extrapulmonary infection can involve virtually any organ. Radiographic manifestations have been reported in the liver, spleen, kidneys, pancreas, lymph nodes, adrenal glands, pleura, and peritoneum. The disease process is characterized pathologically by granuloma formation **(Option (C) is true).** In most cases the granulomas are calcified, resulting in the radiologic demonstration of multiple tiny calcifications. These are seen sonographically as innumerable tiny, highly reflective foci distributed throughout the involved organs (Figure 14-15). Several reported cases of hepatic involvement have shown similar sonographic findings

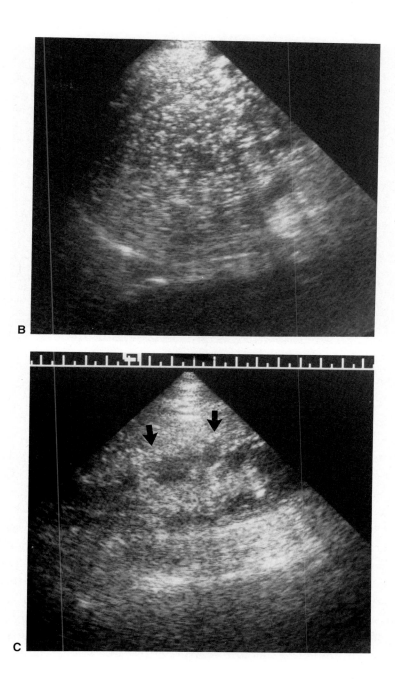

even when the granulomas have not been calcified (presumably representing an early stage of the disease) and when the CT appearance has been normal. Even when present, the calcifications can be very subtle and may not be evident on CT unless noncontrast scans are performed,

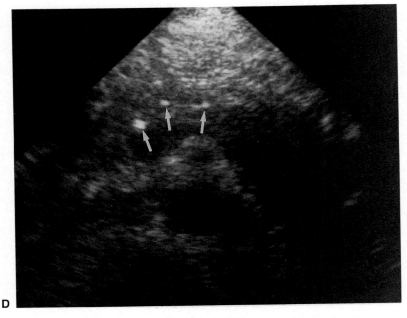

D

Figure 14-15 (Continued). Disseminated *P. carinii* infection. (D) A sonogram shows several calcifications in the pancreas (arrows).

which is not routinely the case. For these reasons, sonography has a higher sensitivity for the detection of this abnormality **(Option (D) is true).** Another interesting aspect of this disease is that the spleen can have a pattern of involvement different from that observed in other organs **(Option (E) is true).** Multiple calcifications like those seen in other organs can be observed (Figure 14-15), but another pattern of discrete masses can be present (Figure 14-16). These focal masses have low attenuation values on CT and appear hypoechoic with cystic areas on sonography. They may develop calcified rims or punctate central calcifications on subsequent examinations. The reason for this different manifestation in the spleen is unknown. Pleural and peritoneal involvement presents with fluid (e.g., pleural effusion or ascites) and can progress to development of pleural or peritoneal calcification.

The sonographic findings in patients with disseminated *P. carinii* infection are fairly distinctive, resulting in a small differential diagnosis. Several case reports have described similar findings in patients with AIDS and disseminated *M. avium-intracellulare* infection. In theory, tuberculosis or other fungal infections in patients with AIDS might result

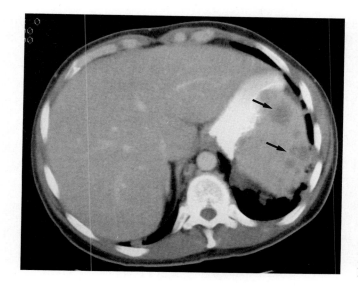

Figure 14-16. Same patient as in Figure 14-1. Disseminated *P. carinii* infection. A CT scan of the liver is normal. However, multiple discrete low-attenution masses are present in the spleen (arrows). These masses are typically hypoechoic on sonography and can appear cystic.

in similar findings, although no patients with this specific appearance have yet been reported.

Gary M. Kellman, M.D.

SUGGESTED READINGS

DISSEMINATED *P. CARINII* AND MYCOBACTERIAL INFECTION

1. Bray HJ, Lail VJ, Cooperberg PL. Tiny echogenic foci in the liver and kidney in patients with AIDS: not always due to disseminated *Pneumocystis carinii*. AJR 1992; 158:81–82
2. Falkoff GE, Rigsby CM, Rosenfield AT. Partial, combined cortical and medullary nephrocalcinosis: US and CT patterns in AIDS-associated MAI infection. Radiology 1987; 162:343–344
3. Feurstein IM, Francis P, Raffeld M, Pluda J. Widespread visceral calcifications in disseminated *Pneumocystis carinii* infection: CT characteristics. J Comput Assist Tomogr 1990; 141:149–151
4. Lubat E, Megibow AJ, Balthazar EJ, Goldenberg AS, Birnbaum BA, Bosniak MA. Extrapulmonary *Pneumocystis carinii* infection in AIDS: CT findings. Radiology 1990; 174:157–160
5. Radin DR. Intraabdominal *Mycobacterium tuberculosis* vs *Mycobacterium avium-intracellula*re infections in patients with AIDS: distinction based on CT findings. AJR 1991; 156:487–491
6. Radin DR, Baker EL, Klatt EC, et al. Visceral and nodal calcification in patients with AIDS-related *Pneumocystis carinii* infection. AJR 1990; 154:27–31

7. Spouge AR, Wilson SR, Gopinath N, Sherman M, Blendis LM. Extrapulmonary *Pneumocystis carinii* in a patient with AIDS: sonographic findings. AJR 1990; 155:76–78

8. Towers MJ, Withers CE, Hamilton PA, Kolin A, Walmsley S. Visceral calcification in patients with AIDS may not always be due to *Pneumocystis carinii*. AJR 1991; 156:745–747

AIDS-RELATED LYMPHOMA

9. Broder S, Karp JE. The expanding challenge of HIV-associated malignancies. CA Cancer J Clin 1992; 42:69–73

10. Safai B, Diaz B, Schwartz J. Malignant neoplasms associated with human immunodeficiency virus infection. CA Cancer J Clin 1992; 42:74–95

11. Townsend RR. CT of AIDS-related lymphoma. AJR 1991; 156:969–974

12. Townsend RR, Laing FC, Jeffrey RB Jr, Bottles K. Abdominal lymphoma in AIDS: evaluation with US. Radiology 1989; 171:719–724

KAPOSI'S SARCOMA

13. Luburich P, Bru C, Ayuso MC, Azon A, Condom E. Hepatic Kaposi sarcoma in AIDS: US and CT findings. Radiology 1990; 175:172–174

14. Moon KL Jr, Federle MP, Abrams DI, Volberding P, Lewis BJ. Kaposi sarcoma and lymphadenopathy syndrome: limitations of abdominal CT in acquired immunodeficiency syndrome. Radiology 1984; 150:479–483

15. Niedt GW, Schinella R. Acquired immunodeficiency syndrome. Clinicopathological study of 56 autopsies. Arch Pathol Lab Med 1985; 109:727–734

16. Towers MJ, Withers CE, Rachlis AR, Pappas SC, Kolin A. Ultrasound diagnosis of hepatic Kaposi sarcoma. J Ultrasound Med 1991; 10:701–703

17. Valls C, Canas C, Turell LG, Pruna X. Hepatosplenic AIDS-related Kaposi's sarcoma. Gastrointest Radiol 1991; 16:342–344

PELIOSIS HEPATIS

18. Maves CK, Caron KH, Bisset GS III, Agarwal R. Splenic and hepatic peliosis: MR findings. AJR 1992; 158:75–76

19. Radin DR, Kanel GC. Peliosis hepatis in a patient with human immunodeficiency virus infection. AJR 1991; 156:91–92

VIRAL HEPATITIS

20. Kurtz AB, Rubin CS, Cooper HS, et al. Ultrasound findings in hepatitis. Radiology 1980; 136:717–723

21. Vieco PT, Rochon L, Lisbona A. Multifocal cytomegalovirus-associated hepatic lesions simulating metastases in AIDS. Radiology 1990; 176:123–124

AIDS: GENERAL AND MISCELLANEOUS

22. Defalque D, Menu Y, Girard PM, Coulaud JP. Sonographic diagnosis of cholangitis in AIDS patients. Gastrointest Radiol 1989; 14:143–147
23. Dolmatch BL, Laing BC, Federle MP, Jeffrey RB, Cello J. AIDS-related cholangitis: radiographic findings in nine patients. Radiology 1987; 163:313–316
24. Federle MP. A radiologist looks at AIDS: imaging evaluation bases on symptom complexes. Radiology 1988; 166:553–562
25. Grumbach K, Coleman BG, Gal AA, et al. Hepatic and biliary tract abnormalities in patients with AIDS. Sonographic-pathologic correlation. J Ultrasound Med 1989; 8:247–254
26. Hamper UM, Goldblum LE, Hutchins GM, et al. Renal involvement in AIDS: sonographic-pathologic correlation. AJR 1988; 150:1321–1325
27. Jeffrey RB Jr, Nyberg DA, Bottles K, et al. Abdominal CT in acquired immunodeficiency syndrome. AJR 1986; 46:7–13
28. Kay CJ. Renal diseases in patients with AIDS: sonographic findings. AJR 1992; 159:551–554
29. Romano AJ, vanSonnenberg E, Casola G, et al. Gallbladder and bile duct abnormalities in AIDS: sonographic findings in eight patients. AJR 1988; 150:123–127
30. Yee JM, Raghavendra BN, Horii SC, Ambrosino M. Abdominal sonography in AIDS. A review. J Ultrasound Med 1989; 8:705–714

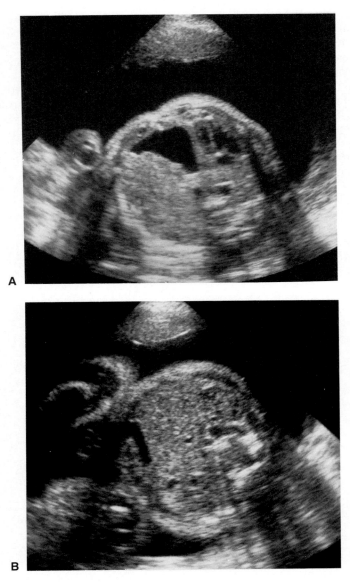

Figure 15-1. This 25-year-old pregnant woman underwent obstetric sonography because of a size-date discrepancy. You are shown transverse sonograms of the fetal thorax (A) and upper abdomen (B) and a longitudinal sonogram of the fetal trunk (C).

Case 15: Diaphragmatic Hernia

Question 63

Which *one* of the following is the MOST likely diagnosis?

(A) Hydrothorax
(B) Cystic adenomatoid malformation
(C) Bronchogenic cyst
(D) Diaphragmatic hernia
(E) Asplenia

The transverse sonogram of the fetal thorax (Figures 15-1A and 15-2A) shows the heart displaced into the right hemithorax by a cystic mass within the left chest. There is no stomach visible on the transverse scan of the upper abdomen (Figures 15-1B and 15-2B). The longitudinal sonogram of the trunk (Figures 15-1C and 15-2C) confirms the displacement of the heart to the right by the cystic mass and the absence of a stomach within the abdomen. This combination of findings is most consistent with congenital diaphragmatic hernia (CDH) **(Option (D) is correct).** The most common type of fetal diaphragmatic hernia results from failure of the posterolateral aspect of the diaphragm to close *in utero*, leading to herniation of abdominal contents through the foramen of Bochdalek. About 80 to 90% of Bochdalek hernias are left-sided. Depending on the size of the defect, left-sided hernias can contain the stomach, small intestine, colon, spleen, liver, and left kidney. Right-sided lesions usually contain the liver and sometimes also contain the gallbladder. The echotexture of the liver and lungs can be similar, making a right-sided lesion more difficult to diagnose with certainty. Several sonographic features of left-sided Bochdalek hernias have been described. The most common findings are demonstrated in the test images, i.e., cardiac displacement by a fluid-containing left chest mass without identification of the stomach in the abdomen. Other reported findings include fluid-filled loops of bowel or peristalsis within the thorax, a small abdominal circumference for gestational age as a result of abdominal-organ displacement into the thorax, an abnormal position of the stomach within the abdomen or

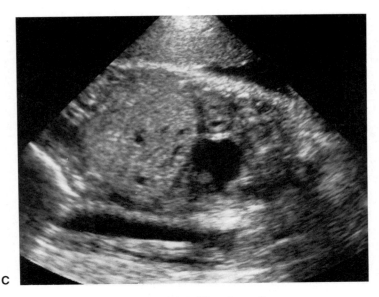

C

Figure 15-1 (Continued)

straddling the diaphragm, pulmonary hypoplasia, and polyhydramnios. The intrathoracic stomach is most often fluid filled, but the herniated bowel infrequently contains visible fluid, and the degree of cardiac displacement appears disproportionate to the size of the fluid-containing "mass." The remaining herniated abdominal content resembles the lung, and the exact size of the hernia is generally impossible to ascertain directly. Failure to identify the stomach within the fetal abdomen from the second trimester onward is quite rare and highly suggestive of a fetal abnormality. In addition to diaphragmatic hernia, the differential diagnosis includes esophageal atresia, swallowing disorders seen with central nervous system disorders or facial clefting, and oligohydramnios.

Infrequently, a hernia occurs through the foramen of Morgagni, where a defect in the anteromedial aspect of the diaphragm allows for herniation of liver and bowel/omentum into the thorax, sometimes specifically into the pericardial sac.

With a significant eventration of the diaphragm, there is a marked thinning of the muscular diaphragm, and superior displacement of the abdominal contents with displacement of the heart and mediastinal structures to the opposite hemithorax can appear identical to a diaphragmatic hernia.

Hydrothorax, or pleural effusion (Option (A)), is characterized by a single contiguous fluid collection surrounding a lung, conforming to the distribution of the pleural space (Figure 15-3). The intrathoracic con-

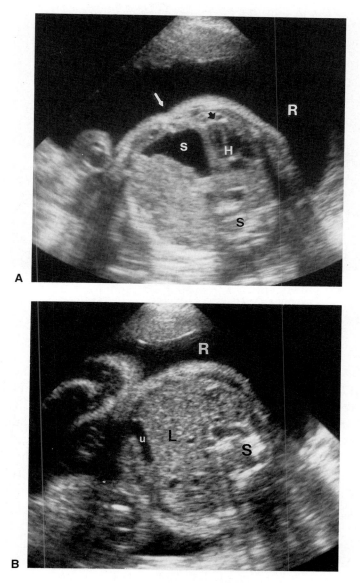

Figure 15-2 (Same as Figure 15-1). Congenital diaphragmatic hernia. (A) A transverse sonogram of the fetal thorax shows the heart (H) displaced into the right hemithorax by a mass containing the stomach (white "s"). The white arrow delineates the midline anteriorly. Black "S" = spine; R = right. Note that the apex (black arrow) of the displaced heart still points toward the left. (B) A transverse sonogram of the fetal upper abdomen shows liver (L) but no stomach. R = right; S = spine. Note the umbilical vein (u) in the liver passing abnormally to the left of the midline.

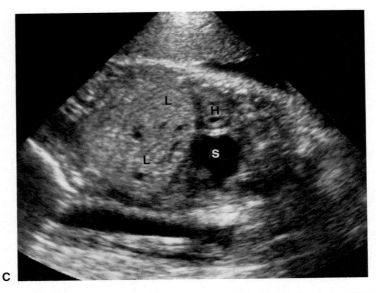

Figure 15-2 (Continued). Congenital diaphragmatic hernia. (C) A longitudinal sonogram shows the intrathoracic stomach (S) displacing the heart (H) to the right. The liver (L), but no stomach, is noted in the abdomen.

tents can be displaced away from the effusion, but the intra-abdominal organs are normal in position and appearance. These findings vary from those in the test images. Fetal hydrothorax is a frequent finding with fetal hydrops, together with ascites and subcutaneous edema. It can be found in association with other congenital anomalies, including CDH. An isolated effusion can result from lymphatic obstruction, intrauterine infection, or, rarely, a cardiac etiology. It has been reported as the only finding in patients with trisomy 21. Some effusions are idiopathic, and instances of spontaneous resolution without apparent sequelae have been reported. When fetal congestive heart failure occurs, ascites, rather than pleural effusion, is usually the first noncardiac manifestation. The fetal heart is right-side dominant, and right-heart failure will elevate systemic rather than pulmonary venous pressures, leading to ascites. If the effusion is isolated and small, the outcome should be favorable. Larger effusions, of course, particularly if bilateral, place the fetus at risk for pulmonary hypoplasia.

Cystic adenomatoid malformation (CAM) (Option (B)) is a hamartomatous malformation of the lung with cystic components; it usually involves an individual lobe but can occasionally involve a whole lung. Three types have been described histologically, depending on the size of

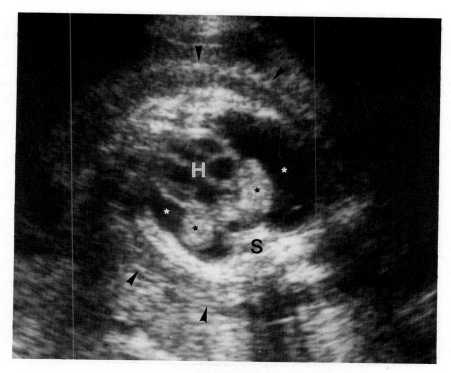

Figure 15-3. Hydrops fetalis with pleural effusions. A transverse sono-gram of the thorax shows large bilateral pleural effusions (white aster-isks) surrounding the collapsed lung (✱). The heart (H) maintains a normal central position. Extensive subcutaneous edema (arrowheads) is also present. S = spine.

cysts seen in the lesion. About 50% are type I lesions, with either a single large cyst or, more often, multiple cysts greater than 2 cm in diameter making up most of the mass. About 40% are type II lesions, with multiple smaller cysts averaging 1 to 2 cm in diameter interspersed with solid ele-ments. The remaining 10% are type III lesions, which are predominantly solid but contain multiple, usually microscopic, cysts. The prognosis of patients with CAM depends on the size of the mass and the resultant degree of pulmonary hypoplasia and on the complications due to associ-ated anomalies. Survival is possible with a solitary lung, but a larger mass can cause significant mediastinal shift such that the contralateral lung is also compromised. Larger masses can also result in possible esophageal compression, as well as cardiac compromise with reduced diastolic return, leading to congestive failure with hydrops (8 to 47% of patients) and polyhydramnios (66%). The presence of polyhydramnios, ascites, and hydrops worsens the outcome. Type I CAM is the most com-

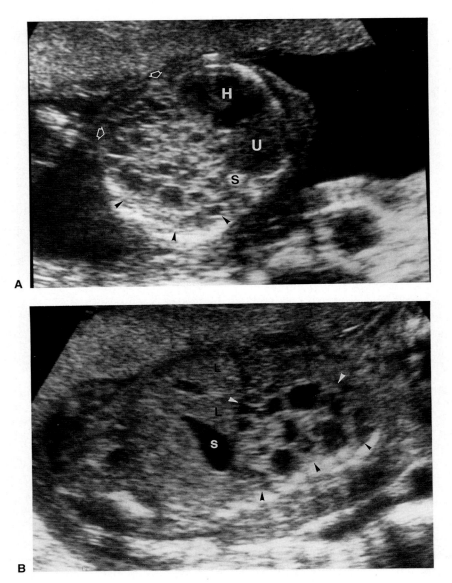

Figure 15-4. Type I cystic adenomatoid malformation. (A) A transverse sonogram of the thorax shows a large mixed echogenic and cystic mass (arrowheads and arrows) displacing the heart (H) into the right hemithorax. Residual right lung (U) is seen posterior to the heart, adjacent to the spine (S). (B) A longitudinal sonogram shows multiple large cystic spaces within the otherwise echogenic mass (arrowheads). The stomach (S) and liver (L) are seen in the abdomen.

mon variety and has the best prognosis. Sonographically, a heterogeneous mass with multiple prominent cystic areas, often causing cardiac

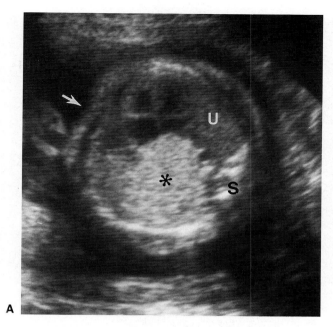

A

Figure 15-5. Type III cystic adenomatoid malformation. (A) A transverse sonogram of the thorax at 22 weeks gestational age shows a large, homogeneous echogenic mass (✱) displacing the heart into the left hemithorax. S = spine; U = left lung. The arrow indicates the anterior midline.

displacement, is seen (Figure 15-4). Associated anomalies are rare, and the postnatal survival rate is about 67%, since most masses are surgically removed successfully following birth. Type II CAM appears sonographically similar to the type I lesion, but the cysts are smaller. About 50% of affected fetuses have other anomalies, which, together with the risk for pulmonary hypoplasia, portends a poor prognosis. Associated anomalies are infrequent in patients with type III (microcystic) CAM, but these lesions are often quite large and exert a significant mass effect on the contralateral lung, resulting in a high morbidity. Sonographically, type III CAM has a uniformly echogenic appearance as a result of the multiple interfaces present with multiple small cysts (Figure 15-5). There are reported cases of spontaneous reduction in size or even apparent spontaneous resolution of a presumed CAM (Figure 15-5). In all patients with CAM, the stomach is found in its normal position. The described features for all three types of CAM, including normal stomach position, are different from those in the test images. The differential diagnosis for the heterogeneous, cyst-containing types I and II CAM includes CDH, sequestration, mediastinal teratoma, bronchogenic cyst,

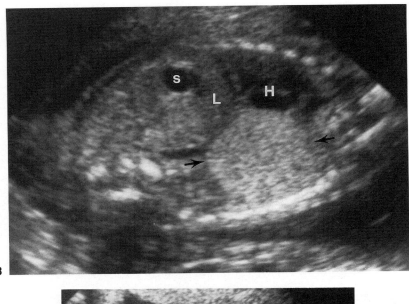

B

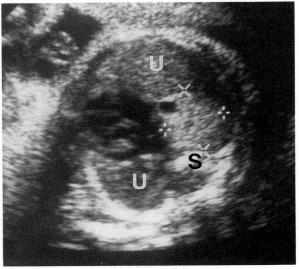

C

Figure 15-5 (Continued). Type III cystic adenomatoid malformation. (B)
A longitudinal sonogram shows that the echogenic chest mass (arrows)
has some mass effect on the upper abdomen. The stomach (S) is identified in the abdomen inferior to the liver (L). H = heart. (C) A follow-up
transverse sonogram of the thorax at 27 weeks gestational age shows a
diminution in the size of the mass (between + and x cursors), relatively
normal cardiac position, and bilateral lung tissue (U). S = spine. (D) At
35 weeks gestational age there has been even further diminution in the
size of the echogenic chest mass (arrowheads), with normal-sized lungs
(U). S = spine. No definite abnormality was seen on neonatal radiographs, and the diagnosis is thus presumptive.

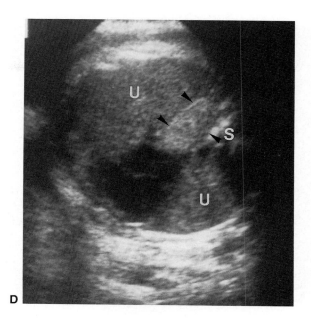

D

neurenteric cyst, and neuroblastoma. The differential diagnosis for a solid, echogenic intrathoracic mass includes, in addition to type III CAM, bronchopulmonary sequestration (especially if at the left base) (Figure 15-6), bronchial atresia, cardiac rhabdomyoma (Figure 15-7), pericardial teratoma, and CDH.

A bronchogenic cyst (Option (C)) results from abnormal development of the fetal foregut, with a cystic outpouching that is generally found centrally in the mediastinum, often close to the bronchial tree or pericardium, but can be seen in the lung. Bronchogenic cyst is one of an embryologically related group of abnormalities termed bronchopulmonary malformations, which include bronchopulmonary sequestration, neurenteric cysts, and tracheoesophageal fistula. The lesion is quite rare. It is classically small to medium in size, ovoid or round, and hypoechoic at sonography. With secondary bronchial obstruction, an accumulation of proteinaceous material can develop within the obstructed lung. Such an obstructed lung has a markedly echogenic echotexture resembling type III CAM or bronchopulmonary sequestration. The intra-abdominal structures are not affected by a bronchogenic cyst. The reported sonographic features of either an isolated bronchogenic cyst or one complicated by bronchial occlusion are not seen in the test images. Dextrocardia has been described in association with a bronchogenic cyst. The test images do not show dextrocardia, which would manifest as a right-side-directed

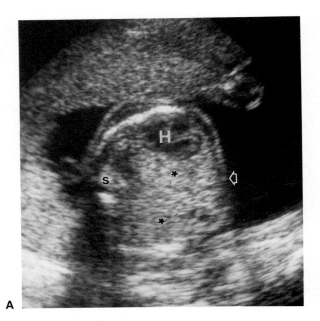

A

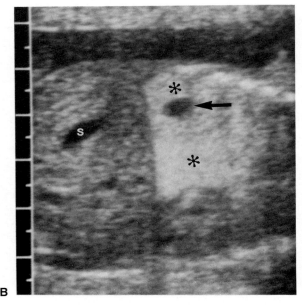

B

Figure 15-6. Broncho-pulmonary sequestration. (A) A transverse sonogram of the thorax shows a large, homogeneous echogenic mass (✱) displacing the heart (H) to the right. s = spine. The arrow indicates the midline. (B) A longitudinal sonogram confirms a left-sided echogenic intrathoracic mass (✱) with one cystic area (arrow). The stomach (s) is in the abdomen. The mass was thought to be a type III CAM. The neonate did well, with initial chest radiographs showing a smaller mass than was suggested by the prenatal sonograms. Sequestration was diagnosed by sonographic detection of a feeding vessel off of the aorta and was confirmed at surgery.

cardiac apex; instead, they show cardiac displacement into the right hemithorax with a left-side-directed apex.

Situs inversus totalis, in which there is a mirror-image reversal of the thoracic and abdominal organs, is infrequently associated with other serious anomalies. This contrasts with partial situs inversus, in which

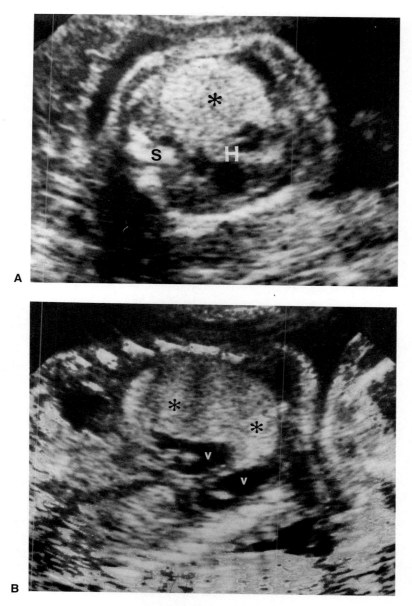

Figure 15-7. Cardiac rhabdomyoma. (A) A transverse sonogram of the thorax shows the heart (H) displaced to the right by a large, homogeneous, echogenic mass (✱). S = spine. (B) A short-axis sonogram of the ventricles (v) clearly shows that the echogenic mass (✱) arises from the free wall of the left ventricle and extends partially into the septum.

complex combinations of non-mirror-image situs abnormalities of thoracic and/or abdominal organs occur and in which associated anomalies

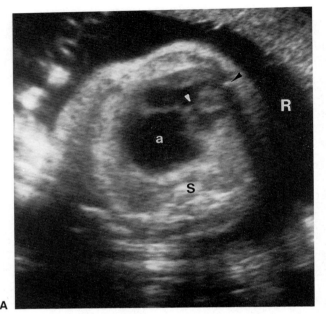

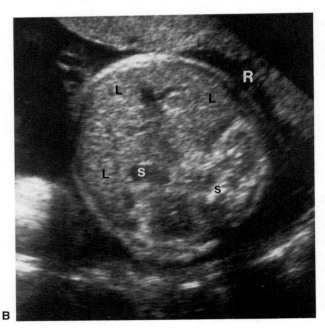

Figure 15-8. Asplenia. (A) A transverse image of the thorax shows dextrocardia with the heart apex (black arrowhead) directed to the right. An AVSD is present, with a common atrium (a) and the VSD (white arrowhead) readily apparent on the frozen image. S = spine; R = right. (B) A transverse sonogram of the abdomen shows a midline and symmetric liver (L), a stomach (white "S") slightly medial in position, and no spleen. Black "S" = spine; R = right.

are frequent. Such cases are recognized by a discordance from the usual pattern of a left-sided cardiac apex aligned with a left-sided stomach. Two such entities, the asplenia (Option (E)) and polysplenia syndromes, share some similarities in the types of situs abnormalities present but also have key differences. In both syndromes, the penetrance of the various defects varies, with complex cardiac disease more frequent in patients with asplenia. In patients with the asplenia syndrome, the classic findings are an absent spleen and a 90% frequency of bilaterally right-sided lungs. In 40% of patients the cardiac apex is directed to the right. Complex cardiac defects including endocardial cushion defect, transposition of the great vessels, single ventricle, pulmonary stenosis/atresia, and total anomalous pulmonary venous return (TAPVR) are present in 60 to 90% of patients (Figure 15-8A). Bilateral superior venae cavae are common, and the aorta and inferior vena cava are either on the same side or juxtaposed. Abdominal malformations include a right-sided or midline stomach in 65% of patients, symmetric or midline liver and gallbladder in 50%, and various degrees of intestinal malrotation (Figure 15-8B). Renal anomalies, including dysplasia, cystic kidneys, and fused kidneys, are seen in 25%. Early mortality is high, most often as a result of complex cyanotic heart disease as well as complications secondary to other anomalies. In patients with asplenia, dextrocardia is not secondary to an intrathoracic mass as in the test patient, and the stomach is identified somewhere in the abdomen, often with a midline liver, features not suggestive of CDH. In contrast to asplenia, the polysplenia syndrome is characterized by multiple spleens and a 65% frequency of bilateral left-sided lungs. About 37% of patients have a right-sided cardiac apex and 70% have TAPVR, but complex cardiac disease is less frequent, with a 40% frequency of endocardial cushion defect and a 10 to 20% frequency of transposition of the great vessels, pulmonary stenosis/atresia, and single ventricle. Also, 50% of patients have bilateral superior venae cavae and 70% have azygos return of the inferior venae cavae. The abdominal findings in patients with polysplenia include a midline to right-sided stomach in 65% and a midline liver in 25%.

Question 64

Concerning fetal diaphragmatic hernia,

(A) with a left-sided hernia, the cardiac axis is usually altered so that the apex is directed to the fetal right
(B) about 30% of fetuses with a prenatal diagnosis will survive
(C) about 30 to 40% of affected fetuses have an associated structural or chromosomal defect
(D) early detection (prior to 24 weeks) improves outcome
(E) there is an 85% mortality rate if polyhydramnios is present

The normal fetal heart is situated slightly to the left of the midline. The cardiac apex is directed to the left side of the fetus, about midway

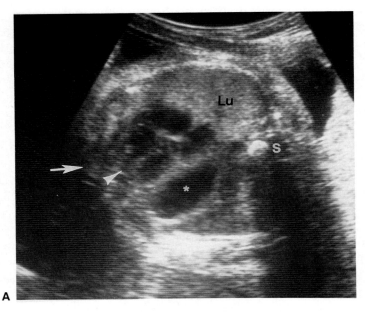

A

Figure 15-9. Congenital diaphragmatic hernia. (A) A transverse sonogram of the thorax shows a left CDH containing the stomach (✳), with
modest displacement of the heart to the right. The cardiac apex (arrowhead) remains pointing to the left. S = spine. The arrow indicates the
anterior midline. Note the large, clearly apparent right lung (Lu). (B) A
transverse sonogram of the abdomen shows the umbilical vein (u) passing from the cord insertion to the left, implying herniation of the liver
into the chest. S = spine. Postnatally the neonate did well, probably
reflecting the large residual normal right lung and modest mediastinal
shift.

between the anterior and lateral aspects of the chest, with a range of
about 20° in either direction. In patients with a left-sided CDH, the heart
is displaced into the right hemithorax; however, in most cases the cardiac
apex remains directed to the left (Figures 15-9 and 15-10) **(Option (A) is
false).** It is important to assess the fetal heart axis when attempting to
differentiate the various potential causes of cardiac malposition. An
intrathoracic mass is not always readily identifiable sonographically.
With a situs abnormality the cardiac apex is generally directed to the
right, whereas a left-sided chest mass merely displaces the entire heart
to the right, maintaining a left-directed cardiac apex. Compression of the
left ventricle has also been found in patients with an intrathoracic mass
but not in those with a situs abnormality.

The overall survival rate for patients with CDH is low, particularly
for those with associated anomalies or chromosomal defects. The mortal-

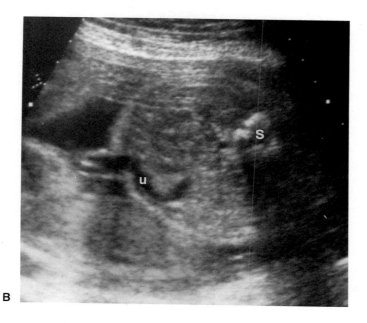

B

ity rate is 75 to 80% for patients with CDH diagnosed *in utero*, and even patients with isolated lesions have a mortality rate of 60 to 70%, despite the best neonatal surgical techniques and support measures that include extracorporeal membrane oxygenation (ECMO) **(Option (B) is true).** ECMO, effectively an external lung, has been used both before and after surgery as a temporary support tool while the patient is otherwise stabilized and intrinsic lung function is maximized. The traditional poor outcome relates to several factors. The primary factor is the underlying deficiency in lung development secondary to the *in utero* mass effect on the developing pulmonary tissues (Figures 15-9A and 15-10). Associated anomalies have an intrinsic morbidity and mortality, too. Several authors have reported a poorer prognosis when there is a reduced left- to right-ventricular-width ratio, with nonsurvivors having a mean value of 0.66 in one series. Presumably, underdevelopment of the left heart secondary to the adjacent mass has an adverse effect on postnatal cardiac function.

In utero surgical repair has been used with some success in selected fetuses. When the hernia contains liver, intrauterine repair is more problematic. Herniation of liver is indicated by a marked alteration in the course of the umbilical vein to the left (Figures 15-1 and 15-9B). Successful fetal surgery is less likely, since vascular compromise may occur secondary to kinking of the umbilical vein when the liver is repositioned into the abdomen.

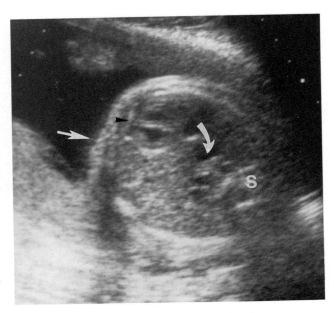

Figure 15-10. Congenital diaphragmatic hernia. A transverse sonogram of the thorax shows marked displacement of the heart into the right hemithorax. The cardiac apex (arrowhead) is still left-directed, however. The stomach (curved arrow) lies in the right hemithorax, posterior to the heart, and little residual right lung could be detected. S = spine. The straight arrow indicates the anterior midline. The changes all indicate a very large mass effect on the developing lungs. Although predicting the outcome of fetuses with CDH is not reliable, a poor outcome was predicted here, and in fact the neonate died despite surgical intervention. Contrast the findings in this fetus with those shown in Figure 15-9.

The reported frequency of associated anomalies and chromosomal defects in fetuses with CDH ranges from about 20 to 50%, with the higher percentage more applicable to the stillborn population **(Option (C) is true).** Cardiovascular defects are frequent, and a dedicated fetal cardiac examination is indicated when CDH is identified. The central nervous system and gastrointestinal and genitourinary tracts should also be carefully evaluated for structural defects. Several chromosomal abnormalities have been noted in association with CDH, with trisomy 18 being the most frequent. The presence of associated structural defects or a karyotypic abnormality precludes consideration for prenatal surgery.

Early prenatal detection of CDH is an unfavorable prognostic sign, since it implies a larger mass, which is more readily detected and hence more likely to develop complications. This is particularly true when a patient is referred for sonography with a history of being "large for dates" and polyhydramnios secondary to CDH is discovered. The earlier the presentation or detection of the mass, the greater the probability that the mass is large and that significant pulmonary hypoplasia will occur **(Option (D) is false).**

When polyhydramnios is associated with any intrathoracic mass, including CDH, it usually results from one or both of the following mechanisms. First, any obstruction to the upper gastrointestinal tract will reduce fetal swallowing of amniotic fluid and result in marked polyhydramnios. Second, cardiac displacement by an intrathoracic mass can mechanically interfere with venous return, which can lead to congestive heart failure and potential further complications of hydrops fetalis and polyhydramnios. Intuitively, polyhydramnios is therefore most likely to be seen with a large CDH, increasing the probability of developing lethal pulmonary hypoplasia and worsening the prognosis. In fact, a large stomach within a CDH suggests gastric outlet obstruction, is usually associated with polyhydramnios, and has a worse than average prognosis. Several of the common associated structural anomalies and chromosomal abnormalities can also contribute to the development of polyhydramnios. Although one recent study found no increased mortality when CDH was associated with polyhydramnios, the survival rate is generally reported to be lower in that circumstance. The anomalies and mechanisms that cause polyhydramnios increase the mortality of CDH beyond the average of about 70% for all affected fetuses to approximately 85% **(Option (E) is true).**

Question 65

Concerning fetal cardiac ultrasonography,

- (A) over 90% of cardiac defects are detected on the four-chamber view
- (B) about 25% of fetuses with a cardiac anomaly detectable on prenatal sonography have a chromosomal abnormality
- (C) pulmonary hypoplasia due to an increased cardiothoracic ratio results from a cardiac abnormality in 75% of cases
- (D) about 50% of fetuses with complete heart block have a structural cardiac defect
- (E) a parallel orientation of the great vessels at the base of the heart is normal

The sonographic evaluation of the fetal heart is an important component of the routine fetal anatomic survey. The cardiovascular system is involved with more serious congenital anomalies than are other systems, with up to 8 in 1,000 live births affected with congenital heart disease. The sonographic examination of the heart is directed toward the detec-

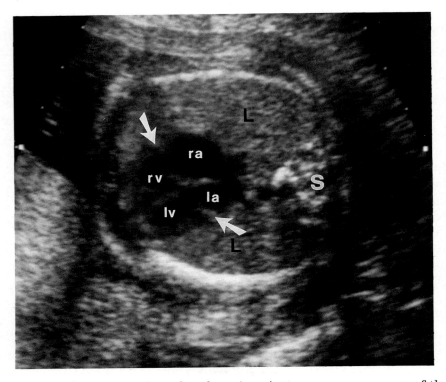

Figure 15-11. Normal four-chamber view. A transverse sonogram of the thorax shows the fetal heart centrally positioned with its apex, as defined by the interventricular septum, directed slightly to the left, here dependent, side. The right ventricle (rv), left ventricle (lv), right atrium (ra), and left atrium (la) are all readily delineated. The AV valves (arrows indicate valve planes) are noted between their respective chambers. Note the large, midlevel echogenic lungs (L) filling the remainder of the thorax. S = spine.

tion of as many structural and functional cardiac abnormalities as possible. The position and axis of the heart within the thorax, as well as the cardiac rate and rhythm, must be initially observed. The current standard for structural cardiac evaluation is the four-chamber view.

The four-chamber view depicts the ventricles, atria, and atrioventricular valves on an axial view of the thorax (Figure 15-11). Abnormalities that directly affect these structures can be detected on this view, as can, potentially, secondary changes from remote defects. Some defects are missed, however, because of the rapid motion inherent to the heart and its small size on early sonograms. In addition, the small size of many ventricular septal defects (VSDs) makes their detection difficult, and the common atrial septal defect (ASD) is routinely overlooked. The great vessels are not imaged on the four-chamber view, and so entities such as transposition of the great vessels (TGV), tetralogy of Fallot, double-outlet right ventricle, and truncus arteriosus are not detected. An early study suggested that up to 90% of cardiac lesions were seen on the four-chamber view, but others have subsequently found that a detection rate of 60 to 70% more accurately reflects the sensitivity of that single image **(Option (A) is false).**

Cardiac defects are found in 8 of 1,000 live births. Of these infants, about 10% manifest a chromosomal abnormality. Stillborn fetuses, however, have both a significantly higher frequency of cardiac defects and a 35% association with a chromosomal defect when a cardiac defect is present. The intrinsic mortality of cardiac defects and the multisystem anomalies seen in fetuses with chromosomal abnormalities result in fetal wastage that is not documented in postnatal studies but is often apparent *in utero*. When a cardiac abnormality is detected on a prenatal sonogram, the frequency of an associated chromosomal abnormality has been found to be 22 to 32% **(Option (B) is true).** Similarly, up to 50% of fetuses with a cardiac defect detected prenatally have other detectable fetal anomalies. Conversely, about 25% of fetuses in whom a noncardiac defect is discovered will also have a cardiac abnormality. Many cardiac defects can be detected *in utero*, although some are harder to detect than others. An atrioventricular septal defect (AVSD) or endocardial cushion defect (Figure 15-8A), isolated VSD, hypoplastic ventricle (Figure 15-12), single ventricle or atrium, and Ebstein's anomaly can all be imaged on a four-chamber view. Images of the great vessels are needed to detect TGV and tetralogy of Fallot. ASDs are classically missed, presumably because of the presence of a natural physiologic defect, the foramen ovale, and the size of the lesion. Similarly, VSDs are often missed because of their small size and their location in a rapidly moving organ. Trisomy 21 is associated with a 40 to 50% frequency of cardiac defects, particularly AVSD or VSD. About 90% of fetuses with trisomy 18 will have a cardiac lesion, especially VSD, AVSD, or aortic and pulmonic valve abnormalities; less often, these fetuses have TGV, tetralogy of Fallot, dextrocardia, or double-outlet right ventricle. A VSD is the most frequent finding in fetuses with trisomy 13, 80 to 90% of whom have a heart defect. Coarctation of the aorta and a bicuspid aortic valve are present in about 20% of fetuses with Turner's syndrome, but both are difficult to visualize prenatally by sonography.

Subjectively, the normal heart occupies about one-quarter to one-third of the cross-sectional area of the thorax. Objectively, the cardiothoracic ratio relates the transverse diameter of the heart on an axial four-chamber view to the transverse diameter of the thorax, with a normal mean of .50 (range .45 to .55). Exact points for the measurement of these

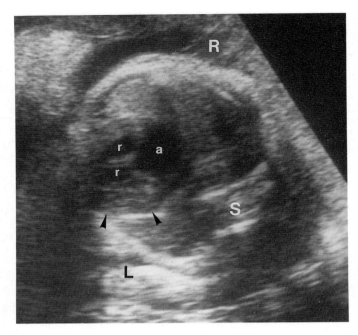

Figure 15-12. Hypoplastic left ventricle. A transverse sonogram of the thorax shows the fetal heart centrally positioned with its apex directed to the left (L = left; R = right; S = spine). The fluid-filled right ventricular chamber (r) is readily seen, traversed by papillary muscle. The left ventricle is seen as a thickened muscle with no detectable lumen (arrowheads). A prominent right atrium (a) is noted with the left atrium diminutive and difficult to image.

diameters have not been elucidated, and this ratio remains useful but somewhat subjective. Absolute values for cardiac and thoracic circumferences from 24 weeks to term have also been described (Figure 15-13). As a rough measure of cardiac and thoracic size, either the cardiothoracic ratio or the specific heart and thorax circumferences may provide useful information in fetal analysis. Mensuration of the thorax should incorporate only the bony thorax so as not to include any skin thickening that might be present in fetuses with pathologic conditions such as skeletal dysplasias or hydrops fetalis. The cardiothoracic ratio is increased when the heart is enlarged, the bony thorax is small, or both. Cardiac enlargement can result from entities such as tricuspid atresia, complex cardiac disease, cardiomyopathy, and congestive failure of any cause. Clinical interest in detecting an abnormal cardiothoracic ratio arises from a desire to predict pulmonary hypoplasia. Although cardiac enlargement can alter the cardiothoracic ratio, it alone is infrequently of a sufficient

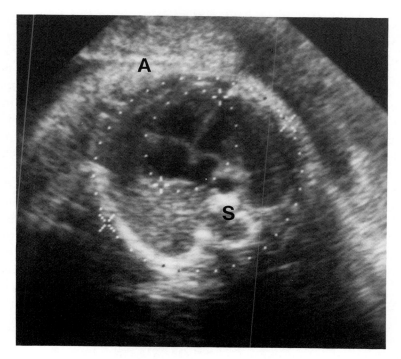

Figure 15-13. Cardiac and thoracic circumference measurements. A transverse sonogram of the thorax shows a normal four-chamber view of the fetal heart. Electronic calipers outline the cardiac (+) and thoracic (x) margins. S = spine; A = anterior.

magnitude to cause pulmonary hypoplasia. Conversely, however, the small thoracic circumference, and hence the increased cardiothoracic ratio, seen with several of the skeletal dysplasias often results in marked pulmonary hypoplasia and subsequent neonatal morbidity and mortality **(Option (C) is false).**

During evaluation of the fetal heart, the cardiac rate and rhythm, as well as the structure, must be examined. The usual fetal heart rate during the second and third trimesters is 120 to 160 beats/min. Transient bradycardia is nonpathologic and can be induced by scanning pressure. In most cases, bradycardia is not related to an underlying structural defect and the outcome is good. Sustained bradycardia below 100 beats/min, with or without hydrops, has in some series been associated with an increased risk of fetal morbidity and death. Complete heart block is the most common cause of sustained bradycardia. With complete heart block there is a clear discordance between the atrial and ventricular rates. This can be documented with M-mode sonography. About half the fetuses with complete heart block will have an underlying cardiac anomaly **(Option (D) is true)**, often an AVSD, either isolated or as a component of more complex cardiac disease, as might be seen in fetuses with the asplenia/polysplenia syndromes. Nonstructural causes of complete heart block often include conduction pathway damage from maternal autoimmune disease such as systemic lupus erythematosus. Tachycardia is an infrequent sonographic finding but, when present, usually occurs at rates exceeding 200 beats/min. It is most often due to supraventricular tachycardia and is less frequently due to atrial flutter/fibrillation. Transient or short bursts usually do not result in significant fetal morbidity or mortality; however, if they are sustained they may lead to fetal congestive heart failure. With the evolution of signs of congestive heart failure and hydrops fetalis, which carries a dire prognosis, therapeutic options should be considered for fetal therapy via maternal adminstration of antidysrhythmic drugs. Maternal side effects can result, however, and prophylactic medication is not advisable prior to the detection of fetal compromise.

The aortic outflow tract and aorta arise from the left ventricle and pass to the right as they ascend in the thorax. In contrast, the pulmonary outflow tract and pulmonary artery pass from the right ventricle toward the left as they ascend in the thorax anterior to the aorta. These vessels are therefore roughly perpendicular to one another as they arise from their respective ventricles **(Option (E) is false).** Cardiac malformations primarily involving the great vessels, including TGV, tetralogy of Fallot, double-outlet right ventricle, and truncus arteriosus, are detected on sonography by examining the great vessels and their relationships to the ventricles and not merely by studying the four-chamber view.

Question 66

Concerning the fetal thorax,

- (A) lung growth continues postnatally with further formation of alveoli
- (B) aveolar growth starts in the early second trimester
- (C) most fetuses with type I (macrocystic) cystic adenomatoid malformation die
- (D) pulmonary hypoplasia is usually secondary to a fetal genitourinary tract anomaly with oligohydramnios
- (E) a unilateral, right-sided pleural effusion is usually secondary to congenital heart disease

The development of the fetal lungs from an outpouching off the pharynx is divided into four stages. In stage 1, between 5 and 16 weeks, the basic bronchial framework is formed. In stage 2, between 16 and 24 weeks, respiratory bronchioles with a few terminal sacs have formed. The terminal sacs are well vascularized and can support respiratory function. In stage 3, from 24 weeks to birth, there is a marked proliferation in the terminal sacs and beginning formation of alveoli. Surfactant is produced during this stage. Stage 4 of lung growth is that of alveolar growth, which starts in the late fetal period **(Option (B) is false)** and continues to about age 8. Only about one-sixth to one-eighth of the adult alveoli are present at birth, and they exist primarily in an immature state. Increasing lung size postnatally results from both the enlargement of maturing alveoli and an increase in the number of new immature alveoli, which have the potential for forming even more alveoli **(Option (A) is true).** The timing of an insult to the developing lung plays a critical role in fetal outcome. A large mass effect during early bronchial branching will result in a marked reduction in the overall framework on which the lung develops, resulting in severe pulmonary hypoplasia and death. Progressively later insults allow for greater lung development on which to build postnatally, increasing the likelihood of survival.

Type I CAM exerts a mass effect on the developing lung but is not associated with an increased frequency of other anomalies. Therefore, as with other isolated masses affecting the thorax, fetuses with this condition have an outcome most directly related to the amount of functional lung. The larger the mass, or the earlier a mass becomes large enough to hinder lung growth, the worse the outcome. CAM often appears to have significant mass effect, but about two-thirds of type I lesions still leave adequate pulmonary development for neonatal survival **(Option (C) is false).**

Normal fetal lung growth depends on several factors, including unimpeded fetal breathing movements, normal amniotic fluid volume, adequate intrathoracic space, and the presence of pulmonary fluid. Pulmonary hypoplasia results from any restriction of lung growth. External factors such as marked oligohydramnios will compress the fetal thorax. Oligohydramnios can occur secondary to ruptured membranes, growth retardation, and fetal genitourinary tract anomalies. About 20 to 25% of cases of pulmonary hypoplasia are due to the last cause **(Option (D) is false).** About half the time, pulmonary hypoplasia is secondary to an intrathoracic process such as a diaphragmatic hernia, CAM, sequestration, pleural effusion, or cardiac enlargement. Occasionally, elevation of the diaphragm by an abdominal mass or marked ascites significantly compromises pulmonary development. Intrinsic restrictions on pulmonary development also occur in fetuses with a small thoracic cage, which is characteristic of several of the lethal skeletal dysplasias such as thanatophoric dysplasia (Figure 15-14).

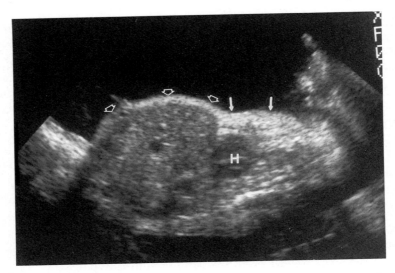

Figure 15-14. Thanatophoric dysplasia with pulmonary hypoplasia. A longitudinal sonogram of the fetal trunk shows an abrupt reduction in the size of the thorax (solid arrows) relative to the abdomen (open arrows). H = heart.

In the fetus, the right heart is the dominant ventricle. In the adult, congestive heart failure often results in pleural effusions as the pulmonary venous pressure rises. Fetal heart failure is a right-sided phenomenon with the elevated venous pressures transmitted to the systemic circulation rather than the pulmonary veins. Ascites is therefore more likely to develop as the first sign of fetal cardiac failure. Isolated fetal pleural effusions are more likely to be chylous, related to abnormalities in the lymphatic system, as with Noonan's syndrome or pulmonary lymphangiectasia **(Option (E) is false).** Of course secondary effusions can be seen as a component of hydrops fetalis, which has multiple etiologies including cardiac disease.

Richard A. Bowerman, M.D.

SUGGESTED READINGS

CONGENITAL DIAPHRAGMATIC HERNIA

1. Adzick NS, Harrison MR, Glick PL, Nakayama DK, Manning FA, deLorimier AA. Diaphragmatic hernia in the fetus: prenatal diagnosis and outcome in 94 cases. J Pediatr Surg 1985; 20:357–361

2. Adzick NS, Vacanti JP, Lillehei CW, O'Rourke PP, Crone RK, Wilson JM. Fetal diaphragmatic hernia: ultrasound diagnosis and clinical outcome in 38 cases. J Pediatr Surg 1989; 24:654–658
3. Comstock CH. The antenatal diagnosis of diaphragmatic anomalies. J Ultrasound Med 1986; 5:391–396
4. Jurcak-Zaleski S, Comstock CH, Kirk JS. Eventration of the diaphragm. Prenatal diagnosis. J Ultrasound Med 1990; 9:351–354
5. Sharland GK, Lockhart SM, Heward AJ, Allan LD. Prognosis in fetal diaphragmatic hernia. Am J Obstet Gynecol 1992; 166:9–13
6. Stolar C, Dillon P, Reyes C. Selective use of extracorporeal membrane oxygenation in the management of congenital diaphragmatic hernia. J Pediatr Surg 1988; 23:207–211

FETAL HYDROTHORAX

7. Castillo RA, Devoe LD, Falls G, Holzman GB, Hadi HA, Fadel HE. Pleural effusions and pulmonary hypoplasia. Am J Obstet Gynecol 1987; 157:1252–1255
8. Mahony BS, Filly RA, Callen PW, Chinn DH, Golbus MS. Severe nonimmune hydrops fetalis: sonographic evaluation. Radiology 1984; 151:757–761

CYSTIC ADENOMATOID MALFORMATION

9. Fine C, Adzick NS, Doubilet PM. Decreasing size of a congenital cystic adenomatoid malformation *in utero*. J Ultrasound Med 1988; 7:405–408
10. Johnson JA, Rumack CM, Johnson ML, Shikes R, Appareti K, Rees G. Cystic adenomatoid malformation: antenatal demonstration. AJR 1984; 142:483–484
11. Johnston RJ, McGahan JP, Hanson FW, Lindfors KK. Type III congenital cystic adenomatoid malformation associated with elevated maternal serum alpha-fetoprotein. J Perinatol 1988; 8:222–224
12. Stocker JT, Madewell JE, Drake RM. Congenital cystic adenomatoid malformation of the lung. Classification and morphologic spectrum. Hum Pathol 1977; 8:155–171

BRONCHOGENIC CYST

13. Albright EB, Crane JP, Shackelford GD. Prenatal diagnosis of a bronchogenic cyst. J Ultrasound Med 1988; 7:90–95
14. Young G, L'Heureux PR, Krueckeberg ST, Swanson DA. Mediastinal bronchogenic cyst: prenatal sonographic diagnosis. AJR 1980; 152:125–127

ASPLENIA/POLYSPLENIA SYNDROMES

15. Chitayat D, Lao A, Wilson RD, Fagerstrom C, Hayden M. Prenatal diagnosis of asplenia/polysplenia syndrome. Am J Obstet Gynecol 1988; 158:1085–1087
16. Jones KL. Smith's recognizable patterns of human malformation. Philadelphia: WB Saunders; 1988:543–544

FETAL LUNG

17. Johnson A, Callan NA, Bhutani VK, Colmorgen GH, Weiner S, Bolognese RJ. Ultrasonic ratio of fetal thoracic to abdominal circumference: an association with fetal pulmonary hypoplasia. Am J Obstet Gynecol 1987; 157:764–769
18. Lawrence S, Rosenfeld CR. Fetal pulmonary development and abnormalities of amniotic fluid volume. Semin Perinatol 1986; 10:142–153
19. Mayden KL, Tortora M, Chervenak FA, Hobbins JC. The antenatal sonographic detection of lung masses. Am J Obstet Gynecol 1984; 148:349–351
20. Page DV, Stocker JT. Anomalies associated with pulmonary hypoplasia. Am Rev Respir Dis 1982; 125:216–221

FETAL HEART

21. Benacerraf BR, Sanders SP. Fetal echocardiography. Radiol Clin North Am 1990; 28:131–147
22. Comstock CH. Normal fetal heart axis and position. Obstet Gynecol 1987; 70:255–259
23. Copel JA, Cullen M, Green JJ, Mahoney MJ, Hobbins JC, Kleinman CS. The frequency of aneuploidy in prenatally diagnosed congenital heart disease: an indication for fetal karyotyping. Am J Obstet Gynecol 1988; 158:409–413
24. Copel JA, Pilu G, Green J, Hobbins JC, Kleinman CS. Fetal echocardiographic screening for congenital heart disease: the importance of the four-chamber view. Am J Obstet Gynecol 1987; 157:648–655
25. DeVore GR, Horenstein J, Platt LD. Fetal echocardiography. VI. Assessment of cardiothoracic disproportion—a new technique for the diagnosis of thoracic hypoplasia. Am J Obstet Gynecol 1986; 155:1066–1071
26. McGahan JP. Sonography of the fetal heart: findings on the four-chamber view. Radiology 1991; 156:547–553
27. Wladimiroff JW, Stewart PA, Sachs ES, Niermeijer MF. Prenatal diagnosis and management of congenital heart defect: significance of associated fetal anomalies and prenatal chromosomal studies. Am J Med Genet 1985; 21:285–290

THORAX/HEART MEASUREMENTS

28. Filkins KA, Brown TF, Levine OR. Real time ultrasonic evaluation of the fetal heart. Int J Gynaecol Obstet 1981; 19:35–39
29. Nimrod C, Davies D, Iwanicki S, Harder J, Persaud D, Nicholson S. Ultrasound prediction of pulmonary hypoplasia. Obstet Gynecol 1986; 68:495–498

Notes

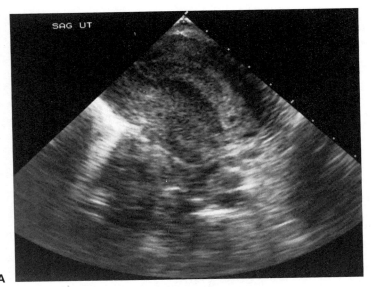

A

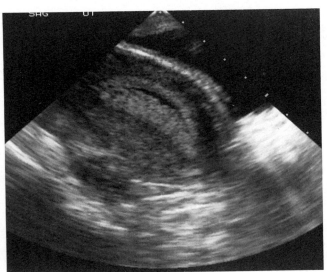

B

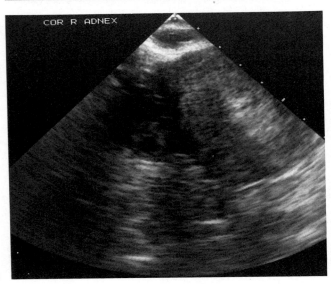

C

Figure 16-1. This 23-year-old woman presented to the emergency room with a history of pelvic pain and irregular vaginal bleeding. You are shown sagittal (A and B) and coronal (C) transvaginal sonograms of the lower pelvis.

could explain the history of pelvic pain in the test patient. The cystic teratoma acts as a fulcrum to potentiate partial or complete rotation of the ovarian pedicle on its axis. Typically, the ovary is enlarged and congested from the circulatory impairment. The uterus in such patients is normal. Therefore, the prominent decidual reaction and endometrial fluid in the test patient preclude ovarian dermoid as the most likely diagnosis.

Question 68

Concerning acute pelvic inflammatory disease,

(A) it affects 1% of women between 15 and 39 years of age
(B) the "indefinite uterus sign" (poorly defined uterine border) is a specific sonographic sign
(C) tubo-ovarian abscesses are commonly unilocular
(D) the ovaries are involved in only the most severe cases
(E) tubo-ovarian abscess is easily distinguished from appendiceal abscess by transvaginal sonography

Acute pelvic inflammatory disease (PID) reached epidemic proportions in this country during the mid 1960s. This disease exclusively affects sexually active females. Over 1 million cases occur annually, and the disease affects approximately 1% of women between 15 and 39 years of age **(Option (A) is true).**

The most common organisms responsible for PID are *Neisseria gonorrhoeae* and *Chlamydia trachomatis*. These organisms, which are introduced vaginally, incite an inflammatory response in the uterus initially. The sonographic appearance is extremely variable and can be nonspecific. In the earliest stages of the disease process, endometritis can be evident as mild uterine enlargement, mild thickening of the endometrial stripe (Figure 16-9), and either increased or decreased endometrial echogenicity. In patients who present during the secretory phase of the menstrual cycle, it is not possible to discern whether any apparent thickening is due to endometritis or physiologic changes. A hypoechoic rim around the stripe, similar to the halo effect seen just before ovulation, can occur. In patients with very severe cases, fluid can resemble the pseudogestational sac occasionally seen with ectopic pregnancy. These inflammatory uterine abnormalities correspond at laparoscopy to findings of erythema, edema, periuterine exudate, and adhesions. With progression of the inflammatory disease, the fallopian tubes become involved; this is usually evident on sonography as peritubular or cul-de-sac fluid. More severe infection can cause occlusion of the tubal ostium, resulting in pyo- or hydrosalpinx. The ovaries are relatively resistant to

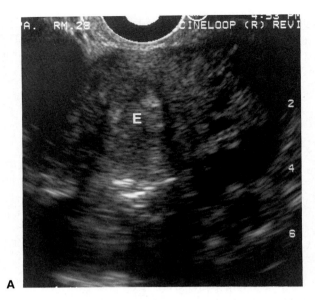

Figure 16-9. Endometritis. (A) A coronal transvaginal sonogram of thickened endometrium (E) in a patient with discharge and cultures positive for *N. gonorrhoeae.* (B) Sagittal sonogram of normal-sized left ovary with follicles. Note the slightly irregular contour (arrows).

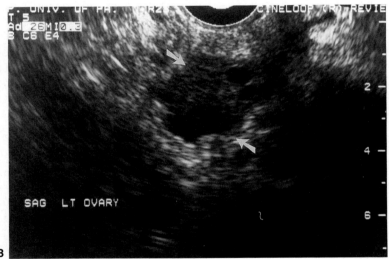

infection and are involved in only the most severe cases **(Option (D) is true).**

Inflamed ovaries typically are enlarged, have indistinct borders, and are associated with periovarian fluid collections (Figure 16-10). These sonographic findings correlate with peritoneal adhesions and periovarian exudate at laparoscopy. The tubo-ovarian abscess is by definition a complex mass consisting of an inflamed fallopian tube and ovary that are often fixed, thereby appearing as an ill-defined and enlarged adnexal

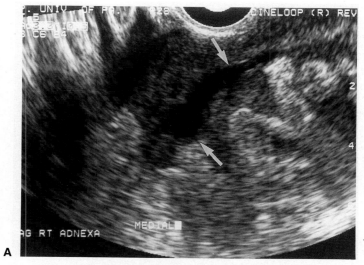

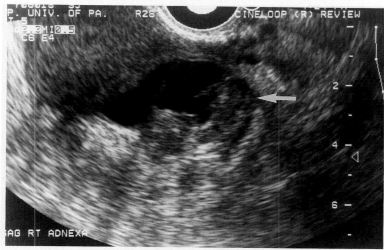

Figure 16-10. Tubo-ovarian abscess. (A) A sagittal sonogram of the right adnexus shows a thick-walled hydrosalpinx (arrows). (B) A sagittal sonogram of the right adnexus shows a multiloculated, complex mass (arrow) compatible with abscess.

mass in which it is not possible to distinguish between the two structures. The diffuse inflammatory changes that involve numerous pelvic structures in patients with acute PID tend to produce a multilocular rather than a unilocular mass on sonography **(Option (C) is false).**

The resulting adnexal or cul-de-sac masses are usually complex, with both cystic and solid components. Septations of variable thickness and

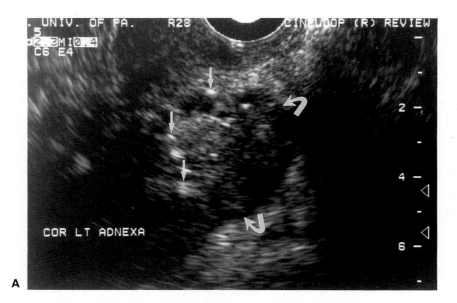

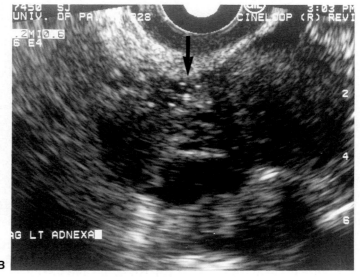

Figure 16-11. Abscess with adhesions. (A) A coronal sonogram of the left adnexus demonstrates a complex mass with punctate, bright reflectors (straight arrows) and a thin rim of normal ovarian stroma (curved arrows). (B) Sagittal sonogram of the mass (arrow) that at surgery represented a tubo-ovarian abscess with extensive adhesions and inflammation involving the bowel.

fluid-debris levels have been described (Figure 16-11). Areas of acoustic shadowing can occur beyond air pockets within adherent loops of bowel.

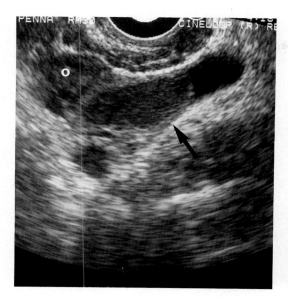

Figure 16-12. Pyosalpinx. A sagittal sonogram shows a dilated right fallopian tube (arrow) filled with purulent echogenic material. o = ovary.

Purulent exudates may be evident as simple or complex fluid collections in and around the pelvic organs (Figure 16-12). The sonographic detection of ill-defined uterine, ovarian, and tubal contours is a nonspecific finding that has been described as the "indefinite uterus sign." It can be seen in both acute and chronic PID, chronic ectopic pregnancy, endometriosis, and virtually any disease that causes a pelvic inflammatory response **(Option (B) is false).**

Transvaginal sonography is an adjunctive tool, which can be used to demonstrate the response of the pelvic viscera to palpation under direct real-time visualization. For example, peristalsis can be readily induced in normal fluid and gas-filled bowel loops, in contrast to the more fixed appearance of inflamed, adherent bowel. Similarly, the normal uterus and ovaries are sharply marginated with well-defined borders on sonography. Once these structures become involved with inflammatory exudate and adhesions, the normal distinct tissue planes are lost. This is more easily identifiable on transvaginal scans than on transabdominal scans. Swayne et al. correlated the sonographic and pathologic findings in 65 patients with PID. The most frequent pattern on transabdominal scans was total pelvic disorganization (41%), followed by focal extrauterine masses (37%). Both findings have been described in appendicitis with perforation, although involvement of the entire pelvis is quite unusual. However, it is difficult to differentiate appendiceal abscess with or without rupture from acute PID with tubo-ovarian abscess by transvaginal sonography alone **(Option (E) is false).** This can be done only if the

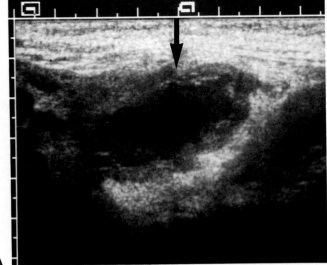
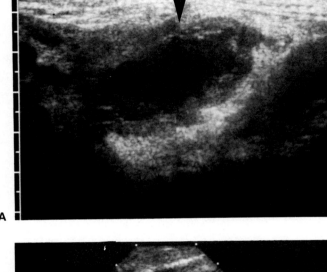

A

B

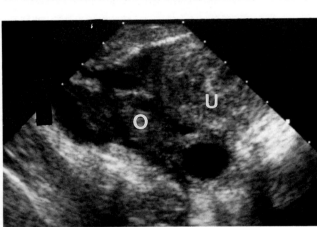

Figure 16-13. Severe salpingitis mimicking appendicitis. (A) A sagittal transabdominal sonogram shows a tubular, thick-walled mass (arrow) in a patient with right lower quadrant pain and peritoneal signs. (B) A sagittal transvaginal sonogram shows the uterus (U) and adjacent right ovary (O) with a small follicle. (C) A transvaginal sonogram shows an inflamed fallopian tube (arrow) in an unusual location, superior to the uterus and ovary. A moderate quantity of pus was present in the abdomen at surgery.

abscess cavity is shown to be clearly within the confines of the ovary. In patients with possible appendiceal abscess, it is preferable to also use a high-frequency linear transabdominal probe with graded compression. Even if both techniques are performed, misdiagnoses still occur.

In patients with severe salpingitis, the size and appearance of the inflamed tube can mimic the inflamed appendix on both sonographic and gross pathologic examination (Figure 16-13). In patients with gangrenous appendicitis complicated by rupture, there is spillage of purulent exudate from the right lower quadrant to the dependent pouch of Douglas. The involvement of the uterus and one or both adnexa by direct

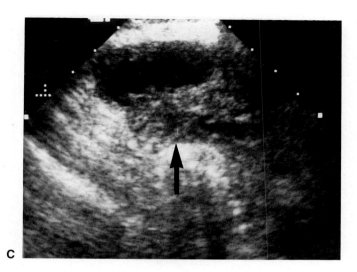

C

extension can be difficult to distinguish from sexually transmitted acute PID. The depiction of separate normal ovaries on transvaginal or transabdominal sonography virtually excludes a diagnosis of severe PID, but rare exceptions do occur (Figure 16-13).

Question 69

Concerning the pseudogestational sac of ectopic pregnancy,

(A) it is characterized by fluid within the endometrial cavity
(B) it can be located within any segment of the uterus
(C) it is due to sloughing decidua
(D) it has a single surrounding echogenic wall
(E) it occurs in approximately 30% of ectopic pregnancies

Before the advent of transvaginal sonography, direct identification of ectopic gestation was relatively uncommon. The main role of transabdominal sonography in a patient with suspected ectopic pregnancy was to diagnose intrauterine gestation, thereby effectively excluding ectopic pregnancy. The double-decidual sac sign was described as a means of distinguishing an early intrauterine gestation, prior to the development of a fetal pole, from a pseudogestational sac of ectopic pregnancy. The estimated frequency of pseudogestational sac in ectopic pregnancy has been reported as 10 to 20% **(Option (E) is false).**

The pseudogestational sac represents a collection of fluid or blood within the decidualized endometrium **(Option (A) is true),** rarely simu-

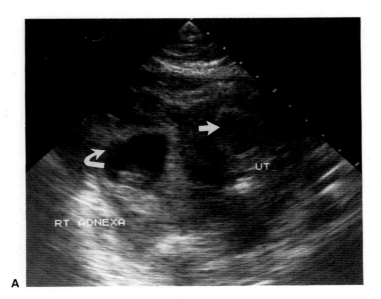

A

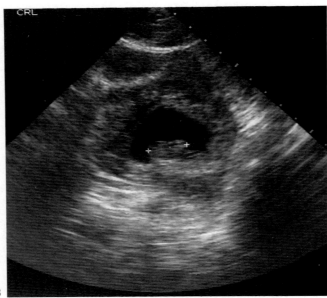

B

Figure 16-14.
Live ectopic pregnancy. (A) A coronal transvaginal sonogram shows the uterus (UT) containing a pseudogestational sac with debris (straight arrow) and a right ectopic pregnancy (curved arrow). (B) A sagittal sonogram shows a live ectopic pregnancy. Cursors denote the length of the early embryo.

lating the appearance of a normal gestational sac; in most cases, it actually resembles an abnormal early sac. In contradistinction to normal intrauterine gestational sacs, the pseudogestational sac is created by sloughing decidua **(Option (C) is true).** It is believed that hemorrhage beneath the necrotic decidua and the inner myometrium is the initiating event. This amorphous fluid collection often lacks the spherical shape

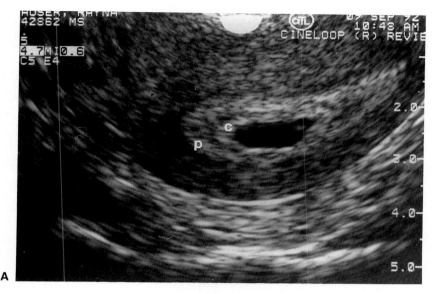

A

Figure 16-15. Normal early pregnancy. (A) A sagittal transvaginal sonogram of the uterus demonstrates the double-decidual-sac sign with two
echogenic rings representing the decidual capsularis (c) and the decidual
parietalis (p). (B) A coronal transvaginal sonogram shows a complex
right adnexal mass (arrows) due to an early hemorrhagic corpus luteum
cyst. This mass could easily be mistaken for a tubal ring, but the presence of the double-decidual-sac sign is strong confirmatory evidence of an
early intrauterine pregnancy.

and well-defined margins of a normal gestational sac (Figure 16-14). The
pseudogestational sac is positioned centrally within the endometrial cavity, whereas a normal gestational sac implants eccentrically within the
myometrium. It can be located within any segment of the uterus **(Option (B) is true).**

The normal early gestational sac is surrounded by two concentric
echogenic rings thought to represent the decidua parietalis adjacent to
the inner decidual capsularis (Figure 16-15). The base of the gestational
sac is bordered by a single layer, the decidua basalis. The decidual layers
lining the endometrium are usually closely apposed with a small space
between them, representing the endometrial cavity. This space can enlarge or widen when there is bleeding within the endometrial cavity. The
pseudogestational sac of ectopic pregnancy is composed of a single decidual layer due to separation of the endometrial lining. Sonography in
these patients demonstrates a single concentric echogenic line of variable thickness and echogenicity **(Option (D) is true).** Any pregnant pa-

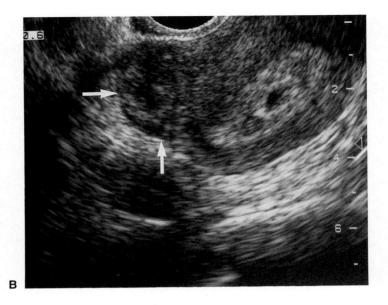

B

tient with this type of intrauterine fluid collection must be considered at risk for an ectopic gestation, with an abnormal intrauterine pregnancy as the main differential diagnosis. Careful attention to the extrauterine findings and close clinical correlation with history and laboratory data serve to narrow the diagnosis further. Transvaginal sonography has decreased the likelihood that the pseudogestational sac will be confused with a true sac. Early reports suggest that color and duplex Doppler sonography will be helpful in distinguishing these entities. The pseudogestational sac lacks chorionic villi and so lacks the increased intratrophoblastic flow of the normal intrauterine gestational sac (Figure 16-16) and the increased peritrophoblastic venous flow that has been described as a feature of the abnormal intrauterine sac.

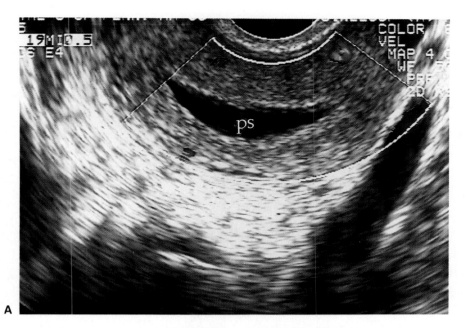

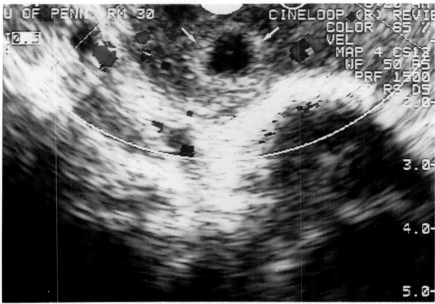

Figure 16-16. Pseudogestational sac. This patient presented with a history of prior spontaneous abortion 7 weeks ago. She had experienced no bleeding since that time and had a quantitative beta-human chorionic gonadotropin level greater than 4,000 units. (A) A coronal sonogram of the uterus demonstrates a fluid collection (ps) without increased peritrophoblastic flow. (B) A sagittal sonogram of the right adnexal area demonstrates an extrauterine gestational sac (arrows).

Question 70

Concerning ectopic pregnancy,

    (A) transvaginal sonograms usually provide more information than transabdominal scans do

    (B) a live extrauterine fetus is identifiable sonographically in fewer than 25% of cases

    (C) isthmic pregnancies tend to rupture latest

    (D) in a patient with a positive pregnancy test, the finding of particulate cul-de-sac fluid strongly suggests the diagnosis

    (E) in a patient with a positive pregnancy test, a tubal ring usually represents an unruptured ectopic pregnancy

The exact etiology of ectopic pregnancy is not completely understood. Even multiparity does not preclude development of an ectopic pregnancy in subsequent pregnancies. Ectopic pregnancies can occur in a number of extrauterine locations. There is a high frequency of tubal implantation, estimated at approximately 95% of all ectopic pregnancies. This has proved valuable in identifying many patients at greatest risk, for example, those with a history of tubal inflammation, manipulation, or surgery. The ampullary portion of the fallopian tube is the most common site of implantation outside the uterus, and the isthmic portion is the second most common site. Rarely, implantation occurs in the abdomen, cervix, or ovary (Figure 16-17). The isthmus of the fallopian tube is very narrow; therefore, ectopic pregnancies in this location tend to rupture early **(Option (C) is false).** Cornual pregnancies in the interstitial portion of the tube are partially enveloped by myometrium and therefore rupture late, with the greatest risk of maternal morbidity and mortality.

Transvaginal sonography has significantly improved the ability to diagnose ectopic pregnancy definitively in its earliest stages. The morphologic features of normal intrauterine gestations can now be depicted at least 1 week earlier than was possible with transabdominal sonography. The higher-frequency vaginal probe utilized in close proximity to the pelvic structures confers advantages over the transabdominal technique by enabling the earlier recognition of an ectopic pregnancy. Thorsen et al., in a series of 60 proven ectopic pregnancies, reported direct visualization of the ectopic gestational sac in 38% of cases with transvaginal scans compared with 22% with transabdominal scans. All 83 intrauterine pregnancies were identified with transvaginal scans, compared with only 34 identified with transabdominal sonography. Kivikoski et al., in a smaller series of 25 ectopic pregnancies, described adnexal findings as highly suspicious in 84% with vaginal sonograms and 68% with abdominal sonograms. In addition, improved visualization of the endometrial tissues with transvaginal sonography decreases the likelihood that pseudo-

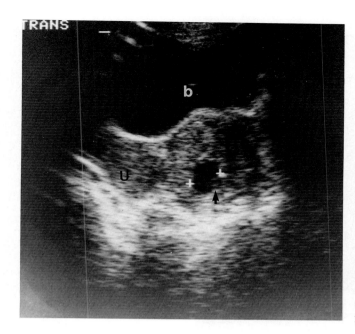

Figure 16-17. Ovarian ectopic pregnancy. A transabdominal sonogram shows a thick-walled adnexal mass, which is larger than the uterus (U). The chorionic cavity is delineated by cursors. Note the early yolk sac (arrow). b = bladder.

gestational sacs will be misconstrued as normal or abnormal intrauterine pregnancies **(Option (A) is true).** The use of higher-frequency vaginal probes in close proximity to the pelvic structures allows very accurate depiction of the adnexal and cul-de-sac abnormalities associated with ectopic pregnancy (Figure 16-18).

The most specific sonographic sign of an ectopic gestation is a live extrauterine embryo. Before the advent of transvaginal sonography, this was considered a relatively rare finding. Recent studies with the transvaginal technique have reported this finding in 15 to 21% of cases **(Option (B) is true).**

A tubal or adnexal ring has been observed more frequently than a live extrauterine gestation. The actual percentage is likely to vary with different populations. The frequency in this author's experience is far below that reported by Cacciatore (>60%). The adnexal ring represents the actual ectopic gestation that has burrowed into the endosalpinx of the fallopian tube (Figure 16-19). It appears as a central cystic region surrounded by a hyperechoic rim of trophoblastic tissue. It can be difficult to visualize because of surrounding gas-containing bowel or hemorrhage. The sonographic identification of this ring as a structure truly separate from the ovary and uterus is considered by most authorities to represent a very specific sign of ectopic gestation (Figure 16-20). It has been shown at laparoscopy to correlate consistently with an unruptured

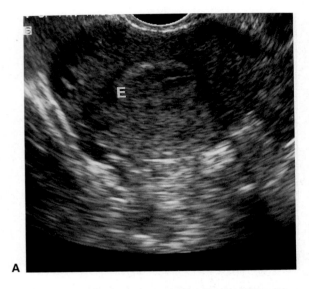

A

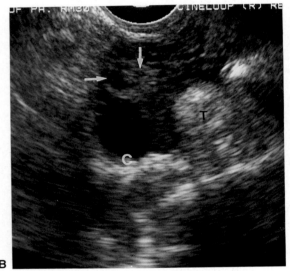

B

Figure 16-18. Ipsilateral ectopic pregnancy, corpus luteum cyst, and benign cystic teratoma. (A) A coronal transvaginal sonogram shows an empty uterus with a thickened endometrial stripe (E) in an asymptomatic patient. (B) A coronal sonogram of the left adnexus demonstrates a corpus luteum cyst (C), benign cystic teratoma (T), and an unruptured ectopic pregnancy (arrows). (C) Color Doppler imaging demonstrates characteristic peritrophoblastic flow (arrow).

ectopic pregnancy, with positive predictive values reported as high as 100% **(Option (E) is true).** However, other pelvic masses occasionally mimic the appearance of a tubal ring (Figure 16-21). Preliminary results also suggest that the introduction of color Doppler imaging has further increased the sensitivity and specificity of transvaginal sonography in the diagnosis of ectopic pregnancy. With color Doppler sonography, the prominent peritrophoblastic vascularity creates a ring of increased color

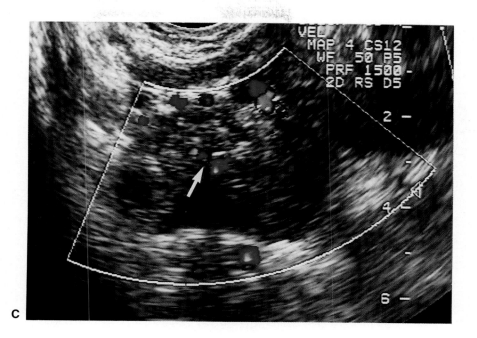

C

flow signal that can be very helpful in confirming suspicious cases and in clarifying confusing cases (Figures 16-18, 16-22, and 16-23). The ring of increased color flow has been called the "ring of fire."

The presence of a moderate to large amount of free peritoneal fluid is known to indicate a high likelihood of ectopic pregnancy, although it is a less specific sign. Physiologic amounts of fluid, 5 mL or less, can be seen in normal or abnormal intrauterine pregnancy or ectopic pregnancy. Detection of this small quantity of fluid is not useful in limiting the differential diagnosis. In patients with ectopic pregnancy, free peritoneal fluid usually represents blood or, less often, serous fluid produced mainly by hormonally stimulated secretions from the ovary. The most common cause of hemoperitoneum in ectopic pregnancy is leakage of blood from the fimbriated end of the tube. Actual tubal rupture is uncommon, with a reported frequency of 10 to 15%. Intraperitoneal fluid is more common in ectopic (40 to 83%) than in intrauterine (10 to 23%) pregnancies. Particulate fluid correlates with hemoperitoneum at surgery. It has been reported in 25 to 50% of patients with ectopic pregnancy, with a positive predictive value of 93% **(Option (D) is true).** Patients with intrauterine pregnancy generally have anechoic fluid, except in unusual cases where the pregnancy is complicated by appendiceal abscess or ruptured corpus luteum cyst (Figure 16-24).

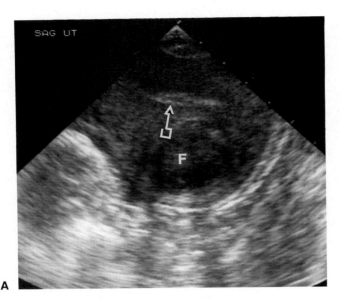

A

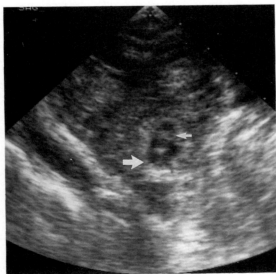

B

Figure 16-19. Leaking
ectopic pregnancy. (A) A
sagittal transvaginal
sonogram shows a normal
thin endometrial stripe
(arrow) and an intramu-
ral fibroid (F) in this patient with a palpable
mass and a positive se-
rum pregnancy test.
(B) A sagittal transvagi-
nal sonogram of the left
adnexus demonstrates a
tubal ring (large arrow)
with a tiny yolk sac
(small arrow).

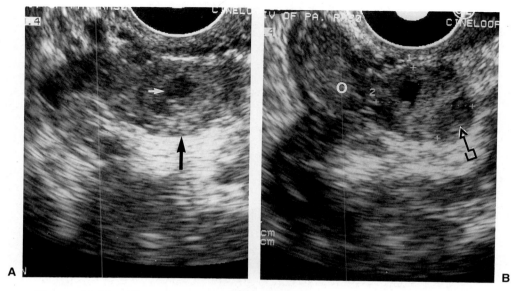

Figure 16-20. Unruptured ectopic pregnancy. (A) A coronal transvaginal sonogram of the right adnexus demonstrates a well-defined thick-walled echogenic mass (long arrow) with an irregular hypoechoic center (short arrow). (B) A coronal sonogram angled to the right pelvic sidewall demonstrates a normal ovary (O) lateral to the tubal pregnancy (arrow); the border of the tubal pregnancy is indicated by the electronic cursors.

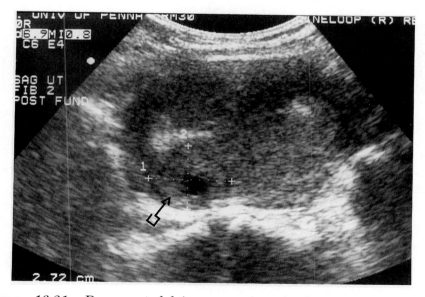

Figure 16-21. Degenerated leiomyoma. A sagittal transvaginal sonogram of the uterus demonstrates an irregular posterior contour and a small intramural mass (cursors) with a thickened echogenic rim (arrow) and a hypoechoic center.

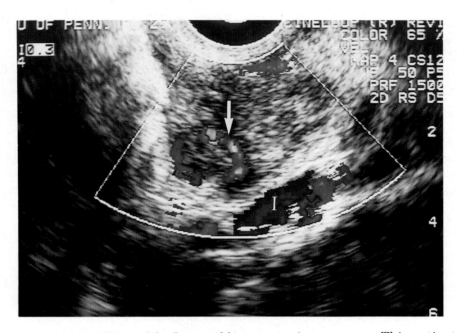

Figure 16-22. "Ring of fire" caused by an ectopic pregnancy. This patient presented to the emergency department with a history of vague cramps and irregular menses. A vaginal sonogram demonstrated a small solid adnexal mass adjacent to the left ovary. Color Doppler imaging shows an area of circumferential increased flow (arrow) at the site of a small unruptured ectopic pregnancy. I = iliac vessels.

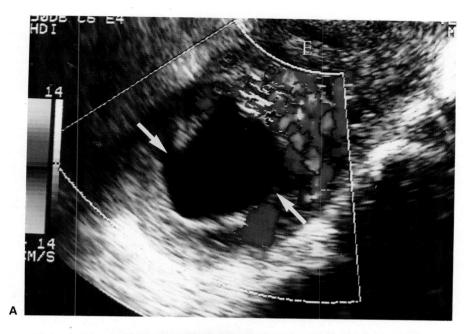

A

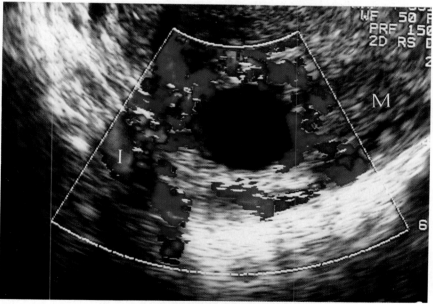

B

Figure 16-23. Cornual ectopic pregnancy. This patient presented with a history of size less than menstrual dates, which projected her gestation to approximately 17 weeks. (A) Sagittal color Doppler images of the uterus demonstrated a large eccentric gestational sac (arrows). E = endometrium. (B) A coronal sonogram shows this cornual ectopic pregnancy to be adjacent to the iliac vessels (I) without normally intervening myometrium (M).

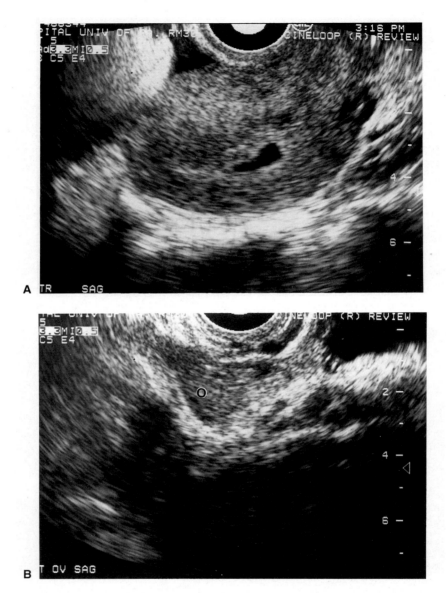

Figure 16-24. Ruptured corpus luteum cyst. This patient presented
emergently with abdominal pain, bleeding, and a quantitative beta-
human chorionic gonadotropin level exceeding 3,800 units. (A) A sagittal
transvaginal sonogram of the uterus demonstrates a small irregular
intrauterine fluid collection, which represented an early abnormal pregnancy. (B) Sagittal sonogram of the right ovary (O). (C) A coronal sonogram of the left adnexal region shows a large quantity of free fluid (F)
and a thick-walled, predominantly cystic mass (arrow). (D) Color Doppler imaging shows hypervascularity in the wall of this cyst. A large
quantity of free peritoneal blood was noted at surgery.

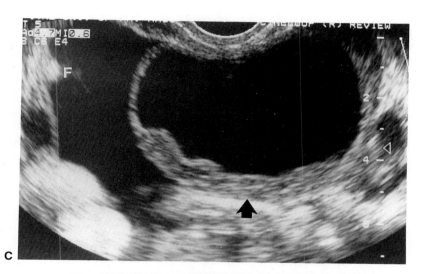

C

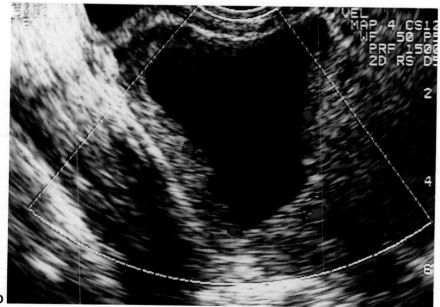

D

Question 71

Concerning early intrauterine pregnancy,

(A) threatened abortion occurs in approximately 25% of pregnancies
(B) embryonic cardiac motion is consistently identifiable on transvaginal scans by 46 menstrual days in all normal gestations
(C) a disproportionately low serum human chorionic gonadotropin (β-hCG) level usually indicates incomplete abortion
(D) most abnormal gestations cease development before a recognizable embryo is formed
(E) weak choriodecidual echogenicity is a criterion of an abnormal gestational sac

Complications occurring early in pregnancy pose diagnostic challenges for both obstetrician and radiologist. Abdominal pain and bleeding are symptoms that frequently herald an abnormality interrupting the normal development of an early gestation (Figure 16-8). Spontaneous abortion (the natural expulsion of an intrauterine gestation prior to 20 weeks) has commonly been quoted as occurring in 10% of all pregnancies. This frequency is difficult to determine precisely, because there is not agreement regarding when a pregnancy actually begins or ends. The frequency of abortion would clearly be lower if the diagnosis depended on histologic documentation of villi rather than on laboratory confirmation of decreasing serum β-hCG levels. Many investigators have identified a substantial loss rate very early in pregnancy. Most of these abnormal gestations cease development before a recognizable embryo is formed **(Option (D) is true)**. The morphologic findings in these early spontaneous abortions frequently include abnormalities of the developing embryo or, occasionally, the placenta. Chromosomal abnormalities, whether anomalies of number or of structure, are quite common in these early abortuses. Many other factors that can affect the embryo and the intrauterine environment place the conceptus at risk. These include viral syndromes, chemicals, radiation, underlying maternal diseases, congenital abnormalities of the reproductive organs, and the presence of an intrauterine contraceptive device.

Threatened abortion is a clinical term that refers to vaginal bleeding that occurs in the first 20 weeks of a potentially live gestation. Aching in the lower back and abdominal cramps can also be present. Bleeding is typically scanty and variable in coloration. By definition, the cervix is closed and no tissue has been passed. This is a relatively frequent complication, occurring in approximately 25% of pregnancies **(Option (A) is true)**. At most 50% of these patients will abort despite all therapeutic measures. Sonography has a pivotal role in evaluating this condition because of its ability to demonstrate an embryo with or without cardiac

A 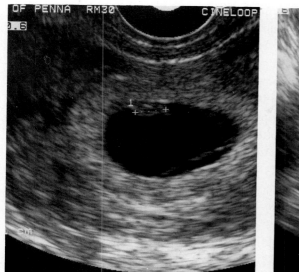 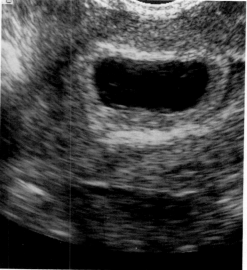 B

Figure 16-25. Early embryonic demise. (A) A coronal transvaginal sonogram of the uterus demonstrates an early embryo (cursors) approximately 7 mm long. There was no embryonic cardiac motion. However, the patient requested a follow-up scan before consenting to dilation and evacuation. (B) A coronal sonogram of the uterus approximately 48 hours later demonstrates reabsorption of the previously seen embryo and a decrease in overall sac size.

activity. When cardiac motion is unequivocally absent, dilation and evacuation should be scheduled since spontaneous expulsion is often delayed (Figure 16-25). Failure to expel a nonviable fetus can be associated with complications of infection and prolonged bleeding. The sonographic finding of cardiac motion confirms the presence of a live embryo and predicts a favorable outcome in many cases; however, it is not an absolute indicator of normality. Transvaginal sonography demonstrates the intrauterine embryo, embryonic cardiac motion, and the yolk sac more often and more clearly than transabdominal sonography does. Cardiac pulsations can be identified with transvaginal sonography as early as 40 menstrual days and can be identified consistently in all normal gestations by 46 menstrual days **(Option (B) is true).** Our ability to diagnose a live intrauterine pregnancy earlier than ever before means that we are probably imaging a finite percentage of pregnancies that will inevitably abort.

The differential diagnosis of absence of a normal living embryo during early pregnancy includes recent spontaneous complete or incomplete abortion, blighted ovum, embryonic demise, early hydatidiform degeneration, and ectopic pregnancy. Incomplete abortion generally refers to the retention of some products of conception within the uterus after most of the gestational tissue has been expelled. The sonographic findings vary with the approximate gestational age at the time of the event and with the amount of tissue passed. Abortions occurring before week 10 of gestation often result in the expulsion of the embryo and placenta together. Retention of all or part of the placenta in abortions that occur after this period is usually heralded by the onset of vaginal bleeding. Embryonic demise refers to an embryo retained in the uterine cavity with absent cardiac activity. This can be reliably diagnosed by transvaginal sonography after the embryo is visualized, especially after it exceeds 5 mm in length. The sonographic findings in missed abortion vary depending on the time elapsed between the sonogram and the fetal demise. The gestational sac can appear unremarkable with a well-formed chorion frondosum, a normal quantity of amniotic fluid, and a distinct embryo. This usually occurs relatively early in the process, whereas later the gestational sac becomes distorted in morphology and position, the amniotic fluid decreases in amount, and the choriodecidual reaction decreases in echogenicity and overall thickness **(Option (E) is true).** The nonviable embryo often lies in a fixed dependent position. In the later stages of the process, an early embryo that has not been expelled may be recognizable only as a distorted clump of echoes (Figure 16-26). Retained second-trimester fetuses can have recognizable anatomic structures with specific features such as overlapping of the fetal skull bones.

The proper evaluation of any patient with suspected ectopic pregnancy requires correlation of the sonographic findings with biochemical assays. The improved sensitivity of both the radioimmunoassay for the serum β subunit of hCG and the enzyme-linked immunosorbent assay for β-hCG in urine permit the diagnosis of pregnancy as early as 3.5 menstrual weeks. There are several approaches to correlation of the sonographic results with hCG levels. These levels are known to double every several days in normal pregnancies, so high-risk patients can be monitored by repeated quantitative measurements of serum hCG levels. Serial determinations of β-hCG levels are indicated in other patients in whom transvaginal sonography is not diagnostic. Ectopic pregnancies generally produce less hCG than do intrauterine pregnancies of the same gestational age. Whether this difference is due to the site of implantation or to decreased proliferation of trophoblasts is uncertain. A decrease, plateau, or smaller than normal increase in hCG concentration is indicative of an abnormal intrauterine or extrauterine pregnancy and is not specific for incomplete abortion **(Option (C) is false).**

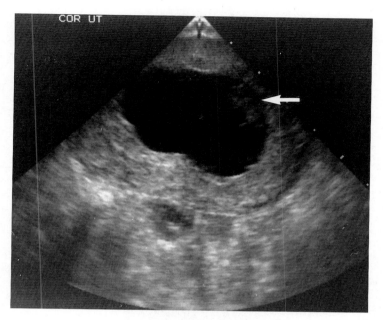

Figure 16-26. Embryonic demise. A coronal transvaginal sonogram of the uterus demonstrates a very large chorionic cavity, which contained an ill-defined clump of echoes (arrow). The gestational sac is surrounded by a very thin wall with absence of the normal thick, echogenic, trophoblastic decidual reaction.

Question 72

Concerning the corpus luteum cysts of pregnancy,

    (A) they form in the ovary at the site of a ruptured follicle
    (B) they are similar in size to follicular cysts
    (C) they are typically both unilocular and unilateral
    (D) they are prone to intermittent hemorrhage and rupture
    (E) most resolve by 6 weeks

Pelvic masses complicating pregnancy are often incidentally discovered on sonography or at the time of routine bimanual examination. In the vast majority of cases, a palpable adnexal mass in the first trimester represents a corpus luteum cyst (Figure 16-27). Transvaginal sonography is a rapid, simple means of confirming this diagnosis. The corpus luteum cyst of menstruation forms in the ovary at the site of a ruptured

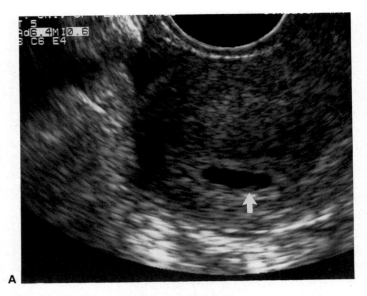

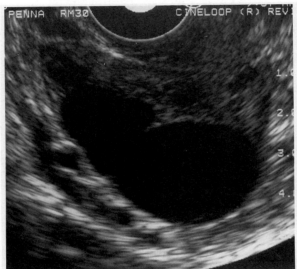

Figure 16-27. Early
intrauterine preg-
nancy. (A) A sagittal
sonogram of the
uterus demonstrates a
very early intrauter-
ine gestational sac (ar-
row). (B) A coronal
sonogram of the right
adnexus demonstrates
a thin-walled, multi-
lobular corpus luteum
cyst projecting from an
enlarged ovary.

follicle. After fertilization occurs, the cyst becomes the corpus luteum of
pregnancy **(Option (A) is true).** The cyst produces progesterone, which
sustains the decidualized endometrium during the early first trimester.
These simple cysts rarely exceed 4 cm in diameter. Excessive bleeding
into the corpus luteum or failure of absorption following discharge of the
oocyte can result in a much larger cyst, which exceeds 10 cm in diameter.
Follicular cysts, which form when a mature follicle fails to ovulate or

involute, are much smaller **(Option (B) is false).** Follicular cysts cannot be differentiated from normal follicles until they reach several centimeters in size. Both follicular and corpus luteum cysts are thin-walled, sharply marginated, round or oval, anechoic, unilateral, and unilocular structures that exhibit enhanced through transmission **(Option (C) is true).** They are only occasionally bilateral. Most follicular and luteal cysts are asymptomatic. Large corpus luteum cysts can induce vague complaints of pain, pelvic pressure, and lower backache. They are prone to hemorrhage and rupture **(Option (D) is true).** Transvaginal sonography can be helpful when symptoms arise from such complications. Bleeding within an unruptured cyst can be apparent sonographically as solid contents, mural nodularity, septations, focal wall thickening, or fluid-debris levels. Hemorrhagic luteal cysts have variable characteristics because of the temporal sequence of clot formation, retraction, and lysis (Figure 16-28). They can appear similar to ovarian neoplasms, endometriomas, abscesses, ectopic pregnancies, and cystic teratomas. Intraperitoneal hemorrhage following rupture can be evident either as simple or particulate cul-de-sac fluid. Surgical excision of the luteal cyst is required in some instances. Corpus luteum cysts tend to reach their maximum size by approximately 8 to 10 weeks, and most have resolved by 16 weeks **(Option (E) is false).** Any masses that persist beyond this menstrual age should be further evaluated. Operative intervention, if deemed necessary, is preferably performed in the second trimester because of a lower fetal loss rate than in first-trimester surgery (2 and 35%, respectively).

Beverly G. Coleman, M.D.

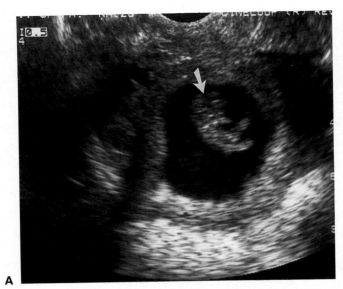

Figure 16-28. Hemorrhagic corpus luteum cyst. (A) A coronal transvaginal sonogram shows early intrauterine pregnancy with identifiable embryonic crown (arrow). (B) A sagittal sonogram shows a complex adnexal mass (solid arrow) due to hemorrhage within a corpus luteum cyst. Note the fluid-debris level (open arrows).

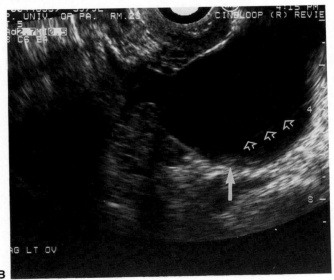

SUGGESTED READINGS

ECTOPIC PREGNANCY

1. Atri M, Bret PM, Tulandi T. Spontaneous resolution of ectopic pregnancy: initial appearance and evolution at transvaginal US. Radiology 1993; 186:83–86

2. Cacciatore B. Can the status of tubal pregnancy be predicted with trans-vaginal sonography? A prospective comparison of sonographic, surgical, and serum hCG findings. Radiology 1990; 177:481–484

3. Emerson DS, Cartier MS, Altieri LA, et al. Diagnostic efficacy of endovaginal color Doppler flow imaging in an ectopic pregnancy screening program. Radiology 1992; 183:413–420

4. Fleischer AC, Pennell RG, McKee MS, Wang KY. Ectopic pregnancy: features at transvaginal sonography. Radiology 1990; 174:375–378

5. Kivikoski AI, Martin CM, Smeltzer JS. Transabdominal and transvaginal ultrasonography in the diagnosis of ectopic pregnancy: a comparative study. Am J Obstet Gynecol 1990; 163:123–128

6. Nyberg DA, Hughes MP, Mack LA, Wang KY. Extrauterine findings of ectopic pregnancy at transvaginal US: importance of echogenic fluid. Radiology 1991; 178:823–826

7. Nyberg DA, Mack LA, Jeffrey RB Jr, Laing FC. Endovaginal sonographic evaluation of ectopic pregnancy: a prospective study. AJR 1987; 149:1181–1186

8. Pellerito JS, Taylor KJ, Quedens-Case C, et al. Ectopic pregnancy: evaluation with endovaginal color flow imaging. Radiology 1992; 183:407–411

9. Thorsen MK, Lawson TL, Aiman EJ, et al. Diagnosis of ectopic pregnancy: endovaginal vs transabdominal sonography. AJR 1990; 155:307–310

PELVIC INFLAMMATORY DISEASE

10. Dallabetta G, Hook EW III. Gonococcal infections. Infect Dis Clin North Am 1987; 1:25–54

11. Jeffrey RB Jr, Laing FC, Lewis FR. Acute appendicitis: high-resolution real-time US findings. Radiology 1987; 163:11–14

12. Patten RM, Vincent LM, Wolner-Hanssen P, Thorpe E Jr. Pelvic inflammatory disease. Endovaginal sonography with laparoscopic correlation. J Ultrasound Med 1990; 9:681–689

13. Swayne LC, Love MB, Karasick SR. Pelvic inflammatory disease: sonographic-pathologic correlation. Radiology 1984; 151:751–755

14. Terry J, Forrest T. Sonographic demonstration of salpingitis. Potential confusion with appendicitis. J Ultrasound Med 1989; 8:39–41

15. Tessler FN, Perrella RR, Fleischer AC, Grant EG. Endovaginal sonographic diagnosis of dilated fallopian tubes. AJR 1989; 153:523–525

16. Westrom L, Mardh PA. Acute pelvic inflammatory disease (PID). In: King K, Holmes KK, Mardh PA, et al. (eds), Sexually transmitted diseases, 2nd ed. New York: McGraw-Hill; 1990:593–613

COMPLICATIONS OF EARLY PREGNANCY

17. Cashner KA, Christopher CR, Dysert GA. Spontaneous fetal loss after demonstration of a live fetus in the first trimester. Obstet Gynecol 1987; 70:827–830

18. Coleman BG. Transvaginal sonography in extrauterine and intrauterine pregnancy. Semin Roentgenol 1991; 26:63–74

19. Coleman BG, Arger PH. Ultrasound in early pregnancy complications. Clin Obstet Gynecol 1988; 31:3–18

20. Kier R, McCarthy SM, Scoutt LM, Viscarello RR, Schwartz PE. Pelvic masses in pregnancy: MR imaging. Radiology 1990; 176:709–713

21. Levi CS, Lyons EA, Lindsay DJ. Early diagnosis of nonviable pregnancy with endovaginal US. Radiology 1988; 167:383–385

22. Nyberg DA, Laing FC, Filly RA. Threatened abortion: sonographic distinction of normal and abnormal gestation sacs. Radiology 1986; 158:397–400

23. Nyberg DA, Mack LA, Laing FC, Jeffrey RB. Early pregnancy complications: endovaginal sonographic findings correlated with human chorionic gonadotropin levels. Radiology 1988; 167:619–622

24. Pennell RG, Baltarowich OH, Kurtz AB, et al. Complicated first-trimester pregnancies: evaluation with endovaginal US versus transabdominal technique. Radiology 1987; 165:79–83

25. Wilcox AJ, Weinberg CR, O'Connor JF, et al. Incidence of early loss of pregnancy. N Eng J Med 1988; 319:189–194

26. Wilson RD, Kendrick V, Wittmann BK, McGillivray B. Spontaneous abortion and pregnancy outcome after normal first-trimester ultrasound examination. Obstet Gynecol 1986; 67:352–355

Notes

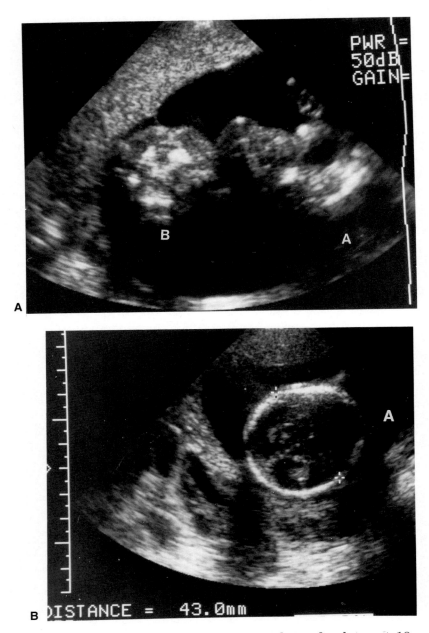

Figure 17-1. This 31-year-old woman was large for dates at 18 weeks gestation. You are shown sonograms of a twin gestation. The fetuses are labeled A and B.

Case 17: Twin-Twin Transfusion Syndrome

Question 73

Which *one* of the following is the MOST likely diagnosis?

(A) Duodenal atresia in twin A
(B) Twin-twin transfusion syndrome
(C) Intrauterine growth retardation in twin B
(D) Monoamniotic twinning
(E) Normal twins with idiopathic polyhydramnios

The test sonograms (Figure 17-1) show a twin intrauterine gestation with marked polyhydramnios (Figure 17-2). Twin A is surrounded by excessive amniotic fluid, and twin B is closely apposed to the uterine wall in a non-gravity-dependent fashion. The sonograms of the head and abdomen of both fetus A (Figure 17-1B and C) and fetus B (Figure 17-1D and E) reveal the biometric parameters of fetus B to be considerably delayed relative to those of fetus A, a finding consistent with early intrauterine growth retardation (IUGR). Specifically, the biometric parameters for fetus A are a biparietal diameter of 43 mm (18.3 weeks) and an abdominal circumference of 123 mm (17.5 weeks) (Figure 17-1B and C). Note the gravity-dependent position of the fetus and the marked polyhydramnios again evident in Figure 17-1C. Biometric parameters for fetus B are a biparietal diameter of 36 mm (16 weeks) and a calculated abdominal circumference (average abdominal diameter multiplied by 3.14) of 83 mm (14.2 weeks) (Figure 17-1D and E). Note the non-gravity-dependent position of fetus B, held anteriorly. Marked oligohydramnios is inferred, with the tightly apposed amniotic membrane fixing the fetus to the placenta. The abdominal circumference of fetus B is below the 5th percentile, and the biparietal diameter is below the 10th percentile for gestational age, indicating severe growth retardation. This combination of findings is most consistent with the twin-twin transfusion syndrome (TTTS) **(Option (B) is correct).**

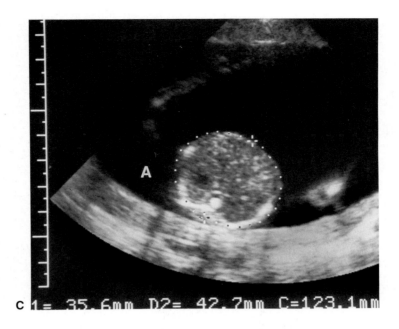

C 1= 35.6mm D2= 42.7mm C=123.1mm

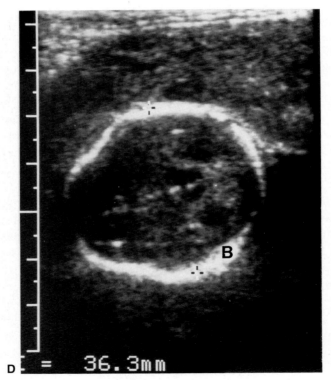

D = 36.3mm

Figure 17-1 (Continued)

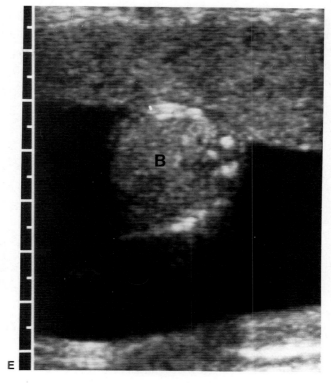

Figure 17-1 (Continued)

TTTS occurs almost universally when there is a monochorionic placentation. In this circumstance a shared placenta is present, within which exist multiple vascular communications between the two fetal circulations. Blood passes from one twin to the other, resulting in a characteristic pattern. The donor twin becomes anemic, hypovolemic, and growth retarded. Reduced urine output results in oligohydramnios, which, if marked, leads to a "stuck twin" appearance of the fetus positioned tightly against the uterine wall, restricted by the amniotic membrane, which is not easily visible. The recipient twin becomes plethoric and hypertensive and develops organomegaly. Increased urine output leads to polyhydramnios, often marked in degree. Hydrops fetalis is an occasional finding in either the donor or recipient fetus. There is a 70% perinatal mortality for all affected fetuses, with donor and recipient fetuses having similar risk. The prognosis is worst for those diagnosed earliest, since these tend to have larger shunts and more serious complications. The key sonographic features for a diagnosis of TTTS are a

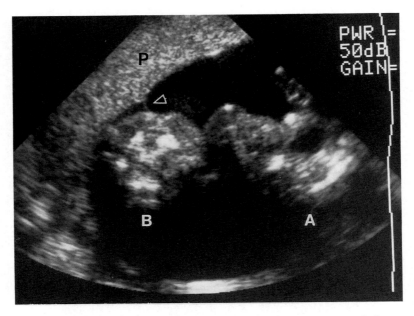

Figure 17-2 (Same as Figure 17-1A). A transverse image of the uterus shows a twin gestation at 18 weeks, with polyhydramnios. Fluid extends entirely around fetus A, whereas fetus B is anterior and close to the edge of the amniotic cavity. A short segment of a thin membrane (arrowhead) extends from the placenta (P) to wrap closely around fetus B.

discrepancy in amniotic fluid volume, intertwin growth differences exceeding either 18 mm in abdominal circumference or 25% in estimated fetal weight, and evidence of monochorionicity. Documentation of separate placentas or different fetal gender rules out a monochorionic gestation. A thick, clearly visible membrane suggests a dichorionic pregnancy, whereas a thin membrane that is not easily visible or an absent membrane indicates monochorionic twins (Figure 17-3).

Therapeutic options are limited. Serial sonograms are needed, however, to assess fetal growth and condition. In mild TTTS, expectant management may be appropriate. Serial amniocentesis to reduce polyhydramnios has increased the survival rate in some series, by unknown mechanisms. Selective feticide has been suggested, although theoretical problems exist. An acute and significant transfusion from the living (high-pressure) to dead (low-pressure) system could have adverse effects, as would passage of embolic or thromboplastic products from the dead fetus. Fetoscopic laser ablation has been successfully used to cauterize the placenta between the two cord insertions, obliterating the

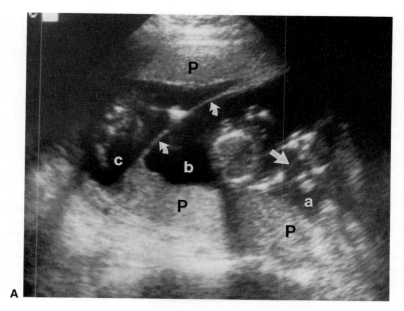

A

Figure 17-3. Triplet gestation. (A) A longitudinal image of the uterine cavity reveals three fetuses in separate sacs (denoted as a, b, and c). P = placental tissue. A single anterior placenta is seen with gestation c, while a posterior placenta is shared by gestations a and b. A thick membrane (curved arrows) composed of both chorion and amnion separates gestations b and c, whereas a thin, difficult-to-identify membrane (straight arrow) composed only of amnion separates gestations a and b. Gestations a and b are therefore monochorionic and monozygotic, with a common placenta. Gestations c and a/b as a unit can be considered dichorionic and could have arisen on either a dizygotic or monozygotic basis. Gestations a and b are at risk for TTTS, which did not occur during pregnancy, since growth parameters were normal. Intrauterine death of fetus a shortly before birth, however, resulted in an apparent peripartum "transfusion" from fetus b to fetus a, causing a plethoric appearance of the dead triplet at birth and a pale, anemic twin b. Anastomoses were clearly present across their common placenta that were balanced while they were both alive. With the death of fetus a, pressure gradients changed, allowing the acute twin transfusion to occur.

shunt vessels and halting the transplacental transfusion and its complications.

Although fetus A has marked polyhydramnios, which is associated with duodenal atresia (Option (A)), there is no evidence for a double-bubble sign or dilated stomach within the fetal abdomen, excluding this diagnosis. Marked polyhydramnios of any cause within one gestational sac can potentially result in a stuck twin appearance in the other sac

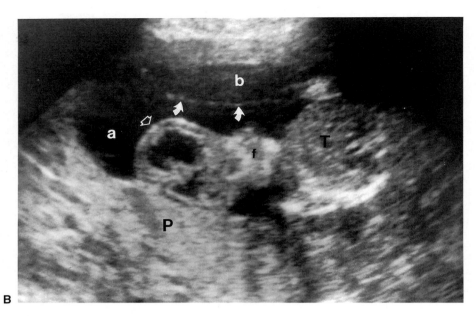

Figure 17-3 (Continued). Triplet gestation. (B) A coronal image of fetus a shows the fetal trunk (T) and face (f). No ossified calvarium is present, and a distorted brain with dilated ventricles protrudes superior to the face (open arrow). Acrania associated with amniotic band syndrome was diagnosed following delivery. Note the contiguity between the placenta (P) and the anomalous brain, as entanglement in the membranes has occurred. There is an increased frequency of anomalies in monozygotic pregnancies. Note the thin membrane (solid arrows) between sacs a and b.

(Figure 17-4). By a mechanism that is unknown but may be related to increased pressure from the polyhydramnios, amniotic fluid is restricted in the second sac, resulting in oligohydramnios and restriction of fetal movement. However, this would not result in the severe growth retardation seen in fetus B in the test case. The appearance of a stuck twin could also be seen with marked oligohydramnios secondary to absent fetal urine production, as with renal agenesis, but the polyhydramnios in the other sac in the test case would not be explained.

IUGR of one twin (Option (C)) can lead to a growth discrepancy between twins and to oligohydramnios. It is uncommon at the early gestational age seen in the test case, most often being a third-trimester occurrence. When IUGR is present in the second trimester, a chromosomal abnormality, intrauterine infection, or underlying maternal disease or teratogen exposure should be suspected. IUGR with oligohy-

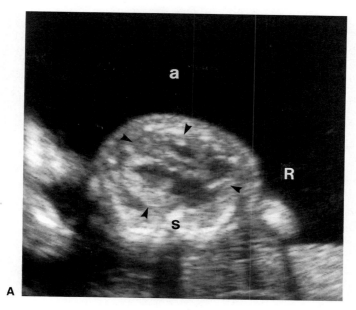

Figure 17-4. Cardiac anomaly in twin gestation with polyhydramnios and oligohydramnios, simulating twin-twin transfusion syndrome. (A) A transverse image of the thorax of fetus A shows marked cardiac enlargement (arrowheads) and severe polyhydramnios (a). R = right; s = spine. In contrast to the findings in this fetus, a normal heart would occupy about one-third of the cross-sectional area of the thorax on a four-chamber view.

dramnios involving fetus B in the test case would fail to explain the marked polyhydramnios in sac A.

With monoamniotic twins (Option (D)), a single gestation sac is present with no internal membrane. Fewer than 1% of twins show this configuration. Fetal mortality is about 50% in these cases, in large part because the fetuses are free to mingle within the single amniotic cavity. Entanglement of the cords is possible, often ending with cord occlusion and death of one or both twins (Figure 17-5). In the test case, one fetus is clearly restricted and unable to move, being fixed in a nondependent position. Only a very short segment of membrane is identified in the test images because of its otherwise close apposition to the fetus, secondary to marked oligohydramnios, but its presence is inferred. Therefore, this diagnosis is excluded. Monoamniotic pregnancies are monochorionic and hence are at risk for developing TTTS. Growth discrepancy between the twins would be apparent, but the oligohydramnios-polyhydramnios relationship would not be seen because of the absence of a separating membrane.

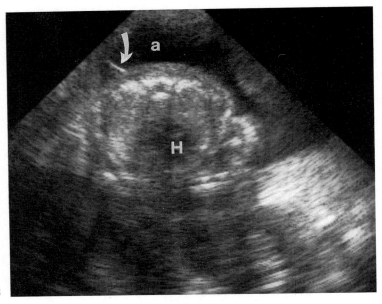

B

Figure 17-4 (Continued). Cardiac anomaly in twin gestation with polyhydramnios and oligohydramnios, simulating twin-twin transfusion syndrome. (B) A transverse image of the thorax of fetus B shows marked
oligohydramnios, with the fetus held tight to the edge of myometrium
and only a short segment of membrane delineated (arrow). H = heart.
The only amniotic fluid near fetus B is in the sac of fetus A (a). The
marked discrepancy in fluid volume between the sacs initially suggested
TTTS. Careful attention to the fetal anatomic survey revealed a complex
cardiac anomaly as the cause for the pronounced polyhydramnios, which
secondarily compressed the other sac and resulted in oligohydramnios.
Therapeutic amniocentesis of sac a resulted in a rapid reaccumulation of
fluid around fetus B, a finding that would be unusual in TTTS with
chronic oligohydramnios from IUGR. (C) A 4-week follow-up transverse
image of fetus A shows worsening cardiomegaly and interval development of hydrops fetalis with subcutaneous edema (✱) and pericardial
effusion (+). Polyhydramnios is again noted (a). s = spine.

Multiple gestations are associated with polyhydramnios, as are
many other fetal and nonfetal conditions. Polyhydramnios in twin gestations can be idiopathic (Option (E)) or can have diverse causes including
TTTS and intrinsic fetal anomalies (Figure 17-4). Idiopathic polyhydramnios in normal twins is clearly incorrect since the marked growth
discrepancy excludes a diagnosis of normal twins. Additionally, although
polyhydramnios in sac A could be idiopathic and presumably nonpathologic, the oligohydramnios in the other sac suggests significant fetal compromise.

514 / *Diagnostic Ultrasonography II*

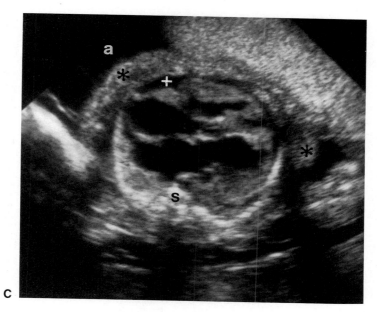

Figure 17-4 (Continued)

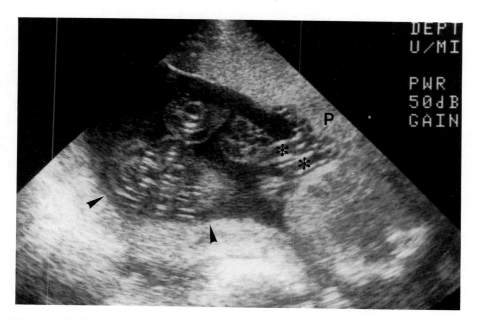

Figure 17-5. Monoamniotic, monochorionic gestation. Two umbilical cords (✳) can be seen arising side by side from the placenta (P). The cords are free to intermingle within the single amniotic cavity (arrowheads). No intervening membrane is seen, although scanning in multiple planes and from different orientations is necessary to exclude a very thin membrane.

Question 74

Concerning twin-twin transfusion syndrome,

    (A) the most common sonographic sign is a discrepancy in amniotic fluid volume between gestational sacs

    (B) all monozygotic twins are at risk of developing it

    (C) percutaneous umbilical blood sampling is useful in differentiating it from other causes of a "stuck twin"

    (D) multiorgan vascular insults occur in both donor and recipient twins

The transplacental shunting of blood in TTTS results in anemia, hypovolemia, and reduced urine output in the donor and in polycythemia, hypervolemia, and increased urine output in the recipient. If these changes are of a significant magnitude, oligohydramnios will result around the donor twin, with severe cases resulting in a stuck twin appearance, and polyhydramnios, often marked, will develop in the recipient sac. Sonographically, abnormal fluid volume is the most consistently detected finding that suggests the presence of TTTS in essentially all subsequently proven cases **(Option (A) is true).** In most cases, oligohydramnios and polyhydramnios will coexist in the same twin gestation (Figure 17-6). The acute development of polyhydramnios in a twin gestation is particularly suspicious for TTTS. In some instances, abnormal fluid volumes will be the earliest findings, predating significant growth discrepancies. Discrepancy in fetal size, manifested as a difference of at least 25% in estimated fetal weight or 18 mm in abdominal circumference, is somewhat less frequently detected sonographically but is also critical to confirming the final pathologic diagnosis.

TTTS can occur only when blood is shunted from one twin to the other through vascular communications in a single placenta, which occurs only with monochorionic gestations. All dizygotic twins have separate placentas, are dichorionic, and are therefore not at risk. Monozygotic pregnancies have different chorionicity and amnionicity, however, depending on the timing of blastomere cleavage. Early cleavage in one-third of monozygotic pregnancies results in a dichorionic gestation similar to dizygotic gestations, which is therefore not at risk for TTTS. Later cleavage results in a monochorionic gestation in all cases and a diamniotic gestation in nearly 99% of cases. About two-thirds of monozygotic gestations are monochorionic and are therefore at risk for developing TTTS **(Option (B) is false).** Vascular communications occur across essentially all monochorionic placentas (98%) but are seen only rarely (1.5%) in dichorionic, fused placentas. For all practical purposes, TTTS can be presumed to be a phenomenon of monochorionic and not dichorionic twins. Vascular communications can be superficial, deep, or both.

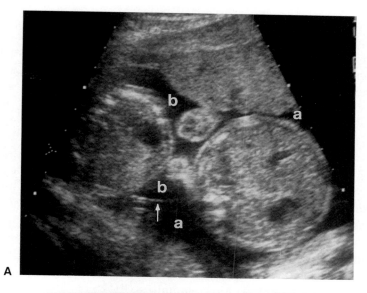

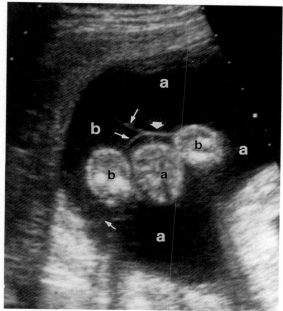

Figure 17-6. Twin-twin transfusion syndrome without "stuck twin." (A) A sonogram showing a transverse image of both fetal abdomens confirms an obvious growth discrepancy. A thin, monochorionic membrane (arrow) separates sacs a and b, with fluid clearly still apparent around fetus B. (B) Marked polyhydramnios is apparent in sac a (white a), as is an extremity of fetus A (black a). Sac b (white b) is clearly oligohydramniotic, but that twin is not yet stuck to the side wall. The monochorionic membrane is thin (thin arrows) where it is a single thickness and appears thicker (thick arrow) where a double layer is apposed because an extremity (black b) is trapped. A monochorionic membrane is most readily imaged when it lies perpendicular to the sound beam.

Superficial communications are most often artery to artery, vein to vein, or artery to vein, as well as combinations of the above. Such superficial anastomoses permit blood to shift in response to pressure and volume changes, allowing fluxes that typically do not by themselves result in TTTS. The deep communications most frequently involve an arteriovenous shunt through one or more cotyledons that are supplied by an artery of one twin but drained by a vein from the other twin. These vascular communications, if unbalanced by superficial connections, are believed to be most responsible for the development of TTTS. Clearly, not all monochorionic pregnancies develop TTTS. Most evolve normally. Some develop only mild cases. Depending on unknown factors, up to 5 to 30% of monochorionic gestations develop a significant transfusion. In some instances there may be a spontaneous improvement of a previously compromised pregnancy. Often, however, one or both twins will die *in utero* or shortly following birth.

Percutaneous umbilical blood sampling (PUBS) is a sonographically guided interventional procedure whereby a needle is introduced into the umbilical vein, usually in the cord close to the placenta, for the purpose of withdrawing fetal blood for laboratory evaluation. Hematocrit, platelet count, oxygen saturation, antibody levels to infectious or blood elements, and rapid karyotyping are some of the tests performed. When evaluating a stuck twin, PUBS can be used to assess fetal hemoglobin levels, with discrepant values necessary to establish the diagnosis of TTTS. Other causes of a stuck twin should not be associated with a difference in the fetal hematocrits **(Option (C) is true).** Fetal blood sampling can also confirm the diagnosis of TTTS when blood-grouping studies are performed on both fetuses. Theoretically, the severity of anemia in the donor could be assessed and a fetal blood transfusion performed. However, it is unclear how this would affect the already polycythemic recipient twin.

Anemia, hypovolemia, and hypotension all subject the donor twin to the risk of ischemic injury, whereas polycythemia, hypervolemia, and hypertension can result in hemorrhagic damage in the recipient **(Option (D) is true).** Intrauterine fetal death of either fetus can rapidly alter the existing pressure gradient across the vascular bed between the twins (Figure 17-3). A rapid transfusion from the high-pressure living twin to the low-pressure dead twin has been seen and may be the cause of ischemic damage in the living twin. Vascular insults in a surviving twin have also been postulated secondary to passage of thromboplastin-rich blood from a dead twin, with resultant thrombotic complications.

Question 75

Concerning intrauterine growth retardation,

(A) uteroplacental dysfunction accounts for 75% of fetuses that fall below the 10th-percentile weight for gestational age
(B) the sonographic diagnosis depends on an accurate estimation of gestational age
(C) the head-to-abdomen circumference ratio is useful for detecting "asymmetric" growth retardation
(D) the head-to-abdomen circumference ratio is age independent
(E) the femur length-to-abdomen circumference ratio is useful for detecting "symmetric" growth retardation
(F) the umbilical artery Doppler waveform shows increased diastolic flow

There is considerable variation in the criteria used by different investigators to define IUGR. Definitions range from a fetal weight below the 3rd percentile for gestational age to the more commonly used fetal weight below the 10th percentile for age. With all of the many suggested diagnostic methods, relatively poor sensitivity and specificity are noted. For instance, about 75% of fetuses with weight that falls below the 10th percentile for gestational age are merely small for gestational age, manifesting a limited yet intrinsically normal growth potential **(Option (A) is false)**. About 20% of fetuses that fall below the 10th-percentile-weight cutoff have growth retardation secondary to nonfetal etiologies, including maternal disease states, smoking, and malnutrition and placental insufficiency. Another 5% of fetuses in this group are small because of intrinsic fetal abnormality that may be due to a chromosomal abnormality, congenital anomaly, or an early *in utero* insult such as infection or teratogen exposure.

IUGR has been loosely classified as symmetric and asymmetric. With the latter, the abdominal size lags behind that of the head, presumably resulting in relative brain sparing at the expense of other organs and fat stores. In this circumstance, a growth disturbance is suggested by a discrepancy in the dating parameters. With symmetric IUGR, most often seen with the early and severe insults that cause intrinsic fetal abnormality, there is a reduction in all growth parameters. Without accurate knowledge of the gestational age, either by the date of last menstrual period or prior physical examination or by an early sonographic examination, a single sonographic examination on a fetus with symmetric IUGR cannot be appropriately interpreted. The growth parameters are equal, and so an incorrect, low "normal" gestational age could be assigned to a fetus that was in reality more advanced yet growth retarded **(Option (B) is true)**. All pregnancies at risk for IUGR should have accurate baseline dating provided by a sonographic examination as early as possible in the gestation.

The head-to-abdomen circumference ratio (HC:AC) has long been used as a predictor of IUGR. About 80% of cases of IUGR result from uteroplacental insufficiency, manifested primarily in the third trimester as reduced growth of the fetal abdomen. With asymmetric IUGR, head growth remains normal with relative brain sparing and the abdominal size becomes diminished as liver stores of glycogen and soft tissue fat are expended. In such cases, the HC:AC will be abnormally large for a given gestational age, suggesting the diagnosis **(Option (C) is true).** Appropriate use of the HC:AC does require knowledge of the true gestational age, however, because HC:AC is not independent of gestational age. There is differential growth of the head and abdomen, resulting in a declining ratio as pregnancy continues **(Option (D) is false).** At 16 weeks the HC:AC is about 1.2, the head being clearly larger than the abdomen. Abdominal growth slowly but surely outpaces head growth throughout the rest of pregnancy, with the HC:AC falling to 1.0 at about 36 weeks and below 1.0 as term is approached.

The femur length-to-abdominal circumference ratio (FL:AC) has a constant normal value of 0.20 to 0.24 (95% confidence interval) after 21 weeks gestational age. As an age-independent measure, the FL:AC can suggest small or large abdominal circumferences even if the precise gestational age is not known. This is in contradistinction to the HC:AC, for which the gestational age must be known. Elevation of the FL:AC beyond 0.235 (90th percentile) suggests a small fetal abdomen relative to the femur, a common finding with asymmetric growth retardation. Problems with the ratio, however, include relatively poor sensitivity and specificity for IUGR. In particular, symmetric IUGR is not detected by this ratio, since all fetal parameters are reduced equally and the ratio remains normal **(Option (E) is false).**

The umbilical artery Doppler waveform reflects blood flow from the fetus to the placenta during both fetal systole and diastole. As normal pregnancies progress, there is a decrease in placental vascular resistance as new arterial channels are formed within the villi. As a result, increased diastolic flow relative to systolic flow is apparent in the umbilical artery waveform. Such a low-resistance circuit within the placenta is critical to nutrient and oxygen delivery from mother to fetus, especially in the third trimester. Most IUGR is believed to be caused by uteroplacental insufficiency, which reduces blood flow to the fetus. This presumably arises from elevated placental vascular resistance, which may be caused by obliteration of small placental vessels or by unknown mechanisms. This leads directly to a reduction in diastolic flow within the

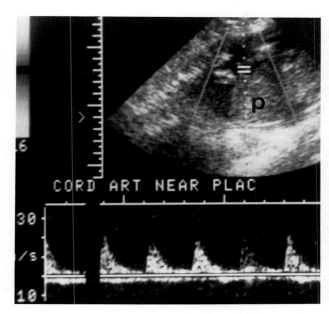

Figure 17-7. Intrauterine growth retardation with abnormal Doppler waveform. Sampling near the placenta (p) from a cord umbilical artery in a fetus with sonographic signs of IUGR shows a reduction in the diastolic flow relative to the systolic flow. Such findings suggest increased vascular resistance within the placenta, which has resulted in poor delivery of nutrients and oxygen to the fetus.

umbilical arteries, indicating reduced fetal to placental perfusion (Figure 17-7) **(Option (F) is false).**

Question 76

Concerning polyhydramnios,

(A) the most common fetal cause of severe polyhydramnios is a central nervous system abnormality

(B) when associated with fetal small bowel obstruction, the obstruction is usually proximal

(C) when present with intrauterine growth retardation, it suggests a congenital anomaly or chromosomal defect

(D) it is found in about 25% of patients with fetal hydrops

Polyhydramnios is diagnosed in about 0.5 to 3.5% of pregnancies. The volume of amniotic fluid increases until about 34 weeks gestation, at which time it gradually diminishes until term, with a wide variation at any particular gestational age. Strict criteria for a sonographic diagnosis of polyhydramnios have been difficult to derive because of the variability in normal fluid volume during pregnancy. Subjective evaluation is often used, with obvious limitations. An objective standard has been suggested by evaluation of the single largest amniotic fluid pocket, with a vertical pocket exceeding 8 cm considered positive. The amniotic fluid index (AFI) has gained popularity, being calculated as the sum of the measurements of the deepest vertical pocket of amniotic fluid in each quadrant of the gravid uterus. A normal AFI from 36 to 42 weeks is 12.9 ± 4.6 cm. Values have also been derived for earlier gestations and have proven useful in the diagnosis of both polyhydramnios and oligohydramnios.

Regardless of the basis for the diagnosis of polyhydramnios, however, the etiologies are multiple. It is idiopathic in 33 to 66% of cases, with major associations in other cases being maternal diabetes, fetal anomalies, and multiple gestations. The fetus plays a major role in amniotic fluid dynamics. Fluid is constantly swallowed and then absorbed in the fetal small bowel. Fetal urine is subsequently excreted into the amniotic fluid. Any break in this circuit will alter the amniotic fluid volume, often dramatically. With severe polyhydramnios, the organ systems most commonly involved, in order of frequency, are the central nervous system (CNS) **(Option (A) is true),** gastrointestinal tract, cardiovascular system, musculoskeletal system, and genitourinary tract. Presumed mechanisms for CNS-caused polyhydramnios include impaired swallowing and direct fluid transudation across exposed membranes. Obstruction of the gastrointestinal tract proximal to the level where significant amniotic fluid resorption has occurred will also result in polyhydramnios. This level is not strictly defined but definitely includes all obstructions at or above the proximal jejunum. More distal small bowel obstructions show variable degrees of polyhydramnios. Most gastrointestinal tract obstructions reported in cases of polyhydramnios involve the proximal gastrointestinal tract **(Option (B) is true),** including duodenal atresia, esophageal atresia, diaphragmatic hernia, and anterior wall defects.

IUGR is most often caused by conditions external to the fetus and is detected in the third trimester. Oligohydramnios is often a concomitant feature. A proposed mechanism for the development of IUGR-associated oligohydramnios is that chronic fetal hypoxia results in redistribution of fetal cardiac output away from the kidneys and to the fetal brain, resulting in reduced fetal urine output. An association of IUGR with polyhydramnios is distinctly unusual and suggests the presence of growth restriction due to an intrinsically abnormal fetus. A chromosomal abnormality, fetal anomaly, or severe early insult such as a congenital infection should be suspected in such a circumstance **(Option (C) is true).** IUGR related to intrinsic fetal abnormality also tends to occur at an unusually early gestational age.

Fetal hydrops results from both immune, i.e., rh isoimmunization, and nonimmune causes. Nonimmune causes now outnumber immune causes by a significant margin and include a multitude of etiologies.

Commonly seen features in fetuses with hydrops include ascites, pleural and pericardial effusions, and subcutaneous edema, in addition to any specific findings related to the underlying abnormality. Polyhydramnios is seen in about 50 to 75% of cases **(Option (D) is false)**. Presumed mechanisms for formation of polyhydramnios include high-output cardiac failure with excess urine production and low-output cardiac failure with both reduced lung resorption and general transudation of fluid from the compromised and edematous fetus (Figure 17-3).

Question 77

Concerning twin gestations,

(A) dizygotic pregnancies are always dichorionic
(B) about 10% of dichorionic/diamniotic twins are monozygotic
(C) with monoamniotic twinning, the fetal mortality is about 20%
(D) in most cases, the demise of one twin in the first trimester has no untoward effects on the surviving twin
(E) overall, they are associated with a threefold-greater frequency of fetal anomalies than are singleton pregnancies

Each zygote will at a minimum result in one placenta, one chorion, and one amnion. Therefore, a dizygotic twin gestation will always have two separate placentas, each with its own amnion and chorion **(Option (A) is true)**. A dizygotic pregnancy can result in more than two embryos, of course, if there is further cleavage of one or both zygotes. This could result in several different patterns of chorionicity, amnionicity, and number of placentas, depending on the number of cleavages and embryos that result. These possibilities are rare, however, and are excluded in the test case, which involves a twin gestation.

The rate of monozygotic twinning is fairly stable among different world populations, but considerable variability exists in the frequency of dizygotic twinning. As a general guide, about two-thirds of twins are dizygotic, becoming dichorionic/diamniotic pregnancies. The remaining one-third of twins are monozygotic, with variable chorionicity and amnionicity based on the timing of separation of the developing zygote. In about one-third of these, division of the blastomere within the first 3 days results in complete duplication with two placentas, which may be separate or fused, and dichorionic/diamniotic membranes. Such dichorionic, monozygotic gestations, which account for about 11% of all twins **(Option (B) is true)**, cannot be differentiated sonographically from dizygotic twins. Most of the remaining two-thirds of monozygotic gestations divide between days 3 and 8, resulting in a single placenta and

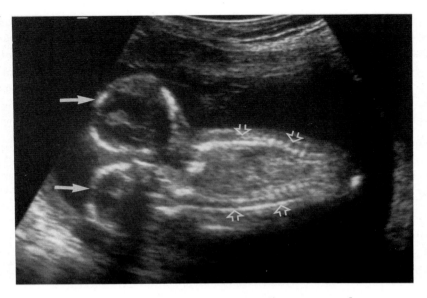

Figure 17-8. Conjoined twins. A longitudinal sonogram shows separate heads (solid arrows) but fusion of the soft tissues of the fetal bodies from the upper thorax to the sacrum. Entire separate spines are noted (open arrows).

monochorionic/diamniotic membranes; this occurs in about 21% of all twins. In fewer than 1% of twins, late division of the blastomere (between days 8 and 13) leads to a single amniotic cavity with monochorionic/monoamniotic membranes. The latest possible, and exceedingly rare, division of a monozygotic gestation involves the inner cell mass, or embryonic disc, which, when split between days 13 and 15, will result in conjoined twins within a monoamniotic/monochorionic sac (Figure 17-8).

Monoamniotic twinning is rare, occurring in less than 1% of all twin gestations. The presence of both twins within a single sac leads to increased risks beyond those of both singletons and twins in general. All monozygotic twins have an increased risk of fetal anomalies, and the subset of monochorionic gestations are at risk for TTTS and its complications. Added to these significant risk factors are complications peculiar to monoamniotic pregnancies. Conjoined twins occur only in monoamniotic pregnancies. The major contributing factor to fetal morbidity, though, is the potential for cord-related accidents involving one or both fetuses. The combined risk of fetal mortality in this population is about 50% **(Option (C) is false).**

Many more twin gestations are diagnosed in the first trimester than come to delivery. The term "vanishing twin" has been applied to such fetal loss. Early estimates suggested the occurrence of this phenomenon in 13 to 78% of cases, although certainly fluid collections not representative of a true gestational sac were included in some of these cases. Twin gestation should not be diagnosed without the benefit of detecting fetal structures in duplicate, preferably two heartbeats or potentially two clearly separate yolk sacs. With stricter criteria, the incidence of a vanishing twin has been adjusted to 21%. The term vanishing twin refers to the apparent resorption of the early embryo and sac. In the first trimester, the survival rate for the remaining twin generally parallels that for singleton gestations of the same age **(Option (D) is true).** Prior to the development of fetal bones, the entire embryo and sac tend to resorb. When osseous structures have formed in the late first trimester, fetal demise may not result in complete resorption of fetal tissue, which instead becomes shrunken and compressed as the amniotic fluid is resorbed around it. This process often results in a fetus papyraceus, wherein residual fetal parts are "mummified" (Figure 17-9). Careful examination at delivery sometimes reveals a firm residual mass of tissue, containing identifiable fetal osseous parts, attached to the membranes of the surviving twin. In contrast, with demise of a twin in the second or third trimester, disseminated intravascular coagulation resulting from release of thromboplastic substances from the dead twin can result in organ damage within the survivor. Such a pathologic process tends to occur in monochorionic gestations, which represent about 21% of all twin gestations, in which vascular communications exist between the fetal circulations.

About 1% of singleton fetuses have a fetal anomaly. Twin gestations are associated with a threefold increase in malformations over singleton pregnancies **(Option (E) is true).** The increased rate of fetal malformations in twins is for monozygotic, not dizygotic, pregnancies. A significant increase in neural tube and cardiac defects has been documented in twins, but anomalies of any organ system in a singleton pregnancy can also be seen with twins (Figure 17-3). Certain malformations are, however, also unique to monozygotic twins. With an acardiac monster, a grotesquely anomalous fetus is perfused, via placental anastomoses, from the normal "pump" twin, which is eventually at risk for developing congestive failure. Rarely, conjoined twins, which occur only in monoamniotic gestations, are seen (Figure 17-8). Union at the chest is most common, often extending to include the abdomen as well. Involvement of the pelvis and cranium is less frequent.

Richard A. Bowerman, M.D.

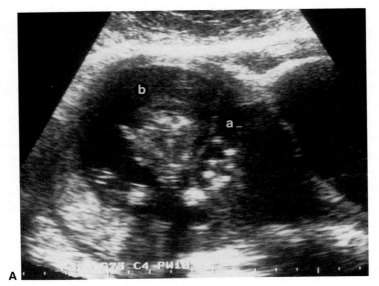

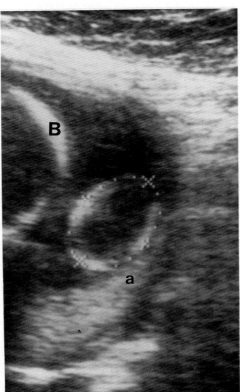

Figure 17-9. Intrauterine twin demise with fetus papyraceus. (A) A longitudinal sonogram shows a normal fetus in sac b. Oligohydramnios and a nonliving fetus were present in sac a. (B) Within sac a, the head circumference of fetus A is seen to be small but still ovoid. B = calvarium of fetus B. (C) A scan 5 weeks later confirmed continued growth of fetus B. Fetus A is now compressed against the anterior uterine wall, with only the deformed skull (solid arrowhead) and spine (open arrowheads) seen. At delivery, a small firm mass adherent to the membranes and containing fetal osseous structures was recovered. B = calvarium of fetus B.

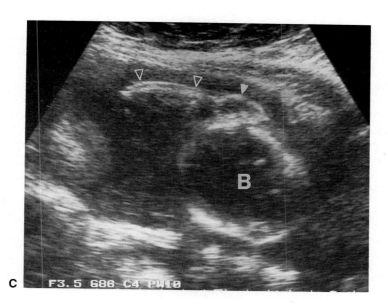

C   F3. 5 G86 C4 PW10

SUGGESTED READINGS

TWIN-TWIN TRANSFUSION SYNDROME

1. Aherne W, Strong SJ, Corney G. The structure of the placenta in the twin transfusion syndrome. Biol Neonat 1968; 12:121–135
2. Arts NFT, Lohman AHM. The vascular anatomy of monochorionic diamniotic twin placentas and the transfusion syndrome. Eur J Obstet Gynecol 1971; 1:85–93
3. Blickstein I. The twin-twin transfusion syndrome. Obstet Gynecol 1990; 76: 714–722
4. Brown DL, Benson CB, Driscoll SG, Doubilet PM. Twin-twin transfusion syndrome: sonographic findings. Radiology 1989; 170:61–63
5. Caballero P, Del Campo L, Ocon E. Cystic encephalomalacia in twin embolization syndrome. Radiology 1991; 178:892–893
6. De Lia J, Cruikshank DP, Keye WR Jr. Fetoscopic neodymium:YAG laser occlusion of placental vessels in severe twin-twin transfusion syndrome. Obstet Gynecol 1990; 75:1046–1053
7. Elliot JP, Urig MA, Clewell WH. Aggressive therapeutic amniocentesis for treatment of twin-twin transfusion syndrome. Obstet Gynecol 1991; 77: 537–540
8. Fusi L, McFarland P, Fisk N, Nicolini U, Wigglesworth J. Acute twin-twin transfusions: a possible mechanism for brain-damaged survivors after intrauterine death of a monochorionic twin. Obstet Gynecol 1991; 78: 517–520
9. Hurst RW, Abbitt PL. Fetal intracranial hemorrhage and periventricular leukomalacia: complications of twin-twin transfusion. AJNR 1989; 10: S62–S63

10. Mahony BS, Petty CN, Nyberg DA, Luthy DA, Hickok DE, Hirsch JH. The "stuck twin" phenomenon: ultrasonographic findings, pregnancy outcome, and management with serial amniocenteses. Am J Obstet Gynecol 1990; 163:1513–1522

11. Patten RM, Mack LA, Nyberg DA, Filly RA. Twin embolization syndrome: prenatal sonographic detection and significance. Radiology 1989; 173:685–689

12. Rausen AR, Seki M, Strauss L. Twin transfusion syndrome. J Pediatr 1965; 66:613–628

13. Szymonowicz W, Preston H, Yu VY. The surviving monozygotic twin. Arch Dis Child 1986; 61:454–458

14. Wieacker P, Wilhelm C, Prömpeler H, Petersen KG, Schillinger H, Breckwoldt M. Pathophysiology of polyhydramnios in twin transfusion syndrome. Fetal Diagn Ther 1992; 7:87–92

INTRAUTERINE GROWTH RETARDATION

15. Benson CB, Doubilet PM. Doppler criteria for intrauterine growth retardation: predictive values. J Ultrasound Med 1988; 7:655–659

16. Benson CB, Doubilet PM, Saltzman DH, Jones TB. FL/AC ratio: poor predictor of intrauterine growth retardation. Invest Radiol 1985; 20:727–730

17. Bruinse HW, Sijmons EA, Reuwer PJ. Clinical value of screening for fetal growth retardation by Doppler ultrasound. J Ultrasound Med 1989; 8:207–209

18. Campbell S, Thoms A. Ultrasound measurement of the fetal head to abdomen circumference ratio in the assessment of growth retardation. Br J Obstet Gynaecol 1977; 84:165–174

19. Giles WB, Trudinger BJ, Baird PJ. Fetal umbilical artery flow velocity waveforms and placental resistance: pathologic correlation. Br J Obstet Gynaecol 1985; 92:31–38

20. Hadlock FP, Deter RL, Harrist RB, Roecker E, Park SK. A date-independent predictor of intrauterine growth retardation: femur length/abdominal circumference ratio. AJR 1983; 141:979–984

21. Hadlock FP, Deter RL, Rossavik IK. Detection of abnormal fetal growth patterns: intrauterine growth retardation and macrosomia. In: Athey PA, Hadlock FP (eds), Ultrasound in obstetrics and gynecology. St. Louis: CV Mosby; 1985:38–59

22. Manning FA, Hohler C. Intrauterine growth retardation: diagnosis, prognostication, and management based on ultrasound methods. In: Fleischer AC, Romero R, Manning FA, Jeanty P, James AE (eds), The principles and practice of ultrasound in obstetrics and gynecology. Norwalk, CT: Appleton & Lange; 1991:331–347

POLYHYDRAMNIOS

23. Moore TR. Superiority of the four-quadrant sum over the single-deepest-pocket technique in ultrasonographic identification of abnormal amniotic fluid volumes. Am J Obstet Gynecol 1990; 163:762–767

24. Moore TR, Cayle JE. The amniotic fluid index in normal human pregnancy. Am J Obstet Gynecol 1990; 162:1168–1173

25. Phelan JP, Smith CV, Broussard P, Small M. Amniotic fluid volume assessment with the four-quadrant technique at 36–42 weeks' gestation. J Reprod Med 1987; 32:540–542

TWINS—GENERAL

26. Anderson RL, Golbus MS, Curry CJ, Callen PW, Hastrup WH. Central nervous system damage and other anomalies in surviving fetus following second trimester antenatal death of co-twin. Report of four cases and literature review. Prenat Diagn 1990; 10:513–518

27. Barss VA, Benacerraf BR, Frigoletto FD Jr. Ultrasonographic determination of chorion type in twin gestation. Obstet Gynecol 1985; 66:779–783

28. Benirschke K, Kaufman P. Pathology of the human placenta. New York: Springer-Verlag; 1990:636–753

29. Benson CB, Doubilet PM. Ultrasound of multiple gestations. Semin Roentgenol 1991; 26:50–62

30. Coleman BG, Grumbach K, Arger PH, et al. Twin gestations: monitoring of complications and anomalies with US. Radiology 1987; 165:449–453

31. D'Alton ME, Dudley DK. The ultrasonographic prediction of chorionicity in twin gestation. Am J Obstet Gynecol 1989; 160:557–561

32. Landy HJ, Weiner S, Corson SL, Batzer FR, Bolognese RJ. The "vanishing twin": ultrasonographic assessment of fetal disappearance in the first trimester. Am J Obstet Gynecol 1986; 155:14–19

33. Schinzel AA, Smith DW, Miller JR. Monozygotic twinning and structural defects. J Pediatr 1979; 95:921–930

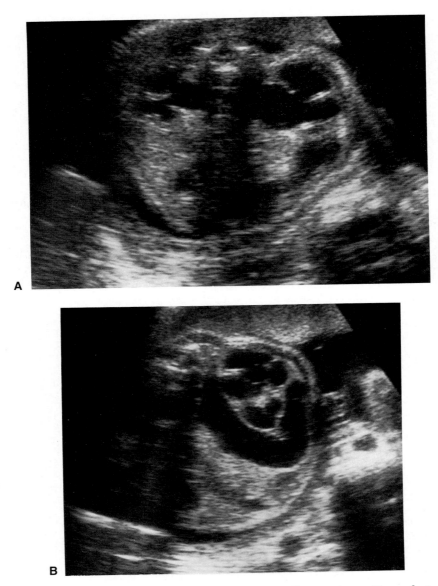

Figure 18-1. This 25-year-old woman underwent routine obstetric sonography at 28 weeks gestation. You are shown transverse images of the fetal upper abdomen (A) and mid-abdomen (B) and a longitudinal image of the fetal trunk (C).

Case 18: Obstructed Duplex Kidney

Question 78

Which *one* of the following is the MOST likely diagnosis?

(A) Duplication anomaly with obstruction
(B) Prune belly syndrome
(C) Multicystic renal dysplasia
(D) Posterior urethral valves
(E) Autosomal recessive polycystic disease

The transverse sonogram of the fetal upper abdomen (Figure 18-1A) shows bilateral hydronephrosis, greater on the left than on the right (Figure 18-2). On the mid-abdominal sonogram (Figure 18-1B), a prominent, tubular, fluid-filled structure is seen extending around the hydronephrotic kidney. The longitudinal image (Figure 18-1C) shows the heart within the fetal thorax, the abdomen containing the stomach, and the bladder inferiorly in the pelvis. Within the bladder is a prominent, curvilinear structure, contiguous with the bladder wall inferiorly in the trigonal region. This combination of findings is consistent with a duplex left collecting system with marked hydroureteronephrosis of the left upper pole system, secondary to ectopic distal ureteral insertion with a ureterocele **(Option (A) is correct).** Duplication can be partial or complete. Partial duplication is generally of no consequence, since fusion of the partially split upper tract occurs proximally to a single ureter inserting normally into the bladder. No increased incidence of obstruction, incontinence, or ascending infection will occur. With complete duplication there are two separate ureters, with the one from the upper pole inserting ectopically. Embryologically, the ureter is formed from the ureteric bud, which starts as an outgrowth from the mesonephric duct, or primitive kidney. The mesonephric duct, together with the primitive digestive tract, enters the cloaca in close proximity to other developing pelvic organs. Abnormal splitting or migration of the ureteric bud, as occurs with a duplication anomaly, leads most often to aberrant ureteral insertion into the bladder, at a site more distal and more medial than usual

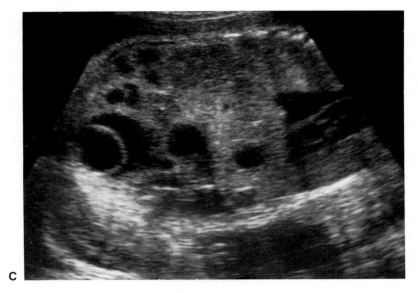

C

Figure 18-1 (Continued)

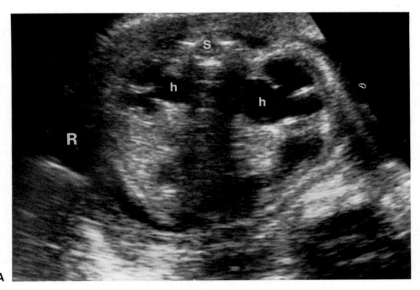

A

Figure 18-2 (Same as Figure 18-1).   Obstructed duplication anomaly in a fetus at 28 weeks gestation. (A) A transverse image through the upper abdomen shows bilateral hydronephrosis (h), greater on the left than on the right (R). The dilated left system is the upper-pole moiety. S = spine. (B) A transverse image lower in the abdomen shows dilatation of the left lower pole collecting system (h) and a markedly dilated and somewhat tortuous left upper pole ureter (u). S = spine; R = right. (C) A coronal image of the fetus shows the bladder (b) deep in the pelvis, with an internal curved structure representing the wall of a urine-distended ectopic ureterocele (u). S = stomach; H = heart. Note portions of tortuous, dilated left upper pole ureter seen in transverse section between the stomach and bladder.

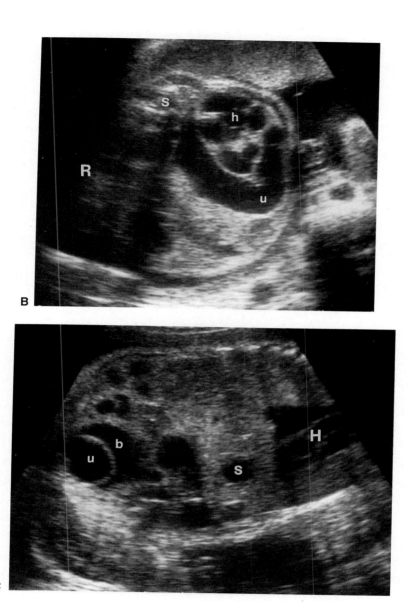

(Wiegert-Meyer rule). Other sites of ectopic insertion include the proximal or distal urethra in either sex; the vestibule, uterus, or vagina in a female; and the seminal vesicle or vas deferens in a male. With distal obstruction secondary to a ureterocele, pronounced dilatation of the upper-pole intrarenal collecting system will occur (Figure 18-3A). The ureter becomes similarly dilated and can become very tortuous, even

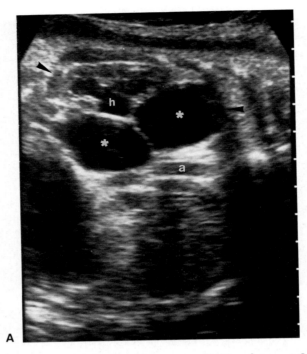

Figure 18-3. Obstructed duplication anomaly in a fetus at 30 weeks. (A) A longitudinal sonogram of the left kidney (arrowheads) in a fetus with a duplex system shows marked dilatation of the upper-pole collecting system and pelvis (asterisks), and mild dilatation of the lower-pole collecting system (h). a = aorta. (B) A transverse image of the mid-abdomen shows the dilated left ureter extending all the way to the right (R) abdominal wall before passing to the pelvis. i = iliac crest; L = liver. (C) A longitudinal scan of the pelvis shows ectopic ureterocele (u) distended with urine and seen as a filling defect in the bladder (b). T = thigh.

extending well across the midline (Figure 18-3B). The lower-pole moiety is often dilated, as in the test case, as a result of reflux from distortion of its ureteral orifice into the bladder by the ectopically inserted ureter (Figure 18-3A). As noted in the test case, an ectopic ureterocele occasionally enlarges and dissects submucosally such that the opposite trigone is affected, causing obstruction or reflux of the contralateral kidney.

Prune belly syndrome (Option (B)), also known as the Eagle-Barrett syndrome, is characterized by dilatation of the urinary tract, essentially absent musculature of the abdominal wall, and, in male patients, undescended testes. The most notable urinary tract finding is megacystis, with variable degrees of hydroureter and hydronephrosis (Figure 18-4). No intraluminal filling defect is present in the bladder. These features do

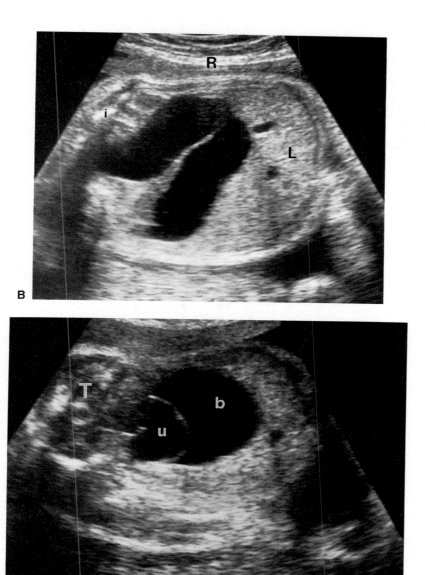

not match those of the test case. The markedly thinned abdominal wall in prune belly syndrome contains little or no residual muscle. The etiology of these findings is unknown. Classic teaching suggests an intrinsic abnormality of the musculature of the affected structures. However, recent work suggests that early *in utero* distension of the abdominal wall destroys the developing musculature. Such distension could arise from outlet obstruction of the fetal bladder or from marked ascites of any

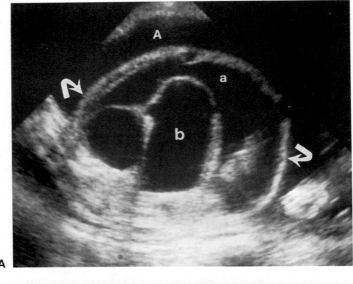

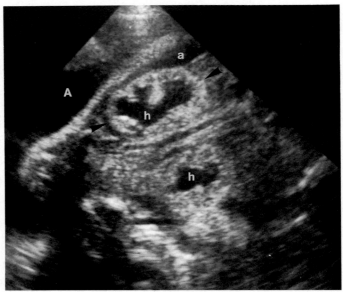

Figure 18-4. Prune belly syndrome in a fetus at 26 weeks. (A) A transverse image of the fetal abdomen just above the umbilicus reveals a large bladder (b) and ascites (a), which has distended the fetal abdomen (arrows), with an abdominal circumference measurement appropriate for 39 weeks. The volume of amniotic fluid (A) is increased. (B) A longitudinal image of the fetal abdomen nicely delineates the echogenic right kidney (arrowheads) and bilateral hydronephrosis (h). Ascites (a) and amniotic fluid (A) are noted. Following delivery, typical abdominal features of prune belly syndrome were noted, and no urethral obstruction was delineated. High-output renal failure with no evidence of renal concentrating ability was observed, with gradual improvement in function over the first week of life. Presumably this case represents a relieved bladder outlet obstruction that had caused dilatation of the bladder and upper tracts with enough renal damage to result in high-output failure and polyhydramnios. However, relief of the obstruction, perhaps both at the urethral level and by the development of urine ascites, prevented irreversible renal damage.

cause. In the former circumstance, residual findings of urinary tract dilatation could also be explained. However, at birth, most neonates with the thin, redundant abdominal wall typical of prune belly syndrome have no outlet obstruction. Perhaps in these cases the obstruction was relieved *in utero*, in contrast to those with continued obstruction or ascites that manifest thinning of the abdominal wall and continued marked distension by the ascites or due to a dilated bladder. Only in cases associated with outlet obstruction would oligohydramnios be expected.

Sonographically, a multicystic dysplastic kidney (Potter type II) (Option (C)) will contain multiple cysts of various sizes that are not connected but replace essentially all renal parenchyma (Figure 18-5). The kidney can be large, normal sized, or, occasionally, small. These features differ from those in the test case. There are two theories about the formation of multicystic dysplastic kidney. Embryologically, the ureteric bud develops into the ureter, renal pelvis, calyces, and collecting tubules and induces development of the renal parenchyma from the metanephric blastema. According to the first theory, failure of the ureteric bud to form properly or induce renal development results in a totally nonfunctional kidney, composed of multiple cysts with no parenchyma and lacking a renal pelvis. The second theory indicates that, with partial or late failure of the inductive process, minimal early development of the kidney can occur but inadequate connections between the developing collecting system and kidney lead to obstruction and secondary cystic dysplasia. Segmental multicystic dysplastic kidney, created by the same mechanisms, has also been reported in association with a duplex kidney. Multicystic dysplastic kidney is usually a unilateral process with normal fluid volume and a good prognosis. However, bilateral multicystic dysplastic kidney is uniformly fatal because of the nonfunctional status of the affected kidneys. Contralateral renal anomalies are present in 20 to 40% of fetuses with multicystic dysplastic kidney; these include renal agenesis, ureteropelvic junction (UPJ) obstruction, and multicystic dysplastic kidney. Amniotic fluid volume depends on the status of the contralateral kidney.

Posterior urethral valves (Option (D)) obstruct the prostatic urethra in the male fetus, resulting in a dilated proximal urethra and bladder (Figure 18-6). The degree of bladder outlet obstruction can vary, and this is reflected in the sonographic features associated with valves. About half of the affected fetuses have sonographically evident hydroureteronephrosis of some degree, secondary to reflux or obstruction. In some cases the kidneys are small or echogenic or contain cysts, all of which are signs suggesting cystic renal dysplasia (Figure 18-6C). Cystic renal dysplasia (Potter type IV) occurs secondary to an *in utero* obstruction, resulting in reduced or absent renal function depending on the severity of the dys-

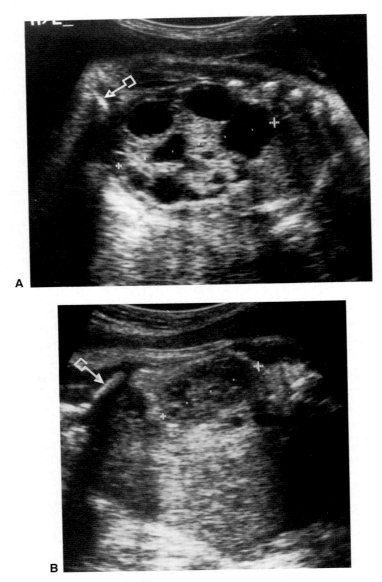

Figure 18-5. Multicystic dysplastic kidney (Potter type II) in a fetus at 32 weeks. (A) A longitudinal sonogram shows an enlarged (5.8-cm) left kidney containing multiple noncommunicating cystic structures of various sizes (+ calipers), typical for multicystic dysplastic kidney. Intervening echogenic tissue is also dysplastic pathologically. Typically, no functional renal tissue will be present (one exception being segmental multicystic dysplastic changes in the upper pole of a duplicated kidney). (B) Normal, 4.0-cm right kidney for comparison, imaged on the same scale as in panel A. Iliac crest is indicated by an arrow.

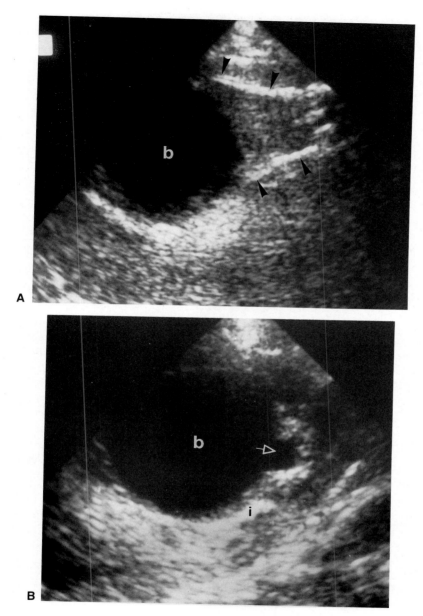

Figure 18-6. Posterior urethral valves in a fetus at 15 weeks. (A) A longitudinal scan through the fetus shows a huge abdominopelvic fluid structure consistent with a dilated bladder (b). The mass impinges on the thorax and splays the ribs (arrowheads). Note the complete lack of amniotic fluid. (B) A longitudinal scan of the distended bladder (b) shows the dilated proximal urethra extending from the trigonal region (arrow), sometimes termed the keyhole deformity. This sign is not specific for posterior urethral valves but can be seen with any entity that obstructs the urethra or causes megacystis. i = iliac crest.

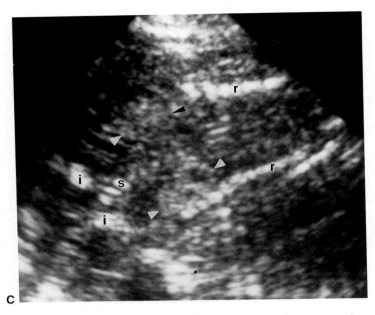

C

Figure 18-6 (Continued). Posterior urethral valves in a fetus at 15 weeks. (C) A longitudinal image shows the fetal kidneys (arrowheads) to be abnormally echogenic. One of the kidneys contains cystic changes. The development of small, echogenic, and particularly cystic changes in the kidneys of fetuses with bladder outlet obstruction is suggestive of irreversible renal dysplasia (Potter type IV). r = ribs; s = spine; i = iliac crests.

plastic changes. Moderate to severe oligohydramnios is present in over 50% of cases. Urine ascites can develop from transudation across a dilated bladder wall, frank rupture of the bladder, or unknown mechanisms. Any affected fetus is at risk for development of pulmonary hypoplasia secondary to oligohydramnios, urine ascites, or marked megacystis (Figure 18-6A). The features of posterior urethral valves, particularly megacystis without filling defect, are not present in the test case. Bladder outlet obstruction can also be caused by a urethral stricture, urethral agenesis, and a persistent cloaca. The findings in fetuses with a stricture can be identical to those in fetuses with valves. In fetuses with urethral atresia and sometimes in those with cloacal persistence, there is complete bladder outlet obstruction, leading to massive megacystis, severe oligohydramnios, variable but severe upper tract findings, and pulmonary hypoplasia. These features are incompatible with survival. Prune belly syndrome, described above, can have similar sonographic features and is probably etiologically related to frank outlet obstruction in most cases.

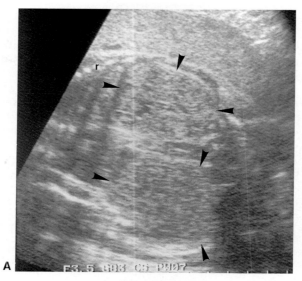

Figure 18-7. Autosomal recessive polycystic disease (Potter type I) in a fetus at 28 weeks. (A) An angled coronal sonogram of the upper abdomen shows bilateral, markedly enlarged, and moderately echogenic kidneys (arrowheads). r = ribs. Marked oligohydramnios is present.

The typical sonographic features of prenatally detected autosomal recessive (infantile) polycystic disease (Potter type I) (Option (E)) are bilateral, markedly enlarged, and echogenic kidneys, associated with oligohydramnios and a small bladder (Figure 18-7). These features are quite different from those in the test case. The abnormal renal enlargement and echogenicity arise from a proliferation and dilatation of renal tubules, creating a multiplicity of sonic interfaces. The cystic tubules are usually too small to resolve as discrete cysts. Affected fetuses usually develop severe pulmonary hypoplasia secondary to oligohydramnios and impingement of the huge kidneys on the thorax. The antenatal diagnosis of autosomal recessive polycystic disease has been made as early as 17 weeks. Some fetuses with autosomal recessive polycystic disease have less-severe or later-onset renal involvement, however, and typical prenatal sonographic features may be absent or less obvious or may appear later in gestation in these cases.

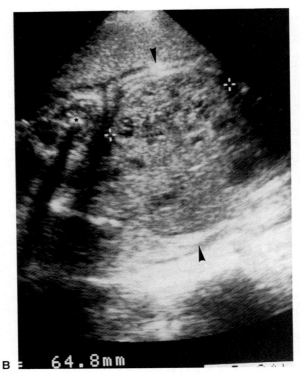

B 64.8mm

Figure 18-7 (Continued). Autosomal recessive polycystic disease (Potter type I) in a fetus at 28 weeks. (B) A longitudinal image of one kidney (+ calipers) confirms enlargement (6.5 cm) and echogenic texture. Several sonolucent areas are consistent with small cysts. Usually the kidneys are large and echogenic, as a result of the multitude of dilated, small collecting tubules creating many echo-reflective interfaces. Occasionally cysts large enough to resolve are seen. Arrowheads indicate abdominal wall, and the asterisk indicates a femur.

Question 79

Concerning fetal hydronephrosis,

(A) in the second trimester, the normal renal pelvis measures no more than 5 mm in its anteroposterior dimension
(B) ureteropelvic junction obstruction is associated with polyhydramnios
(C) fetal interventional therapy for posterior urethral valves should be considered if the amniotic fluid volume is normal
(D) ureteropelvic junction obstruction is bilateral in about 20% of cases
(E) decompression of the obstruction with formation of urine ascites is a favorable prognostic sign

The normal fetal intrarenal collecting system often contains a small amount of urine, even in the second trimester (Figure 18-8). Hydronephrosis manifests as a dilated renal pelvis, whether secondary to obstruction of the urethra, distal ureter, or UPJ. Some overlap clearly exists between the sonographic appearance of the normal and obstructed

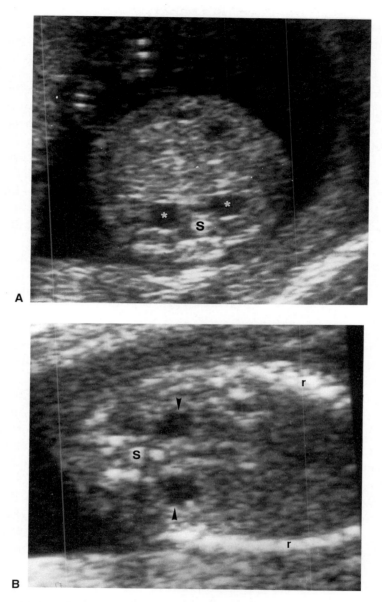

Figure 18-8. Physiologic prominence of the renal pelvis in a fetus at 17 weeks. Transverse (A) and coronal (B) images through the kidneys show bilaterally prominent renal pelves (asterisks, arrowheads) measuring 5 mm in anteroposterior diameter. The fluid-filled pelves are well seen because of their inherent subject contrast with surrounding structures, but the renal parenchyma is poorly visualized. S = spine; r = ribs. Follow-up fetal sonograms showed no progression in renal pelvis size, and post-natal evaluation revealed no obstruction or reflux.

renal pelvis. Criteria have been proposed for the normal anteroposterior dimension of the renal pelvis, with false-positive and false-negative rates determined by the cutoff value. Early work suggested that reasonable standards for maximum normal dimensions were 5 mm in the second trimester **(Option (A) is true)** and 10 mm in the third trimester. Such standards appear to detect most significant dilatations, but strict statistical analysis has not been applied. More rigorous recent work concluded that to avoid any false-negative diagnoses, since hydronephrosis may have significant morbidity if missed, the normal anteroposterior renal pelvis measurement should be below 4 mm for gestational ages up to 33 weeks and below 7 mm beyond that point. This approach of course yields a high false-positive rate, from about 21% beyond 33 weeks to as high as 55% below 23 weeks. Increased sensitivity for the detection of obstruction can be derived by the detection of calyceal distension in addition to that of the renal pelvis alone.

Oligohydramnios is classically associated with severe genitourinary tract anomalies that either result in failure to produce urine or obstruct its passage from the fetus. Paradoxically, both unilateral and bilateral UPJ obstruction can be associated with increased amniotic fluid volume (Figure 18-9) **(Option (B) is true)**. The mechanism for this is not known, but it may be based on a chronic or pronounced obstruction that damages the ability of the kidney(s) to concentrate urine, resulting in a high-output renal failure.

The degree of outlet obstruction and the resultant effect on the upper tracts are variable in fetuses with posterior urethral valves. Amniotic fluid volume should be monitored since it is an indicator of both renal function and the degree of obstruction. When amniotic fluid volume is in the normal range, it is presumed that adequate renal function and urine output are being maintained, and no interventional measures are indicated **(Option (C) is false)**. If the amniotic fluid volume is reduced, fetal renal function can be further evaluated to determine whether the fetus would benefit from interventional therapy. Such an evaluation includes a quantification of amniotic fluid volume, a sonographic assessment of the kidneys for signs of potentially irreversible renal dysplasia, and an evaluation of urine electrolytes and hourly fetal urine output. These tests are generally performed at centers experienced in fetal interventional techniques, since they require withdrawal of urine percutaneously from the fetal bladder. For fetuses thought to have adequate renal function, percutaneous placement of a vesicoamniotic shunt is an option.

Most UPJ obstructions are unilateral. The contralateral kidney should be examined, however, since there is a 10 to 30% frequency of bilateral UPJ obstruction **(Option (D) is true)**. Contralateral renal agenesis or multicystic dysplastic kidney also occurs, and oligohydram-

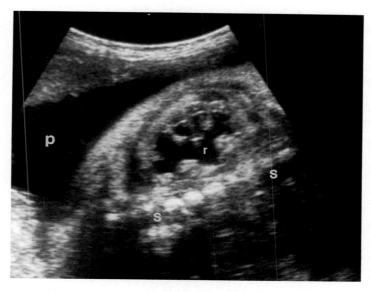

Figure 18-9. Ureteropelvic junction obstruction with polyhydramnios in a fetus at 31 weeks. A longitudinal image of the fetal kidney shows clear dilatation of the renal pelvis (r) and multiple calyces. A normal bladder was noted, and no ipsilateral ureter was detected, making the findings most consistent with a UPJ obstruction. s = spine. Moderate polyhydramnios (p) was present. Either unilateral or bilateral UPJ obstruction can be associated with polyhydramnios, presumably as a result of high-output renal insufficiency.

nios is possible in any of these circumstances when the UPJ obstruction is severe.

Urine ascites is seen in about 15% of fetuses with urethral obstruction. In about half of affected fetuses, no anatomic site of perforation can be determined. Ruptures at the level of the bladder or kidney are responsible for the remainder. When initial extravasation is extraperitoneal, as with a perirenal urinoma, subsequent transudation across an intact peritoneum, or a peritoneal tear, will allow for accumulation of urine acites. Early relief of renal obstruction might spare the kidneys from dysplastic changes, but other effects often portend a poor fetal outcome. Obstruction of this severity has generally resulted in oligohydramnios, which, if present and unrelieved from early in the second trimester, will lead to pulmonary hypoplasia and neonatal demise. Also, the accumulation of a large quantity of ascitic fluid itself impedes lung development **(Option (E) is false).** In most cases, urine ascites develops in the second trimester in association with urethral obstruction, but it occasionally evolves in the third trimester. In such cases, the late development of oligohydramnios and urine ascites postdates considerable lung development, and severe pulmonary hypoplasia would not be expected.

Question 80

Concerning fetal renal cystic disease,

- (A) cystic renal dysplasia is secondary to obstruction in 90% of cases
- (B) in fetuses with an obstructive uropathy, sonographic detection of renal cysts indicates irreversible cystic renal dysplasia (Potter type IV)
- (C) about 30% of fetuses with a multicystic dysplastic kidney have a significant contralateral renal anomaly
- (D) the kidneys in fetuses with autosomal recessive polycystic disease are both large and hypoechoic
- (E) about 30% of fetuses with trisomy 13 have renal cysts

Renal dysplasia, which is indicative of irreversible renal damage, arises from anomalous development of the kidney. About 90% of cases result from an early and severe urinary tract obstruction during induction of the metanephric blastema by the ureteric bud **(Option (A) is true).** The sonographic appearance of kidneys in fetuses with cystic renal dysplasia is quite varied (Figure 18-6C). They are often small but may be of normal size or even large. Such kidneys frequently demonstrate increased echogenicity, but this is not always the case. Additionally, other renal abnormalities can exhibit increased echotexture. Clearly, evaluation of renal echotexture is useful but is often not diagnostic for renal dysplasia. The presence of small cortical cysts in the setting of urinary tract obstruction, however, is considered essentially pathognomonic for the diagnosis **(Option (B) is true).** When the renal cysts are too small to detect sonographically, a definitive diagnosis is again not possible.

Contralateral renal anomalies, including renal agenesis, UPJ obstruction and multicystic dysplastic kidney, are present in 20 to 40% of fetuses with multicystic dysplastic kidney **(Option (C) is true).** Careful scanning of the contralateral renal fossa and evaluation of amniotic fluid volume should be performed. The amniotic fluid volume depends on the status of the contralateral kidney; oligohydramnios associated with some of the above-mentioned combinations will indicate a lethal outcome.

The classic sonographic feature of autosomal recessive polycystic disease is bilateral large, echogenic kidneys (Figure 18-7) **(Option (D) is false).** The cysts are actually dilated collecting tubules, which are too small to resolve sonographically as individual fluid-containing struc-

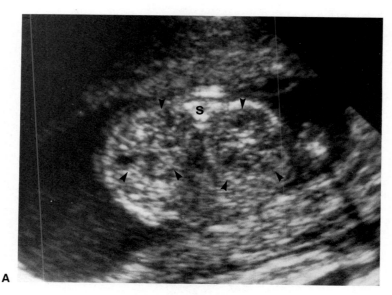

A

Figure 18-10. Meckel-Gruber syndrome in a fetus at 18 weeks. (A) A transverse image of the upper abdomen shows markedly enlarged and heterogeneous kidneys (arrowheads). Multiple small cysts can be identified. s = spine. The kidney circumference is normally about 27 to 30% of the abdominal circumference, a figure clearly exceeded here, where the ratio is about 0.44. Mild oligohydramnios is present.

tures. Instead, they appear echogenic because of the multiplicity of interfaces present. The kidney can be huge. Oligohydramnios is generally present. Neonatal morbidity is high, secondary to pulmonary hypoplasia and renal failure.

Fetal renal cysts are rarely seen, except in fetuses with the primary renal cystic dysplasias. Renal cysts do occur, however, in association with many rare syndromes, including tuberous sclerosis, Jeune's syndrome (asphyxiating thoracic dystrophy), and Zellweger (cerebro-hepato-renal) syndrome, and can potentially be detected *in utero*. Meckel-Gruber syndrome is a rare, lethal, autosomal recessive disorder with histologic features that closely resemble cystic renal dysplasia but are not related to obstruction (Figure 18-10). Large, echogenic kidneys with some evidence of cystic components are typical, along with oligohydramnios. The vast majority also have an encephalocele, and polydactyly is common. Renal cysts are also associated with trisomy 13 in over 30% of cases **(Option (E) is true)** and with trisomy 18 less frequently. Detection of renal cysts necessitates a thorough fetal survey for other anomalies that might be related to a chromosomal anomaly or other syndrome.

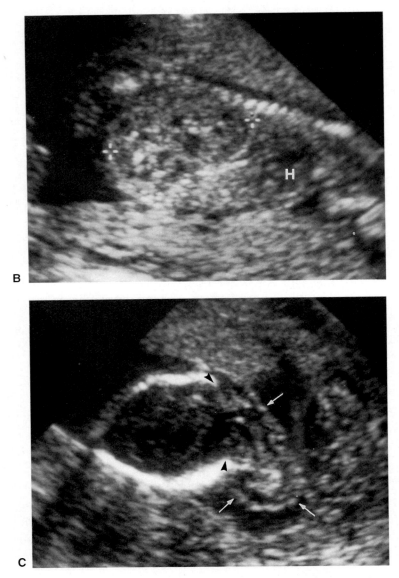

Figure 18-10 (Continued). Meckel-Gruber syndrome in a fetus at 18 weeks. (B) A longitudinal image confirms marked enlargement of the kidney (+ calipers) with multiple small cysts. H = heart. (C) A transverse image of the calvarium reveals a posterior osseous defect (arrowheads) with a large occipital encephalocele (arrows). The combination of cystic renal dysplasia and encephalocele suggests this syndrome, a rare lethal abnormality. Polydactyly is often also present and was suspected at real-time scanning and confirmed at autopsy. (Case courtesy of Murray Howe, M.D., The Toledo Hospital, Toledo, Ohio.)

Question 81

Concerning fetal renal sonography,

(A) the normal range of the ratio of kidney circumference to abdominal circumference is 0.38 to 0.42

(B) normal amniotic fluid volume at 14 weeks gestational age excludes bilateral renal agenesis

(C) a solid renal mass associated with polyhydramnios is most probably due to a congenital Wilms' tumor

(D) about 50% of fetuses with a single umbilical artery have a renal abnormality

Examination of the fetal kidneys is included in the American Institute of Ultrasound in Medicine guidelines for routine obstetric ultrasonography. The normal fetal kidneys are identified sonographically as paired hypoechoic paraspinal structures, normally first delineated between 15 and 18 weeks gestational age. Confirmation of normal renal size, usually performed subjectively, can be evaluated objectively with known standards for circumference, length, diameter, and volume.

Fetal renal sonography can readily detect many renal anomalies, including renal cystic dysplasias, renal agenesis, and obstruction. Abnormalities of renal size, echotexture, and size of the collecting system can all suggest a specific entity. Concomitant oligohydramnios indicates a significant reduction in fetal renal function or an obstruction to fetal urine excretion.

There are several ways to confirm normal renal size *in utero*. In one study, renal length ranged from 24 mm at 24 weeks gestational age to 38 mm at term. Renal length in millimeters roughly correlates with gestational age in weeks. A useful measurement is the ratio of the renal circumference to the abdominal circumference, which maintains a constant value of 0.27 to 0.30 throughout gestation **(Option (A) is false)**. Documentation of abnormal renal size may suggest significant renal abnormality.

Fetal kidneys begin urine production between 11 and 13 weeks gestational age. Before that time, amniotic fluid is formed entirely by transudation of maternal and fetal serum across the placenta and membranes and by other poorly understood mechanisms. The fetal contribution to the amniotic fluid gains significance with the development of increasing renal function; fetal urine production becomes the primary source of amniotic fluid from about 13 to 16 weeks until term. Even without any fetal urine production, the amniotic fluid volume may appear relatively normal until about 14 to 15 weeks, but beyond that point the loss of fluid without fetal replacement is marked by oligohydramnios **(Option (B) is false)**. Renal agenesis occurs when the ureteric bud fails to induce devel-

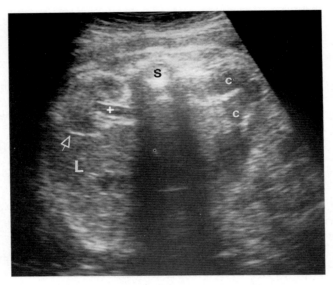

Figure 18-11. Unilateral renal agenesis. A transverse image through the renal beds reveals a normal-appearing right kidney (arrow), including the renal pelvis (+). L = liver; S = spine. No kidney was identified in the left renal fossa. Only a loop of colon (c) was present. Fluid volume is normal in this circumstance because the remaining kidney is functioning. Unilateral renal agenesis can be detected only by directly scanning each renal fossa. Failure to identify a kidney in the normal position should prompt a search for an ectopic kidney.

opment of the kidney from the metanephric blastema. Unilateral renal agenesis (Figure 18-11) occurs in 1 in 600 newborns and is often associated with genital tract abnormalities. Bilateral renal agenesis occurs in about 1 in 3,500 newborns. In fetuses without kidneys there is severe oligohydramnios, pulmonary hypoplasia, and death shortly after birth. Sonographically, severe oligohydramnios makes fetal evaluation difficult. No bladder is noted even on extended scanning, kidneys are not seen, and prominent adrenal glands resembling kidneys are present (Figure 18-12).

Polyhydramnios is associated with a multitude of fetal abnormalities from many different organ systems. It is infrequently seen in association with genitourinary tract anomalies, however. As noted above, causes of renal obstruction such as UPJ obstruction can result in high-output renal failure and polyhydramnios. Solid fetal renal masses are rare. A solid mass is usually a mesoblastic nephroma, a benign hamartoma that for unknown reasons is often seen with polyhydramnios (Figure 18-13).

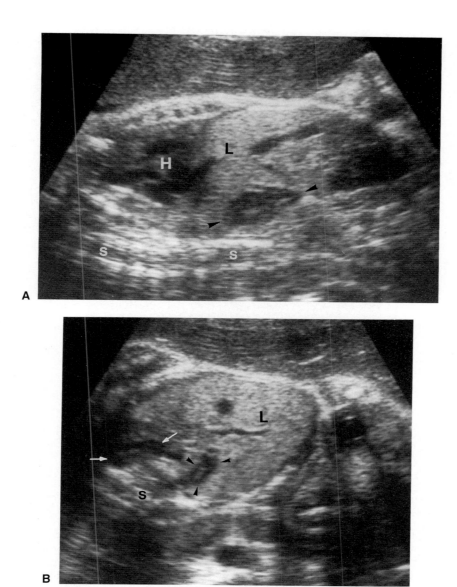

Figure 18-12. Bilateral renal agenesis in a fetus at 30 weeks. (A) A longitudinal image of the fetal trunk shows a reniform structure (arrowheads), which is a prominent adrenal gland. When the kidney is absent, the normally prominent fetal adrenal gland can assume a more reniform and less conical shape. No amniotic fluid is present. L = liver; s = spine; H = heart. (B) A transverse image through the upper abdomen shows both adrenal glands (arrowheads, arrows) as more typical, ovoid, hypoechoic structures with a linear, echogenic centrum. No kidneys are seen. The abdominal contour is distorted by the extreme oligohydramnios typical of bilateral renal agenesis. s = spine; L = liver.

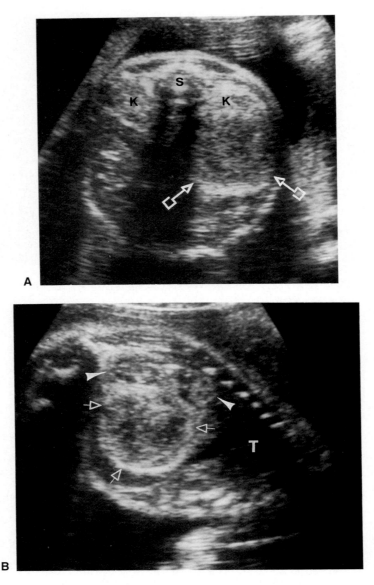

Figure 18-13. Mesoblastic nephroma in a fetus at 32 weeks. (A) A transverse image of the kidneys (K) shows a large solid mass (arrows) anteriorly on the left, with poor definition of the left kidney. S = spine. (B) A longitudinal image shows the left kidney (arrowheads) compressed posteriorly by the well-defined, heterogeneous solid mass (arrows). T = thorax. Polyhydramnios is often associated with a fetal mesoblastic nephroma but was not seen in this case.

Neonatal Wilms' tumor is quite rare, and although it could potentially be diagnosed *in utero*, no cases have been reported **(Option (C) is false).**

A single umbilical artery (SUA) is present in about 1% of pregnancies. Associated malformations have been reported in 8 to 50% of fetuses with a SUA. Any organ system can be affected, and multiple anomalies can be seen in a single fetus. Musculoskeletal and genitourinary anomalies are most frequent, followed by gastrointestinal tract, cardiovascular system, and central nervous system anomalies. Renal anomalies, though relatively frequent, are seen in only a fraction of involved fetuses **(Option (D) is false).** Detection of a SUA with gray-scale sonography can be difficult or even impossible in the first half of the second trimester. The use of color Doppler sonography increases the sensitivity for detection of the umbilical arteries, either directly within the cord or as they pass from the umbilicus lateral to the bladder within the fetal pelvis. Other entities associated with SUA include intrauterine growth retardation, which can be seen without other anomalies, and trisomy 18, which is usually associated with additional structural defects.

Richard A. Bowerman, M.D.

SUGGESTED READINGS

HYDRONEPHROSIS

1. Arger PH, Coleman BG, Mintz MC, et al. Routine fetal genitourinary tract screening. Radiology 1985; 156:485–489
2. Bosman G, Reuss A, Nijman JM, Wladimiroff JW. Prenatal diagnosis, management and outcome of fetal uretero-pelvic junction obstruction. Ultrasound Med Biol 1991; 17:117–120
3. Corteville JE, Gray DL, Crane JP. Congenital hydronephrosis: correlation of fetal ultrasonographic findings with infant outcome. Am J Obstet Gynecol 1991; 165:384–388
4. Harrison MR, Filly RA. The fetus with obstructive uropathy: pathophysiology, natural history, selection, and treatment. In: Harrison MR, Golbus MS, Filly RA (eds), The unborn patient. Philadelphia: WB Saunders; 1990:328–393
5. Hoddick WK, Filly RA, Mahony BS, Callen PW. Minimal fetal renal pyelectasis. J Ultrasound Med 1985; 4:85–89
6. Nussbaum AR, Dorst JP, Jeffs RD, Gearhart JP, Sanders RC. Ectopic ureter and ureterocele: their varied sonographic manifestations. Radiology 1986; 159:227–235

PRUNE BELLY SYNDROME

7. Adzick NS, Harrison MR, Flake AW, deLorimier AA. Urinary extravasation in the fetus with obstructive uropathy. J Pediatr Surg 1985; 20:608–615

8. Meizner I, Bar-Ziv J, Katz M. Prenatal ultrasonic diagnosis of the extreme form of prune belly syndrome. JCU 1985; 13:581–583

9. Woodhouse CR, Ransley PG, Innes-Williams D. Prune belly syndrome—report of 47 cases. Arch Dis Child 1982; 57:856–859

RENAL CYSTIC DISEASE

10. Beck AD. The effect of intra-uterine urinary obstruction upon the development of the fetal kidney. J Urol 1971; 105:784–789

11. Bernstein J. The morphogenesis of renal parenchymal maldevelopment (renal dysplasia). Pediatr Clin North Am 1971; 18:395–407

12. Madewell JE, Hartman DS, Lightenstein JE. Radiologic-pathologic correlations in cystic disease of the kidney. Radiol Clin North Am 1979; 17:261–279

13. Mahony BS, Callen PW, Filly RA, Golbus MS. Progression of infantile polycystic kidney disease in early pregnancy. J Ultrasound Med 1984; 3:277–279

14. Mahony BS, Filly RA, Callen PW, Hricak H, Golbus MS, Harrison MR. Fetal renal dysplasia: sonographic evaluation. Radiology 1984; 152:143–146

15. Osathanondh V, Potter EL. Pathogenesis of polycystic kidneys: type 4 due to urethral obstruction. Arch Pathol 1964; 77:502–509

16. Reuss A, Wladimiroff JW, Niermeyer MF. Sonographic, clinical and genetic aspects of prenatal diagnosis of cystic kidney disease. Ultrasound Med Biol 1991; 17:687–694

17. Sanders RC, Hartman DS. The sonographic distinction between neonatal multicystic kidney and hydronephrosis. Radiology 1984; 151:621–625

18. Stuck KJ, Koff SA, Silver TM. Ultrasonic features of multicystic dysplastic kidney: expanded diagnostic criteria. Radiology 1982; 143:217–221

BLADDER OUTLET OBSTRUCTION

19. Avni EF, Thoua Y, Van Gansbeke D, et al. Development of the hypodysplastic kidney: contribution of antenatal US diagnosis. Radiology 1987; 164:123–125

20. Barth RA, Filly RA, Sondheimer FK. Prenatal sonographic findings in bladder exstrophy. J Ultrasound Med 1990; 9:359–361

21. Glazer GM, Filly RA, Callen PW. The varied sonographic appearance of the urinary tract in the fetus and newborn with urethral obstruction. Radiology 1982; 144:563–568

22. Hayden SA, Russ PD, Pretorius DH, Manco-Johnson ML, Clewell WH. Posterior urethral obstruction. Prenatal sonographic findings and clinical outcome in fourteen cases. J Ultrasound Med 1988; 7:371–375

23. Mahony BS, Callen PW, Filly RA. Fetal urethral obstruction: US evaluation. Radiology 1985; 157:221–224

24. Meizner I, Bar-Ziv J. *In utero* prenatal ultrasonic diagnosis of a rare case of cloacal exstrophy. J Clin Ultrasound 1985; 13:500–502

25. Richards DS, Langham MR Jr, Mahaffey SM. The prenatal ultrasonographic diagnosis of cloacal exstrophy. J Ultrasound Med 1992; 11:507–510

RENAL AGENESIS

26. Potter EL. Bilateral absence of ureters and kidneys: a report of 50 cases. Obstet Gynecol 1965; 25:3–12
27. Schmidt W, Kubli F. Early diagnosis of severe congenital malformations by ultrasonography. J Perinat Med 1992; 10:233–241
28. Sherer DM, Thompson HO, Armstrong B, Woods JR Jr. Prenatal sonographic diagnosis of unilateral renal agenesis. JCU 1990; 18:648–652

KIDNEYS—GENERAL

29. Bertagnoli L, Lalatta F, Gallicchio R, et al. Quantitative characterization of the growth of the fetal kidney. JCU 1983; 11:349–356
30. Cohen HL, Cooper J, Eisenberg P, et al. Normal length of fetal kidneys: sonographic study in 397 obstetric patients. AJR 1991; 157:545–548
31. Graham D, Sanders RC. Amniotic fluid. Semin Roentgenol 1982; 17:210–218
32. Grannum P, Bracken M, Silverman R, Hobbins JC. Assessment of fetal kidney size in normal gestation by comparison of ratio of kidney circumference to abdominal circumference. Am J Obstet Gynecol 1980; 136:249–254
33. Patten RM, Mack LA, Wang KY, Cyr DR. The fetal genitourinary tract. Radiol Clin North Am 1990; 28:115–130
34. Sanders RC. *In utero* sonography of genitourinary anomalies. Urol Radiol 1992; 14:29–33

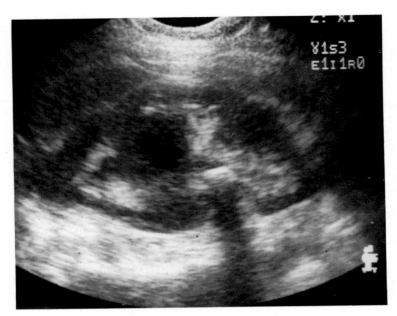

Figure 19-1

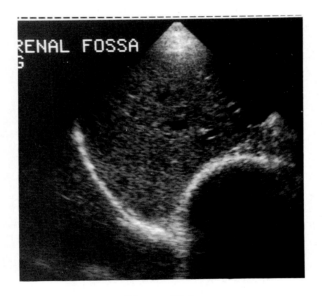

Figure 19-2

The architectural distortion present in kidneys of patients with XGP enables this disease to be differentiated sonographically from pyonephrosis, a distinction that may be difficult to make in the absence of a staghorn calculus. Renal tuberculosis and renal neoplasms also should be considered in the differential diagnosis of this sonographic appearance.

Figure 19-2 is a longitudinal sonogram of the right renal fossa. Normal liver is seen anterior to a highly echogenic, smoothly curved interface with sharply marginated posterior acoustic shadowing (Figure 19-6). This appearance suggests diffuse calcification of the underlying structure, which should be the kidney. No normal renal parenchyma is visualized. Diffuse parenchymal calcification resulting from extensive cortical nephrocalcinosis is the primary diagnostic consideration. Of the options given, only oxalosis is associated with this appearance, which results from deposition of calcium oxalate crystals in the renal tubules **(Option (C) is the correct answer to Question 83).** The abdominal radiograph of the patient whose sonogram is shown in Figure 19-2 (Figure 19-6C) demonstrates abnormal, bilateral increased renal cortical density with central calculi.

Air surrounding the kidney and diffuse fatty infiltration of the kidney are the main considerations for the differential diagnosis of the findings in Figure 19-2. Air within the renal parenchyma or in the perinephric space, as seen in patients with emphysematous pyelonephritis, should produce "dirty" shadowing, with visualization of portions of the kidney in most cases. Intraparenchymal gas can be distinguished from diffuse calcification on a conventional radiograph.

Fatty infiltration of the kidneys with architectural distortion can occur in patients with extensive angiomyolipomas, resulting in a sonographic appearance similar to that seen in Figure 19-2 of a highly echogenic structure in the renal fossa (Figure 19-7). However, diffuse parenchymal infiltration with fat does not produce the posterior acoustic shadowing seen with diffuse parenchymal calcification. An abdominal radiograph or CT scan can confirm the diagnosis.

Primary hyperoxaluria (oxalosis) is a rare hereditary autosomal recessive disorder caused by an inborn error of glyoxalate (type I) or hydroxypyruvate (type II) metabolism. Consequent excess production and urinary excretion of oxalate result in oxalate crystalluria, calcium oxalate nephrocalcinosis, and nephrolithiasis due to calcium oxalate calculi early in childhood followed by progressive renal failure and death in adolescence. In patients with advanced disease, calcium oxalate crystals are deposited in many solid organs. Acute renal failure from oxalosis is rare in infancy.

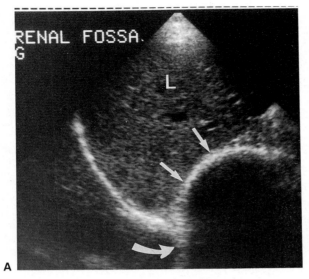

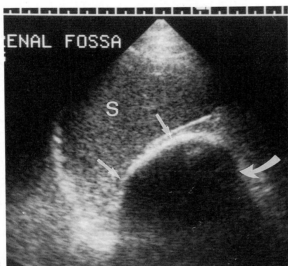

Figure 19-6. Oxalosis. (A [Same as Figure 19-2] and B) Longitudinal sonograms of right (A) and left (B) renal fossae. The location is confirmed by visualization of the liver (L) and spleen (S), respectively. Smooth-contoured, curved, echogenic bands (straight arrows) are seen; note the sharp margins (curved arrows) of the posterior acoustic shadow. (C) A radiograph demonstrates radiopaque renal cortex bilaterally (cortical nephrocalcinosis) and collecting-system calculi. (Courtesy of William D. Middleton, M.D., Mallinckrodt Institute of Radiology, St. Louis, Mo.)

Secondary hyperoxaluria is most commonly the result of increased intestinal absorption of dietary oxalate as a result of small bowel disease, ileal resection, or bypass, but it can also be caused by dietary increase in oxalates, pyridoxine deficiency, ethylene glycol poisoning, and methoxyflurane anesthesia. Nephrolithiasis or nephrocalcinosis, usually cortical in distribution, can also be caused by the secondary form.

Calcification begins at the corticomedullary junction and characteristically involves both the renal cortex and the medullary pyramids. The

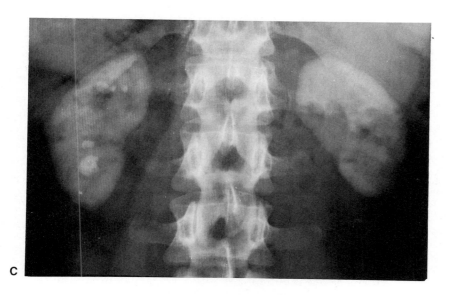

C

CT appearance of oxalosis includes calcification of the entire cortex and global calcification of both cortex and medulla. Sonographically, cortical echogenicity is increased by calcium oxalate deposition; the corticomedullary junction is obliterated. Renal size remains normal. With extensive calcification the renal bed can be obscured sonographically, as in Figure 19-2. The sonographic differential diagnosis includes cortical nephrocalcinosis associated with acute cortical necrosis; hypercalcemia related to malignancy; and severe increased cortical echogenicity seen with end-stage renal disease, in which case the renal size is usually small and posterior shadowing is absent. Brennan et al. found the magnitude of increased parenchymal echogenicity in oxalosis, which is greater than that of mesenteric fat, helpful in differentiating oxalosis from other diseases that cause increased parenchymal echogenicity.

Figure 19-3, a longitudinal sonogram of the right kidney, demonstrates discrete, nonshadowing foci of increased parenchymal echogenicity confined to the medullary pyramids, with a ringlike configuration in the upper pole (Figure 19-8A). The renal cortex and contour appear normal. This appearance is characteristic of medullary nephrocalcinosis. Of the options given, only renal tubular acidosis (RTA) is associated with medullary nephrocalcinosis **(Option (B) is the correct answer to Question 84).**

Nephrocalcinosis is a broad term indicating renal parenchymal calcium deposition, which may be predominantly cortical or medullary or can involve both regions. Fan-shaped clusters of stippled echogenic

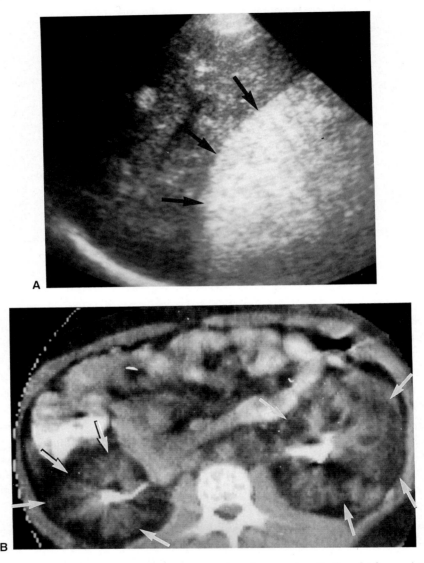

Figure 19-7. Angiomyolipomatous involvement of the kidney in a patient with tuberous sclerosis. (A) A longitudinal sonogram through the right renal fossa demonstrates a highly echogenic structure with smooth contour (arrows) and no posterior acoustic shadowing. Normal renal parenchyma is not seen. This constellation of findings suggests diffuse parenchymal infiltration by fat, rather than cortical calcification. (B) A CT scan of the kidneys demonstrates diffuse fatty infiltration throughout the renal parenchyma (arrows).

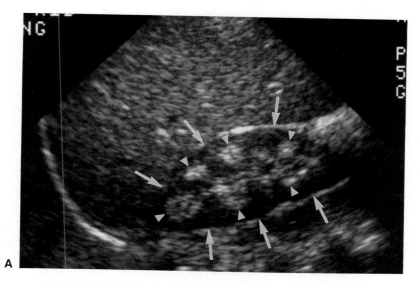

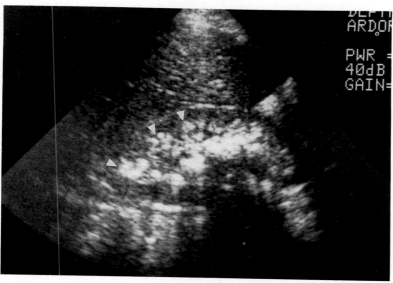

Figure 19-8. Medullary nephrocalcinosis. (A) Same as Figure 19-3. A longitudinal scan of the right kidney shows that the renal cortex (arrows) is appropriately hypoechoic compared with the liver and that the renal contours are normal. Ringlike foci of increased echogenicity (arrowheads) are confined to the medullary pyramids, consistent with medullary nephrocalcinosis. The etiology in this case was renal tubular acidosis. (Courtesy of Gary M. Kellman, M.D., Fairfax, Va.) (B) A longitudinal sonogram of the right kidney in a patient with Lesch-Nyhan's syndrome demonstrates similar but more prominent echogenic medullary rings (arrowheads), associated with early medullary nephrocalcinosis. Central echogenic structures with posterior acoustic shadowing represent pelvic calculi. (Courtesy of Christine M. Dudiak, M.D., Loyola University Medical Center, Chicago, Ill.)

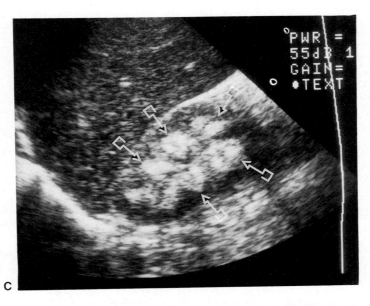

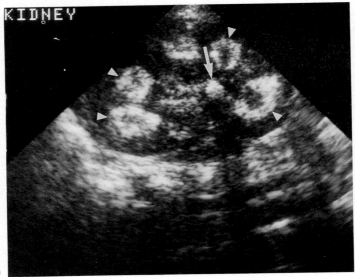

Figure 19-8 (Continued). Medullary nephrocalcinosis. Longitudinal sonograms of the right (C) and left (D) kidneys in an infant with a history of long-term diuretic therapy. Echogenic medullary rosettes (arrowheads) are characteristic of medullary nephrocalcinosis. A nonobstructing pelvic calculus (arrows) is also seen on the left. (Courtesy of Aruna Vade, M.D., Loyola University Medical Center, Chicago, Ill.)

reflectors in the periphery of the medullary pyramids (Figure 19-8B through D) are a very early sonographic manifestation of nephrocalcinosis and are detectable before other radiographic or biochemical abnormalities. Shadowing is inconsistent and is frequently absent; the renal cortex usually appears normal.

Medullary nephrocalcinosis indicates a metabolic abnormality usually associated with hypercalciuria and hypercalcemic states. It can also be seen with medullary sponge kidney and papillary necrosis *in situ*. According to Banner, 40% of cases are secondary to primary hyperparathyroidism and 20% are secondary to RTA, with the remaining 40% divided among multiple other etiologies.

In patients with RTA, abnormal renal tubular function results in chronic systemic acidosis and urine alkalosis. Proximal (type II) RTA, characterized by excessive urinary loss of bicarbonate, is not associated with the formation of renal calculi. In distal (type I) RTA, impaired hydrogen ion transfer into the urine can result in stone formation, usually apatite. The reported frequency of medullary nephrocalcinosis and lithiasis is approximately 30% in infants and 70% in adults with primary or idiopathic RTA. Delayed skeletal maturation and osteomalacia are seen in affected children.

Secondary RTA with nephrocalcinosis and lithiasis can develop in patients with other processes that affect hydrogen ion excretion from the distal tubule; these processes include medullary sponge kidney (distal RTA), Wilson's disease, Fanconi's syndrome, hyperglobulinemias, use of nephrotoxic drugs, and acetazolamide administration.

Cortical nephrocalcinosis is usually bilateral and diffuse. Unilateral or focal cortical calcification is usually due to tumor or infection; infection can also produce diffuse calcification. The most common causes of diffuse bilateral cortical calcification are hypercalcemic states associated with malignancy, hyperparathyroidism, or vitamin D intoxication; acute cortical necrosis (ACN); and chronic glomerulonephritis.

ACN (Figure 19-9) is a rare cause of acute renal failure; it is precipitated by renal injury secondary to shock, hemorrhage, sepsis, myocardial infarction, burns, renal vein thrombosis, hemolytic-uremic syndrome, toxemia of pregnancy with placental abruption, or severe dehydration. The proposed mechanism of injury is ischemic necrosis due to hypoperfusion, vasospasm, capillary damage, or intravascular thrombosis. Histologically, there is acute ischemic infarction of the renal cortex, necrosis of the tubular cells and glomeruli, arteriolar thrombosis, and cellular infiltration into the peripheral interstitium. The medulla and a thin rim of subcapsular cortex are spared. Radiologically detectable calcifications have been reported as early as 24 hours after the insult. They occur at

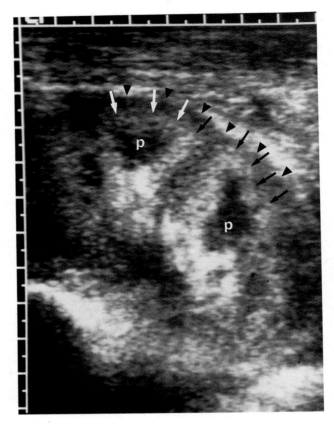

Figure 19-9. Acute cortical necrosis. A longitudinal renal sonogram demonstrates increased cortical echogenicity (arrows). There is preservation of normal echogenicity in the medullary pyramids (p) and in a thin subcapsular band of cortex (arrowheads).

the junction between viable and necrotic tissue or diffusely throughout the cortex.

Sonographically, the renal cortex can initially appear hypoechoic. Increased cortical echogenicity develops, sparing a thin rim of subcapsular cortex and the medulla. Progressive decrease in renal size occurs. In patients with diffuse calcification, the entire kidney and renal fossa can be obscured by shadowing, an appearance similar to that of chronic glomerulonephritis and oxalosis. The diagnosis is made on the basis of clinical features, with radiographic identification of diffuse cortical calcification suggesting ACN.

In patients with AIDS, diffuse infection and renal calcification (Figure 19-10) can be caused by *Pneumocystis carinii* infection and have been reported to occur in association with *Mycobacterium avium-intracellulare* (MAI) infection. In patients with MAI infection, an unusual pattern of "partial nephrocalcinosis" has been described in which there is asym-

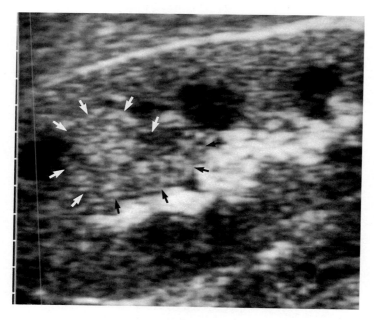

Figure 19-10. Renal involvement in AIDS. A magnified sonogram of the kidney demonstrates a subtle irregular area of increased parenchymal echogenicity in the distribution of a renal septum (arrows). There is no acoustic shadowing. Adjacent areas of normal-appearing parenchyma are also seen. A patchy distribution of nephrocalcinosis involving the cortex and medulla has been described in patients with AIDS, in association with MAI and *P. carinii* infection. (Courtesy of Christine M. Dudiak, M.D.)

metric, patchy, heterogeneous distribution of delicate calcifications involving both cortex and medulla. Diffuse and focal cortical nephrocalcinosis have been reported to occur in patients with multiorgan involvement by *P. carinii*. Focal segmental glomerulosclerosis, a common renal manifestation of AIDS, results in diffusely increased cortical echogenicity with preservation of corticomedullary differentiation.

Sonographically, it can be difficult to differentiate extensive nephrocalcinosis or large renal calculi (staghorn calculi) from air. Intrarenal gas, seen in patients with emphysematous pyelonephritis (EP) (Option (A)) (Figure 19-11), results in sonographic visualization of highly echogenic reflectors with posterior shadowing in the parenchyma, central sinus, or both, similar to calculi. The acoustic shadow seen with gas typically appears "dirtier" than that seen with calcifications because of low-level echoes within the acoustic shadow caused by reverberation artifact. Shadowing from extensive intraparenchymal gas can obscure

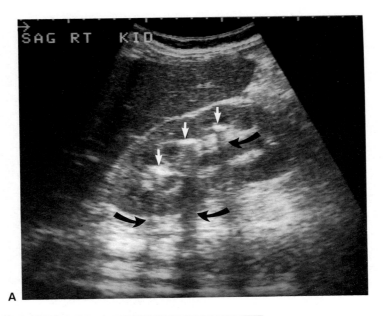

A

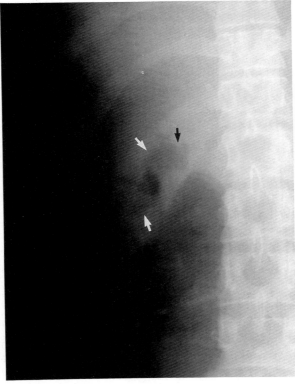

B

Figure 19-11. Emphysematous pyelonephritis. (A) A sagittal sonogram of the right kidney demonstrates highly echogenic foci (straight arrows) conforming to the contour of the collecting system. The margins of the posterior acoustic shadows are indistinct (curved arrows). This appearance is suggestive of intrarenal air. (B) A corresponding radiograph shows air outlining the collecting system of the right kidney (arrows).

the renal bed and can be indistinguishable from bowel gas associated with intestinal ileus. This will hamper sonographic evaluation and create a confusing image. In these cases a conventional radiograph is valuable for distinguishing between air and calculi. CT is most effective in demonstrating both intrarenal involvement and perinephric extension.

EP is a fulminant, necrotizing, life-threatening renal inflammatory process characterized by the bacterial production of gas within the renal parenchyma. It is usually unilateral. EP is seen most commonly in diabetic patients, immunosuppressed patients (especially those with renal transplants), or patients with urinary tract obstruction or neoplasm. Impaired host immunity and ischemia, resulting in poor response to antibiotics, are exacerbating factors. *E. coli* infection is common; *Klebsiella*, *Proteus*, and *Aerobacter* infections are also associated but are less common. Mortality rates as high as 35 to 50% are reported. Patients are typically acutely ill, although symptoms can be mild compared with the severity of the disease. There is often bacteriuria, bacteremia, leukocytosis, hyperglycemia, or azotemia. Management is typically surgical. Percutaneous nephrostomy with relief of obstruction and aggressive antibiotic therapy have been reported to be successful in a few patients.

Other causes of intrarenal air include bronchial, enteric, or cutaneous fistulae; air within a well-localized abscess; and reflux from the bladder or ileal diversion.

Figure 19-4 is a longitudinal sonogram of a normal right kidney **(Option (D) is the correct answer to Question 85)**. The cortex is smooth with normal echogenicity, similar to that of the liver. The renal pyramids are represented by triangular structures oriented with the base peripheral and the apex central, bordering the echogenic central sinus and hypoechoic relative to the adjacent cortex. Cortical septa interposed between the pyramids also extend to the central sinus. Within the central sinus, small, echogenic nonshadowing foci represent segmental arteries and veins. Deep to and posterior to the kidney, slightly curved echogenic structures with sharply defined posterior shadowing represent either the cortices of ribs or transverse processes (Figure 19-12).

The kidney can be divided into three regions: the cortex, the medulla, and the central sinus. The renal cortex is normally of uniform thickness and is less echogenic than the adjacent liver and spleen in adults. Renal echogenicity equivalent to that of the liver is a nonspecific finding. Platt et al., in a prospective study, found that 72% of 153 patients in whom the right kidney was isoechoic with the liver had no clinical or laboratory evidence of renal disease. Echogenicity can vary as a function of the scan plane (with increased echogenicity observed on transverse images) and the type of transducer used. With increasing age, there is thinning of the

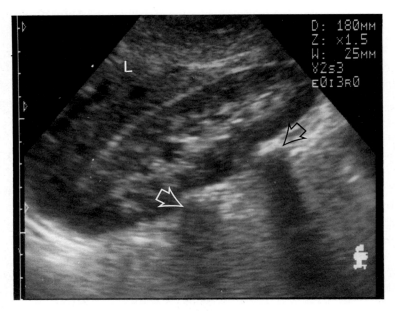

Figure 19-12 (Same as Figure 19-4).   Normal kidney. The renal cortex has a smooth contour and is isoechoic to the adjacent liver (L). The medullary pyramids have apices oriented centrally. Renal cortical septa are interposed between the pyramids. The central sinus contains echogenic nonshadowing foci, representing segmental vessels. Sonic shadows deep to the kidney are caused by posterior ribs (arrows).

renal parenchyma with a concurrent increase in the amount of renal sinus fat.

Several developmental variations can mimic abnormal renal masses or parenchymal scarring sonographically. "Pseudomasses" include "dromedary humps" and prominent columns of Bertin (Figure 19-13). Apparent duplication of the upper renal pole, more common on the left and in obese individuals, can result from sonic-beam refraction between the lower pole of the spleen (or liver) and adjacent fat. Junctional cortical defects and interlobular grooves can be mistaken for parenchymal scars. Remnants of fetal lobulation (lobation) are represented by more subtle indentation of the cortical outline.

The renal medulla, containing the collecting tubules, is sonographically represented by the triangular pyramids, which are normally less echogenic than adjacent cortex. The pyramids can be identified by their shape, location peripheral to the central sinus, and separation laterally by cortical septa. Arcuate vessels, seen in 25% of patients, appear as intense echogenic foci at the corticomedullary junction and can simulate

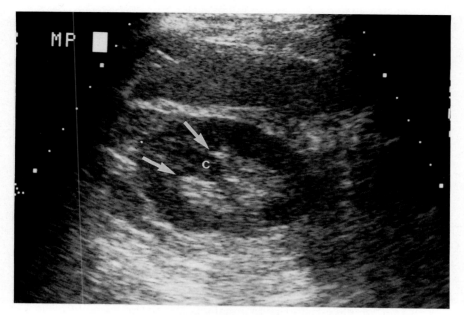

Figure 19-13. Column of Bertin. A transverse sonogram of a normal kidney demonstrates a prominent mass of renal tissue representing a column of Bertin (c). It is isoechoic with adjacent cortex, does not distort the renal contour, and is invaginated by central sinus fat (arrows).

small calculi. The cortex and medulla are differentiated sonographically in approximately half of all adult patients, depending on habitus and transducer frequency.

The central sinus is composed of fat, calyces, infundibula, renal pelvis, and vessels. Its intense echogenicity is attributed mainly to hilar fat, with secondary contributions from fibrous septa, blood vessels, and lymphatics. The calyces appear as sonolucent structures within the central sinus.

Question 86

Concerning renal stones,

    (A) the presence of acoustic shadowing depends on chemical composition

    (B) they are more accurately detected by sonography than by abdominal radiography

    (C) they are reliably distinguished from pelvic blood clots by sonography

    (D) detection of acoustic shadowing depends on the focal zone of the transducer

    (E) normal renal structures simulate small stones sonographically

More than 80% of kidney stones contain some form of calcium. Commonly encountered calculi include those composed of calcium oxalate, calcium phosphate, or a combination of the two; magnesium ammonium calcium phosphate (struvite-apatite or triple-phosphate stones); uric acid; and cystine. Calcium oxalate/phosphate stones account for most calculi found in several published series.

The sonic shadow posterior to a stone is due to the large difference in acoustic impedance at the interface of the crystalline surface of the stone and adjacent tissue (Figure 19-14). In general, there is no significant correlation between stone composition and detection of a posterior acoustic shadow **(Option (A) is false).** Stafford et al. demonstrated no effect of calculus composition on detection of human renal calculi of different compositions implanted into porcine kidneys. All stones are visualized sonographically as echogenic foci. Calculi create an acoustic shadow, regardless of their radiographic opacity, whereas other filling defects, such as tumor, thrombi, or sloughed papilla, do not **(Option (C) is true).**

Rare nonshadowing matrix "stones" have been reported. These are composed partially of urinary matrix, a mucoprotein, and are found more frequently in women than in men. They are associated with the presence of urea-splitting bacteria, typically *Proteus vulgaris* and *P. mirabilis*, and may coexist with crystalline calculi. Lack of shadowing of matrix calculi is attributed to the similarity in acoustic impedance and absorption coefficients of the urinary matrix and renal parenchyma.

Magnesium ammonium phosphate (struvite) calculi usually result from urinary tract infection by a urea-splitting bacteria, usually *P. mirabilis*, and are associated with alkaline urine. Pure struvite stones are of low radiodensity, are rare, and are less echogenic than other more commonly encountered calculi. Struvite stones are frequently laminated with denser calcium salts; the laminations reflect recurrent infection and changes in urine pH. Staghorn calculi (Figure 19-15) most commonly contain struvite-apatite.

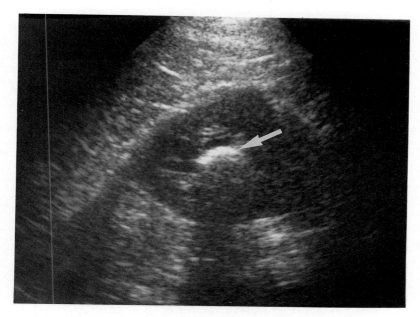

Figure 19-14. Nephrolithiasis. A transverse sonogram of the right kidney demonstrates a curved, strongly echogenic structure in the expected location of the collecting system (arrow); note the sonic shadowing. The appearance suggests a pelvic calculus.

Sonography is more sensitive than abdominal radiography for stone detection **(Option (B) is true);** CT is the most sensitive of available imaging modalities, depicting even radiographically nonopaque calculi as foci with high attenuation values. Studies by Middleton et al. and Vrtiska et al. found that sonography was more sensitive than abdominal radiography for stone detection in patients who had undergone extracorporeal shock wave lithotripsy but was slightly inferior to a combination of abdominal radiography and renal tomography. The overall sensitivities of sonography, considering only radiopaque calculi, were 95 and 93% in these two studies, respectively. Specificity for stone detection was somewhat lower (89%), with false-positive interpretations being due to catheters, renal arterial calcifications, and normal echogenic structures within the renal sinus. In the study by Middleton et al., the ability to detect stones was independent of stone location and patient size.

Sonography and radiography/tomography are complementary modalities in the evaluation of renal calculi. Sonography can demonstrate noncalcified stones, such as uric acid calculi, which are not detected on radiography/tomography. In certain clinical settings, such as in thin patients

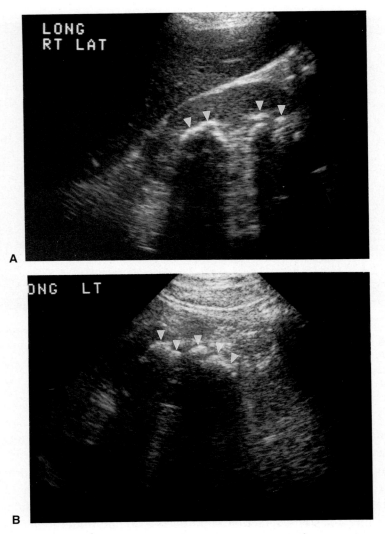

Figure 19-15. Bilateral staghorn calculi. Longitudinal sonograms of the right (A) and left (B) kidneys demonstrate highly echogenic curved structures (arrowheads) in the region of each renal pelvis. Note the well-defined zones of sonic shadowing obscuring the pelvicalyceal anatomy. (C) An abdominal radiograph confirms the presence of bilateral staghorn calculi.

with faintly opaque stones and in patients with scoliosis, sonography is more helpful than radiography/tomography. Sonography is more accurate in the detection of hydronephrosis and segmental caliectasis. However, sonography has significantly decreased accuracy when there is air or a stent within the collecting system, if there is marked renal scarring,

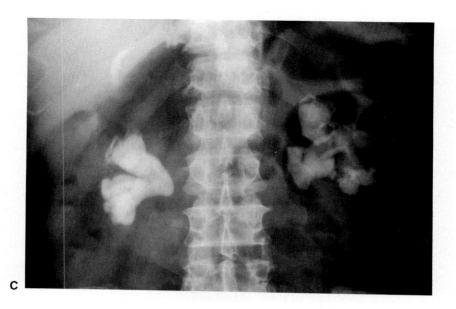

C

or in the presence of postoperative changes including surgical clips and other metallic devices.

Sonographic detection of calculi depends on stone size and on transducer frequency and focal zone **(Option (D) is true).** Stone size is the most important variable; intervening tissue and focal-zone placement also affect imaging. The stone must be the same size as or larger than the width of the beam profile, usually at least 4 to 5 mm in diameter in the clinical setting. In the studies of Middleton et al., Vrtiska et al., and others, most of the stones missed sonographically were smaller than 5 mm in diameter.

Sonographic detection of a renal calculus requires identification of a highly echogenic focus with posterior acoustic shadowing. Very small calculi may not produce the expected shadowing. The perceived size of the stone can change with depth from the transducer (as a result of deterioration of lateral-beam resolution) and stone composition. Higher-frequency (5- and 7.5-MHz) transducers are more accurate in stone size determination than are lower-frequency (3.5-MHz) transducers.

Small stones located beyond the nominal transducer focal zone may not exhibit shadowing because of their size and the width of the sonic beam, whereas those within the focal zone will produce shadowing (Figure 19-16). Reverberation artifacts may fill in the acoustic shadow of larger calculi, especially those with smooth surfaces. Distortion of the

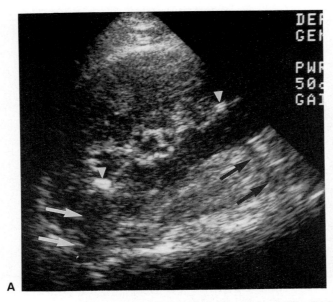

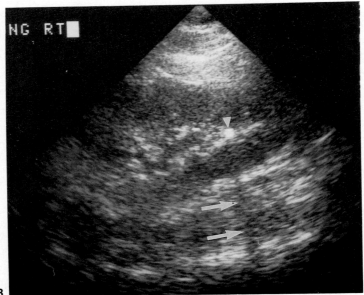

Figure 19-16.
Nephrolithiasis. (A
and B) Longitudinal
sonograms in two
different patients
with small renal cal-
culi demonstrate
bright echogenic
foci (arrowheads)
caused by the
stones. Sonic shad-
owing (arrows) is
subtle.

beam profile by the rib cage can cause differing beam profiles between
scans, resulting in variable acoustic shadowing.

Adequate patient hydration accentuates renal obstruction and hydronephrosis and aids in stone visualization by providing a full urinary
bladder through which to visualize the distal ureters and the ureteroves-

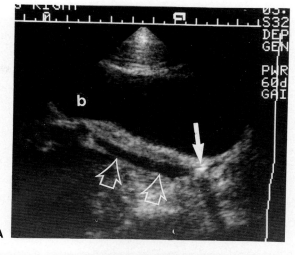

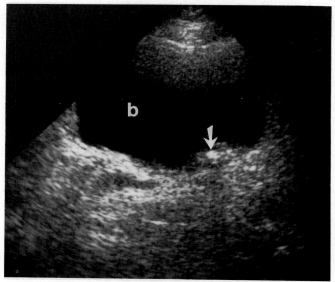

Figure 19-17. Distal ureteral stone. (A) A sagittal sonogram demonstrates a sonolucent tubular structure (open arrows) deep to the distended urinary bladder (b). This corresponds to a fluid-filled distal right ureter. An echogenic shadowing structure (arrow) just proximal to the ureterovesical junction represents an obstructing calculus. (B) A transverse sonogram of the distended urinary bladder (b) in another patient demonstrates an echogenic shadowing structure (arrow) at the ureterovesical junction, compatible with an obstructing calculus. The soft tissue mass surrounding the stone represents periureteral edema.

ical junction, the most common site for obstruction by a stone (Figure 19-17). An aperistaltic, fluid-filled ureter can be observed, with peri-

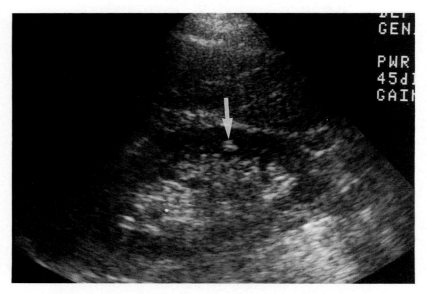

Figure 19-18. Angiomyolipoma. A longitudinal renal sonogram demonstrates a small focus of increased parenchymal echogenicity (arrow). This could be mistaken for a stone. However, a calculus of this size should produce acoustic shadowing, which is absent in this image. The echogenicity is similar to that of the central sinus, suggesting the presence of fat and the diagnosis of a small angiomyolipoma.

ureteric edema surrounding the obstructing calculus. Visualization of ureteric jets into the bladder implies lack of complete obstruction.

Normal structures that can mimic small calculi sonographically include pericalyceal fat and vessels **(Option (E) is true).** Renal arterial calcifications, submucosal calyceal plaques, milk of calcium in a calyceal diverticulum, and air bubbles or stents within the collecting system can also simulate nephrolithiasis. CT or conventional radiography will differentiate intraparenchymal or collecting system air from calculi.

Echogenic, nonshadowing masses found within a dilated collecting system include blood clots, pyogenic debris, sloughed papillae, fungus balls, tumors, very small stones, and matrix stones. A normal renal papilla projecting into a dilated calyx can appear as a nonshadowing filling defect. It can be recognized by demonstrating its continuity with the adjacent normal renal parenchyma.

An echogenic, nonshadowing intraparenchymal renal mass can represent a small infarct, angiomyolipoma, renal cell carcinoma, hemangioma, oncocytoma, or metastasis. Angiomyolipomas (Figure 19-18) vary in their sonographic appearance; most of the lesions in the 1981 study of

Hartman et al. were more echogenic than renal cortex and similar in appearance to the central sinus, although lesions of mixed or relatively low echogenicity were also found. Renal cell carcinomas are generally less echogenic than angiomyolipomas, but Charboneau et al. found that 4% of renal cell carcinomas in their study population were highly echogenic and comparable in appearance to angiomyolipoma.

Question 87

Concerning xanthogranulomatous pyelonephritis,

(A) renal sonograms commonly demonstrate renal stones
(B) most patients are asymptomatic
(C) it is associated with a syndrome of reversible hepatic dysfunction
(D) renal involvement is usually focal
(E) it is frequently associated with renal cell carcinoma

XGP is an uncommon, severe, chronic suppurative renal parenchymal infection usually affecting women in the fourth through seventh decades. Contributory factors include chronic urinary tract obstruction with or without a calculus, ineffectively treated chronic urinary sepsis, alteration of lipid metabolism, vascular compromise, and altered immune response. Common complaints include recurrent low-grade fevers, back or flank pain, weight loss, chills, and dysuria. In a study of 16 cases of XGP by Hartman et al., pain was the presenting symptom in 81% of cases, a mass in 56%, and weight loss in 38%. The duration of symptoms can be acute (days) or subacute to chronic (weeks to months or even years) **(Option (B) is false)**. *P. mirabilis, E. coli,* and *Pseudomonas, Klebsiella,* and *Staphylococcus* species are frequently found on urine culture. Leukocytosis, anemia, elevated serum alpha and gamma globulin levels, and an elevated erythrocyte sedimentation rate are common. Most patients have pyuria and proteinuria; some have hematuria. Sterile cultures are found in urine samples from up to one-third of patients as a result of complete renal or ureteral obstruction, and culture of renal parenchyma specimens can yield organisms differing from those in the urine. Reversible hepatic dysfunction syndrome, in which there are abnormal liver function tests with or without hepatomegaly that return to normal after nephrectomy, has been found in association with both XGP and renal cell carcinoma **(Option (C) is true)**. Abnormal levels of alkaline phosphatase activity, serum alpha-2 globulin, albumin, serum glutamic-oxaloacetic transaminase, and indirect bilirubin, as well as prolongation of the prothrombin time, are reported. According to Hartman, reversible hepatic dysfunction syndrome occurs in 20 to 40% of patients with diffuse XGP. In their study, Malek and Elder noted reversible hepatic dysfunction in all 13 patients with XGP, whereas Goodman et al. found evidence of hepatic dysfunction in 63% of 19 patients with XGP in whom liver function studies were obtained. In the latter study, hyperglobulinemia was the most common abnormality identified, in 11 of 14 patients. Utz et al. reported this syndrome in 65 patients with non-metastatic renal cell carcinoma.

XGP is nearly always unilateral. Chronic collecting-system obstruction at the calyceal, renal pelvic, or ureteral level is usually present. Fibrosis at the level of obstructing calculus often prevents significant dilatation of the local collecting system, with dilatation limited to the more peripheral collecting-system components. Secondary medullary vascular compromise can cause papillary necrosis. The precise mechanism is not known, but the subsequent granulomatous, rather than acute inflammatory, response is attributed to a failure of host immunity. The inflammatory process extends along the transitional mucosa of the obstructed segment, from the pelvis and calyces to the medulla and cortex, with subsequent destruction, cavitation, or abscess formation. The destroyed renal parenchyma is replaced by lipid laden macrophages ("foam" or "xanthoma" cells). Extrarenal extension of the inflammatory process is common.

Renal involvement can be diffuse or segmental. The diffuse form is seen in up to 80% of patients **(Option (D) is false).** Diffuse XGP is typically associated with a non-functioning kidney on intravenous pyelography, found in 80% of 68 cases studied by Anhalt et al. However, this is not a universal observation; Malek and Elder found non-function in only 27% of 26 cases. A mass is present in up to 62% of patients with focal involvement. Up to 70% of cases of diffuse XGP are associated with obstructing renal stones **(Option (A) is true),** commonly staghorn calculi. Focal XGP affects one renal calyx or pole of a duplication and can be associated with an obstructing calculus. The etiology is thought to be the same as that of diffuse XGP. There is poor renal function in the affected segment, within an otherwise functioning kidney. Focal XGP can be difficult to differentiate from renal cell carcinoma on the basis of either radiographic findings or needle biopsy. The two entities rarely coexist. The first recognized case of focal XGP associated with renal cell carcinoma was reported by Huisman and Sands in 1992. The first known case of bilateral XGP in association with renal cell carcinoma and amyloidosis in the native kidneys of a renal transplant recipient was reported by Akhtar and Qunibi, also in 1992. These authors found only 11 cases of renal cell carcinoma in association with XGP reported in the literature **(Option (E) is false)** and noted that renal parenchymal tumors are not etiologically related to XGP. Conversely, neoplasms with chronic urinary tract

If XGP presents as an intrarenal mass without extrarenal extension or identifiable renal calculi, radiologic distinction from renal neoplasm or tuberculosis can be impossible. The sonographic differential diagnosis for the more common presentation of diffuse XGP includes extensive papillary necrosis and lymphoma. The less common cystic appearance, in the absence of calculi, can be indistinguishable from that of pyonephrosis.

Caryl G. Salomon, M.D.
Thomas L. Lawson, M.D.

SUGGESTED READINGS

OXALOXIS

1. Brennan JN, Diwan RV, Makker SP, Cromer BA, Bellon EM. Ultrasonic diagnosis of primary hyperoxaluria in infancy. Radiology 1982; 145:147–148
2. Wilson DA, Wenzl JE, Altshuler GP. Ultrasound demonstration of diffuse cortical nephrocalcinosis in a case of primary hyperoxaluria. AJR 1979; 132:659–661

NEPHROCALCINOSIS

3. al-Murrani B, Cosgrove DO, Svensson WE, Blaszczyk M. Echogenic rings—an ultrasound sign of early nephrocalcinosis. Clin Radiol 1991; 44:49–51
4. Banner MP. Urolithiasis and nephrocalcinosis. In: Putman CE, Ravin CE (eds), Textbook of diagnostic imaging. Philadelphia: WB Saunders; 1988:1257–1269
5. Falkoff GE, Rigsby CM, Rosenfield AT. Partial, combined cortical and medullary nephrocalcinosis: US and CT patterns in AIDS-associated MAI infection. Radiology 1987; 162:343–344
6. Ginalski JM, Portmann L, Jaeger PH. Does medullary sponge kidney cause nephrolithiasis? AJR 1990; 155:299–302
7. Glazer GM, Callen PW, Filly RA. Medullary nephrocalcinosis: sonographic evaluation. AJR 1992; 138:55–57
8. Green D, Carroll BA. Ultrasound of renal failure. In: Hricak H (ed), Genitourinary ultrasound. New York: Churchill Livingstone; 1986:55–88
9. Huntington DK, Hill SC, Hill MC. Sonographic manifestations of medical renal disease. Semin US CT MR 1991; 12:290–307
10. Rumack CM, Wilson SR, Charboneau JW. Diagnostic ultrasound. Chicago: Mosby-Year Book; 1991:239–241
11. Sefczek RJ, Beckman I, Lupetin A, Dash N. Sonography of acute renal cortical necrosis. AJR 1984; 142:553–554
12. Spouge AR, Wilson SR, Gopinath N, Sherman M, Blendis LM. Extrapulmonary *Pneumocystis carinii* in a patient with AIDS: sonographic findings. AJR 1990; 155:76–78

13. Sty JR, Starshak RJ, Hubbard AM. Acute renal cortical necrosis in hemolytic uremic syndrome. JCU 1983; 11:175–178

NORMAL KIDNEY

14. Carter AR, Horgan JG, Jennings TA, Rosenfield AT. The junctional parenchymal defect: a sonographic variant of renal anatomy. Radiology 1985; 154:499–502
15. Lafortune M, Constantin A, Breton G, Vallee C. Sonography of the hypertrophied column of Bertin. AJR 1986; 146:53–56
16. Mahony BS, Jeffrey RB, Laing FC. Septa of Bertin: a sonographic pseudotumor. JCU 1983; 11:317–319
17. Middleton WD, Melson GL. Renal duplication artifact in US imaging. Radiology 1989; 173:427–429
18. Patriquin H, Lefaivre JF, Lafortune M, Russo P, Boisvert J. Fetal lobation: an anatomy-ultrasonographic correlation. J Ultrasound Med 1990; 9:191–197
19. Platt JF, Rubin JM, Bowerman RA, Marn CS. The inability to detect kidney disease on the basis of echogenicity. AJR 1988; 151:317–319

EMPHYSEMATOUS PYELONEPHRITIS

20. Goldman SM, Fishman EK. Upper urinary tract infection: the current role of CT, ultrasound, and MRI. Semin US CT MR 1991; 12:355–360
21. Piccirillo, M, Rigsby, CM, Rosenfield AT. Sonography of renal inflammatory disease. Urol Radiol 1987; 9:66–78

RENAL CALCULI AND MIMICS

22. Charboneau JW, Hattery RR, Ernst EC III, James EM, Williamson B Jr, Hartman GW. Spectrum of sonographic findings in 125 renal masses other than benign simple cyst. AJR 1983; 140:87–94
23. Choyke PL, Pahira JH, Davros WJ, Nilges E, Dwyer AJ, Mun SK. Renal calculi after shock wave lithotripsy: US evaluation with an *in vitro* phantom. Radiology 1989; 170:39–44
24. Dillard JP, Talner LB, Pinckney L. Normal renal papillae simulating caliceal filling defects on sonography. AJR 1987; 148:895–896
25. Dinsmore BJ, Pollack HM, Banner MP. Calcified transitional cell carcinoma of the renal pelvis. Radiology 1988; 167:401–404
26. Hartman DS, Goldman SM, Friedman AC, Davis CJ Jr, Madewell JE, Sherman JL. Angiomyolipoma: ultrasonic-pathologic correlation. Radiology 1981; 139:451–458
27. King W III, Kimme-Smith C, Winter J. Renal stone shadowing: an investigation of contributing factors. Radiology 1985; 154:191–196
28. Middleton WD, Dodds WJ, Lawson TL, Foley WD. Renal calculi: sensitivity for detection with US. Radiology 1988; 167:239–244
29. Stafford SJ, Jenkins JM, Staab EV, Boyce I, Fried FA. Ultrasonic detection of renal calculi: accuracy tested in an *in vitro* porcine kidney model. JCU 1981; 9:359–363

30. Vrtiska TJ, Hattery RR, King BF, et al. Role of ultrasound in medical management of patients with renal stone disease. Urol Radiol 1992; 14:131–138

31. Zwirewich CV, Buckley AR, Kidney MR, Sullivan LD, Rowley VA. Renal matrix calculus. Sonographic appearance. J Ultrasound Med 1990; 9:61–64

XANTHOGRANULOMATOUS PYELONEPHRITIS

32. Akhtar M, Qunibi W. Bilateral xanthogranulomatous pyelonephritis involving native kidneys in a renal transplant recipient: association with renal cell carcinoma and amyloidosis. Am J Kidney Dis 1992; 20:289–293

33. Anhalt MA, Cawood CD, Scott R Jr. Xanthogranulomatous pyelonephritis: a comprehensive review with report of 4 additional cases. J Urol 1971; 105:10–17

34. Golomb J, Solomon A, Peer G, Merimsky E, Aviram A, Braf Z. Bilateral metachronous xanthogranulomatous pyelonephritis in end-stage renal failure. Urol Radiol 1986; 8:95–97

35. Goodman M, Curry T, Russell T. Xanthogranulomatous pyelonephritis (XGP): a local disease with systemic manifestations. Report of 23 patients and review of the literature. Medicine (Baltimore) 1979; 58:171–181

36. Hartman DS. Radiologic pathologic correlation of the infectious granulomatous diseases of the kidney. Monogr Urol 1985; 6:26–43

37. Hartman DS, Davis CJ Jr, Goldman SM, Isbistes SS, Sanders RC. Xanthogranulomatous pyelonephritis: sonographic–pathologic correlation of 16 cases. J Ultrasound Med 1984; 3:481–488

38. Hayes WS, Hartman DS, Sesterhenn IA. From the Archives of the AFIP. Xanthogranulomatous pyelonephritis. RadioGraphics 1991; 11:485–498

39. Huisman TK, Sands JP. Focal xanthogranulomatous pyelonephritis associated with renal cell carcinoma. Urology 1992; 39:281–284

40. Malek RS, Elder JS. Xanthogranulomatous pyelonephritis: a critical analysis of 26 cases and of the literature. J Urol 1978; 119:589–593

41. Subramanyam BR, Megibow AJ, Raghavendra BN, Bosniak MA. Diffuse xanthogranulomatous pyelonephritis: analysis by computed tomography and sonography. Urol Radiol 1982; 4:5–9

42. Utz DC, Warren MM, Gregg JA, Ludwig J, Kelalis PP. Reversible hepatic dysfunction associated with hypernephroma. Mayo Clin Proc 1970; 45:161–169

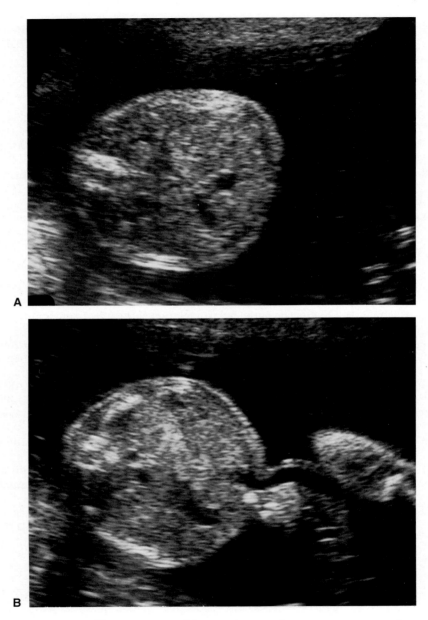

Figure 20-1. This 35-year-old woman underwent routine obstetric sonography at 22 weeks gestational age. You are shown transverse sonograms of the upper (A) and lower (B) fetal abdomen and of the fetal chest (C).

Case 20: Trisomy 18

Question 88

Which *one* of the following is the MOST likely diagnosis?

(A) Down's syndrome
(B) Beckwith-Wiedemann syndrome
(C) Turner's syndrome
(D) Limb-body wall complex
(E) Trisomy 18

The sonogram of the fetal upper abdomen (Figures 20-1A and 20-2A) shows polyhydramnios and absence of the fetal stomach. The image of the fetal lower abdomen (Figures 20-1B and 20-2B) demonstrates a small anterior abdominal wall mass at the umbilical cord insertion, consistent with an omphalocele. The four-chamber view of the heart (Figures 20-1C and 20-2C) reveals a large ventricular septal defect (VSD) and an atrial septal defect (ASD). The finding of multiple congenital anomalies is highly suggestive of a chromosomal defect, the best choice being trisomy 18 **(Option (E) is correct).** Trisomy 18 is the second most common multiple-malformation syndrome, trailing only Down's syndrome (trisomy 21) in incidence. It is present in about 1 of 3,500 to 7,000 live births but is recognized in approximately 1 in 550 pregnancies. This discrepancy is explained by an *in utero* mortality rate of approximately 70% of fetuses with trisomy 18. Of further note, 95% of live-born infants will not survive the first year. A striking association is seen with intrauterine growth retardation (IUGR), which often occurs early, is severe, and affects about 85% of fetuses. Polyhydramnios, rarely seen in fetuses with IUGR, is present in about 30% of fetuses with trisomy 18. A multitude of anomalies affecting all organ systems have been reported. Cardiovascular malformations, present in over 90%, include VSD, aortic and pulmonic valvular defects, ASD, atrioventricular septal defect (AVSD), and double-outlet right ventricle. The hands are held in a clenched position with overlapping digits in about 70% of cases (Figure 20-3A). Other skeletal anomalies include rocker-bottom feet and clubfoot. Abnormalities of the

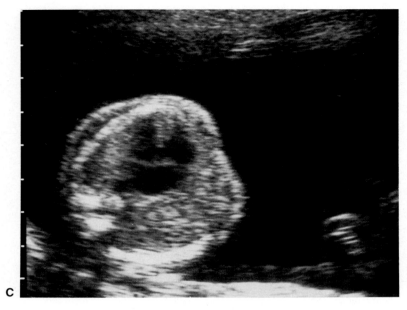

C

Figure 20-1 (Continued)

gastrointestinal tract are present in up to 40% of affected fetuses; they include abdominal-wall defects (omphalocele, hernia), diaphragmatic hernia, and esophageal atresia/tracheoesophageal fistula. Renal anomalies are seen in under 50%; they include horseshoe, ectopic, duplex, and hydronephrotic kidneys (Figure 20-3B). Central nervous system abnormalities are infrequent but include cerebellar hypoplasia, hydrocephalus, and neural tube defects. Choroid plexus cysts are noted in 20 to 30% of fetuses with trisomy 18 (Figure 20-3C), in contrast to the 1% rate in the general population. Until recently, all reported patients with trisomy 18 and choroid plexus cysts also had associated anomalies detected. A few recent reports of isolated choroid plexus cysts as the only finding in a fetus with trisomy 18 lend support to the argument that an amniocentesis should be performed when any choroid plexus cyst is identified. Controversy exists, however, and a prudent philosophy suggests a thorough and complete fetal survey when any fetal anomaly is detected.

Down's syndrome (Option (A)) has an overall live birth incidence of 1 in 660 to 1,000. The risk rises dramatically with advanced maternal age, yet most affected fetuses are found in mothers under 34 years of age. About 20% of fetuses with Down's syndrome are delivered by the 5% of pregnant women beyond 34 years of age. A 25 to 30% intrauterine death rate has been observed. The number and frequency of sonographically

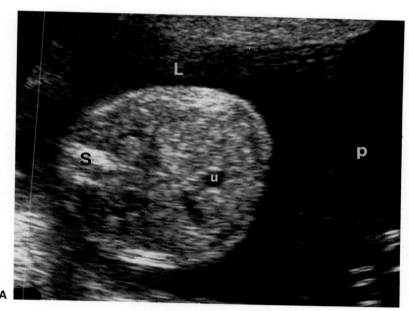

Figure 20-2 (Same as Figure 20-1). Trisomy 18 with multiple congenital anomalies in a fetus at 22 weeks gestational age. (A) A transverse sonogram of the fetal upper abdomen reveals no stomach. Marked polyhydramnios (p) is apparent. S = spine; u = umbilical vein within liver; L = left side of abdomen. (B) A transverse image of the fetal lower abdomen shows a small anterior abdominal wall mass protruding into the base of the umbilical cord (arrow), adjacent to the umbilical vein (u). The echogenic content of the mass appeared to be only bowel. S = spine; p = polyhydramnios. (C) A transverse image of the fetal thorax shows a four-chamber view of the heart with the apex directed toward the left (L). Both a VSD and, more posteriorly, an ASD (arrows) are present. S = spine; p = polyhydramnios.

detectable fetal anomalies are considerably less with trisomy 21 than with trisomy 18. Cardiovascular defects, classically AVSD (AV communis or endocardial cushion defect), VSD, and ASD (Figure 20-4), are present in 40%. Duodenal atresia (Figure 20-5), pleural effusions, and hydrops are seen in fewer than 20%. A short fifth middle phalanx and clinodactyly are present in 50 to 60% of affected fetuses, although sonographic detection of these anomalies is difficult and time-consuming. Affected newborns have a propensity to short stature and excessive soft tissue over the posterior neck, both of which may be identified in 30 to 50% of fetuses *in utero* through measurement of the femur and nuchal region, respectively. Abdominal wall defects are not a feature of trisomy 21. The pattern of anomalies in the test case is less likely to be due to trisomy 21 than trisomy 18.

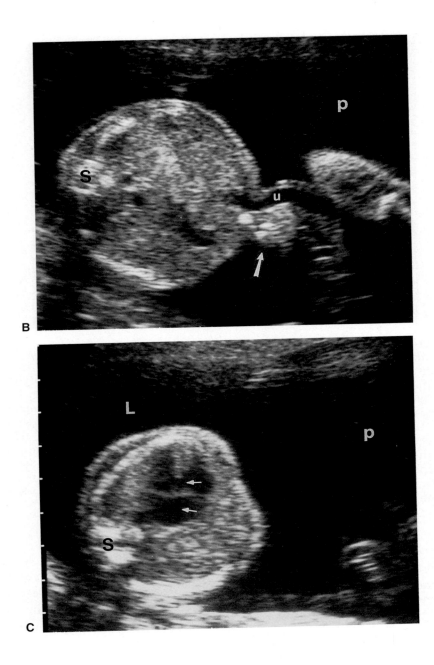

An omphalocele is identified in about 10% of fetuses with the Beck-with-Wiedemann syndrome (Option (B)), but the gastrointestinal tract obstruction and structural cardiac defects present in the test case are not consistent with this diagnosis. Approximately 5 to 10% of all omphalo-

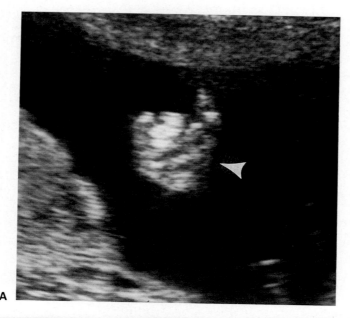

A

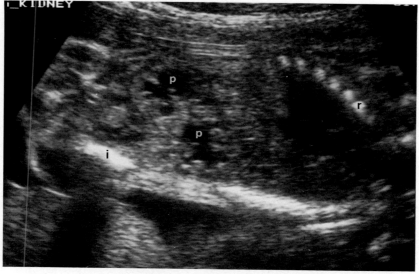

B

Figure 20-3. Same patient as in Figures 20-1 and 20-2. Trisomy 18. (A) An image of a fetal hand shows the clenched-fist appearance typical of this disorder (arrowhead). No change from this position was noted during scanning. (B) Roughly coronal image of the fetal trunk through the ribs (r) and iliac crest (i). There is bilateral renal pelvicaliectasis (p) consistent with ureteropelvic junction obstructions. (C) An off-axis image through the fetal brain shows bilateral choroid plexus cysts (arrowheads). c = cisterna magna.

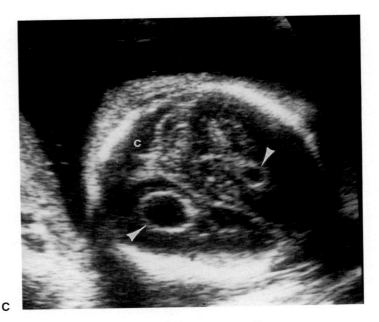

Figure 20-3 (Continued)

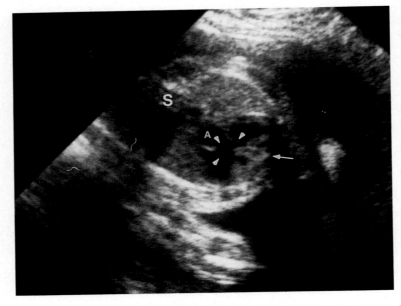

Figure 20-4. Atrioventricular septal defect in a fetus with trisomy 21. A transverse image through the thorax and a four-chamber view of the heart shows wide communication between both atria and ventricles (arrowheads). On real-time imaging, abnormal motion of the AV valves was also apparent. A = left atrium; S = spine. The arrow indicates the cardiac apex and ventricular septum anteriorly.

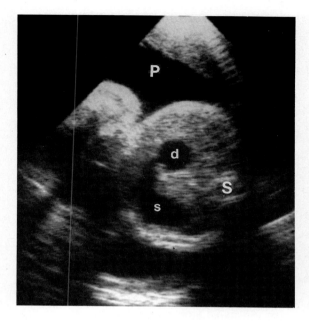

Figure 20-5. Duodenal atresia in a fetus with trisomy 21. A transverse image of the upper abdomen shows the "double bubble" sign with visualization of a fluid-filled stomach (s) and fluid-filled duodenum (d), connected in this plane by the pylorus. Polyhydramnios (P) is present. S = spine.

celes are seen in fetuses with this syndrome, however. Other major associated features that can be detected prenatally include macroglossia, macrosomia, and nephromegaly. Prenatal detection of macroglossia will alert the delivery team to the potential need for airway support.

The major detectable sonographic features of Turner's syndrome (Option (C)) are bilateral cervical cystic hygromas and nonimmune hydrops fetalis; the latter variably manifest as ascites, pleural or pericardial effusions, or subcutaneous edema (Figure 20-6). The incidence of Turner's syndrome is about 1 in 5,000 live births, but it is estimated that fewer than 1% of 45 XO conceptuses survive to live birth. As many as 10% of first-trimester abortuses have an XO karyotype, and for those that survive to the second trimester the high morbidity continues, particularly for fetuses with the larger hygromas and more extensive hydropic change. About 20% of affected fetuses have cardiovascular defects, including aortic coarctation, bicuspid aortic valve, valvular aortic stenosis, and hypoplastic left heart. Only the last of these is detectable on the standard four-chamber view of the heart, and the sensitivity for the others is low even on evaluation of the great vessels. The anomalies apparent in the test case differ from those expected for fetuses with Turner's syndrome.

The body wall defect seen in fetuses with the limb-body wall complex (LBWC) (Option (D)), a uniformly fatal anomaly, is more extensive than

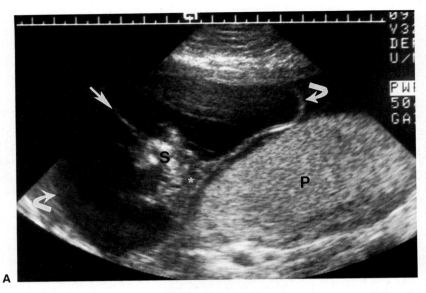

A

Figure 20-6. Turner's syndrome. (A) A transverse image through the fetal neck shows the spine (S), anterior soft tissues (✱), and massive, bilateral, posterolateral cystic hygromas (curved arrows). The midline nuchal ligament, typical of cervical hygromas, is noted (straight arrow). Cervical cystic hygromas can achieve such huge proportions that they may simulate amniotic fluid and can be overlooked on brief perusal, as in this case, where one lateral margin cannot be discerned since it abuts the uterine wall. P = placenta. (B) A transverse image of the abdomen through the stomach (white s) and spine (black S) shows extensive subcutaneous edema (arrows), typical of hydropic change. This case is atypical in that no ascites is present, and such subcutaneous edema is usually the last manifestation of serious hydrops fetalis. This points out the variable appearances possible with fetal hydrops. The association of large bilateral cervical hygromas with fetal hydrops is highly suggestive of Turner's syndrome and usually causes fetal death *in utero.*

a simple omphalocele. It generally involves the lateral as well as the anterior aspect of the abdomen, with herniation of a large component of the abdominal organs (Figure 20-7A and B), and often extends into the thorax. Major fetal disruptions are possible, including limb amputations (Figure 20-7C), marked scoliosis, facial clefts, and exencephaly. The umbilical cord is short or absent, with the anomalous portions of the fetus closely opposed to the placenta and entangled in the membranes, resulting in fetal disruptions similar to those seen with the amnion rupture sequence. A vascular insult to the early developing embryo is thought to play a role in causing the severe defects noted with this entity. None of the features of the LBWC are seen in the test case.

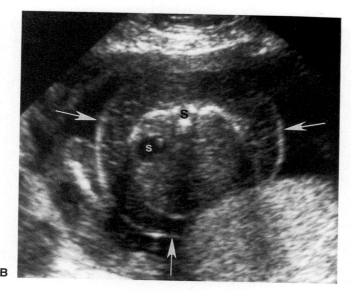

B

Figure 20-6 (Continued)

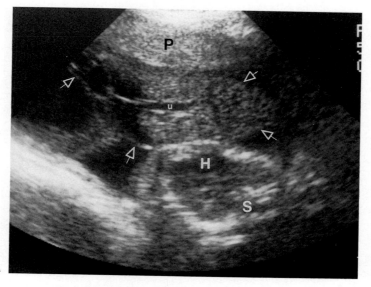

A

Figure 20-7. Limb-body wall complex in a fetus at 16 weeks gestational age. (A) A transverse image of the thorax through the heart (H) and spine (S) shows extensive herniation of liver and adjacent membranes (arrows) anteriorly. The liver and entangling membranes were noted on real-time imaging to be adherent to the placenta (P). u = umbilical vein in liver.

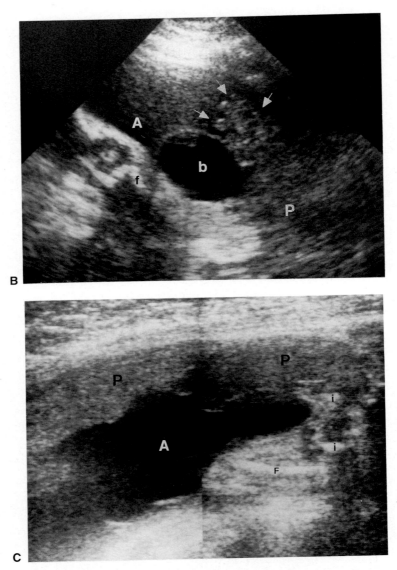

Figure 20-7 (Continued). Limb-body wall complex in a fetus at 16 weeks gestational age. (B) An angled transverse image through the low pelvis (P) and left thigh (f = distal femur) shows a large bladder (b) and loops of bowel (arrows) herniated into the amniotic cavity (A). (C) A transverse image through the low pelvis and thighs shows the left femur (F) and both ischial tuberosities (i). No right lower extremity was present, and the right side of the fetal pelvis was fused to the placenta (P). A = amniotic fluid.

Question 89

Concerning fetal abdominal wall defects,

   (A) gastroschisis is frequently associated with genitourinary tract anomalies

   (B) in up to 60% of cases, omphalocele is associated with other anomalies

   (C) there is a 40 to 50% chance of an underlying chromosomal defect when an omphalocele is found

   (D) a small omphalocele containing no liver has a lower probability of an associated chromosomal anomaly than does one containing liver

   (E) scoliosis is a usual feature of limb-body wall complex

Anterior abdominal wall defects are a relatively common group of disorders, which have widely divergent sonographic features and prognoses. Several of these abnormalities are isolated lesions amenable to postnatal surgical repair and a good quality of life; others have either major intrinsic malformations or associations with other conditions that are fatal or present the utmost challenge to the postnatal surgical and medical teams.

Gastroschisis is a full-thickness defect in the abdominal wall, usually in a right periumbilical locus, through which there is herniation of bowel into the amniotic cavity. It has been suggested that abnormal involution of the embryologic right umbilical vein or interruption of the omphalomesenteric artery leads to a defect in the developing abdominal wall. Gastroschisis is usually not associated with chromosomal abnormalities or other fetal anomalies, except those directly related to the defect **(Option (A) is false).** Ischemia due to torsion or compression of vessels within the herniated segments and inflammatory changes of the bowel wall secondary to chemical irritation from the amniotic fluid are believed to be responsible for the development of gastrointestinal tract complications, including bowel atresias, stenoses, and obstructions, in about 25% of cases (Figure 20-8). Growth retardation is common; together with neonatal sepsis and gastrointestinal tract and operative complications, this results in a 10 to 15% mortality for gastroschisis.

Embryologically, the anterior abdominal wall is formed by the growth and fusion of the paired lateral, caudal, and cephalic folds, which are respectively at, below, and above the level of the umbilicus. Failure of fusion of one or more of these paired structures will result in characteristic anterior-wall defects. An omphalocele results from a failure of lateral-fold fusion with a subsequent defect in the umbilical ring, through which the cord normally inserts to the fetal abdomen. The consequence of failed fusion of the caudal folds is bladder extrophy, with variable degrees of anterior-wall disruption and associated bladder exteriorization. Defects in the cephalic folds, which normally merge superiorly to the umbilicus,

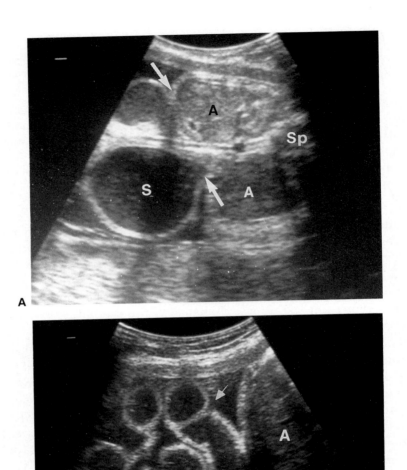

Figure 20-8. Gastroschisis in a fetus at 32 weeks gestational age. (A) A transverse image of the fetal abdomen (A) at the level of the umbilicus shows an extensive anterior-wall defect (arrows) and mass, which contains part of the stomach (S). Sp = spine. The lesion was so large that identification of a separate umbilical cord insertion was not possible. (B) A sonogram of the mass shows multiple thick-walled loops of bowel (arrows) floating free without any covering membrane, a typical feature of gastroschisis. The thickened bowel walls result from inflammatory changes due to a chronic chemical peritonitis from contact with amniotic fluid. A = abdomen.

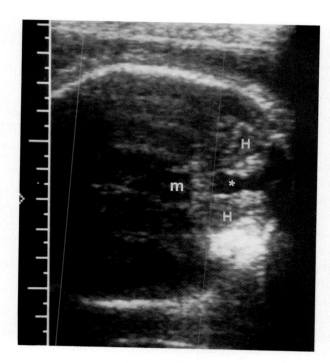

Figure 20-9. Dandy-Walker variant in a patient with omphalocele. An angled transverse image of the posterior fossa shows the hypoechoic cerebellar hemispheres (H) separated by fluid (*) in the midline, where the echogenic vermis should normally be seen. With absence of the vermis, the enlarged fourth ventricle communicates posteriorly with the cisterna magna through the defect. m = brain stem.

result in the most severe abnormalities, with extension into the thorax. Exteriorization of a split sternum, diaphragm, pericardium, and heart, in association with an abdominal wall lesion, is termed the pentalogy of Cantrell. Complex cardiac disease is usually present. Sonographic findings of omphalocele include herniation of bowel, liver, and occasionally stomach into a sac composed of a blended amnionic and peritoneal membrane. Ascitic fluid can be seen within the sac. The umbilical vessels traverse the hernia sac and exit it close to its apex, forming the umbilical cord. In contrast to gastroschisis, the detection of an omphalocele has considerable implications beyond the defect itself. Associated fetal anomalies are common, occurring in 15 to 64% of cases **(Option (B) true).** These frequently include abnormalities of the central nervous system (CNS) (Figure 20-9), heart, genitourinary tract, and skeletal system. From 35 to 58% of fetuses with an omphalocele have a chromosomal abnormality **(Option (C) is true).** A significant majority will have trisomy 18, but occasionally trisomy 13, or, rarely, triploidy are also found. The combined rate of fetal anomalies and/or chromosomal abnormalities associated with an omphalocele is 67 to 88%. Interestingly, the probability of an underlying chromosomal defect is greater for a small omphalocele not containing liver than it is for a larger defect (Figure 20-1B)

(Option (D) is false). Clearly, prenatal sonographic identification of an omphalocele should precipitate a thorough search for other anomalies, as well as an amniocentesis for karyotypic evaluation. About 5 to 10% of neonates with an omphalocele also have Beckwith-Wiedemann syndrome, and 12% of neonates with Beckwith-Wiedemann syndrome have an omphalocele. Affected neonates may have macroglossia, organomegaly, neonatal hypoglycemia, hemihypertrophy, and a propensity for Wilms' tumor.

LBWC is a lethal malformation with an extensive lateral body wall defect that often involves the thorax as well as the abdomen, craniofacial clefting and calvarial defects, and limb amputations. Embryologically, the normal separation of the intraembryonic celom (abdominal cavity) from the extraembryonic celom (chorionic cavity) fails to occur. Since this developmental process is centered about the umbilicus, there is resultant herniation of fetal abdominal organs into the extraembryonic celom, where they are essentially attached to the placenta by either a very short or no umbilical cord. The amnion and chorion also fail to fuse properly and can further entangle other fetal structures, causing the sporadic amputations and craniofacial clefting similar to that seen with the amniotic band syndrome. Uneven traction on the entrapped, developing fetus results in the typical severe and frequently sharply angulated scoliosis **(Option (E) is true).**

Question 90

Concerning the fetal anterior abdominal wall,

(A) the "mass" due to physiologic midgut herniation is not seen after 12 weeks gestational age

(B) an isolated omphalocele has a prognosis similar to that of gastroschisis

(C) maternal serum α-fetoprotein levels are higher with a gastroschisis than with an omphalocele

(D) typical sonographic features of gastroschisis include a right paraumbilical defect containing bowel but no liver

(E) typical sonographic features of omphalocele include a midline mass with a limiting membrane

The normal embryologic development of the fetal abdomen includes a herniation of the midgut into the base of the umbilical cord, presumably to allow adequate room for development of other organs. This herniation can be detected sonographically as a small, echogenic mass at the base of the umbilical cord, simulating a small anterior abdominal wall defect. On transabdominal or transvaginal scanning, midgut herniation can be seen as early as 7 to 8 weeks. When first detectable, the base of the cord where the midgut is located measures about 4 mm in greatest dimension. With fetal growth, this gradually increases to a maximum dimension of 7 mm. The midgut then returns to a more capacious abdominal cavity between 10.5 and 11 weeks gestational age. By 12 weeks gestational age the umbilical cord at the insertion site into the fetus contains only vessels and supporting structures, and any anterior-wall mass is therefore indicative of a pathologic entity **(Option (A) is true).**

The prognosis for a fetus with an omphalocele relates primarily to the complications inherent to the associated anomalies and chromosomal abnormalities that are present in 67 to 88% of cases. With such concurrent abnormalities, mortality exceeds 80%. However, when an isolated omphalocele is present, there is only about a 10% mortality rate, which is due predominantly to complications from sepsis and surgical repair. This approximates the mortality for gastroschisis, which results similarly from surgical complications as well as from ischemic injury to bowel **(Option (B) is true).** The striking difference in the mortality figures for isolated and complicated omphaloceles emphasizes the importance of accurately classifying an anterior-wall lesion to differentiate omphalocele from gastroschisis and, subsequently, to confirm or exclude other significant fetal structural abnormalities.

α-Fetoprotein (AFP) is a fetus-specific protein produced in the fetal liver. Any break in the integrity of the fetal skin, as with an open neural tube defect, will result in an increased transudation of AFP into the amniotic fluid, where it can be readily detected in a fluid sample obtained by amniocentesis. By mechanisms that are not entirely clear, small but measurable quantities of AFP, both normal and abnormal, can be found in the maternal serum. Measurement of the maternal serum AFP (MS-AFP) level has been used primarily as a screening test for the detection of neural tube defects. The MS-AFP level can be elevated for causes other than neural tube defects, however. MS-AFP levels vary with gestational age, and accurate dates must be known to interpret the results properly. In 30 to 40% of cases the MS-AFP level is erroneously thought to be elevated, because of assignment of the wrong dates. Multiple gestations will cause increased production of AFP and are responsible for 10% of high values. Fetal demise, placental hemorrhage, and idiopathic causes also lead to elevated levels. Several other fetal anomalies have been associated with high MS-AFP levels. Abdominal wall defects are the most common, since an obvious defect in the fetal skin allows for transudation of fetal fluids. An omphalocele does have a nominal covering membrane, in contrast to the open communication between amniotic and peritoneal cavities with a gastroschisis; therefore, an omphalocele is associated with lower levels of MS-AFP (which also have more overlap

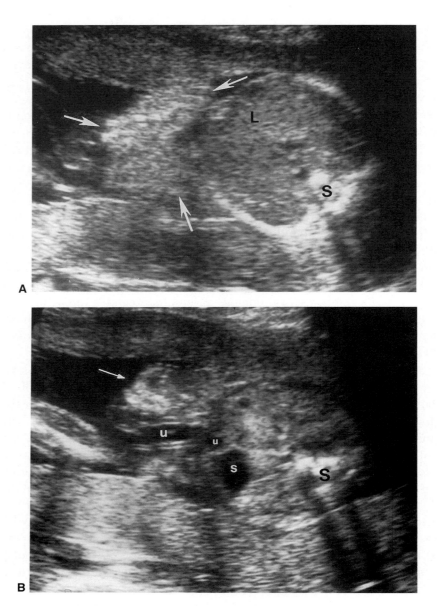

Figure 20-10. Gastroschisis in a fetus at 22 weeks gestational age. (A) A transverse image through the abdomen shows the liver (L) and spine (S), with a large, somewhat irregularly marginated anterior wall mass (arrows). (B) An image of the cord insertion shows the umbilical vein (u) passing from the abdomen to the cord, with the mass (arrow) emerging from the abdomen to the right of the cord insertion site. The left-sided stomach (white "s") and spine (black "S") are noted.

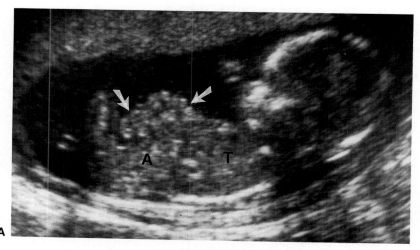

A

Figure 20-11. Gastroschisis in a fetus at 14 weeks gestational age. (A) A longitudinal scan of the fetus through the abdomen (A) and thorax (T) shows a scalloped, nodular-appearing anterior wall mass (arrows). (B) A transverse image through the normal cord insertion (wide arrow) shows the right thigh (T), the spine (S), and right-sided herniation of bowel (thin arrow)

with normal levels) than is a gastroschisis **(Option (C) is true).** Sacrococcygeal teratoma and cystic hygroma can also cause high MS-AFP levels. Low levels of MS-AFP have been associated with trisomy 21, with about 15 to 20% of affected fetuses detected in this way. To reach even this low level of sensitivity, however, amniocentesis must be performed in 7 to 9% of unaffected pregnancies. By using combination screening of maternal serum for AFP, estriol, and human chorionic gonadotropin ("triple test"), the sensitivity for the detection of trisomy 21 increases about threefold over that of the measurement of AFP levels alone.

The typical sonographic features of gastroschisis include a paraumbilical, usually right-sided, full-thickness defect in the abdominal wall through which loops of bowel herniate into the amniotic cavity (Figure 20-10A). A normal cord insertion site can often be identified (Figure 20-10B), especially with Doppler interrogation. The herniated bowel is not limited by a membrane but is free to float within the amniotic cavity, resulting in a scalloped or frankly irregular external margin (Figure 20-11). The variable appearance of the exteriorized bowel becomes more apparent as gestation advances and the bowel elongates. Liver is not generally seen in a gastroschisis; no limiting membrane is present and the cord insertion is normal **(Option (D) is true).**

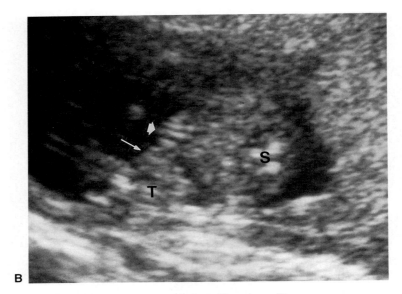

Figure 20-11 (Continued)

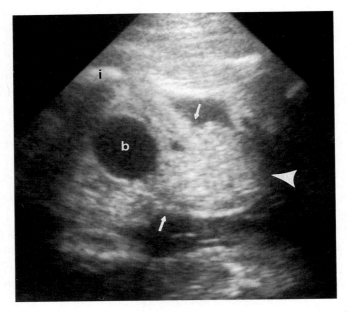

Figure 20-12. Omphalocele in a fetus at 26 weeks gestational age. An angled transverse scan of the pelvis and anterior abdominal wall shows the bladder (b), iliac crest (i), and a broad-based, smoothly marginated, anterior abdominal wall mass (arrowhead) that is herniating through the anterior abdominal wall (arrows). No separate cord insertion site is identified. The homogeneous echotexture of the mass is most consistent with liver.

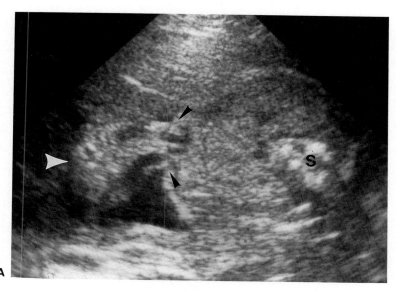

A

Figure 20-13. Omphalocele in a fetus at 24 weeks gestational age. (A) A transverse image through the umbilicus shows a narrow-necked (black arrowheads) anterior-wall mass (white arrowhead), which involves the umbilical cord vessels. This small lesion was believed to contain no liver, increasing the odds of a chromosomal abnormality, but the karyotype was normal. S = spine. (B) A transverse image of the abdomen shows the spine (S) and the anterior-wall mass (white arrowhead). The umbilical vein (U) is marginal in the neck (black arrowheads) of the lesion, potentially simulating a gastroschisis. However, it can be seen to course within the smoothly marginated confines of the mass for several centimeters. (C) A transverse image of the abdomen (A) delineates the smooth-walled omphalocele anteriorly (arrows), with the cord (c), which is mildly enlarged, re-forming at its apex.

The typical sonographic features of an omphalocele include a protruding anterior-wall mass that encompasses the cord insertion (Figure 20-12). It has a smooth, rounded external surface delineated by an enveloping membrane **(Option (E) is true)**, and the cord can be identified arising from the apex of the mass. When the umbilical vein courses in the edge of an omphalocele as it penetrates the abdominal wall, it can simulate a gastroschisis (Figure 20-13A). With careful scanning the umbilical vessels can usually be seen within the sac, however, oriented close to the membrane often for several centimeters before penetrating to re-form the umbilical cord (Figure 20-13B and C). Fluid can accumulate within the sac, optimizing visualization of the surrounding membrane. Bowel is generally noted within an omphalocele, which may or may not

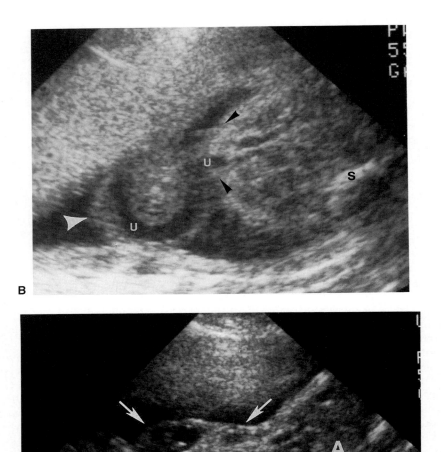

B

C

contain liver. Herniated liver can often be identified by its internal vascular anatomy. Other abdominal organs, including the gallbladder and stomach, are occasionally seen in larger lesions.

Question 91

Concerning fetal chromosomal abnormalities,

(A) the risk of trisomy 18 in a fetus with an isolated choroid plexus cyst is 5 to 10%
(B) karyotyping is indicated following detection of gastroschisis
(C) chromosomal abnormalities are associated with 15% of early spontaneous abortions
(D) identification of more than one anomaly increases the probability of a chromosomal abnormality
(E) the trisomy syndrome most frequently associated with holoprosencephaly is Down's syndrome

There is continuing controversy about the association of choroid plexus cysts with trisomy 18. About 1 to 3% of normal fetuses have one or more choroid plexus cysts (Figure 20-14). They are generally detected in the second trimester and resolve by the beginning of the third trimester. Various studies have found that 20 to 70% of fetuses with trisomy 18 have choroid plexus cysts (Figure 20-3C). In most fetuses with trisomy 18, however, multiple anomalies are identified, even prenatally (Figures 20-1 and 20-3A and B). However, there are reported cases of fetuses with trisomy 18 and isolated choroid plexus cysts without other detectable abnormalities. It is estimated that about 1% of fetuses with choroid plexus cysts also have trisomy 18, and the vast majority of these have other detectable anomalies on detailed fetal survey. The frequency of trisomy 18 in a fetus with an isolated choroid plexus cyst is certainly much lower than 1% **(Option (A) is false).** Large, bilateral cysts are not necessarily more likely to be associated with trisomy 18, and cysts on the order of 3 to 5 mm in diameter have been reported in affected fetuses.

In contrast to omphalocele, which has a 35 to 58% frequency of associated chromosomal abnormality, there is no reported association of gastroschisis with chromosomal abnormalities **(Option (B) is therefore false).**

It has been estimated that up to 43% of pregnancies fail, many before the threshold for clinical detection. About 15% of clinically known pregnancies end in a spontaneous abortion, most prior to 10 weeks gestational age. Such early fetal loss is associated with chromosomal abnormalities in 30 to 60% of cases **(Option (C) is false).** Trisomies, monosomy, triploidy, and tetraploidy, as well as other unusual chromosomal defects not generally associated with stillbirths or term deliveries, are most frequently seen with early pregnancy wastage. Most triploid pregnancies end in first-trimester spontaneous abortions. Occasionally such a fetus survives into the second or third trimester. Multiple congenital anomalies without any particular pattern are the norm (Figure 20-15).

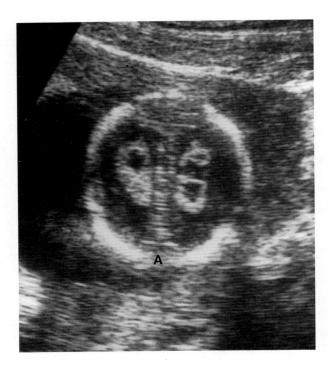

Figure 20-14. Choroid plexus cysts. A transverse image through the cerebral ventricles shows bilateral large choroid plexus cysts. No other anomalies were identified, and the karyotype was normal. A = anterior.

Classically, early and severe growth retardation with oligohydramnios is noted (Figure 20-16). Triploid pregnancies are also generally associated with partial molar changes in the placenta, with less obvious and more-focal hydropic change than is seen with a complete mole (Figure 20-15). In contrast to the very high incidence of chromosomal defects in fetuses that undergo early spontaneous abortion, about 4 to 6% of stillbirths and 0.5% of live births have a chromosomal abnormality.

A single fetal structural defect is usually associated with a multifactoral mode of transmission, including genetic and environmental influences. Chromosomal abnormalities tend to manifest multiple anomalies, however, many of which are readily identifiable by sonographic examination. If a fetal anomaly is detected, there is an 11 to 35% probability that a chromosomal defect is present. In most fetuses ultimately proven to have a chromosomal abnormality, more than one anomaly is detected on careful sonographic examination. It follows that the identification of multiple defects, each with a low independent probability of occurring, are most probably related by some unifying factor, such as a chromosomal abnormality **(Option (D) is true).**

Down's syndrome (trisomy 21) does not manifest major CNS structural defects **(Option (E) is false).** Major CNS structural abnormalities

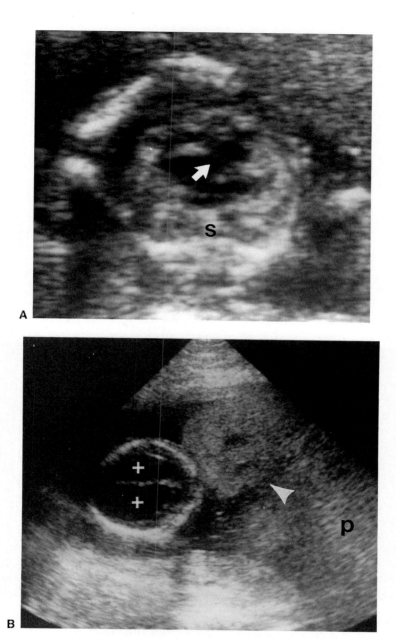

Figure 20-15. Triploidy in a fetus at 18 weeks gestational age. (A) A transverse image of the thorax with an attempted four-chamber view of the heart shows a globular heart with a VSD (arrow). S = spine. (B) A transverse image of the fetal head shows bilateral hydrocephalus (+). The placenta (p) is generally enlarged and contains an area of early hydropic change (arrowhead). Pathologically, the placenta had findings consistent with a partial mole.

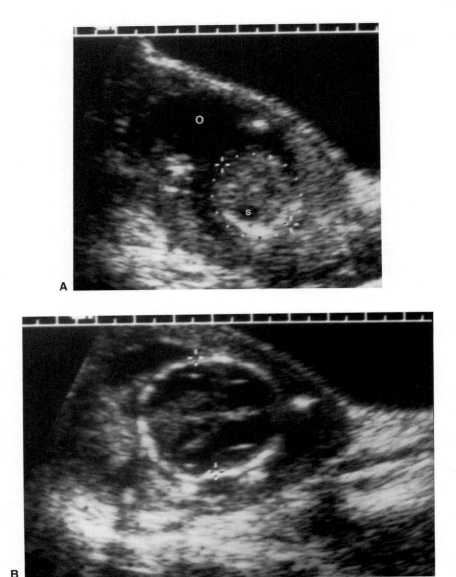

Figure 20-16. Triploidy in a fetus at 15 weeks gestational age. (A) A longitudinal image of the uterine cavity shows oligohydramnios (o) and an abdominal circumference (delineated by markers) consistent with 13 weeks gestational age. s = stomach. Early and severe growth retardation, plus oligohydramnios, suggests serious fetal compromise including chromosomal abnormalities such as triploidy. (B) A transverse image of the head shows a biparietal diameter (delineated by cursors) of 15 weeks, with subtle ventricular dilatation, which was confirmed at autopsy.

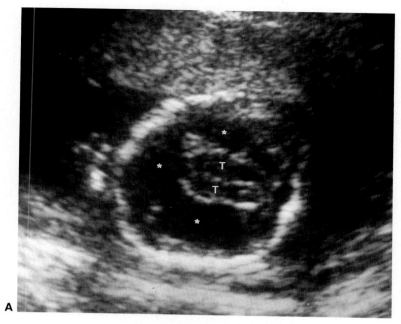

A

Figure 20-17. Trisomy 13 with alobar holoprosencephaly in a fetus at 16 weeks gestational age. (A) A transverse image of the brain shows fused thalami (T) and a unilocular ventricle communicating across the anterior midline (✳). (B) A transverse image of the abdomen at the level of the umbilicus shows the spine (s) posteriorly and an anterior abdominal wall mass (arrows) consistent with an omphalocele.

are seen in fetuses with trisomies 13 and 18 and triploidy, however. About 40 to 60% of fetuses with holoprosencephaly have a chromosomal anomaly. Most have trisomy 13 (Figure 20-17A), but holoprosencephaly can also be seen in fetuses with triploidy and, rarely, 13q– and 18p– syndromes. A multitude of other abnormalities can be identified with trisomy 13; these include microcephaly, microphthalmia, cleft lip and palate, hydrocephalus, cerebellar hypoplasia, polydactyly and syndactyly, radial aplasia, cardiac septal defects, anterior-wall defects (Figure 20-17B), polycystic disease, and hydronephrosis.

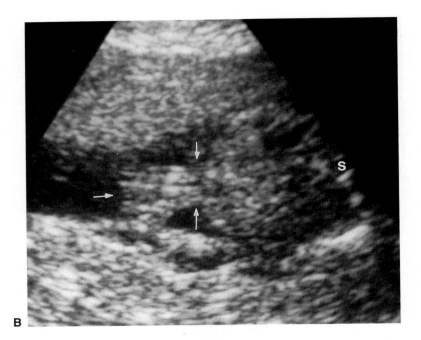

B

Question 92

Concerning Down's syndrome,

    (A) on sonography, affected fetuses usually have short femurs
    (B) about 10% of affected fetuses have duodenal atresia
    (C) it occurs in about 30% of fetuses with duodenal atresia
    (D) it is associated with fetal hydrops
    (E) septal defects are the most frequently imaged cardiac anomalies

Several studies have reported the sonographic detection of short femurs for gestational age in some second-trimester fetuses with Down's
syndrome. In one early study, using a ratio of actual to expected femur
length, values of 0.91 or less were 68% sensitive and 98% specific for detecting trisomy 21. More recent studies have been less optimistic, with
shortened femurs identified in only 10 to 20% of affected fetuses versus
5% of normal fetuses **(Option (A) is false)**. Therefore, sonographic detection of short femur is not by itself a strong positive predictor of Down's
syndrome; however, when taken together with other findings such as
nuchal thickening (Figures 20-18 and 20-19), gastrointestinal tract obstruction, cardiac defects, and clinodactyly, its predictive value rises.

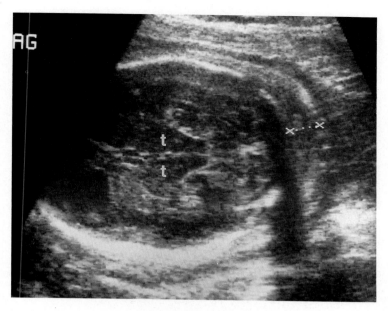

Figure 20-18. Trisomy 21 with nuchal thickening. An angled axial image through the thalami (t) and posterior fossa shows marked nuchal soft tissue thickening (cursors) posterior to the occipital bone.

Gastrointestinal tract lesions are occasionally seen in fetuses with trisomy 21. The most frequent is duodenal atresia, which is present in 8% of affected fetuses **(Option (B) is true).** Esophageal atresia with or without tracheoesophageal fistula (Figure 20-20), anorectal atresia, and omphalocele are also associated. Duodenal obstruction is present in about 1 of 5,000 live births; 75% of these newborns have other anomalies or associations, including Down's syndrome (Figure 20-21), malrotation, tracheoesophageal fistula, and imperforate anus. About one-third of fetuses with duodenal atresia have trisomy 21 **(Option (C) is true).** The prenatal sonographic detection of duodenal atresia with the classic "double bubble" sign of duodenal and gastric distension in association with polyhydramnios is generally not seen until midway through the second trimester at the earliest, making this sign insensitive as an early indicator of Down's syndrome.

Fetal hydrops is a pathologic accumulation of fluid within the fetus, arising from a multitude of causes. Sonographically, it is generally diagnosed initially by the identification of fluid within at least two serous cavities, such as ascites, pleural effusions, or a pericardial effusion. Advanced cases lead to generalized subcutaneous edema with scalp and body wall thickening of greater than 5 mm. Underlying structural abnor-

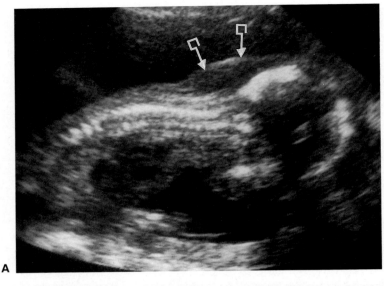

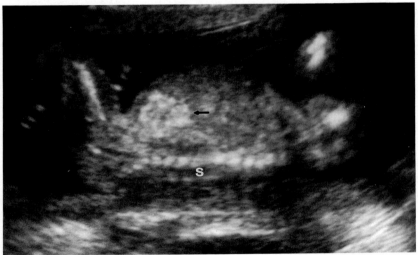

Figure 20-19. Trisomy 21 with nuchal thickening. (A) A parasagittal image shows marked nuchal thickening (arrows) posterior to the cervico-occipital region. (B) No other definite fetal abnormality was detected, but there was a suggestion on this longitudinal image of the fetus that the fetal bowel (arrow) was abnormally echogenic. s = spine. This is a controversial finding, since normal developing bowel is often quite echogenic. However, reports now exist of abnormal, usually markedly echogenic bowel in association with chromosomal abnormalities.

malities are detected in some cases, although up to 40% of cases have no known cause. Chromosomal abnormalities associated with hydrops in-

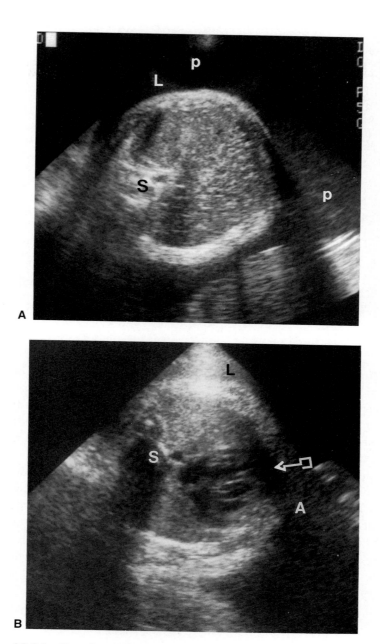

Figure 20-20. Esophageal atresia in a fetus with trisomy 21 at 21 weeks gestational age. (A) A transverse image of the fetal upper abdomen shows no stomach. Polyhydramnios (p) is present. S = spine; L = left side. (B) A transverse image of the thorax shows normal cardiac position, with the apex to the left (arrow), and no intrathoracic mass to suggest diaphragmatic hernia. S = spine; A = anterior; L = left. The combination of abdominal, thoracic, and fluid findings is most consistent with esophageal atresia.

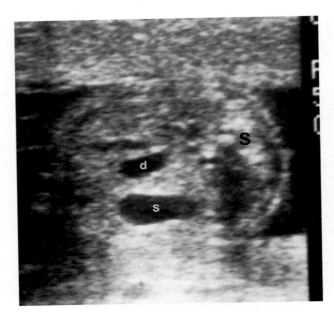

Figure 20-21. Annular pancreas in a fetus with trisomy 21. An axial image of the upper abdomen shows the "double bubble" sign with fluid in both the stomach (s) and the duodenum (d). S = spine. At autopsy, duodenal obstruction secondary to an annular pancreas was discovered.

clude Turner's syndrome (XO); trisomies 13, 18, and 21 **(Option (D) is true);** triploidy; and miscellaneous deletion syndromes. In the setting of an abnormal karyotype, fetal hydrops is most commonly associated with Turner's syndrome, usually with coexistent bilateral, large cervical cystic hygromas. Fetuses with trisomy 21 occasionally manifest identical findings or may have hydrops alone without the hygromas.

About 40% of newborns with Down's syndrome have a cardiovascular abnormality. AVSD is the most common (Figure 20-4), followed by an isolated VSD. The typical large septal defect of an AVSD is readily imaged on a four-chamber view of the heart. The sonographic detection of a VSD depends on its size and position, with an overall sensitivity of about 50% **(Option (E) is true).** ASDs also occur but are very difficult to diagnose *in utero.* A patent ductus arteriosus, not infrequent in neonates, is a normal physiologic structure in the fetus.

Question 93

Concerning fetal hydrops,

(A) the earliest sonographic finding in the fetus is pericardial fluid
(B) approximately 30% of cases are of immunologic etiology
(C) the most common cause of nonimmune hydrops is intrauterine infection
(D) the presence of associated bilateral cervical cystic hygromas suggests Turner's syndrome
(E) the mortality rate in fetuses with nonimmune hydrops exceeds 50%

Fetal hydrops refers to the accumulation of excessive fluid within the fetus. In severe cases fluid can be detected in the peritoneal, pleural, and pericardial cavities, as well as in the subcutaneous tissues (Figure 20-22). Involvement of at least two of these anatomic spaces is necessary to make the diagnosis and to exclude isolated findings not representative of hydrops. In most cases, ascites is the earliest finding and the most reliable predictor that hydrops is evolving. One early study suggested that pericardial fluid was the initial finding with impending hydrops, but this has not been upheld by others. A more recent study of affected fetuses documented several cases of initially isolated ascites, a few cases of ascites with either pleural or pericardial effusions, and several cases in which all three serous cavities were involved. In no case did an isolated pericardial effusion occur **(Option (A) is false)**.

Many entities can be associated with hydrops, although pathophysiologically there are only a limited number of common pathways leading to the end-stage findings. Hydrops fetalis has classically been divided into cases with immune causes and those with nonimmune causes; most recognized cases 40 years ago related to immune disease. Improved recognition and prevention of most of the immune causes of fetal hydrops, predominantly Rh disease, have shifted the current balance such that more than 90% of cases of hydrops are secondary to nonimmune causes **(Option (B) false)**. As Rh antigens have become less problematic due to preventive therapy with Rhogam, a greater percentage of immune hydrops now relates to other antigens including D, E, C, Kell, and Duffy. In fetuses with immune hydrops, maternal antibodies to fetal erythrocytes cause hemolysis and fetal anemia. Subsequently, intrahepatic erythropoiesis causes hepatomegaly with resultant portal hypertension, and hypoproteinemia leads to reduced oncotic pressure. Both these processes promote the development of fetal hydrops and often placentomegaly. The number of postulated mechanisms for development of nonimmune hydrops is greater, but they are often intertwined. Hypoproteinemia, infections, primary cardiac abnormalities, anemia with or without high-output failure, and malformations with mass effect can all

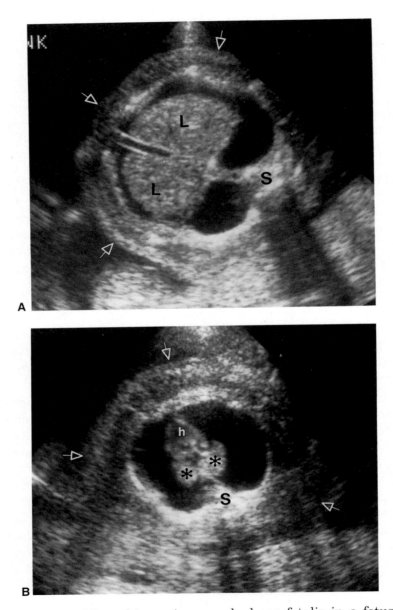

Figure 20-22. Idiopathic nonimmune hydrops fetalis in a fetus at 28 weeks gestational age. (A) A transverse image of the fetal abdomen shows the liver (L) surrounded by ascites. Arrows indicate marked subcutaneous edema. S = spine. (B) A transverse image of the thorax shows the heart (h) and diminutive lungs (✱) surrounded by large bilateral pleural effusions. Arrows indicate marked subcutaneous edema. S = spine.

alter capillary permeability, reduce colloid osmotic pressure, or increase hydrostatic pressure in arteries, veins, or lymphatics; all of these mechanisms can play a role in the pathogenesis of hydrops. Combinations of fetal abnormalities and pathologic mechanisms lead to some variability in the sonographically detected features of nonimmune hydrops. The most common etiology of hydrops is cardiac failure, usually from a conduction or valvular abnormality. Multiple-malformation syndromes or chromosomal abnormalities such as Turner's or Down's syndrome are also leading causes. Fetal anemia can arise for several nonimmune-related reasons, including twin-twin transfusion syndrome and thalassemia. Diminished venous return, which is believed to be secondary to venous obstruction by a thoracic or abdominal mass, is a frequent cause of hydrops. Proven infection is a relatively infrequent cause of hydrops **(Option (C) is false)**, although an undetected antecedent infection is possible in some of the approximately 30 to 40% of hydropic fetuses for which no etiologic diagnosis can be established.

Bilateral posterolateral cervical cystic hygromas, together with hydrops fetalis, are associated with a chromosomal abnormality in about 70 to 75% of cases. Of these, about 75 to 85% have Turner's syndrome (XO) **(Option (D) is true)**, with trisomies 18 and 21 being the other leading associations. Regardless of etiology, there is a near 100% mortality for affected fetuses.

The appearance of nonimmune hydrops usually heralds a significant underlying defect(s) that seriously compromises fetal well-being. This is reflected in the 1 in 700 to 1,000 incidence of prenatal detection of fetuses with nonimmune hydrops versus a 1 in 1,500 to 4,000 frequency at delivery. A significant percentage of affected fetuses die *in utero*, at documented rates of 50 to 90% **(Option (E) is true)**.

Richard A. Bowerman, M.D.

SUGGESTED READINGS

TRISOMY 18

1. Benacerraf BR, Miller WA, Frigoletto FD Jr. Sonographic detection of fetuses with trisomies 13 and 18: accuracy and limitations. Am J Obstet Gynecol 1988; 158:404–409
2. Chan L, Hixson JL, Laifer SA, Marchese SG, Martin JG, Hill LM. A sonographic and karyotypic study of second-trimester fetal choroid plexus cysts. Obstet Gynecol 1989; 73:703–706

3. Chinn DH, Miller EI, Worthy LM, Towers CV. Sonographically detected fetal choroid plexus cysts. Frequency and association with aneuploidy. J Ultrasound Med 1991; 10:255–258

4. Chitkara U, Cogswell C, Norton K, Wilkins IA, Mehalek K, Berkowitz RL. Choroid plexus cysts in the fetus: a benign anatomic variant or pathologic entity? Report of 41 cases and review of the literature. Obstet Gynecol 1988; 72:185–189

5. DeRoo TR, Harris RD, Sargent SK, Denholm TA, Crow HC. Fetal choroid plexus cysts: prevalence, clinical significance, and sonographic appearance. AJR 1988; 151:1179–1181

6. Fitzsimmons J, Wilson D, Pascoe-Mason J, Shaw CM, Cyr DR, Mack LA. Choroid plexus cysts in fetuses with trisomy 18. Obstet Gynecol 1989; 73:257–260

7. Gabrielli S, Reece EA, Pilu G, et al. The clinical significance of prenatally diagnosed choroid plexus cysts. Am J Obstet Gynecol 1989; 160:1207–1210

8. Nadel AS, Bromley BS, Frigoletto FD Jr, Estroff JA, Benacerraf BR. Isolated choroid plexus cysts in the second-trimester fetus: is amniocentesis really indicated? Radiology 1992; 185:545–548

9. Ostlere SJ, Irving HC, Lilford RJ. A prospective study of the incidence and significance of fetal choroid plexus cysts. Prenat Diagn 1989; 9:205–211

10. Perpignano MC, Cohen HL, Klein VR, et al. Fetal choroid plexus cysts: beware the smaller cyst. Radiology 1992; 182:715–717

DOWN'S SYNDROME

11. Adams MM, Erickson JD, Layde PM, Oakley GP. Down's syndrome. Recent trends in the United States. JAMA 1981; 246:758–760

12. Benacerraf BR, Barss VA, Laboda LA. A sonographic sign for the detection in the second trimester of the fetus with Down's syndrome. Am J Obstet Gynecol 1985; 151:1078–1079

13. Benacerraf BR, Laboda LA, Frigoletto FD. Thickened nuchal fold in fetuses not at risk for aneuploidy. Radiology 1992; 184:239–242

14. Perrella R, Duerinckx AJ, Grant EG, Tessler F, Tabsh K, Crandall RF. Second-trimester sonographic diagnosis of Down syndrome: role of femur-length shortening and nuchal-fold thickening. AJR 1988; 151:981–985

15. Peters MT, Lockwood CJ, Miller WA. The efficacy of fetal sonographic biometry in Down syndrome screening. Am J Obstet Gynecol 1989; 161:297–300

16. Weingast GR, Hopper KD, Gottesfeld SA, Manco-Johnson ML. Congenital lymphangiectasia with fetal cystic hygroma: report of two cases with coexistent Down's syndrome. JCU 1988; 16:663–668

ANTERIOR ABDOMINAL WALL—GENERAL

17. Bair JH, Russ PD, Pretorius DH, Manchester D, Manco-Johnson ML. Fetal omphalocele and gastroschisis: a review of 24 cases. AJR 1986; 147:1047–1051

18. Copel JA, Pilu G, Kleinman CS. Congenital heart disease and extracardiac anomalies: associations and indications for fetal echocardiography. Am J Obstet Gynecol 1986; 154:1121–1132

19. Crawford DC, Chapman MG, Allan LD. Echocardiography in the investigation of anterior abdominal wall defects in the fetus. Br J Obstet Gynecol 1985; 92:1034–1036

20. Cyr DR, Mack LA, Schoenecker SA, et al. Bowel migration in the normal fetus: US detection. Radiology 1986; 161:119–121

21. deVries PA. The pathogenesis of gastroschisis and omphalocele. J Pediatr Surg 1980; 15:245–251

22. Ghidini A, Sirtori M, Romero R, Hobbins JC. Prenatal diagnosis of pentalogy of Cantrell. J Ultrasound Med 1988; 7:567–572

23. Kirk EP, Wah RM. Obstetric management of the fetus with omphalocele or gastroschisis: a review and report of one hundred twelve cases. Am J Obstet Gynecol 1983; 146:512–518

24. Lindfors KK, McGahan JP, Walter JP. Fetal omphalocele and gastroschisis: pitfalls in sonographic diagnosis. AJR 1986; 147:797–800

25. Mahony BS, Filly RA, Callen PW, Golbus MS. The amniotic band syndrome: antenatal sonographic diagnosis and potential pitfalls. Am J Obstet Gynecol 1985; 152:63–68

26. Mann L, Ferguson-Smith MA, Desai M, Gibson AA, Raine PA. Prenatal assessment of anterior abdominal wall defects and their prognosis. Prenat Diagn 1984; 4:427–435

27. Mayer T, Black R, Matlak ME, Johnson DG. Gastroschisis and omphalocele. An eight-year review. Ann Surg 1980; 192:783–787

28. Mirk P, Calisti A, Fileni A. Prenatal sonographic diagnosis of bladder extrophy. J Ultrasound Med 1986; 5:291–293

29. Palomaki GE, Hill LE, Knight GJ, Haddow JE, Carpenter M. Second-trimester maternal serum alpha-fetoprotein levels in pregnancies associated with gastroschisis and omphalocele. Obstet Gynecol 1988; 71: 906–909

30. Patten RM, Van Allen M, Mack LA, et al. Limb-body wall complex: *in utero* sonographic diagnosis of a complicated fetal malformation. AJR 1986; 146:1019–1024

31. Petrikovsky BM, Walzak MP Jr, D'Addario PF. Fetal cloacal anomalies: prenatal sonographic findings and differential diagnosis. Obstet Gynecol 1988; 72:464–469

32. Pettenati MJ, Haines JL, Higgins RR, Wappner RS, Palmer CG, Weaver DD. Wiedemann-Beckwith syndrome: presentation of clinical and cyto-genetic data on 22 new cases and review of the literature. Hum Genet 1986; 74:143–154

33. Sermer M, Benzie RJ, Pitson L, Carr M, Skidmore M. Prenatal diagnosis and management of congenital defects of the anterior abdominal wall. Am J Obstet Gynecol 1987; 156:308–312

34. Van Allen MI, Curry C, Gallagher L. Limb body wall complex: I. Pathogenesis. Am J Med Genet 1987; 28:529–548

35. Van Allen MI, Curry C, Walden CE, Gallagher L, Patten RM. Limb-body wall complex: II. Limb and spine defects. Am J Med Genet 1987; 28:549–565

OMPHALOCELE

36. Getachew MM, Goldstein RB, Edge V, Goldberg JD, Filly RA. Correlation between omphalocele contents and karyotypic abnormalities: sonographic study in 37 cases. AJR 1991; 158:133–136

37. Gilbert WM, Nicolaides KH. Fetal omphalocele: associated malformations and chromosomal defects. Obstet Gynecol 1987; 70:633–635

38. Hauge M, Bugge M, Nielson J. Early prenatal diagnosis of omphalocele constitutes indication for amniocentesis. Lancet 1983; 2:507

39. Hughes MD, Nyberg DA, Mack LA, Pretorius DH. Fetal omphalocele: prenatal US detection of concurrent anomalies and other predictors of outcome. Radiology 1989; 173:371–376

40. Nyberg DA, Fitzsimmons J, Mack LA, et al. Chromosomal abnormalities in fetuses with omphalocele. Significance of omphalocele contents. J Ultrasound Med 1989; 8:299–308

GASTROSCHISIS

41. Hoyme HE, Higginbottom MC, Jones KL. The vascular pathogenesis of gastroschisis: intrauterine interruption of the omphalomesenteric artery. J Pediatr 1981; 98:228–231

42. Lenke RR, Hatch EI Jr. Fetal gastroschisis: a preliminary report advocating the use of cesarean section. Obstet Gynecol 1986; 67:395–398

HYDROPS FETALIS

43. Benacerraf BR, Frigoletto FD Jr. Sonographic sign for the detection of early fetal ascites in the management of severe isoimmune disease without intrauterine transfusion. Am J Obstet Gynecol 1985; 152:1039–1041

44. Chinn DH. Ultrasound evaluation of hydrops fetalis. In: Callen PW (ed), Ultrasonography in obstetrics and gynecology, 2nd ed. Philadelphia: WB Saunders; 1988:277–296

45. Chitkara U, Wilkins I, Lynch L, Mehalek K, Berkowitz RL. The role of sonography in assessing severity of fetal anemia in Rh- and Kell-isoimmunized pregnancies. Obstet Gynecol 1988; 71:393–398

46. DeVore GR, Donnerstein RL, Kleinman CS, Platt LD, Hobbins JC. Fetal echocardiography. II. The diagnosis and significance of a pericardial effusion in the fetus using real-time-directed M-mode ultrasound. Am J Obstet Gynecol 1982; 144:693–700

47. Fleischer AC, Killam AP, Boehm FH, et al. Hydrops fetalis: sonographic evaluation and clinical implications. Radiology 1981; 141:163–168

48. Giacoia GP. Hydrops fetalis (fetal edema). A survey. Clin Pediatr 1980; 19:334–339

49. Hansman M, Arabin B. Nonimmune hydrops fetalis. In: Chervenak FA, Isaacson GC, Campbell S (eds), Ultrasound in obstetrics and gynecology. Boston: Little, Brown; 1993:1027–1049

50. Holzgreve W, Curry CJ, Golbus MS, Callen PW, Filly RA, Smith JC. Investigation of nonimmune hydrops fetalis. Am J Obstet Gynecol 1984; 150:805–812

51. Holzgreve W, Holzgreve B, Curry CJ. Nonimmune hydrops fetalis: diagnosis and management. Semin Perinatol 1985; 9:52–67

52. Hutchison AA, Drew JH, Yu VY, Williams ML, Fortune DW, Beischer NA. Nonimmunologic hydrops fetalis: a review of 61 cases. Obstet Gynecol 1982; 59:347–352

53. Mahony BS, Filly RA, Callen PW, Chinn DH, Golbus MS. Severe nonimmune hydrops fetalis: sonographic evaluation. Radiology 1984; 151:757–761

54. Warsof SL, Nicolaides KH, Rodeck C. Immune and non-immune hydrops. Clin Obstet Gynecol 1986; 29:533–542

CHROMOSOMAL ABNORMALITIES—GENERAL

55. Benacerraf BR, Neuberg D, Bromley B, Frigoletto FD Jr. Sonographic scoring index for prenatal detection of chromosomal abnormalities. J Ultrasound Med 1992; 11:449–458

56. Garden AS, Benzie RJ, Miskin M, Gardner HA. Fetal cystic hygroma colli: antenatal diagnosis, significance, and management. Am J Obstet Gynecol 1986; 154:221–225

57. Jones KL. Smith's recognizable patterns of human malformation. Philadelphia: WB Saunders; 1988:10–79

58. Nyberg DA, Mack LA, Bronstein A, Hirsch J, Pagon RA. Holoprosencephaly: prenatal sonographic diagnosis. AJR 1987; 149:1051–1058

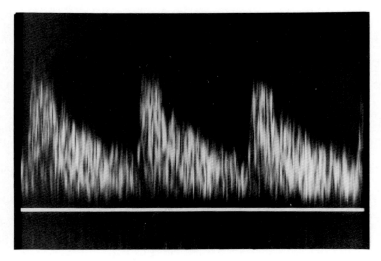

Figure 21-1

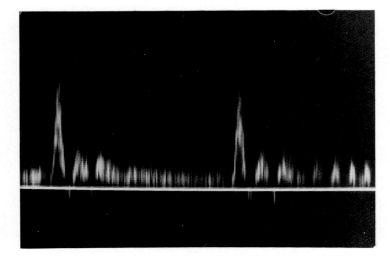

Figure 21-2

Case 21: Doppler Waveforms

Questions 94 through 97

For each of the numbered normal Doppler waveforms listed below (Questions 94 through 97), select the *one* lettered vessel (A, B, C, D, or E) that is MOST closely associated with it. Each lettered vessel may be used once, more than once, or not at all.

94. Figure 21-1
95. Figure 21-2
96. Figure 21-3
97. Figure 21-4

(A) External carotid artery
(B) Internal carotid artery
(C) Superficial femoral artery
(D) Renal arcuate artery
(E) Cavernosal artery

Like other parenchymal organs such as the kidneys, liver, and spleen, the brain has a low vascular resistance. Therefore, the internal carotid artery has a "low resistance"-type Doppler waveform. This is characterized by a broad systolic peak and a gradual diastolic downslope with relatively high levels of end-diastolic flow. The waveform in Figure 21-4 was obtained from the internal carotid artery **(Option (B) is the correct answer to Question 97).**

The external carotid artery, on the other hand, supplies the facial musculature and scalp, which have a high vascular resistance. This is reflected in the Doppler waveform of the external carotid artery, which has a narrow and spiked systolic peak, a rapid diastolic downslope, and relatively little end-diastolic flow. In addition, by tapping the superficial temporal branch of the external carotid artery (located in front of the external auditory meatus), pulsations that are visible on the Doppler waveform can be transmitted into the external carotid artery. Figure 21-2, which was obtained from a normal external carotid, illustrates the

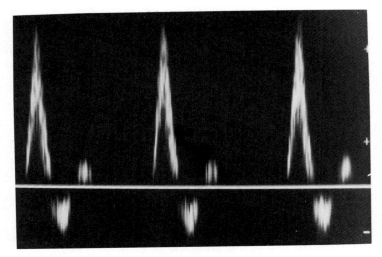

Figure 21-3

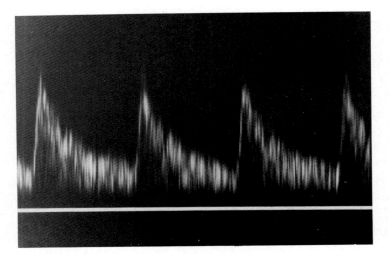

Figure 21-4

low-resistance pattern as well as the pulsations from the temporal tap maneuver **(Option (A) is the correct answer to Question 95).**

Further analysis of the internal carotid artery waveform shows that there is a clear space between the baseline and the actual waveform. This is called the spectral window and is present because the range of blood flow velocities in the center of a normal internal carotid artery is relatively limited, with most velocities grouped near the maximum velocity. This is particularly true during systolic acceleration, when the Doppler waveform is very thin. Figure 21-1, on the other hand, shows a low-resistance waveform similar to that of a normal internal carotid artery except that the spectral window has been filled in by lower-frequency components. This is referred to as spectral broadening. It is frequently seen in images of patients with internal carotid artery stenosis when turbulent flow produces a large range of flow velocities oriented in multiple nonlaminar directions. However, it can also occur in normal small vessels such as the renal arcuate arteries **(Option (D) is the correct answer to Question 94).** In very small vessels, the pulsed Doppler sample gate is larger than the diameter of the vessel. Therefore, erythrocytes from both the center and periphery of the lumen are sampled. Because flow velocities near the vessel wall are very low, a much broader range of velocities are sampled and thus the velocity spectrum is broadened.

The waveform illustrated in Figure 21-3 shows a typical triphasic pattern seen in arteries, such as the superficial femoral artery, supplying the upper or lower extremity **(Option (C) is the correct answer to Question 96).** This pattern reflects a very high vascular resistance. In systole, blood travels in a forward direction, causing distension of the peripheral arteries. In early diastole, there is elastic recoil of the peripheral arteries; because forward flow into the arterioles is limited, the elastic recoil forces blood to flow temporarily in the reverse direction back toward the aorta. Later in diastole, flow temporarily returns to a forward direction as the blood passes through the arterioles and into the venous circulation.

The cavernosal artery (Option (E)) is a small vessel that travels in the middle of the corpora cavernosa. The Doppler waveform normally demonstrates spectral broadening because the cavernosal artery is small. The systolic and diastolic components of the cavernosal artery are dependent on the stage of penile erection. In the flaccid state, resistance to flow in the cavernosal artery is high and the flow may be too slow to detect. When flow is detected, systolic peaks are damped and there is minimal or no diastolic flow. Early in the course of an erection, the waveform has a low-resistance pattern. At full tumescence, the waveform has a high-resistance pattern due to activation of the veno-occlusive mechanism. Unless the exact stage of erection is specified, it is not possible to determine whether a given waveform originated from a cavernosal artery.

Question 98

Concerning postcatheterization arteriovenous fistulas,

(A) they occur more frequently after arterial puncture below the femoral bifurcation than after puncture above it

(B) they are readily detected by gray-scale sonography

(C) they cause decreased diastolic flow in the proximal femoral artery

(D) perivascular tissue vibration is a characteristic finding

(E) venous pulsations are diagnostic

Arteriovenous (AV) fistulas represent an uncommon but well-recognized complication following femoral catheterization. Their frequency after cardiac interventions is estimated to be considerably less than 1%. As with other postcatheterization complications (such as pseudoaneurysms, arterial lacerations, and arterial occlusions), the frequency of AV fistulas increases with increasing invasiveness of the procedure. It is highest for intra-aortic balloon pump placement and cardiac valvuloplasty and lowest for diagnostic cardiac catheterization.

Several factors can increase the risk of developing an AV fistula following catheterization. The most important is performing the femoral puncture below the bifurcation of the common femoral artery into the superficial femoral artery and profunda femoral artery **(Option (A) is true)**. The important vascular anatomy in this region is illustrated in Figures 21-5 and 21-6.

Above the bifurcation, the common femoral artery and common femoral vein lie side by side; puncture of the artery at this level will only rarely disturb the adjacent vein. Immediately below the bifurcation, the femoral vein starts to course deep to the superficial femoral artery. In addition, small venous branches may pass directly between the superficial femoral and profunda femoral arteries. Therefore, puncture below the bifurcation often results in needle passage through both the artery and the underlying vein and thus creates a potential for communication between these two vessels. Additional factors that predispose to formation of AV fistulas are the administration of anticoagulant or thrombolytic agents during or after the catheterization and simultaneous arterial and venous catheterization for left- and right-heart studies.

In the acute period, patients with femoral AV fistulas are usually asymptomatic. If the AV shunting of blood flow is sufficient, high-output cardiac failure can develop. Ischemia may also develop in the lower extremities, especially if there is preexisting vascular disease. With time, the feeding and draining vessels will enlarge and collateral vessels will be recruited to accommodate the increased blood flow.

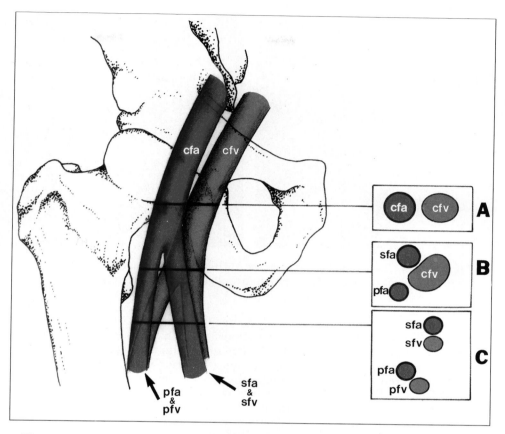

Figure 21-5. Arterial and venous anatomy of the femoral bifurcation. The diagram on the left demonstrates the relationship of the femoral artery bifurcation to the adjacent femoral vein. The inserts on the right demonstrate the cross-sectional anatomy above and below the bifurcation. cfa = common femoral artery; cfv = common femoral vein; sfa = superficial femoral artery; sfv = superficial femoral vein; pfa = profunda femoral artery; pfv = profunda femoral vein. (Reprinted with permission from Middleton [8].)

Hematoma, bruit, and localized pain are the findings that most frequently raise the clinical suspicion of a vascular complication following a cardiac catheterization. Unfortunately, these signs and symptoms are not sensitive or specific enough to form the basis for management decisions. Therefore, imaging becomes extremely important. Gray-scale sonography can detect morphologic abnormalities following femoral puncture, but in most cases AV fistulas produce purely hemodynamic alterations and are not associated with any significant morphologic changes. Therefore, gray-scale sonography is very insensitive to AV fistu-

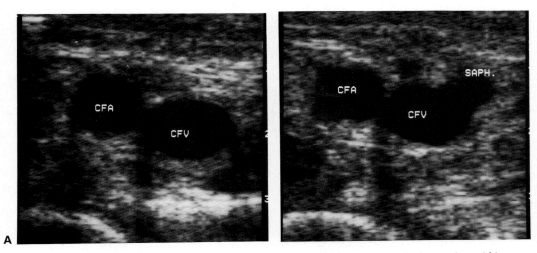

Figure 21-6. Gray-scale appearance of the right femoral bifurcation. (A) Transverse view of the common femoral artery (CFA) and vein (CFV). Note the lack of significant overlap of the two vessels at this level. (B) Slightly inferiorly, the saphenous vein (SAPH.) enters the common femoral vein along the medial side. (C) Slightly more inferiorly, the common femoral artery bifurcates into the superficial femoral artery (SFA) and profunda femoral artery (PFA). The common femoral vein has not yet bifurcated at this level. (D) Slightly more inferiorly, the superficial and profunda femoral arteries are beginning to separate, and a small branch vein (BRANCH) is seen passing between the superficial and profunda femoral arteries and coursing into the common femoral vein. At this level, the lateral aspect of the common femoral vein is positioned deep to the superficial femoral artery. (E) Slightly more inferiorly, the common femoral vein has now bifurcated into the superficial femoral vein (SFV) and profunda femoral vein (PFV). The superficial femoral vein is positioned partially deep to the superficial femoral artery. (F) Slightly more inferiorly, the superficial and profunda femoral veins begin to separate from each other and travel deep to their corresponding arteries.

las **(Option (B) is false).** Duplex Doppler sonography is much better suited to detecting the local hemodynamic alterations associated with AV fistulas, and good results have been obtained with this method. Unfortunately, duplex Doppler sonography requires extensive experience, and good results reported in the literature may not be universally reproducible. However, Doppler analysis of AV fistulas has been greatly facilitated by the use of color Doppler sonography. One recent study documented no false-positive or false-negative color Doppler examinations in a series of 25 patients with and without AV fistulas and pseudoaneurysms. This level of success means that management decisions can be made and sur-

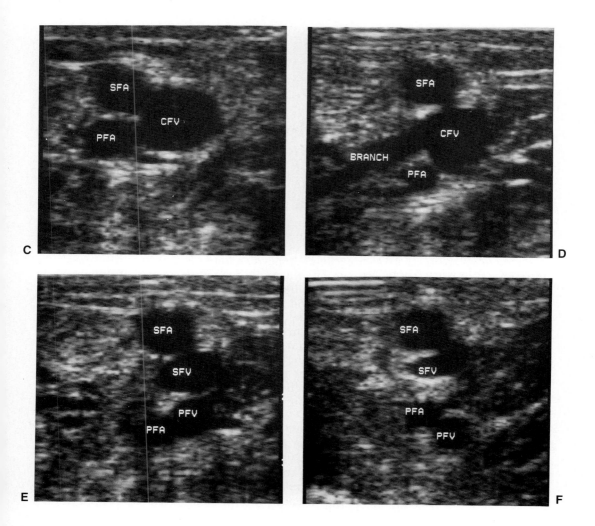

gery can be performed without further studies in the vast majority of patients.

To identify AV fistulas, it is necessary to understand their hemodynamic characterizations. The basic underlying effect of AV fistulas is a direct bypass of the high-resistance vascular bed of the lower extremity into the low-resistance venous system. There is a pressure gradient between the artery and vein throughout the cardiac cycle, and so continuous forward flow is seen in the artery at the site of the AV fistula. Doppler waveform analysis of the artery in this region will show persistent antegrade diastolic flow throughout the cardiac cycle. This increased diastolic flow is usually easily distinguished from the normal absence of

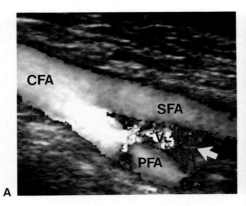 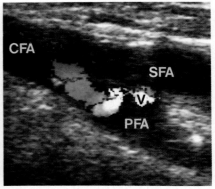

A   B

Figure 21-7. Femoral arteriovenous fistula. (A) A longitudinal color Doppler image of the groin at peak systole demonstrates the common femoral artery (CFA), superficial femoral artery (SFA), and profunda femoral artery (PFA). A region of aliasing is seen at the origin of the profunda femoral artery, and perivascular tissue vibration is seen in the soft tissues between the superficial and profunda femoral arteries (arrow). Prominent flow is also seen in a venous structure (V) located between the superficial and profunda femoral arteries. (B) During diastole, normal absence of flow is seen throughout the femoral bifurcation with the exception of the origin of the profunda femoral artery, where the AV fistula is located. (C) A duplex Doppler waveform from the superficial femoral artery demonstrates normal high-resistance flow with early diastolic flow reversal but no end-diastolic flow. The systolic peaks are varied as a result of a cardiac arrhythmia. (D) A pulsed Doppler waveform from the profunda femoral artery origin demonstrates a low-resistance pattern with abundant diastolic flow. (E) A pulsed Doppler waveform from the vein positioned between the superficial and profunda femoral arteries demonstrates no recognizable pattern. This is probably due to a combination of extremely high flow rates and resulting aliasing as well as vibration caused by marked flow turbulence.

flow in diastole **(Option (C) is false).** On the color Doppler image, the persistent diastolic flow results in continuous intra-arterial color assignment in the immediate region of the AV fistula (Figures 21-7 and 21-8).

Venous flow is also altered in AV fistulas. In some cases, the venous waveform at the site of the AV fistula appears extremely distorted and turbulent (Figure 21-7). In others, arterialization of the waveform occurs (Figure 21-8). In many cases, both waveform alterations are seen, but in different portions of the vein. The presence of venous pulsations that correlate with the cardiac cycle is common in the setting of congestive heart failure or fluid overload states. Such pulsations do not necessarily indicate an AV fistula **(Option (E) is false).** Whenever there is a question about whether venous pulsations are due to a localized AV fistula or to

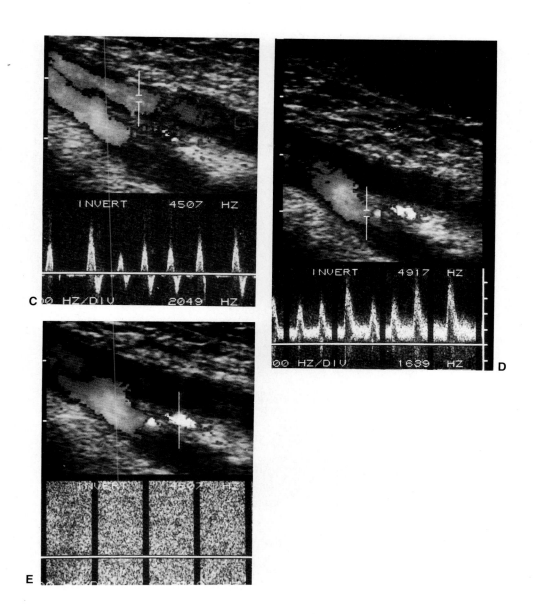

congestive heart failure, evaluation of a contralateral vein is useful (Figure 21-9). If the pulsations are present bilaterally, heart failure or fluid overload is most likely.

In many patients, the turbulent blood flow that occurs with AV fistulas causes intravascular pressure fluctuations that set the vessel wall into vibration. When the wall vibration is sufficiently severe, the perivascular soft tissues will begin to vibrate. This can result in an audible bruit

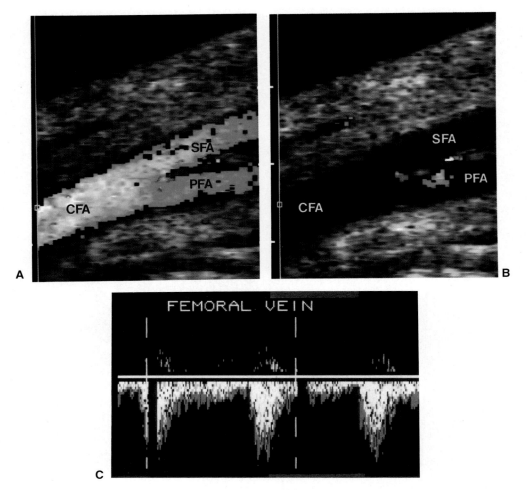

Figure 21-8. Femoral arteriovenous fistula. (A) A longitudinal view of the femoral bifurcation in systole demonstrates normal antegrade flow in the common femoral artery (CFA), superficial femoral artery (SFA), and profunda femoral artery (PFA). (B) During diastole, there is a normal absence of flow throughout the femoral bifurcation, with the exception of the origin of the profunda femoral artery, which was the site of a small AV fistula. (C) A pulsed Doppler waveform from the adjacent common femoral vein demonstrates arterialization of the venous signal.

or even a palpable thrill. On color Doppler imaging, the vibrating tissue interfaces in the perivascular tissue are detected as moving reflectors and are therefore assigned a color. This vibrational motion is randomly directed both toward and away from the transducer, so the color assignment is a random mixture of both red and blue (Figure 21-7A). Perivas-

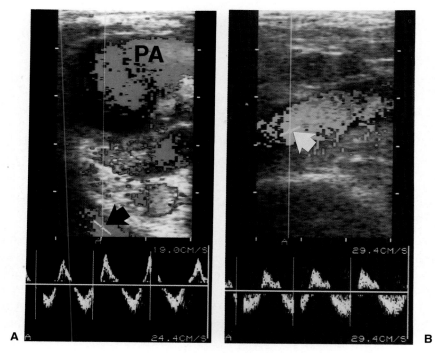

Figure 21-9. Pseudoaneurysm with pulsatile venous flow attributable to
right-sided heart failure. (A) A longitudinal view of the left groin demonstrates a pseudoaneurysm (PA). The pulsed Doppler waveform from the
underlying femoral vein (arrow) demonstrates pulsatile venous flow and
should not be confused with arterial flow caused by an AV fistula. (B) A
pulsed Doppler waveform from the right femoral vein (arrow) shows similar venous pulsations, confirming that this effect is related to the
patient's right-sided heart failure.

cular tissue vibration is frequently the most striking feature of AV fistulas **(Option (D) is true).** The flow turbulence is greatest in peak systole,
and so the perivascular vibration is most intense and extensive during
systole.

Question 99

Concerning Doppler analysis of the neck vessels,

    (A) bidirectional flow in the vertebral artery is seen occasionally in patients with subclavian or innominate artery stenosis

    (B) gray-scale sonography is more reliable than spectral waveform analysis in detecting a stenosis of less than 50% diameter narrowing

    (C) "externalization" of the common carotid artery waveform occurs with occlusion of the external carotid artery

    (D) the accuracy of Doppler velocity calculations is independent of the Doppler angle

    (E) waveform aliasing can be eliminated by using a higher-frequency transducer

Doppler sonographic evaluation of the neck vessels has undergone a number of advances in the past two decades, from the use of continuous-wave Doppler to the use of pulsed Doppler and duplex Doppler and now to the use of color Doppler sonography. Color Doppler imaging has made the examination easier to learn and faster to perform, but the basic principles of analysis learned with continuous-wave and duplex Doppler techniques still apply.

The normal waveform characteristics of the internal and external carotid arteries have already been described. The hemodynamics of the vertebral artery are similar to those of the internal carotid artery, since both supply brain parenchyma. The waveform of the common carotid artery is somewhat variable but generally most closely resembles that of the internal carotid artery since 75 to 80% of common carotid blood flow goes to the internal carotid artery.

The normal flow patterns in the carotid bifurcation are well displayed on color Doppler sonography. In almost all individuals, there is transient flow reversal in the carotid bulb during peak systole and extending for a variable period into diastole. This results in a variably sized and shaped region of blue color assignment pin an otherwise red vessel. In late diastole, this flow reversal is generally replaced by a region of static blood, resulting in a region of no color assignment (Figure 21-10). It is interesting that this region of reversed and static blood flow in the carotid bulb is the precise site where atheromatous plaque tends to originate and predominate. This has led some investigators to propose that the local hemodynamic alterations precipitate plaque formation in this region by either retarding transport of metabolites across the vessel wall or promoting platelet aggregation and subsequent release of atherogenic materials. Regardless of the etiology, when plaque does begin to form in the bulb, it can alter the normal hemodynamics in this region and cause a loss of the normal flow reversal (Figure 21-11). Therefore,

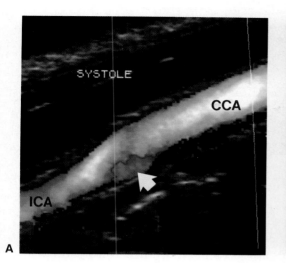

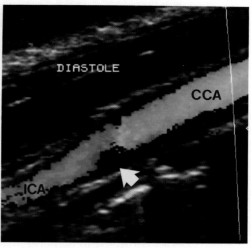

Figure 21-10. Normal flow reversal in the carotid bulb. (A) A longitudinal view of the common carotid artery (CCA) and internal carotid artery (ICA) during peak systole demonstrates a region of flow reversal (arrow) at the carotid bulb. (B) A similar view in diastole demonstrates static blood in the carotid bulb (arrow).

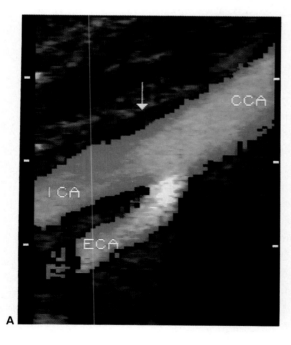

Figure 21-11 (left). Minimal plaque in the carotid bulb. (A) A longitudinal view demonstrates the common carotid artery (CCA) bifurcating into the internal carotid artery (ICA) and external carotid artery (ECA). A small hypoechoic plaque (arrow) is seen in the carotid bulb. This minimal plaque has resulted in loss of the normal flow reversal in this region. (B) A pulsed Doppler waveform from the internal carotid artery just beyond the plaque shows a normal peak systolic velocity of 57 cm/second.

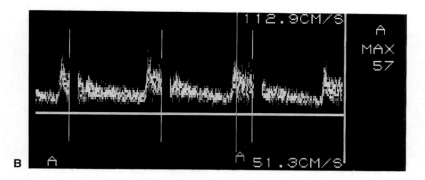

when flow reversal is not seen, a careful investigation for underlying plaque is warranted.

Detection and quantification of carotid stenosis require analysis of several factors. Duplex Doppler sonography relies on the basic principle that blood flow velocity increases in areas of luminal stenosis. For less than 50% diameter stenosis (<75% area stenosis), increases in velocity are mild but sufficient to maintain overall flow volume. When the stenosis causes more than 50% diameter reduction, flow velocities begin to increase more dramatically but overall flow volumes decrease. Therefore, stenosis of greater than 50% diameter reduction is considered hemodynamically significant. As the stenosis reaches a critical level of 90 to 95% diameter reduction, flow velocities start to drop and may in fact return to normal levels. These velocity changes with respect to stenosis are illustrated in Figure 21-12, which shows that it is difficult to detect stenosis of less than 50% diameter narrowing on the basis of velocities determined from spectral waveforms. Fortunately, gray-scale and color Doppler sonography are much more sensitive for detecting these hemodynamically insignificant lesions (Figure 21-11) **(Option (B) is true).**

On the basis of the relatively predictable relationship between blood flow velocity and percent stenosis, numerous investigators have established velocity criteria to estimate degrees of stenosis greater than 50%. The single criterion that has been studied most extensively is the peak systolic velocity at the site of the stenosis. This parameter continues to be the single most accurate means of estimating stenosis.

Another widely used parameter is the ratio between peak systolic velocity in the internal carotid and the ipsilateral common carotid arteries. This parameter was developed to compensate for situations in which the baseline velocities in normal segments of the carotid were either abnormally elevated (for instance, when flow is increased to provide collateral flow for a contralateral internal carotid or common carotid occlu-

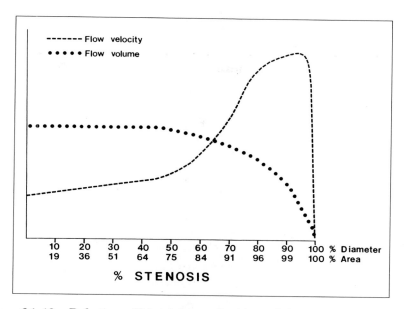

Figure 21-12. Relation of blood flow velocity and flow volume to luminal narrowing. Note that flow volume begins to decrease at 50% diameter stenosis. Flow velocity increases minimally between 0 and 50% stenosis and then increases more dramatically between 50 and 90% stenosis. Stenosis of >95% causes an abrupt fall in flow velocity. (Reprinted with permission from Cardoso and Middleton [15].)

sion) or abnormally depressed (for instance, when cardiac output is decreased).

Both of the above parameters rely on accurate measurement of peak systolic velocity. This requires a Doppler angle of ≤60°. This requirement is a direct result of the Doppler equation. The basic Doppler equation is shown below:

$$F_d = \frac{2F_t V \cos\theta}{C}$$

where F_d is the Doppler frequency shift, F_t is the transducer Doppler frequency, V is the blood flow velocity, C is the speed of sound, and θ is the Doppler angle (between the vessel direction and the Doppler beam). This equation can be solved for the blood flow velocity:

$$V = \frac{F_d C}{2F_t \cos\theta}$$

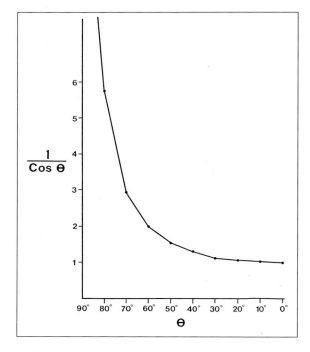

Figure 21-13. Variation in 1/cos θ with respect to the Doppler angle (θ). Between 0 and 60° there is minimal change in the value of 1/cos θ. Above 60°, however, there is a progressively larger variation in the value of 1/cos θ. This marked variation results in difficulties in accurate velocity calculations at the larger Doppler angles.

Therefore, the calculated blood flow velocity is inversely proportional to cos θ (i.e., proportional to 1/cos θ). Figure 21-13 illustrates how 1/cos θ varies at different Doppler angles. As seen, between 0 and 60°, there is little change in the value of 1/cos θ. However, at angles of >60°, 1/cos θ changes very rapidly. If it were always possible to determine the exact Doppler angle, this rapid change in 1/cos θ would not affect velocity calculations. Unfortunately, there is always some inaccuracy in determining the Doppler angle. These slight inaccuracies in angle determination result in major inaccuracies in velocity calculations above 60° but only minor inaccuracies below 60° **(Option (D) is false).** Figure 21-14 illustrates this phenomenon schematically, and Figure 21-15 demonstrates the problem *in vivo*.

Another problem in calculating velocities is aliasing. Aliasing occurs when the Doppler sampling rate (pulse-repetition frequency) is not high enough to display the Doppler frequency shift. This is analogous to the rotation of a stagecoach wheel in a Western movie. As the wheel begins to rotate faster, it reaches a point at which it appears to reverse directions. This occurs when the frame rate of the movie is less than twice the revolutions per minute of the wheel. Similarly, the pulse-repetition frequency must be twice the Doppler frequency shift for the shift to be accurately

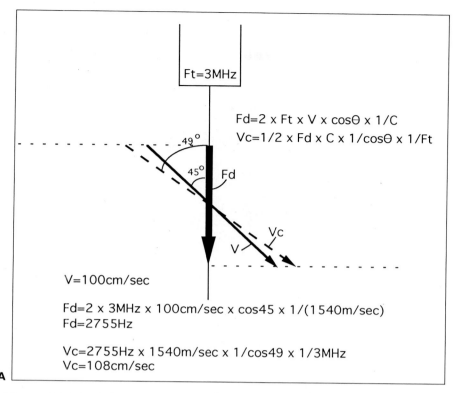

Figure 21-14. Schematic representation of variability of velocity calculations with respect to Doppler angles. (A) If a 3-MHz transducer is used to perform pulsed Doppler analysis of a vessel with blood flow velocity of 100 cm/second (V, represented by the thin arrow) that is traveling at a 45° Doppler angle, the Doppler frequency shift (F_d, represented by the bold arrow) would be 2,755 Hz. If the Doppler angle were estimated at 49° rather than the true 45° (an error of 4°), the calculated velocity (V_c, represented by the dashed arrow) would be 108 cm/seconds, resulting in just an 8-cm/second velocity inaccuracy. (B) At a Doppler angle of 70°, the Doppler frequency shift would be 1,333 Hz. If the Doppler angle were inaccurately estimated to be 74° (an error of 4°), the calculated velocity would equal 124 cm/seconds, resulting in a 24-cm/second velocity inaccuracy. This illustrates the increasing inaccuracies in velocity calculations with Doppler angles above 60°.

displayed. When this does not occur, the higher-frequency shifts in the Doppler waveform will wrap around into the negative half of the scale (Figure 21-16). On color Doppler imaging, aliasing appears as an abrupt change in color from the positive to the negative side (Figure 21-17). With very extensive aliasing, normal flow patterns can appear extremely disordered and turbulent (Figure 21-18).

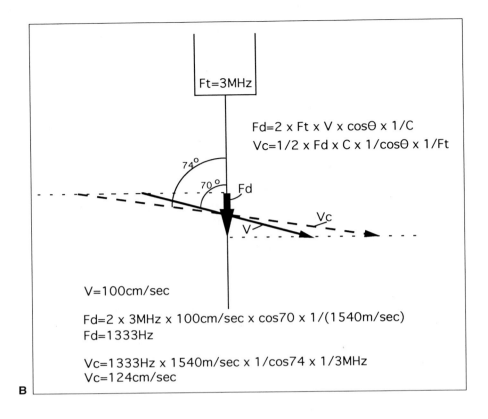

$$Ft=3MHz$$

$$Fd=2 \times Ft \times V \times \cos\theta \times 1/C$$
$$Vc=1/2 \times Fd \times C \times 1/\cos\theta \times 1/Ft$$

74°

70° Fd

Vc

V

$$V=100cm/sec$$

$$Fd=2 \times 3MHz \times 100cm/sec \times \cos70 \times 1/(1540m/sec)$$
$$Fd=1333Hz$$

$$Vc=1333Hz \times 1540m/sec \times 1/\cos74 \times 1/3MHz$$
$$Vc=124cm/sec$$

B

The easiest way to reduce aliasing is simply to increase the pulse-repetition frequency. This is generally accomplished by increasing the Doppler scale. The sacrifice for operating at a high pulse-repetition frequency (high Doppler scale) is a loss of sensitivity. That is why the maximum pulse-repetition frequency is not used routinely. If aliasing is still present after the pulse-repetition frequency has been maximized, then switching to a lower-frequency transducer should be attempted (Figure 21-19). As indicated in the Doppler equation, the Doppler frequency shift is proportional to the transmitted frequency. Decreasing the transmitted frequency with a lower-frequency transducer will lead to a reduction in the Doppler frequency shift, and in some instances this can eliminate aliasing artifacts. Using a higher-frequency transducer will make aliasing worse **(Option (E) is false)**.

In addition to peak systolic velocity and internal carotid artery/common carotid artery velocity ratios, end-diastolic velocities can be used to estimate stenosis. End-diastolic measurements are particularly useful when aliasing artifacts do not allow for accurate calculations of peak systolic velocity.

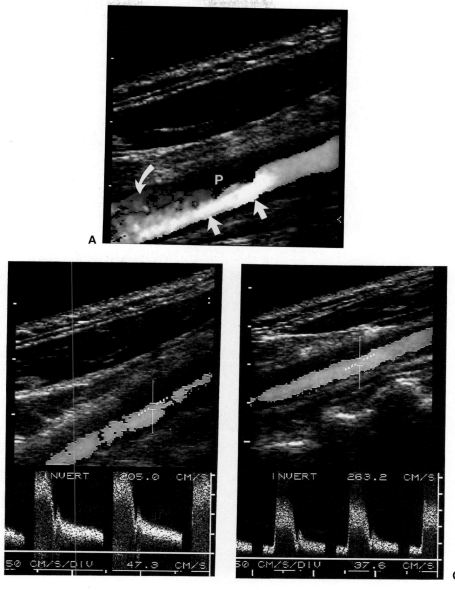

Figure 21-19. Effect of transducer frequency on pulsed Doppler aliasing. (A) A longitudinal color Doppler image of the common carotid artery obtained with a 5-MHz transducer demonstrates focal stenosis due to a hypoechoic plaque (P). The stenosis has resulted in a flow jet (straight arrows) and an abnormal region of flow reversal (curved arrow). (B) A pulsed Doppler waveform from this region obtained with a 7-MHz transducer demonstrates mild aliasing of the systolic peak. (C) A pulsed Doppler waveform obtained with a 5-MHz transducer demonstrates elimination of the aliasing artifact.

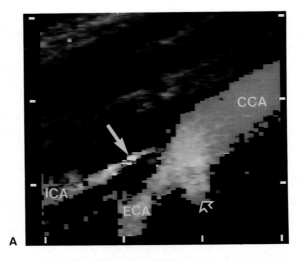

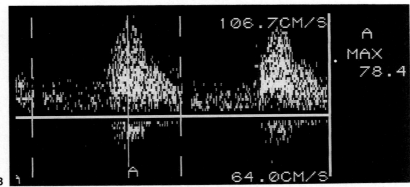

Figure 21-20. High-grade internal carotid artery stenosis with normal flow velocities. (A) A longitudinal view of the carotid bifurcation demonstrates the common carotid artery (CCA), external carotid artery (ECA), external carotid artery branch (open arrow), internal carotid artery (ICA), and high-grade internal carotid artery stenosis (solid arrow). (B) A pulsed Doppler waveform from the stenotic region demonstrates a distorted waveform with marked spectral broadening. However, the peak systolic flow velocity was 78.4 cm/seconds, which is within normal limits.

As mentioned above, when stenosis exceeds approximately 95% diameter reduction, the blood flow velocity actually starts to decrease and at some point may return to the normal range. In such cases, diagnostic error can be avoided by noting the marked reduction in caliber of the flow lumen on color Doppler images (Figure 21-20). In addition, the Doppler waveform will rarely, if ever, appear normal in such cases, despite the normal velocity. As discussed above, turbulent blood flow causes erythrocytes to travel at a broad range of velocities and in multiple nonlaminar directions. This results in a large range of frequency shifts that fill in the normally clear spectral window in the internal carotid artery. This phenomenon is called spectral broadening.

The distinction between subtotal and complete occlusion of the internal carotid is important since patients with a high-grade but subtotal occlusion are candidates for carotid endarterectomy whereas those with a complete occlusion are not. Therefore, optimizing Doppler sensitivity is crucial to detect minimal residual flow in patients with an extremely high-grade stenosis. Accordingly, the Doppler gain should be maximized to the point at which noise starts to appear on the image. The Doppler scale should be lowered as much as possible. Wall filter settings should be minimized to avoid filtering out low-frequency shifts arising from slowly flowing blood. Controls that suppress color Doppler information in image pixels above a certain gray-scale value should also be adjusted so that this suppression is minimized. Finally, transducers operating at different frequencies should be used. If the internal carotid is superficial, switching to a high-frequency transducer can help for two reasons. As the Doppler equation indicates, the Doppler frequency shift is proportional to the transmitted frequency, so that increasing the transmitted frequency will increase the Doppler frequency shift and make residual flow easier to detect. In addition, the magnitude of the echo from small reflectors such as erythrocytes is proportional to the fourth power of the transmitted frequency. Thus, as the transmitted frequency increases, the echo becomes much stronger. Both of these relationships make high-frequency transducers more sensitive, provided the sound pulse can penetrate to the depth of the vessel. If the internal carotid is deep, penetration with high-frequency probes is usually a problem and a lower-frequency transducer with more penetrating power should be used (Figure 21-21).

If all the above maneuvers have been attempted and there is still no detectable flow, one must assume that the vessel is occluded. It then becomes important to prove that the occluded vessel is the internal carotid artery and the patent vessel is the external carotid artery. As described above, the waveforms of the external and internal carotid arteries have characteristic differences that help them to be distinguished (Figure 21-22). The temporal tap maneuver is also useful, as mentioned above. In addition, the external carotid artery is almost always anterior and medial to the internal carotid artery. The external carotid artery also has branches that may be detectable, which can distinguish it from the internal carotid artery.

When the internal carotid artery becomes totally occluded, all of the blood flow in the common carotid artery goes into the external carotid artery. Therefore, the common carotid waveform converts from an appear-

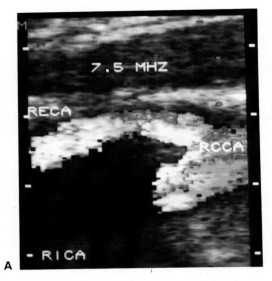

A

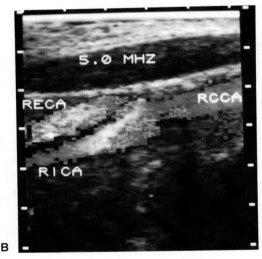

B

Figure 21-21. Pseudo-occlusion of the internal carotid artery. (A) A longitudinal view of the right carotid bifurcation obtained with a 7.5-MHz transducer demonstrates easily detectable flow in the common carotid artery (RCCA) and external carotid artery (RECA). No flow is detected in the internal carotid artery (RICA). (B) A similar view obtained with a 5-MHz transducer shows readily detectable flow in the normal internal carotid artery. This occurred because of the improved penetrating power of the 5-MHz transducer.

ance that primarily mimics the waveform of the internal carotid artery to an appearance that mimics the waveform of the external carotid artery. This is referred to as externalization of the common carotid waveform, and this finding can serve as a clue that the internal carotid artery is occluded (Figure 21-22). Externalization of the common carotid does not occur with external carotid artery occlusion **(Option (C) is false).**

Although the estimation of percent stenosis is an extremely important part of sonographic evaluation of the neck vessels, some investigators believe that it is just as important to evaluate plaque morphology.

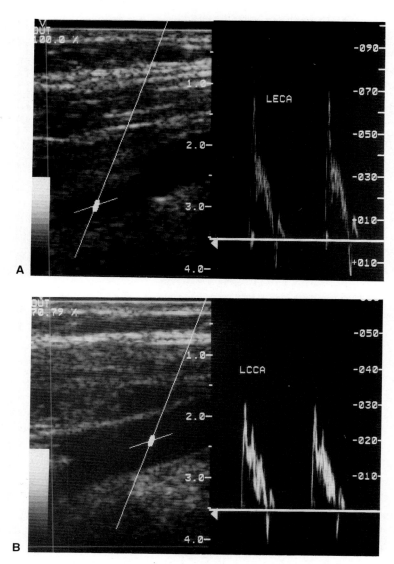

Figure 21-22. Internal carotid artery occlusion. (A) A pulsed Doppler waveform from the left external carotid artery (LECA) demonstrates a high-resistance pattern with a sharp systolic peak and no diastolic flow. (B) A pulsed Doppler waveform from the left common carotid artery (LCCA) demonstrates an identical waveform consistent with externalization of the common carotid artery.

Several studies have indicated that heterogeneous regions within plaque, particularly hypoechoic and anechoic zones, correspond to intraplaque hemorrhage (Figure 21-23). Such hemorrhage can erode through

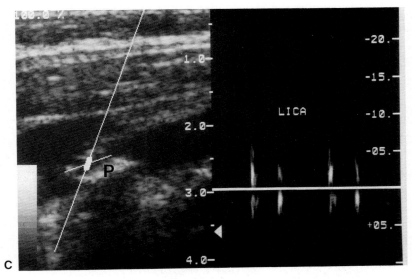

Figure 21-22 (Continued). Internal carotid artery occlusion. (C) A pulsed Doppler waveform from the left internal carotid artery (LICA) demonstrates motion artifact but no effective blood flow. An echogenic plaque (P) is identified in the internal carotid artery origin on the gray-scale image.

the intimal surface of a plaque and result in embolic disease. Therefore, when prominent hypoechoic or anechoic defects are identified, they should be brought to the attention of the referring physician since the plaque may be unstable. Large plaque ulcerations also can be detected by gray-scale and color Doppler sonography (Figure 21-24). Small plaque ulcerations and minimal disruptions in the intimal surface are difficult to detect by any current imaging modality.

Doppler evaluation of the neck vessels should include visualization of the vertebral arteries as well as the carotid arteries. The vertebral arteries travel through the foramina in the transverse processes of the cervical spine. They are best seen in the spaces between the transverse processes (Figure 21-25). Reversal of flow in the vertebral arteries is referred to as a subclavian steal syndrome. It results when there is a stenosis or occlusion at the origin of the subclavian or innominate artery such that blood flow to the ipsilateral upper extremity is derived at least partially from the circle of Willis via retrograde flow in the vertebral artery. As expected, manuevers that alter blood flow to the affected extremity will also alter flow in the ipsilateral vertebral artery. For instance, inflation of a blood pressure cuff above systolic pressure will decrease the amount of blood being siphoned from the vertebral artery.

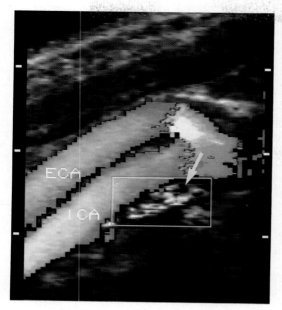

Figure 21-23 (left). Intra-plaque hemorrhage. A longitudinal color Doppler view of the internal carotid artery (ICA) and external carotid artery (ECA) shows a predominantly echogenic plaque at the origin of the internal carotid artery (within the green box). Post-processing has been performed and has accentuated a hypoechoic defect (arrow) within the plaque. This type of defect may represent intraplaque hemorrhage.

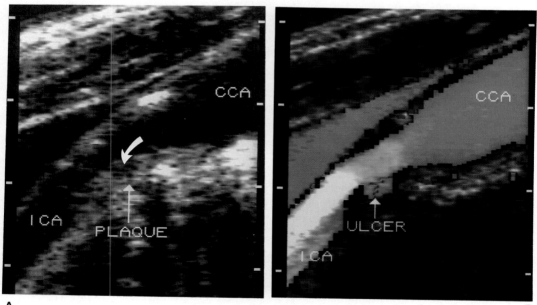

A   B

Figure 21-24. Plaque ulceration. (A) A longitudinal gray-scale image of the common carotid artery (CCA) and internal carotid artery (ICA) demonstrates a smoothly marginated plaque (straight arrow) in the carotid bulb. A hypoechoic region (curved arrow) is identified within the plaque. (B) A longitudinal color Doppler image demonstrates narrowing of the flow lumen by the plaque. Swirling blood flow is identified within the hypoechoic defect, confirming that this represents an ulcer crater as opposed to intraplaque hemorrhage.

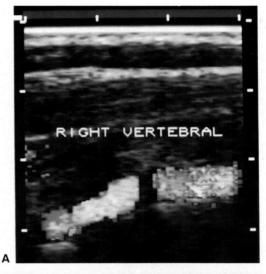

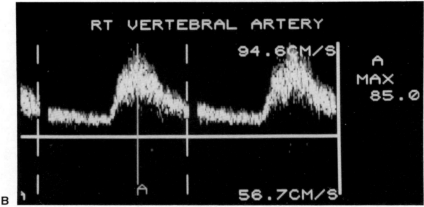

Figure 21-25. Subclavian steal syndrome. (A) A longitudinal color Doppler image of the right vertebral artery demonstrates normal antegrade flow, color coded in red. A portion of the vertebral artery is not seen because of shadowing from the overlying transverse process. (B) A pulsed Doppler waveform from the right vertebral artery demonstrates normal low-resistance antegrade arterial flow, seen above the baseline. (C) A longitudinal color Doppler image of the left vertebral artery demonstrates reversed blood flow, color coded in blue. (D) A pulsed Doppler waveform from the left vertebral artery demonstrates high-resistance retrograde flow, seen below the baseline. The high-resistance pattern reflects the fact that the vertebral artery is now supplying flow to the left upper extremity rather than to the brain. The peak systolic velocity is 45.2 cm/second. (E) A pulsed Doppler waveform from the left vertebral artery obtained after release of a blood pressure cuff on the left upper extremity. The postischemic hyperemia that occurs in the left upper extremity results in decreased vascular resistance to the left upper extremity and increased diastolic flow in the left vertebral artery. The peak systolic velocity has also increased to 61.9 cm/second.

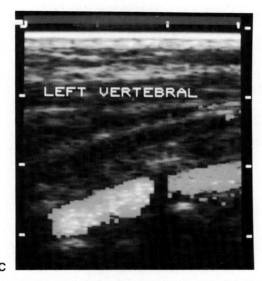

C

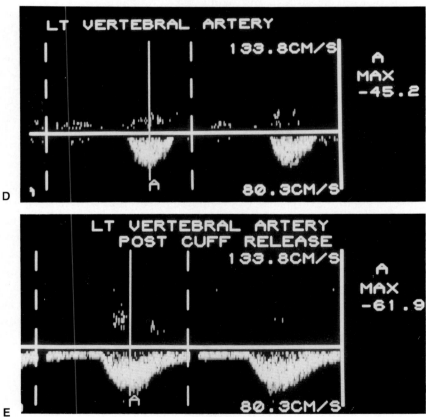

D

E

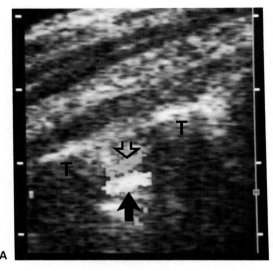

A

Figure 21-26. Subclavian steal syndrome. (A) A longitudinal color Doppler view of the vertebral artery (solid arrow) demonstrates retrograde flow. Flow in the vertebral artery is in the same direction as in the overlying vertebral vein (open arrow), and therefore both vessels are color coded in blue. Shadowing from the overlying transverse processes (T) results in segmental visualization of these vessels. (B) A pulsed Doppler waveform from the left vertebral artery demonstrates retrograde flow during systole, seen as a systolic peak below the baseline. During diastole, flow returns to the normal antegrade direction. This indicates that some blood flow is entering the vertebral artery from its origin at the subclavian artery and thus indicates that the subclavian artery is stenotic but not completely occluded.

On the other hand, exercise or postischemic hyperemia will increase the amount of retrograde vertebral blood flow (Figure 21-25). This siphoning of blood from the circle of Willis via the vertebral artery may result in persistently reversed flow throughout all phases of the cardiac cycle when the subclavian or innominate artery is completely occluded (Figure 21-25). When the origin of the subclavian or innominate artery is stenotic but patent, the waveform from the vertebral artery may be reversed only during systole but may travel in a normal direction during diastole (Figure 21-26) **(Option (A) is true).**

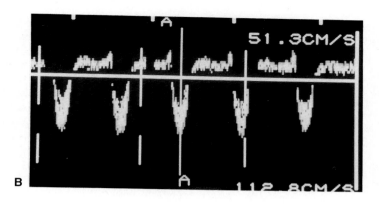

B

Question 100

Concerning postcatheterization pseudoaneurysm,

- (A) swirling intraluminal blood flow is typical
- (B) "to and fro" blood flow in its neck is typical
- (C) surgical repair is necessary
- (D) it is often indistinguishable from a hematoma by gray-scale sonography
- (E) it generally communicates with the artery via a wide neck

Pseudoaneurysms are another complication of femoral artery catheterization. They form when blood leaks from an injured artery and the resulting hematoma maintains a communication with the artery. Initially the hematoma is walled-off by adjacent structures, but with time, a fibrous capsule forms. Because the wall of the aneurysm does not contain normal components of an arterial wall, it is called a pseudoaneurysm. The factors that predispose to AV fistula formation also predispose to pseudoaneurysms. Clinical suspicion of a pseudoaneurysm is usually raised when a mass is palpated in the groin following a femoral puncture. The major differential diagnosis is a hematoma, although other groin masses such as hernias and adenopathy are occasionally encountered.

On gray-scale sonography, both pseudoaneurysms and hematomas appear as fluid collections in the vicinity of the femoral artery. Occasionally, pseudoaneurysms can be seen to expand during systole and contract during diastole. This is unusual, however, and generally it is impossible to distinguish pseudoaneurysms from hematomas on the basis of gray-scale imaging alone **(Option (D) is true)**. Duplex Doppler sonogra-

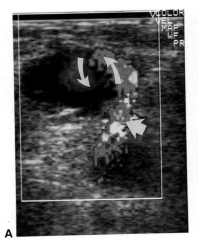

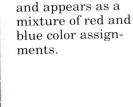

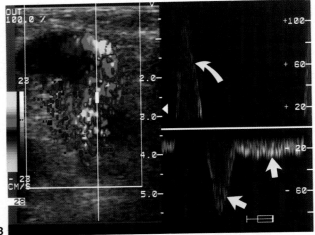

Figure 21-27. Pseudoaneurysm. (A) A transverse view of the right groin demonstrates a small pseudoaneurysm containing a swirling pattern of internal blood flow (curved arrows). The narrow neck of the pseudoaneurysm is also identified (straight arrow). (B) A transverse color Doppler image and a pulsed Doppler waveform demonstrate the typical to-and-fro pattern of flow within the pseudoaneurysm neck, with antegrade flow into the pseudoaneurysm during systole (curved arrow) and retrograde flow out of the pseudoaneurysm in diastole (straight arrows). Tissue vibration is also identified in the soft tissues around the pseudoaneurysm neck and appears as a mixture of red and blue color assignments.

phy is much better suited to distinguishing between pseudoaneurysms and hematomas. A fluid collection showing pulsatile flow that varies with the cardiac cycle is the most common finding in pseudoaneurysms. The most specific finding detected by duplex Doppler sonography is the "to and fro" pattern of flow seen at the neck of the pseudoaneurysm **(Option (B) is true).** This appears as forward flow during systole, when flow from the artery enters the pseudoaneurysm, and as reverse flow during diastole, when flow exits the pseudoaneurysm and reenters the artery (Figure 21-27). The to-and-fro pattern is harder to detect by duplex Doppler sonography because a pseudoaneurysm neck is usually too narrow to be visualized by gray-scale sonography **(Option (E) is false).** Therefore, the region between the pseudoaneurysm lumen and the adjacent

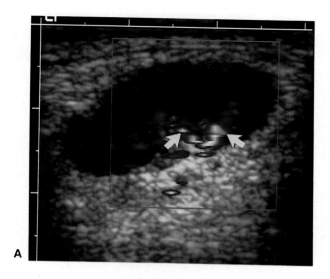

A

Figure 21-28. Inguinal lymph node. (A) A transverse color Doppler image of the groin demonstrates a hypoechoic lymph node that could simulate a complex fluid collection. Near the hilum of the lymph node, pairs of arteries and veins are identified (arrows). This branching pattern of flow is very different from the swirling pattern seen in a pseudoaneurysm. (B) A pulsed Doppler waveform from one of these vessels demonstrates typical arterial flow above the baseline and venous flow below the baseline. The typical to-and-fro pattern seen in pseudoaneurysm necks could not be identified at any point within or adjacent to this lymph node.

artery must be searched for blindly with the pulsed Doppler sample volume. Color Doppler greatly facilitates the identification of the pseudoaneurysm neck and thus allows for more frequent detection of the to-and-fro pattern. It also readily displays the swirling intraluminal blood flow distinctive of pseudoaneurysms **(Option (A) is true).**

Pseudoaneurysms are usually easily diagnosed by color Doppler imaging, but potential pitfalls do exist. Enlarged, inflamed inguinal lymph nodes can simulate fluid collections on gray-scale sonography. They can also generate internal arterial signals that can simulate the pulsatile flow in a pseudoaneurysm lumen (Figure 21-28). However, careful inspection of the flow pattern on color Doppler sonography shows that it is a fanlike appearance of branching arteries entering the mass and veins exiting the mass rather than the swirling pattern seen with pseudoaneurysms. In addition, the artery supplying the lymph node does not have the to-and-fro pattern typical of pseudoaneurysm necks.

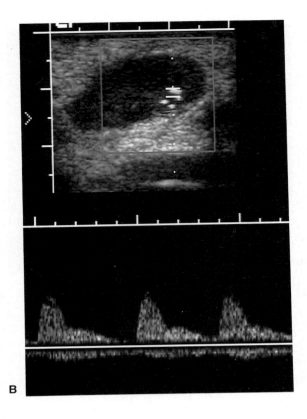

B

Another potential pitfall is ascites-filled femoral hernias. Fluid can enter and exit the hernia through the defect in the abdominal wall, and hence it can simulate the to-and-fro waveform at the site of communication and can generate a swirling pattern of internal flow. However, the communication is with the abdominal cavity and not the arterial system, so that the pulsations vary with the respiratory cycle, not the cardiac cycle (Figure 21-29).

In the past, diagnosis of a pseudoaneurysm was rapidly followed by surgical repair because of the fear of rupture. This is no longer the case **(Option (C) is false).** In the past 4 to 5 years, it has become clear that many pseudoaneurysms detected by color Doppler sonography will thrombose spontaneously. It has also been shown that pseudoaneurysms can be effectively treated by sonography-guided compression. The success rate for this treatment is approximately 75%.

William D. Middleton, M.D.

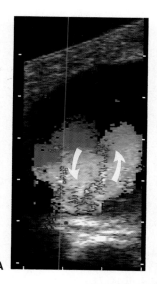

Figure 21-29. Ascites-filled femoral hernia simulating a pseudoaneurysm. (A) A longitudinal view of the groin demonstrates a fluid collection that contains a swirling pattern of internal flow (curved arrows). This pattern exactly mimics that seen in pseudoaneurysms. (B) A pulsed Doppler waveform near the base of the fluid collection demonstrates a pattern somewhat mimicking the to-and-fro pattern seen in pseudoaneurysms, with flow above the baseline (straight arrows) as well as below the baseline (curved arrows). However, the pulsations occurred approximately once every 4.5 seconds, which corresponded to the respiratory cycle and not the cardiac cycle. This suggests communication with the abdominal cavity rather than with the arterial system.

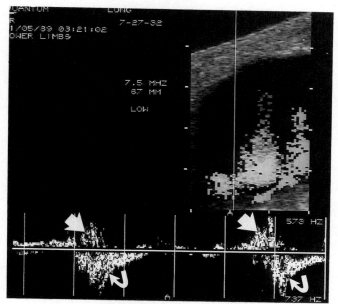

SUGGESTED READINGS

PSEUDOANEURYSM AND ARTERIOVENOUS FISTULAS

1. Altin RS, Flicker S, Naidech HJ. Pseudoaneurysm and arteriovenous fistula after femoral artery catheterization: association with low femoral punctures. AJR 1989; 152:629–631

2. Dorfman GS, Cronan JJ. Postcatheterization femoral artery injuries: is there a role for nonsurgical treatment? Radiology 1991; 178:629–630

3. Fellmeth BD, Roberts AC, Bookstein JJ, et al. Postangiographic femoral artery injuries: nonsurgical repair with US-guided compression. Radiology 1991; 178:671–675

4. Helvie MA, Rubin J. Evaluation of traumatic groin arteriovenous fistulas with duplex Doppler sonography. J Ultrasound Med 1989; 8:21–24

5. Helvie MA, Rubin JM, Silver TM, Kresowik TF. The distinction between femoral artery pseudoaneurysms and other causes of groin masses: value of duplex Doppler sonography. AJR 1988; 150:1177–1180

6. Igidbashian VN, Mitchell DG, Middleton WD, Schwartz RA, Goldberg BB. Iatrogenic femoral arteriovenous fistula: diagnosis with color Doppler imaging. Radiology 1989; 170:749–752

7. Kotval PS, Khoury A, Shah PM, Babu SC. Doppler sonographic demonstration of the progressive spontaneous thrombosis of pseudoaneurysms. J Ultrasound Med 1990; 9:185–190

8. Middleton WD. Duplex and color Doppler sonography of postcatheterization arteriovenous fistulas. Semin Intervent Radiol 1990; 7:192–197

9. Rapoport S, Sniderman KW, Morse SS, Proto MH, Ross GR. Pseudoaneurysm: a complication of faulty technique in femoral arterial puncture. Radiology 1985; 154:529–530

10. Ross RS. Arterial complications. Circulation 1968; 37(Suppl):39–41

11. Sheikh KH, Adams DB, McCann R, Lyerly HK, Sabiston DC, Kisslo J. Utility of Doppler color flow imaging for identification of femoral arterial complications of cardiac catheterization. Am Heart J 1989; 117:623–628

12. Skillman JJ, Kim D, Baim DS. Vascular complications of percutaneous femoral cardiac interventions. Incidence and operative repair. Arch Surg 1988; 123:1207–1212

DOPPLER ANALYSIS OF THE NECK VESSELS

13. Bluth EI, Kay D, Merritt CR, et al. Sonographic characterization of carotid plaque: detection of hemorrhage. AJR 1986; 146:1061–1065

14. Bluth EI, Stavros AT, Marich KW, Wetzner SM, Aufrichtig D, Baker JD. Carotid duplex sonography: a multicenter recommendation for standardized imaging and Doppler criteria. RadioGraphics 1988; 8:487–506

15. Cardoso TJ, Middleton WD. Duplex and color Doppler ultrasound of the carotid arteries. Semin Intervent Radiol 1990; 7:1–8

16. Carroll BA. Carotid sonography. Radiology 1991; 178:303–313

17. Erickson SJ, Mewissen MW, Foley WD, et al. Color Doppler evaluation of arterial stenoses and occlusions involving the neck and thoracic inlet. RadioGraphics 1989; 9:389–406

18. Hunink MG, Polak JF, Barlan MM, O'Leary DH. Detection and quantification of carotid artery stenosis: efficacy of various Doppler velocity parameters. AJR 1993; 160:619–625

19. Merritt CR, Bluth EI. The future of carotid sonography. AJR 1992; 158:37–39

20. O'Leary DH, Polak JF. High-resolution carotid sonography: past, present, and future. AJR 1989; 153:699–704

21. Zwiebel WJ. Duplex sonography of the cerebral arteries: efficacy, limitations, and indications. AJR 1992; 158:29–36

Notes

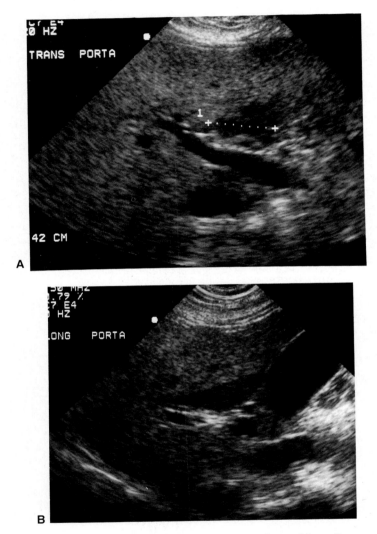

Figure 22-1. This 51-year-old woman was evaluated by ultrasonography because of elevated liver function tests. You are shown transverse (A) and longitudinal (B) images through the region of the porta hepatis.

Case 22: Fatty Infiltration

Question 101

Which *one* of the following is the MOST likely diagnosis?

(A) Metastases
(B) Cavernous hemangioma
(C) Fatty infiltration
(D) Focal nodular hyperplasia
(E) Lymphoma

Figure 22-1 shows a focal region of apparently decreased echogenicity in the hepatic parenchyma located anterior to the porta hepatis (see Figure 22-2). The visualized borders of the region are geographic in shape on the transverse image and straight on the longitudinal image. The location and shape of this zone of decreased echogenicity are very characteristic of focal parenchymal sparing in a liver that has otherwise undergone diffuse fatty infiltration **(Option (C) is correct).**

Fatty infiltration of the liver occurs in a number of situations. Obesity is probably the most common predisposing factor in this country. Alcohol abuse and other toxic injuries such as those due to carbon tetrachloride can cause fatty infiltration as well. Chemotherapy, diabetes mellitus, total parenteral nutrition, malnutrition, and steroids are also common causes. Fatty infiltration causes an increased fine parenchymal echogenicity that may be diffuse and homogeneous or patchy and heterogeneous in distribution. Fatty infiltration can also appear nodular and be focal or multifocal. Frequently, in patients with diffuse fatty infiltration, a small region anterior to the porta hepatis is spared. This small zone of normal hepatic parenchyma appears hypoechoic compared with the surrounding hyperechoic fat-infiltrated parenchyma. The end result is that the normal, spared region appears abnormal and the remainder of the liver appears normal.

Potentially, any type of focal hepatic lesion could be confused with focal sparing. Metastatic disease to the liver (Option (A)) is very common, and so it is the most serious diagnosis to exclude. In the test

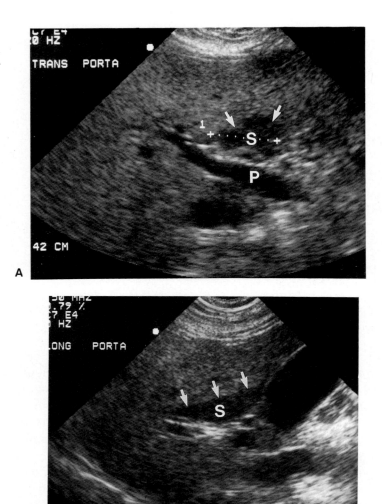

Figure 22-2 (Same as Figure 22-1).   Fatty infiltration with focal parenchymal sparing anterior to the porta hepatis. (A) A transverse sonogram
of the porta hepatis demonstrates a hypoechoic zone of spared normal
hepatic parenchyma (S) surrounded by more echogenic fat-infiltrated
liver. The hypoechoic zone of normal hepatic parenchyma is located anterior to the portal vein (P). Its margins (arrows) are somewhat geographic. (B) A longitudinal sonogram of the liver again demonstrates a
focal region of spared hypoechoic hepatic parenchyma (S) that has a very
straight anterior margin (arrows).

patient, the lack of other lesions, the geographic margins of the hypoechoic region, and the typical location anterior to the porta hepatis make

metastatic disease much less likely than focal sparing. Hepatic lymphoma (Option (E)) and focal nodular hyperplasia (FNH) (Option (D)) are unlikely for similar reasons. Hepatic lymphoma is often diffusely infiltrative and undetectable with sonography. When lymphoma produces focal intrahepatic masses, they tend to be hypoechoic. Occasionally, non-Hodgkin's lymphoma will produce a target appearance with a hyperechoic or isoechoic center and a hypoechoic rim. FNH is a benign tumor composed of normal-appearing but abnormally arranged hepatocytes, bile ducts, blood vessels, and Kupffer cells. FNH has a varied sonographic appearance. It may be hypoechoic, isoechoic, hyperechoic, or mixed or have a target appearance. The central stellate scar, which is typical pathologically, is uncommonly seen sonographically. Cavernous hemangioma (Option (B)) is even less likely than the other possibilities because it is usually a well-defined hyperechoic lesion.

Question 102

Concerning metastatic disease to the liver,

    (A) calcification occurs most frequently in metastases from colon carcinoma
    (B) target lesions imply a squamous cell origin
    (C) intraoperative sonography is more sensitive than MRI in its detection
    (D) perihepatic ascites is an absolute contraindication to sonographically guided percutaneous biopsy
    (E) sonographic detection of focal lesions in livers that are diffusely heterogeneous as a result of cirrhosis usually indicates regenerating nodules

Metastases are the most common cause of focal and multifocal hepatic lesions. The sonographic appearance of hepatic metastases varies greatly. In fact, hepatic metastases from the same primary tumor in the same patient can appear different. It is not possible to confidently predict histology on the basis of the sonographic appearance, but certain trends can be useful in patient management.

Hyperechoic metastases tend to arise from the gastrointestinal tract. Colon cancer in particular tends to produce hyperechoic metastases and is the most likely primary tumor in patients with calcified metastases (Figure 22-3) **(Option (A) is true)**. Calcified metastases can also result from mucinous cystadenocarcinomas of the ovaries, breast, and stomach; osteosarcoma; chondrosarcoma; and neuroblastoma.

Cystic metastases can result from cystic primary tumors such as cystadenocarcinomas of the pancreas and ovary. Tumor necrosis can also produce cystic components in hepatic metastases. This occurs most frequently in patients with squamous cell carcinomas (Figure 22-4), sarco-

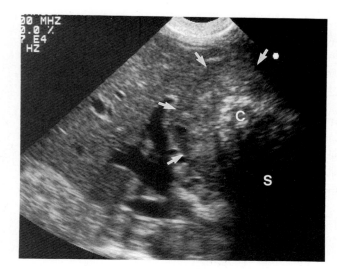

Figure 22-3 (left). Calcified hepatic metastasis from colon carcinoma. A transverse sonogram of the liver demonstrates a large mass (arrows) with a calcified center (C) that casts an acoustic shadow (S).

Figure 22-4 (right). Necrotic, partially cystic metastasis. A transverse sonogram of the liver demonstrates a hypoechoic mass with an irregular cystic space centrally secondary to metastasis from squamous cell carcinoma of the esophagus. (Case courtesy of Sharlene A. Teefey, M.D., University of Washington, Seattle.)

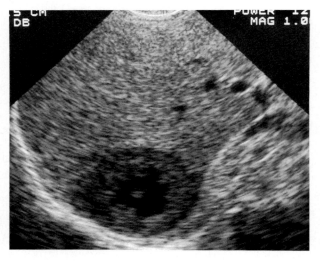

mas (especially leiomyosarcoma), and carcinoid tumors (Figure 22-5) but is also seen with carcinoma of the colon and lung and with malignant melanoma.

Many different primary tumors result in hepatic metastases that have a target appearance composed of an echogenic center and a hypoechoic rim (Figure 22-6). This pattern does not imply any particular cell type **(Option (B) is false),** but a recent study has shown that the target appearance is much more likely to indicate a malignant lesion than a benign lesion. It is particularly helpful in distinguishing metastases

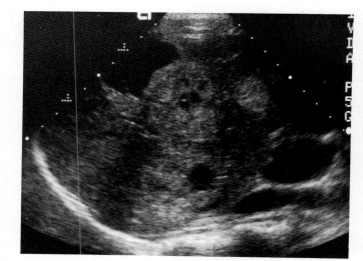

Figure 22-5 (left). Metastatic carcinoid tumor. A longitudinal sonogram of the liver demonstrates several hyperechoic masses with various degrees of cystic necrosis.

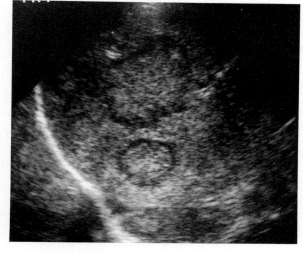

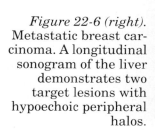

Figure 22-6 (right). Metastatic breast carcinoma. A longitudinal sonogram of the liver demonstrates two target lesions with hypoechoic peripheral halos.

from hemangiomas, since it is quite unusual for hemangiomas to have a hypoechoic halo. It is less helpful in distinguishing metastases from other hepatic masses, since hepatocellular carcinoma (Figure 22-7), FNH, and adenomas frequently have a hypoechoic halo. Non-Hodgkin's lymphomas and *Candida* abscesses can also have a target appearance. Pathologic correlation has shown that the hypoechoic halo arises most often from a peripheral zone of proliferating tumor cells and less often from compressed adjacent hepatic parenchyma.

Another pattern of hepatic metastases is diffuse heterogeneity and coarsening of the hepatic parenchyma (Figure 22-8). In the absence of

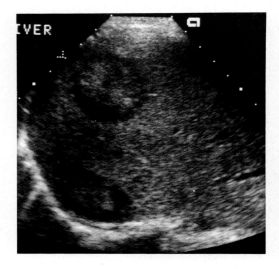

Figure 22-7 (left). Multifocal hepatocellular carcinoma. A transverse sonogram of the liver demonstrates two target lesions similar in appearance to those seen in Figure 22-6.

detectable focal lesions, this appearance is nonspecific and can also be seen in patients with cirrhosis, fatty infiltration, and diffuse hepatocellular carcinoma. In patients with known cirrhosis and diffuse heterogeneity, sonographic detection of hepatic tumors is quite difficult (sensitivity, approximately 50%). However, the specificity of sonography in this setting is very high (approximately 98%). Therefore, the presence of focal masses in a background of diffuse heterogeneity should be viewed with a great deal of concern since most are malignant (either metastatic disease [Figure 22-9] or hepatocellular carcinoma) **(Option (E) is false).**

As in other organs, lymphoma can involve the liver diffusely or can produce multiple focal lesions (Figure 22-10); therefore, it should be considered in the differential diagnosis of hepatic metastases. The uniform histologic nature of lymphoma results in very few acoustic interfaces in these masses, which tend to be very hypoechoic. In fact, on occasion they are anechoic and very closely simulate simple hepatic cysts (Figure 22-11). The degree of increased through transmission behind a lymphomatous mass should be less than that behind a cyst of the same size, and this difference can be of value in distinguishing these two types of lesions. In addition, the margins of lymphomatous nodules tend to be less well defined than do those of cysts.

When focal or multifocal lesions are detected in the liver, sonographically guided biopsy is a valuable technique for determining their histologic type. The three contraindications for sonographically guided biopsy are uncontrollable coagulopathy, lack of a safe biopsy path that avoids vital structures, and inability of the patient to cooperate with the procedure. The presence of perihepatic ascites was once thought to be a

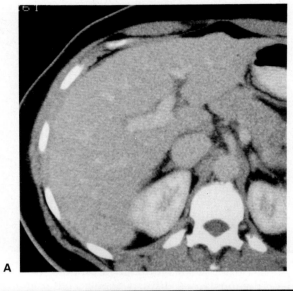

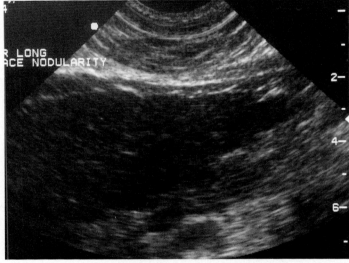

Figure 22-8. Metastatic breast carcinoma diffusely infiltrating the liver and producing a "pseudocirrhotic" appearance. (A) A postcontrast CT scan of the liver demonstrates a normal appearance without identifiable focal lesions. (B) A longitudinal sonogram of the left lobe of the liver demonstrates nodularity of the liver surface, closely mimicking hepatic cirrhosis. No focal lesions were identified sonographically. Several random liver biopsies were performed, and all biopsy specimens revealed metastatic breast carcinoma.

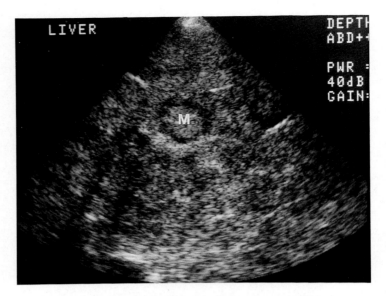

Figure 22-9. Metastatic transitional cell carcinoma. A transverse sonogram of the liver demonstrates diffuse hepatic heterogeneity with one focal hepatic mass (M) producing a target appearance. A biopsy specimen of this lesion was positive for transitional cell carcinoma.

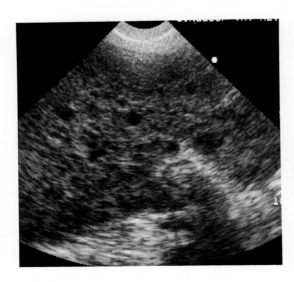

Figure 22-10 (left). Hepatic lymphoma. A transverse sonogram of the liver demonstrates multiple small, hypoechoic hepatic lesions and diffuse heterogeneity and coarsening of the hepatic parenchymal echogenicity secondary to diffuse lymphoma.

contraindication to percutaneous hepatic biopsy, but Murphy et al. have shown that the risk of complications is no greater in patients with ascites than in patients without ascites **(Option (D) is false).** The accuracy of

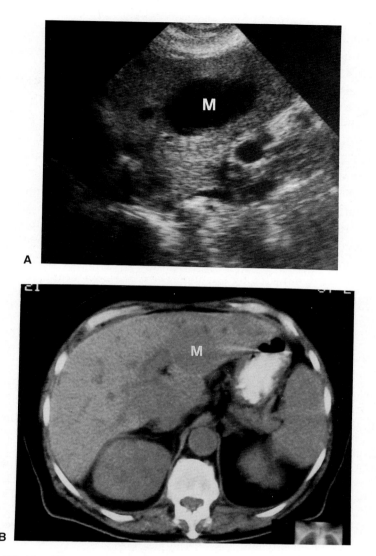

Figure 22-11. Hepatic lymphoma simulating a cyst. (A) A longitudinal sonogram of the left lobe of the liver demonstrates an anechoic mass (M) with increased through transmission. This differs from a simple hepatic cyst only in the lack of sharp demarcation between the margins of the lesions and the adjacent hepatic parenchyma. (B) A CT scan of the same patient demonstrates a low-attenuation but solid mass (M) in the left lobe of the liver. (Case courtesy of Mary A. Middleton, M.D., Mallinckrodt Institute of Radiology, Barnes West Hospital, St. Louis, Mo.)

sonographically guided liver biopsy in establishing the diagnosis of hepatic metastases when lesions are less than 3 cm in size is approximately 95%.

Intraoperative ultrasonography is extremely valuable in patients who are undergoing partial hepatic resection for metastatic disease. It is more sensitive than any preoperative imaging test including MRI and CT arterial portography **(Option (C) is true).** This is based on data showing that CT arterial portography is superior to MRI, with respective sensitivities of 81 to 85% versus 57 to 68%, and on more recent data showing that the sensitivity of ultrasonography is 96%, as opposed to 91% for CT arterial portography. In addition to detecting unsuspected masses that could make the tumor unresectable or could alter the extent of the resection, intraoperative ultrasonography can determine the anatomic relationship of the masses to the hepatic vessels. This information is useful in planning the resection. Intraoperative ultrasonography is very sensitive, but it is not specific enough to definitively distinguish benign from malignant lesions. Therefore, when new lesions that would alter surgery are detected by intraoperative ultrasonography, sonographically guided biopsy may be necessary.

Question 103

Concerning cavernous hemangiomas of the liver,

    (A) they typically exhibit blood flow in multiple vessels on color Doppler ultrasonography
    (B) there is no sex predisposition
    (C) large lesions are easier to characterize sonographically than are small lesions
    (D) scintigraphy with Tc-99m erythrocytes is more sensitive than MRI in detecting them
    (E) in about 25% of cases, percutaneous biopsy results in hemoperitoneum requiring transfusion

Hemangiomas are the most common benign hepatic neoplasms and are second only to metastases as a cause of hepatic masses. They occur in up to 7% of the population in autopsy series. Approximately 10% are multiple, and these are typically small (less than 3 cm in diameter). From 70 to 90% occur in women **(Option (B) is false).** Hemangiomas are frequently located in a subcapsular position, more often in the right lobe posteriorly. They occur in all age groups but are most common in adults.

Cavernous hemangiomas can be thought of as spongelike tumors filled with blood. They consist of tiny spaces lined with a single layer of endothelium and separated by fibrous septa. The multiple acoustic inter-

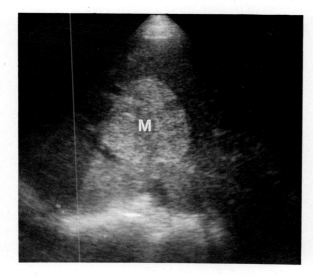

Figure 22-12. Cavernous hemangioma with typical sonographic features. A transverse sonogram of the liver demonstrates a round, well-marginated hyperechoic mass (M) with increased through transmission.

faces between the blood-filled spaces produce the typical hyperechoic appearance on sonography.

The vast majority of hemangiomas are asymptomatic. Occasionally, large lesions cause abdominal discomfort because of the mass effect. Spontaneous hemorrhage, although reported, is extremely rare. Sequestration and destruction of platelets within giant hemangiomas have been reported to result in thrombocytopenia and consumptive coagulopathy; this is called the Kasabach-Merritt syndrome.

The characteristic sonographic appearance of hemangiomas is a spherical, well-defined, homogeneous hyperechoic mass with posterior acoustic enhancement (Figure 22-12). Increased through transmission has been reported in up to 77% of hemangiomas, but its occurrence is variable. In addition, other solid lesions occasionally have increased through transmission, so this finding has limited practical diagnostic value.

Approximately 70% of hemangiomas are hyperechoic, and approximately 70% of these are homogeneous. Fibrosis, thrombosis, and hemorrhagic necrosis cause the remainder of hemangiomas to be either hypoechoic, isoechoic, or mixed in echogenicity (Figure 22-13). These atypical appearances tend to be more common in larger lesions (Figures 22-14 and 2-15) **(Option (C) is false).** Hemangiomas can also appear to have decreased echogenicity when the hepatic parenchymal echogenicity is increased, as in patients with fatty infiltration.

Moody and Wilson have recently shown that many "atypical" hemangiomas actually have a characteristic appearance consisting of a hypo-

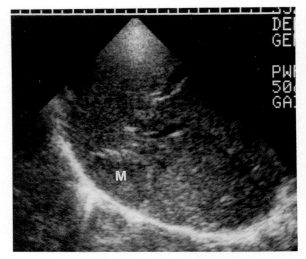

Figure 22-13 (left). Cavernous hemangioma with atypical sonographic features. A transverse sonogram of the liver demonstrates an isoechoic mass (M) with a hyperechoic rim. This was proven to represent a hemangioma by Tc-99m erythrocyte scintigraphy.

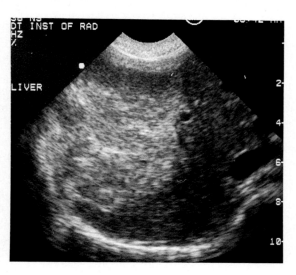

Figure 22-14 (right). Large cavernous hemangioma with atypical sonographic appearance. A transverse sonogram of the liver demonstrates a 7-cm predominantly hyperechoic but heterogeneous mass in the right lobe; this mass was proven to represent a hemangioma by its typical CT appearance.

echoic center and a hyperechoic rim. This pattern was present in 27 of 29 cases of atypical hemangiomas reviewed retrospectively. When this pattern was studied prospectively, 14 of 15 lesions seen over a 6-month period were hemangiomas and only 1 was a malignant mass (leiomyosarcoma of the cava).

Despite the vascular nature of hemangiomas, they rarely have detectable blood flow on color Doppler sonography **(Option (A) is false).** This is because the flow velocities in the lesions are extremely low and are below the threshold for Doppler detectability. If arterial flow is

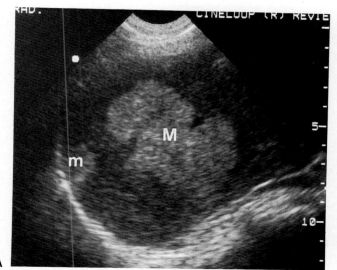

A

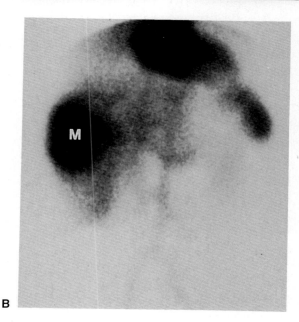

B

Figure 22-15.
Large lobulated
cavernous heman-
gioma. (A) A trans-
verse sonogram of
the liver demon-
strates a large, ho-
mogeneous, hyper-
echoic mass (M)
with a lobulated
external contour. A
second, smaller
mass (m) is seen
adjacent to the
hemidiaphragm.
(B) A delayed ante-
rior Tc-99m eryth-
rocyte scintigram
demonstrates a
mass (M) with increased
blood-pool activity in the
right lobe of the liver corresponding to the large, lobulated, hyperechoic mass
seen on sonography. The
smaller mass seen on
sonography was also
proven to be a hemangi-
oma.

detected within a mass, this greatly decreases the likelihood that it is a
hemangioma.

Hemangiomas are usually stable in both size and sonographic
appearance. However, approximately 8% change size (2% enlarge, 6%
regress partially or completely), and 10% change appearance (become

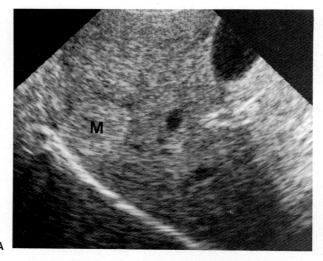

A

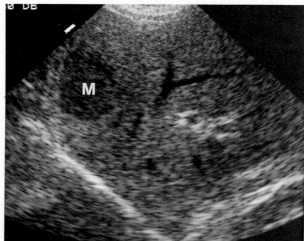

B

Figure 22-16.
Changing appearance of a cavernous hemangioma over time. (A) A transverse sonogram of the liver demonstrates a homogeneous hyperechoic mass (M) in the liver, adjacent to the hemidiaphragm. (B) A follow-up examination performed 3 years later demonstrated stable size of the mass (M) but a change from a hyperechoic to a hypoechoic appearance. (Case courtesy of Sharlene A. Teefey, M.D.)

less echogenic) (Figure 22-16). Hemangiomas have also been reported to enlarge during pregnancy and during estrogen therapy.

The appropriate workup for a suspected hemangioma depends on a number of factors. When a typical-appearing hemangioma is detected in a patient with normal liver function tests, no history of malignancy, and no conditions predisposing to hepatocellular carcinoma, some radiologists would argue that no further evaluation is necessary. Others would recommend a follow-up sonogram in 6 months to ensure lesion stability. A third approach would be to perform another correlative imaging study. In patients with a high risk of either a hepatic malignancy or a potentially symptomatic benign lesion (e.g., adenoma or FNH), obtaining another correlative examination is very important. Scintigraphy with Tc-99m erythrocytes has a specificity of almost 100% for hemangiomas and is the most appropriate next study for most patients. However, Birnbaum et al. have shown that its sensitivity in detecting small (<2 cm) hemangiomas is lower than that of MRI (58% versus 83%) **(Option (D) is false);** therefore, small lesions are probably better evaluated by MRI since it is both very sensitive and relatively specific for hemangioma. The actual size threshold at which MRI should be used instead of scintigraphy is not universally agreed. Certainly, lesions less than 1 cm in diameter should be evaluated by MRI and lesions greater than 3 cm should be evaluated by scintigraphy. The appropriate choice for lesions between 1 and 3 cm depends on the availability of SPECT imaging, on the location of the lesion relative to other blood-pool spaces such as the heart and major hepatic vessels, and on the experience of the radiologist interpreting the MR and scintigraphic studies. Birnbaum et al. suggest that MRI should be used for lesions less than 2.0 cm that are remote from the heart and hepatic vessels and for lesions less than 2.5 cm that are adjacent to these vascular structures.

The vast majority of hemangiomas can be correctly diagnosed noninvasively by a combination of ultrasonography, CT, scintigraphy, and MRI. Therefore it is rarely necessary to perform percutaneous biopsy of hemangiomas. However, the correct diagnosis may not be considered when a hemangioma is atypical, and the next step may be biopsy rather than other imaging tests. Despite the vascular nature of hemangiomas, complications following biopsy are rare (Figure 22-17) **(Option (E) is false).** In the series of 15 hemangiomas biopsied by Cronan et al., there were no complications and there was 100% success in diagnosis from biopsies performed with 20-gauge cutting needles. In the series of 33 hemangiomas biopsied by Solbiati et al., no complications were encountered but there was only a 27% success in diagnosis from biopsies performed with a 22-gauge aspiration needle. To maintain a low complication rate, it is advisable to direct the needle through normal liver parenchyma before it enters the lesion.

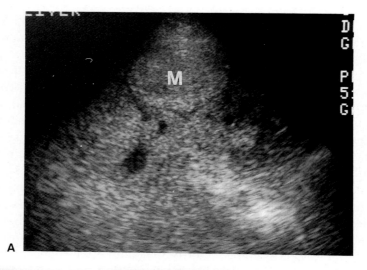

A

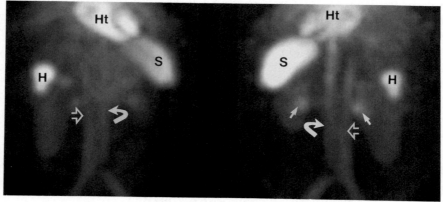

B

Figure 22-17. Hemangioma. This patient with gallstone pancreatitis had an incidental hepatic mass detected sonographically. (A) A transverse sonogram of the liver demonstrates a slightly hyperechoic mass (M) with a thin hypoechoic halo. This appearance was thought to be nonspecific but atypical for a hemangioma. Therefore, a CT scan was obtained and demonstrated a low-attenuation mass with minimal uniform concentric peripheral enhancement, also thought to be atypical for a hemangioma. Because of this, percutaneous fine-needle aspiration biopsy was performed. The aspirate consisted predominantly of blood with little cellular material, and no diagnosis could be obtained. The patient experienced no complications from the biopsy procedure. (B) Volume-rendered SPECT reprojection images (anterior view on right, posterior view on left) obtained from a Tc-99m erythrocyte scintigram demonstrate a focal area of increased activity typical of hemangioma (H). Also seen are the heart (Ht), spleen (S), right and left renal pelves (solid straight arrows), aorta (curved arrow), and inferior vena cava (open arrows).

SUGGESTED READINGS

FATTY INFILTRATION

1. Garra BS, Insana MF, Shawker TH, Russell MA. Quantitative estimation of liver attenuation and echogenicity: normal state versus diffuse liver disease. Radiology 1987; 162:61–67
2. Quinn SF, Gosink BB. Characteristic sonographic signs of hepatic fatty infiltration. AJR 1985; 145:753–755
3. Wang SS, Chiang JH, Tsai YT, et al. Focal hepatic fatty infiltration as a cause of pseudotumors: ultrasonographic patterns and clinical differentiation. JCU 1990; 18:401–409
4. White EM, Simeone JF, Mueller PR, Grant EG, Choyke PL, Zeman RK. Focal periportal sparing in hepatic fatty infiltration: a cause of hepatic pseudomass on US. Radiology 1987; 162:57–59
5. Yates CK, Streight RA. Focal fatty infiltration of the liver simulating metastatic disease. Radiology 1986; 159:83–84
6. Yoshikawa J, Matsui O, Takashima T, et al. Focal fatty change of the liver adjacent to the falciform ligament: CT and sonographic findings in five surgically confirmed cases. AJR 1987; 149:491–494

HEPATIC METASTASES

7. Dodd GD III, Miller WJ, Baron RL, Skolnick ML, Campbell WL. Detection of malignant tumors in end-stage cirrhotic livers: efficacy of sonography as a screening technique. AJR 1992; 159:727–733
8. Heiken JP, Weyman PJ, Lee JK, et al. Detection of focal hepatic masses: prospective evaluation with CT, delayed CT, CT during arterial portography, and MR imaging. Radiology 1989; 171:47–51
9. Marn CS, Bree RL, Silver TM. Ultrasonography of liver. Technique and focal and diffuse disease. Radiol Clin North Am 1991; 29:1151–1170
10. Murphy FB, Barefield KP, Steinberg HV, Bernardino ME. CT- or sonography-guided biopsy of the liver in the presence of ascites: frequency of complications. AJR 1988; 151:485–486
11. Nelson RC, Chezmar JL, Sugarbaker PH, Bernardino ME. Hepatic tumors: comparison of CT during arterial portography, delayed CT, and MR imaging for preoperative evaluation. Radiology 1989; 172:27–34
12. Reading CC, Charboneau JW, James EM, Hurt MR. Sonographically guided percutaneous biopsy of small (3 cm or less) masses. AJR 1988; 151:189–192
13. Soyer P, Levesque M, Elias D, Zeitoun G, Roche A. Detection of liver metastases from colorectal cancer: comparison of intraoperative US and CT during arterial portography. Radiology 1992; 183:541–544
14. Wernecke K, Henke L, Vassallo P, et al. Pathologic explanation for hypoechoic halo seen on sonograms of malignant liver tumors: an *in vitro* correlative study. AJR 1992; 159:1011–1016
15. Wernecke K, Vassallo P, Bick U, Diederich S, Peters PE. The distinction between benign and malignant liver tumors on sonography: value of a hypoechoic halo. AJR 1992; 159:1005–1009

16. Birnbaum BA, Weinreb JC, Megibow AJ, et al. Definitive diagnosis of hepatic hemangiomas: MR imaging versus Tc-99m-labeled red blood cell SPECT. Radiology 1990; 176:95–101

17. Bree RL, Schwab RE, Glazer GM, Fink-Bennett D. The varied appearances of hepatic cavernous hemangiomas with sonography, computed tomography, magnetic resonance imaging and scintigraphy. RadioGraphics 1987; 7:1153–1175

18. Cronan JJ, Esparza AR, Dorfman GS, Ridlen MS, Paolella LP. Cavernous hemangioma of the liver: role of percutaneous biopsy. Radiology 1988; 166:135–138

19. Gibney RG, Hendin AP, Cooperberg PL. Sonographically detected hepatic hemangiomas: absence of change over time. AJR 1987; 149:953–957

20. Marsh JI, Gibney RG, Li DK. Hepatic hemangioma in the presence of fatty infiltration: an atypical sonographic appearance. Gastrointest Radiol 1989; 14:262–264

21. Moody AR, Wilson SR. Atypical hepatic hemangioma: a suggestive sonographic morphology. Radiology 1993; 188:413–417

22. Nelson RC, Chezmar JL. Diagnostic approach to hepatic hemangiomas. Radiology 1990; 176:11–13

23. Solbiati L, Livraghi T, DePra L, Ierace T, Masciadri N, Ravetto C. Fine-needle biopsy of hepatic hemangioma with sonographic guidance. AJR 1985; 114:471–474

Notes

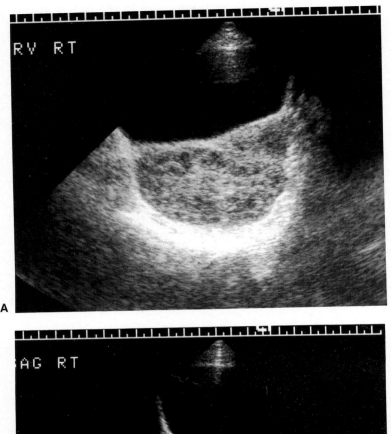

A

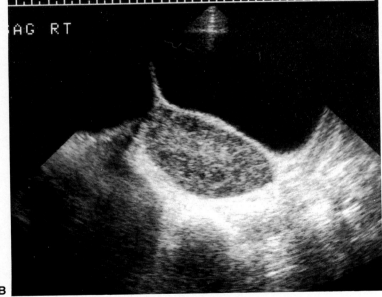

B

Figure 23-1. This 19-year-old woman presented with pelvic pain. You are shown transverse (A) and sagittal (B) sonograms of the right ovary. The left ovary appeared normal.

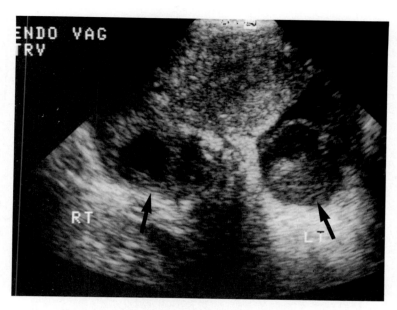

Figure 23-6. Bilateral tubo-ovarian abscesses. An endovaginal sonogram shows bilateral cystic masses (arrows) containing debris and exhibiting through transmission.

A hemorrhagic ovarian cyst (Option (E)) usually presents as a cystic ovarian mass with enhanced through transmission but with internal echoes and, occasionally, internal septations and wall thickness (Figure 23-7). The appearance is similar to a typical endometrioma of the ovary. This is not surprising since both are related to hemorrhage. Occasionally, there is a great deal of hemorrhage within an ovarian cyst, which results in a very echogenic mass, but even in these cases there is almost always enhanced through transmission, indicating the cystic nature of the lesion. In the test images, there is no evidence that the mass is cystic; therefore, hemorrhagic ovarian cyst is a very unlikely possibility.

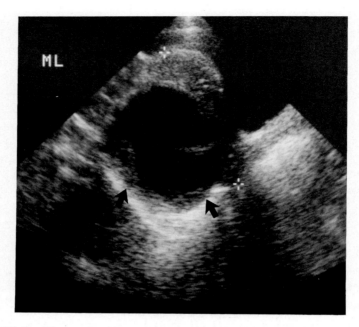

Figure 23-7. Hemorrhagic ovarian cyst. A longitudinal sonogram shows a cystic mass (arrows) exhibiting through transmission and containing some echogenic material.

Question 106

Concerning polycystic ovarian disease,

    (A) most patients have the Stein-Leventhal syndrome
    (B) the ovaries are usually normal in size
    (C) it is usually bilateral
    (D) the follicles are usually greater than 1 cm in diameter

    Polycystic ovarian disease is a highly complicated endocrine disorder characterized by a wide spectrum of clinical symptoms that occurs in women in their reproductive years. The original description was that of the Stein-Leventhal syndrome, which consists of amenorrhea, sterility, and hirsutism and is associated with bulky polycystic ovaries. However, it soon became apparent that most women with polycystic ovarian disease do not have the entire constellation of clinical findings indicative of the Stein-Leventhal syndrome **(Option (A) is false).**

The features that are most characteristic of polycystic ovarian disease are the presence of chronic anovulation and its association with endocrine abnormalities, particularly androgen excess. These functional aberrations account directly or indirectly for the other features of the syndrome. In addition, most patients have high levels of luteinizing hormone (LH) with low or decreased levels of follicle-stimulating hormone (FSH). Therefore, the LH/FSH ratio is elevated. The normal menstrual cycle is disrupted because of the imbalance between these two hormones. Both of these hormones are necessary for normal follicular maturation. In patients with this entity, the ovary continues to produce follicles but does not progress to follicle maturation and ovulation. The LH levels remain high, so the ovarian stroma is hyperstimulated, leading to excessive ovarian androgen levels. The end result of this is follicular atrophy.

The significant spectrum in the endocrine imbalance means that there is also variation in symptoms and in ovarian abnormalities. This is well documented in the surgical literature. The classic description is that of an enlarged white or grayish ovary with a "thickened capsule," but there are a number of reports of ovaries that are normal in size or only mildly enlarged. Follicles tend not to mature as a result of a lack of hormonal balance; therefore, numerous small follicles are frequently present.

The sonographic features of polycystic ovarian disease are variable, reflecting the spectrum of the ovarian abnormalities and the fact that most studies have used transabdominal ultrasonography, which is less precise than endovaginal ultrasonography. In a report by Yeh et al. of 104 patients with polycystic ovarian disease, only 30% of the ovaries were of normal size; this was also true for 29% of the 28 patients studied by Hann et al. Therefore, although the ovaries can be normal in size, they are usually enlarged (Figure 23-8) **(Option (B) is false).**

In the study by Yeh et al., the most important sonographic feature of polycystic ovarian disease was the bilaterally increased number of developing follicles **(Option (C) is true).** They were usually between 0.5 and 0.8 cm in diameter **(Option (D) is false),** and more than five follicles were present in each ovary. Parisi et al. studied 26 patients, 19 of whom had numerous small ovarian follicles. However, in the study by Hann et al., only 39% of the patients had discrete follicles less than 10 mm in size. The other patients had no definite follicles. The ovaries were hypoechoic or had a texture that was isoechoic to the uterus. This discrepancy could reflect the difficulty in imaging ovaries by transabdominal ultrasonography. Also, some of these studies are not recent, and current technology was not used. Ovaries in patients with polycystic ovarian disease are less likely to have maturing follicles (>1.5 cm) than are normal ovaries. This is a reflection of the hormonal imbalance that precludes follicular devel-

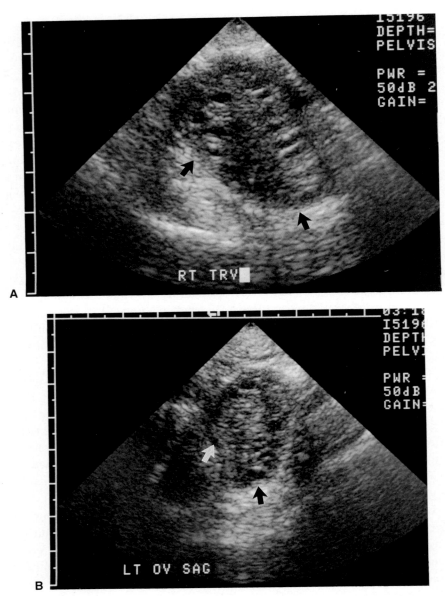

Figure 23-8. Polycystic ovarian disease. Endovaginal sonograms of the right (A) and left (B) ovaries (arrows) show ovarian enlargement. In each ovary, numerous small follicles and increased stromal echogenicity are observed.

opment in these patients. Endovaginal sonography allows for better evaluation of the ovaries. However, few reports have addressed the appear-

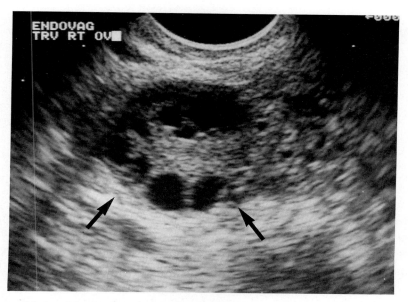

Figure 23-9. Normal ovary with follicles. An endovaginal sonogram shows a number of developing follicles in a normal ovary (arrows).

ance of polycystic ovaries by this technique. Pache et al. found that the stromal echogenicity was markedly increased in over 90% of their 52 patients (Figure 23-8). This was believed to be the greatest discriminator between normal and polycystic ovaries. However, as the authors state, echogenicity is subjective and might be difficult to use as the definitive diagnostic feature. It was also believed that there was a wide overlap between the sizes of the normal and polycystic ovaries. The authors recommended that the use of a number of parameters was the most sensitive and suggested that the combination of follicular size and ovarian volume be used. They used a multivariate logistic discriminant analysis of these two parameters to determine the likelihood of polycystic ovarian disease being present. This is difficult to employ in clinical practice, however.

During endovaginal scanning it is not unusual to see a fairly large number of small, developing follicles in normal ovaries at the appropriate time of the menstrual cycle (Figure 23-9). Therefore, there probably is considerable overlap between the appearance of normal ovaries and that of ovaries in some patients with polycystic ovarian disease. However, the consistent presence of only small follicles, and no dominant follicles, may be a constant finding. Additional studies by endovaginal ultrasonography will be necessary to further define the criteria for the sonographic diagnosis of this entity.

Question 107

Concerning ovarian torsion,

    (A) it does not occur in normal ovaries
    (B) it occurs most commonly in prepubertal girls
    (C) the most typical appearance is an enlarged ovary with cortical follicles
    (D) the sonographic appearance is frequently normal
    (E) it is associated with fluid in the cul-de-sac

Ovarian torsion is a relatively rare but well-recognized clinical and sonographic entity that is caused by partial or complete rotation of the ovarian pedicle on its axis. When this occurs, the lymphatic, venous, and arterial supplies are compromised, eventually leading to ischemia and infarction. If partial obstruction occurs, which is not common, there is massive congestion of the ovarian parenchyma, resulting in a very large ovary. This has been referred to as massive ovarian edema. More commonly, however, the obstruction becomes complete; this results in ischemia and infarction unless there is surgical intervention. Torsion does occur in normal ovaries **(Option (A) is false),** but it is more common in abnormal ovaries, i.e., those that contain cysts or other masses that potentiate the torsion. The ovary in the test patient contained a large cystic mass (Figures 23-2 and 23-10).

Ovarian torsion has been reported in patients at all ages. It is not unusual in children, but it is most common in young women **(Option (B) is false).** The reason for this may be that potentiating masses such as follicular cysts are more common in this age group. The clinical picture is one of lower-quadrant pain on the side of the affected ovary; the pain can last for several days. It is sometimes accompanied by gastrointestinal symptoms, such as nausea, vomiting, constipation, and diarrhea. Of the 26 patients in the study reported by Helvie and Silver, 25 had pelvic or abdominal pain, 18 had nausea or vomiting, and 13 had leukocytosis.

It is entirely possible that the symptoms will resolve spontaneously as a result of detorsion of the supportive ligaments. However, in such cases, the patient is prone to develop torsion subsequently. This is particularly true in children, who are probably at increased risk for repetitive events since torsion in this age group is most probably due to excessive mobility resulting from long supportive ligaments. If a child undergoes surgery for torsion of one ovary, it has been recommended that an oophoropexy (shortening of the ligamentous support) should be performed on the other ovary to prevent subsequent torsion.

The right adnexus is more frequently involved than the left (approximately 60% of cases), probably because the sigmoid colon interferes with twisting of the left adnexus. Because ovarian torsion occurs more fre-

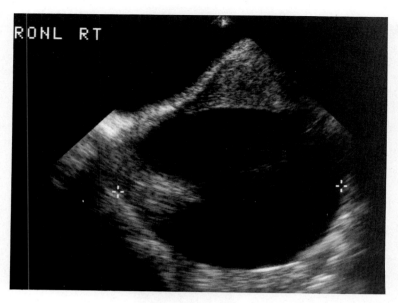

Figure 23-10. Same patient as in Figures 23-1 and 23-2. Ovarian torsion. A transverse sonogram shows a large ovarian cyst that contains some echoes. This was on the cephalic surface of the ovary as seen in Figures 23-1B and 23-2B, and it potentiated the torsion.

quently on the right side and is associated with pelvic or abdominal pain, appendicitis is a prominent consideration in the clinical differential diagnosis. Entities that also must be considered are bowel diseases (including regional enteritis and acute gastroenteritis), urinary tract infection, and other gynecologic conditions.

The sonographic findings in ovarian torsion are variable and depend on whether the torsion has occurred in an abnormal ovary containing a mass that has potentiated the torsion (Figure 23-11) or in a normal ovary (Figure 23-12). A specific sonographic appearance of torsion has been reported by Graif and Itzchak. Of 11 patients with surgically proven torsion, 8 had an obviously enlarged ovary with multiple enlarged follicles in the periphery. This appearance is thought to be typical for this entity (Figures 23-1 and 23-2) **(Option (C) is true)** and is most likely to occur in the absence of underlying ovarian pathology. In that series, seven cases occurred in normal ovaries. The enlarged follicles have been attributed to the congestive changes within the ovary, causing fluid accumulation within the follicles.

If the ovary is abnormal and contains a cystic or solid mass that has potentiated the torsion, the mass usually predominates as the main sonographic finding. In the study by Helvie and Silver of 26 patients with

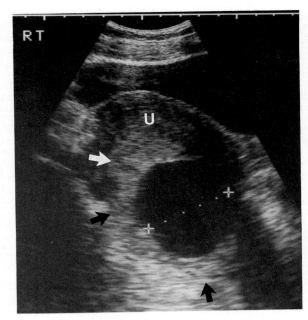

Figure 23-11 (left). Ovarian torsion. A longitudinal sonogram shows a large mass (arrows) with a cystic portion (between calipers) representing an edematous ovary with a cyst that potentiated the torsion. The uterus (U) is anterior.

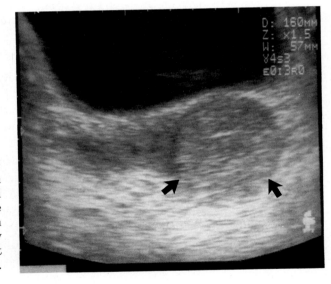

Figure 23-12 (right). Ovarian torsion in a previously normal ovary. A transverse sonogram shows an enlarged ovary (arrows) in the left adnexus.

torsion, of whom 13 had undergone preoperative ultrasonography, only 1 sonogram had the typical appearance described above. In 9 of the 13 patients, the ovary had underlying abnormalities, which were reflected by the sonographic features. In that series, the sonographic appearance was quite variable. The masses were large, ranging from approximately

4 to 10 cm, and as they enlarged, they tended to be midline. They were predominantly cystic, mixed cystic and solid, or predominantly solid. An abnormal sonographic appearance was demonstrated in all patients in both of these series **(Option (D) is false).** Cul-de-sac fluid has been reported in some patients with ovarian torsion. In the series by Helvie and Silver, only 1 of 13 patients had this finding, but other reports have suggested that cul-de-sac fluid is present in a larger percentage of patients **(Option (E) is true).**

In some patients, particularly those without underlying ovarian abnormalities, the sonographic appearance is typical of ovarian torsion and one is therefore able to suggest a specific diagnosis. If there is a cystic or solid mass that has potentiated the torsion, the mass will predominate and the sonogram can have a nonspecific appearance. However, ovarian torsion should be included in the differential diagnosis of such masses when the clinical presentation suggests torsion.

Color Doppler sonography of the ovaries could play a very important role, as further experience with this technique develops, in assessing the blood supply to the ovary. Torsion is unlikely in patients in whom normal ovarian flow can be demonstrated by duplex Doppler or color Doppler sonography. The reliability of Doppler methods is less clear in patients in whom no signal is demonstrated.

Question 108

Concerning hemorrhagic ovarian cysts,

- (A) most appear as heterogeneous masses
- (B) about 20% appear completely anechoic
- (C) more than 90% have increased through transmission
- (D) they can generally be distinguished from other masses with a similar sonographic appearance by follow-up examination
- (E) about 25% of affected patients have recurrent or concomitant ovarian cysts

Ovarian cysts are the most common masses seen on pelvic sonography. They are anechoic, have a thin wall, and can be identified as originating in the ovary, making the diagnosis obvious. However, hemorrhage into the cyst, a known complication, can lead to a variety of sonographic appearances. Depending on the appearance and clinical presentation, a large number of entities may have to be considered. Thus, hemorrhagic ovarian cyst must be distinguished from more serious lesions that require immediate treatment. In a series of patients with hemorrhagic ovarian cysts evaluated by Baltarowich et al. and in another series by Reynolds et al., most of the patients presented with acute pelvic or ab-

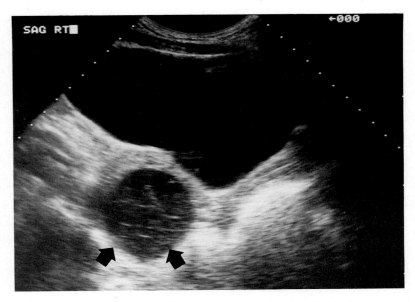

Figure 23-13. Hemorrhagic ovarian cyst. A longitudinal sonogram demonstrates a cystic mass (arrows) with increased through transmission in the left adnexus. The mass contains a number of echoes, including small clumps of echoes and linear fibrin strands.

dominal pain, a palpable adnexal mass, or some combination of these symptoms. However, it is common to discover these lesions as incidental findings on pelvic ultrasonography performed for other reasons on asymptomatic patients, particularly if there is only minor hemorrhage into the cyst.

Hemorrhagic ovarian cysts have a particularly wide spectrum of sonographic appearances because blood can appear different depending on the time elapsed between the actual bleeding and the sonographic study. The sonographic appearance of blood changes with clot formation and clot lysis. In addition, long-standing lesions tend to contain hemorrhagic debris or fibrin strands. Hemorrhagic ovarian cysts, like simple ovarian cysts, can almost always be separated from the uterus and are round and usually well defined. The wall can be either thin or thickened. As demonstrated by the study by Baltarowich et al., the most common appearance is that of a heterogeneous mass **(Option (A) is true).** Usually these are cystic masses that contain some heterogeneous echogenicity (Figure 23-13) and have clumps of echogenic debris (Figure 23-14). Hemorrhagic cysts sometimes appear to be entirely filled with homogeneous echoes (Figure 23-15). The echoes may be hyperechoic and resemble the echogenicity of a dermoid cyst containing fatty material; alterna-

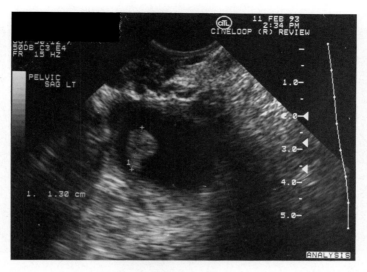

Figure 23-14. Hemorrhagic ovarian cyst. An endovaginal sonogram shows a cystic mass with through transmission and a solid clump of echoes (between calipers). The sonographic findings could mimic the appearance of a dermoid cyst, but the mass was found to have resolved on a subsequent examination.

tively, they may be hypoechoic. Internal septations and fluid-debris levels have also been reported. Hemorrhagic ovarian cysts are almost never totally anechoic **(Option (B) is false)**. In the study by Baltarowich et al., 92% of the lesions had through transmission, as did 93% of the lesions in the series reported by Reynolds et al. **(Option (C) is true).** This is most important since it confirms the cystic nature of the lesion regardless of the number of internal echoes and thus excludes such entities as solid ovarian carcinomas and exophytic or pedunculated uterine fibroids.

The differential diagnosis of hemorrhagic ovarian cysts includes other ovarian cystic lesions. Cystadenomas (Figure 23-16), teratomas, endometriomas (Figure 23-4), and occasionally tubo-ovarian abscesses (Figure 23-6) can appear similar. However, the clinical history may be sufficient to separate a number of these entities. In addition, the other sonographic features that suggest tubo-ovarian abscesses (as discussed above) or ovarian teratomas (such as acoustic shadowing or fat-fluid level) should not be present. A most important point in the diagnosis of hemorrhagic ovarian cysts is that their natural history is the same as that of simple ovarian cysts; i.e., they will involute completely over time. This usually occurs within two menstrual cycles, but in some cases three

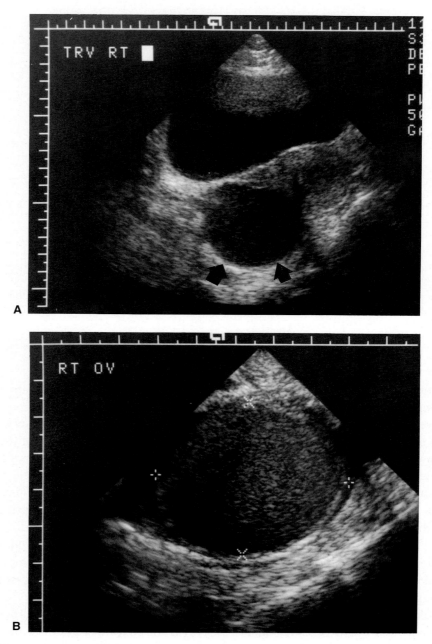

Figure 23-15. Hemorrhagic ovarian cyst. (A) A transverse sonogram shows a hypoechoic homogeneous mass (arrows) with increased through transmission. (B) An endovaginal sonogram shows homogeneous low-level echoes.

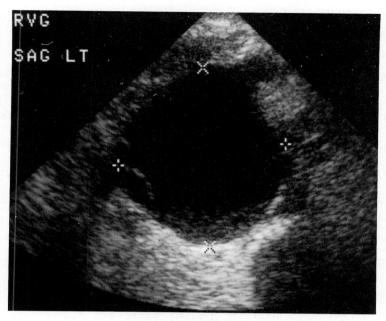

Figure 23-16. Cystadenoma. An endovaginal sonogram shows the cystic mass (between calipers) with septations.

cycles are necessary. No other entity exhibits this pattern **(Option (D) is true)**.

If the hemorrhagic ovarian cyst ruptures, there will be fluid in the cul-de-sac. If there is bleeding as well as rupture, there could be echoes within the fluid, or it may be primarily echogenic because of clot formation. In most cases the fluid is anechoic. Culdocentesis can differentiate a ruptured ovarian cyst from pelvic inflammatory disease, in which purulent fluid would be aspirated. The presence of bloody fluid would not distinguish a hemorrhagic ovarian cyst from a ruptured ectopic pregnancy, but a negative pregnancy test excludes the latter possibility.

A diagnosis of hemorrhagic ovarian cyst is important to the subgroup of patients who tend to have concurrent or recurrent ovarian cysts. In the study by Baltarowich et al., 26% of their patients fell into this category **(Option (E) is true)**. Therefore, as they suggest, conservative therapy in these women is important so that repeated and unnecessary laparoscopies or operations are not performed.

Michael A. Sandler, M.D.
Gary M. Kellman, M.D.

Case 23 / 711

SUGGESTED READINGS

OVARIAN TORSION

1. Bider D, Mashiach S, Dulitzky M, Kokia E, Lipitz S, Ben-Rafael Z. Clinical, surgical and pathologic findings of adnexal torsion in pregnant and non-pregnant women. Surg Gynecol Obstet 1991; 173:363–366
2. Davis AJ, Feins NR. Subsequent asynchronous torsion of normal adnexa in children. J Pediatr Surg 1990; 25:687–689
3. Graif M, Itzchak Y. Sonographic evaluation of ovarian torsion in childhood and adolescence. AJR 1988; 150:647–649
4. Helvie MA, Silver TM. Ovarian torsion: sonographic evaluation. JCU 1989; 17:327–332
5. Siegel MJ. Pediatric gynecologic sonography. Radiology 1991; 179:593–600

POLYCYSTIC OVARIAN DISEASE

6. Hann LE, Hall DA, McArdle CR, Seibel M. Polycystic ovarian disease: sonographic spectrum. Radiology 1984; 150:531–534
7. Katz M, Cohen BM. Polycystic ovarian disease. Curr Probl Obstet Gynecol 1984; 7:5–25
8. Pache TD, Wladimiroff JW, Hop WC, Fauser BC. How to discriminate between normal and polycystic ovaries: transvaginal US study. Radiology 1992; 183:421–423
9. Parisi L, Tramonti M, Derechi LE, Casciano S, Zurli A, Rocchi P. Polycystic ovarian disease: ultrasonic evaluation and correlations with clinical and hormonal data. JCU 1984; 12:21–26
10. Yeh HC, Futterweit W, Thornton JC. Polycystic ovarian disease: US features in 104 patients. Radiology 1987; 163:111–116

HEMORRHAGIC OVARIAN CYSTS

11. Baltarowich OH, Kurtz AB, Pasto ME, Rifkin MD, Needleman L, Goldberg BB. The spectrum of sonographic findings in hemorrhagic ovarian cysts. AJR 1987; 148:901–905
12. Reynolds T, Hill MC, Glassman LM. Sonography of hemorrhagic ovarian cysts. JCU 1986; 14:449–453
13. Wu A, Siegel MJ. Sonography of pelvic masses in children: diagnostic predictability. AJR 1987; 148:1199–1202

Notes

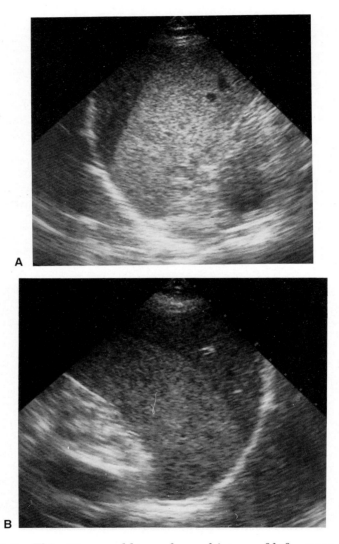

Figure 24-1. This 45-year-old man has a history of left-upper-quadrant pain. You are shown left-upper-quadrant longitudinal (A) and transverse (B) sonograms.

Case 24: Splenic Pseudolesion

Question 109

Which *one* of the following is the MOST likely diagnosis?

(A) Normal variant
(B) Splenic subcapsular hematoma
(C) Left pleural effusion
(D) Left subphrenic fluid collection
(E) Splenic infarct

Longitudinal and transverse sonograms (Figure 24-1) demonstrate a relatively hypoechoic, lenticular mass between the diaphragm and the spleen (Figure 24-2). The spleen has a relatively homogeneous echogenic texture and a normal appearance. The location of the mass between the diaphragm and the spleen might suggest a hematoma; the echogenicity is compatible with this diagnosis. However, there appears to be a small tubular structure within the mass. Its appearance suggests that it may represent a blood vessel coursing through the parenchyma of a normal structure. In fact, it is a portal venous radicle located within a long, lenticular lateral segment of the left lobe of the liver, a normal variant of hepatic configuration (Figure 24-3) **(Option (A) is correct).** Careful scanning should have shown the connection of this perisplenic "mass" with the remainder of the liver, thus confirming its identity. Doppler sonography would also help to confirm that this is an organ and not a fluid collection by demonstrating blood flowing through parenchymal blood vessels (Figure 24-4). Scanning in full inspiration and expiration can also demonstrate that the structure changes in shape or position with respiration, a finding that would also be more likely with normal liver than with a splenic lesion or mass.

Splenic subcapsular hematoma (Option (B)) could have an appearance similar to that in the test patient. A subcapsular hematoma is usually a round or ovoid fluid collection adjacent to the spleen and can be located between the spleen and the left hemidiaphragm. The echogenicity of hematomas is heterogeneous and depends on the age of the lesion.

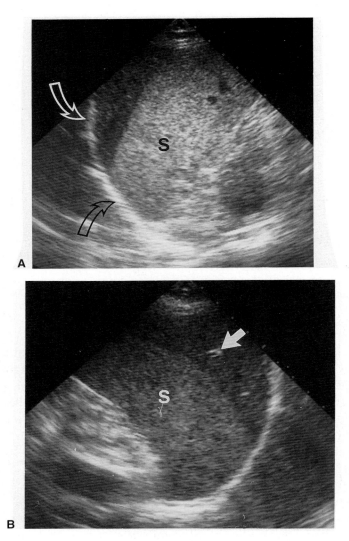

Figure 24-2 (Same as Figure 24-1). Splenic pseudolesion caused by the normal left lobe of the liver. Longitudinal (A) and transverse (B) sonograms demonstrate a lenticular "mass" representing the lateral segment of the left lobe of the liver lying between the left hemidiaphragm (curved arrows) and the normal spleen (S). A small tubular structure (straight arrow), representing a segmental portal venous radicle, is seen within the liver.

In the acute phase, a hematoma can be quite echogenic because of the multiple reflecting interfaces caused by the clot (Figures 24-5 and 24-6). As the clotted blood ages and starts breaking down, lakes of serum create relatively hypoechoic zones (Figure 24-7). These relatively hypoechoic

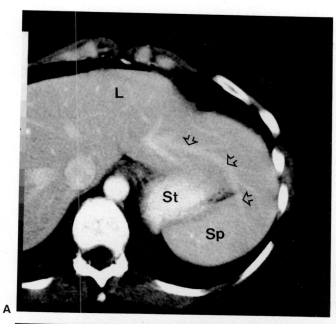

A

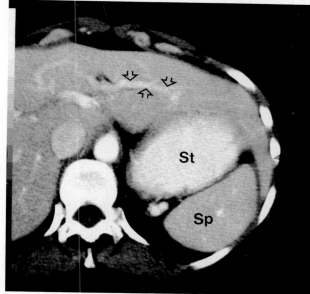

B

Figure 24-3. Lateral segment of the left lobe of the liver adjacent and lateral to the spleen. Postcontrast CT scans of the left upper quadrant demonstrate the lateral segment of the left lobe of the liver extending lateral to the spleen (Sp). Correlate the appearance of this normal variant on CT to the sonographic appearance shown in the test case (Figures 24-1 and 24-2). Note the enhancing portal venous radicles within the liver parenchyma (open arrows). L = liver; St = stomach.

fluid collections can be subcapsular or within the spleen. When large, they will displace adjacent organs, especially the stomach (Figure 24-8).

It can be difficult to identify an acute splenic hematoma sonographically, even when the lesion is obvious on contrast-enhanced CT. This is probably due to several factors. First, the hematoma can be relatively echogenic and similar in echotexture to normal splenic tissue. Second,

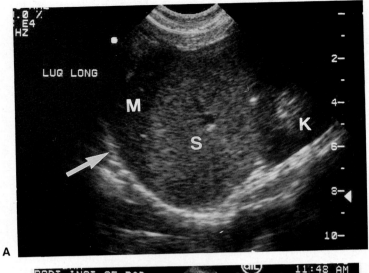

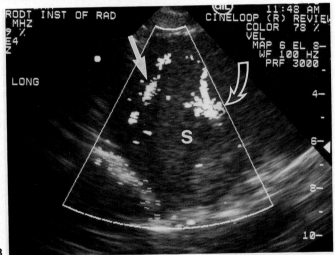

Figure 24-4. Doppler evaluation of a splenic pseudolesion caused by the left lobe of the liver. (A) A longitudinal sonogram of the left upper quadrant demonstrates a relatively hypoechoic lenticular mass (M) below the diaphragm (arrow) and adjacent to the spleen (S). This represents the left lobe of the liver. K = kidney. (B) A color Doppler sonogram (displayed in black and white) of the same area demonstrates blood flow in the splenic artery and vein within the splenic hilum (curved arrow), as well as in a segmental portal vein within the liver (straight arrow). S = spleen.

the spleen can be difficult to image because of overlying ribs and the near-field transducer artifact, which obscure portions of the spleen.

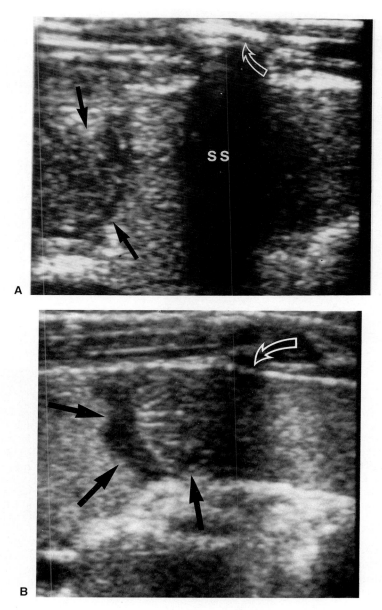

Figure 24-5. Posttraumatic splenic hematoma in a child. (A) An initial longitudinal sonogram demonstrates a vague, poorly defined mass that is relatively isoechoic to the spleen (straight arrows). The appearance mimics normal splenic echotexture. A rib (curved arrow) with a sonic shadow (SS) partially obscures the spleen, making imaging difficult. (B) On a follow-up sonogram, the splenic hematoma is more obvious (straight arrows). This is probably due to breakdown of the hematoma with a secondary collection of serum, which is relatively hypoechoic. A shadow caused by a rib (curved arrow) obscures a portion of the spleen.

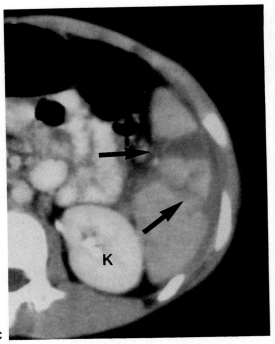

C

Figure 24-5 (Continued [left]). Posttraumatic splenic hematoma in a child. (C) A postcontrast CT confirms the diagnosis of splenic hematoma (arrows). K = kidney.

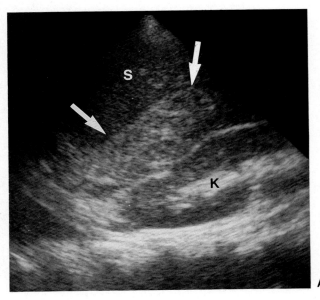

A

Figure 24-6 (right). Acute splenic hematoma. (A) A longitudinal sonogram demonstrates an echogenic mass (arrows) in the dorsal aspect of the spleen that represents an acute hematoma. (B) Postcontrast CT confirms the diagnosis of a splenic hematoma (arrows). S = spleen; K = kidney.

Scanning in full inspiration and expiration can be helpful as respiratory excursion may change the position of the organ and mass relative to

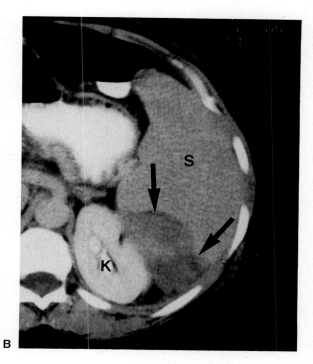

B

Figure 24-6 (Continued)

Figure 24-7. Three-week-old splenic hematoma. A longitudinal sonogram of the spleen (S) demonstrates a subcapsular fluid collection (black arrows) that represents a chronic subcapsular hematoma. Note the linear echogenic areas, probably representing residual blood clot (white arrows).

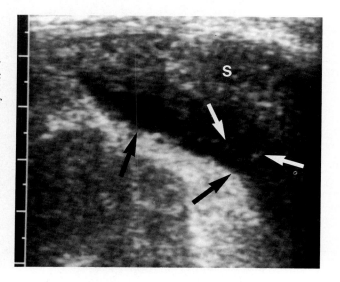

overlying ribs, providing a better sonic window or view. In the test patient, the echotexture pattern of the mass and identification of blood vessels within the mass suggested normal liver rather than hematoma.

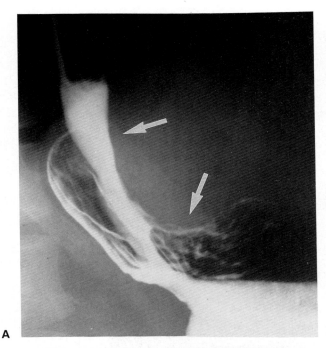

A

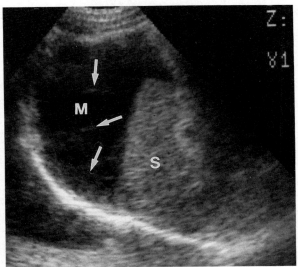

B

Figure 24-8. Three-month-old splenic hematoma. (A) An erect radio-graph from an upper gastrointestinal examination demonstrates an extrinsic mass deforming the gastric cardia (arrows). Following the upper gastrointestinal examination, sagittal (B) and left coronal (C) sonograms of the left upper quadrant were obtained. They demonstrate a loculated cystic perisplenic mass (M). Fibrous strands are seen within the lesion (arrows). (D) A postcontrast CT scan confirms the location of the mass (M) and the displacement of the stomach and left lobe of the liver. Based on the history of significant trauma 3 months earlier, the mass location, and the appearance, a diagnosis of chronic splenic hem-atoma was made. ST = stomach; S = spleen; L = liver.

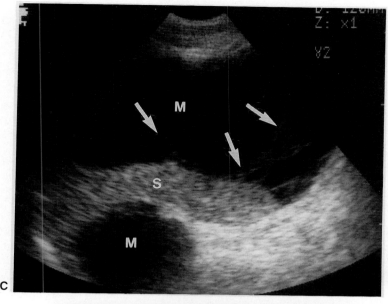

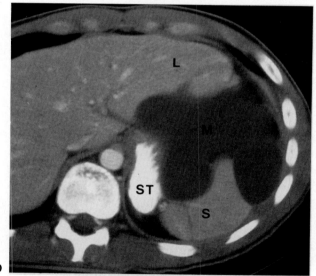

Splenic hematomas usually resolve. However, they can persist and present later in life as cystic lesions (Figure 24-9). Approximately 80% of simple splenic cystic lesions seen in adults are secondary to prior trauma. The remaining 20% are due to inflammatory causes or are true epithelial cysts.

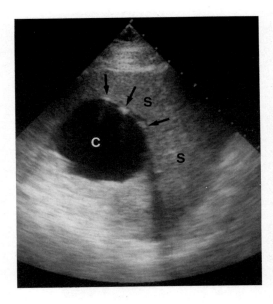

Figure 24-9. Posttraumatic splenic cystic lesion. A longitudinal sonogram demonstrates an echo-free, round cystic lesion (C) in the periphery of the spleen (S). Focal echogenic areas of calcification (arrows) are present in the wall of the lesion and cause associated ring-down artifacts. The patient had a history of significant left-upper-quadrant trauma approximately 5 years previously.

Left pleural effusions (Option (C)) are seen above the diaphragm. On long-axis sagittal or coronal sonograms of the left upper quadrant, pleural effusions are seen craniad to the echogenic curvilinear left hemidiaphragm (Figure 24-10). With larger effusions, atelectatic lung is seen surrounded by the pleural effusion. Rarely, the atelectatic lung can mimic a diaphragm, in which case an erroneous diagnosis of combined pleural effusion and ascites may be made. On axial sonograms through the left upper quadrant, the pleural effusion is seen behind or dorsal to the left hemidiaphragm. The spleen and upper pole of the left kidney are located in a more ventral position (Figure 24-10). The mass in the test patient is clearly below or caudal to the left hemidiaphragm. At the time of the examination, real-time observation of the diaphragm and diaphragmatic motion would have confirmed the location of the mass.

A left subphrenic fluid collection such as an abscess or a pancreatic pseudocyst (Option (D)) can be loculated and could mimic the appearance seen in the test case. Pseudocysts and abscesses are usually round or ovoid. They can have variable echogenicity, depending on the presence of internal debris. Usually, such fluid collections are hypoechoic centrally with a peripheral rim of variable echogenicity and sharpness (Figure 24-11). Both an abscess and a pancreatic pseudocyst can be perisplenic or intrasplenic. It is thought that the pseudocysts gain entry into the spleen via the tail of the pancreas, which extends to the splenic hilum. The hilum has no capsule and therefore lacks a barrier to the spread of released pancreatic enzymes. Echogenicity of intrasplenic pseudocysts

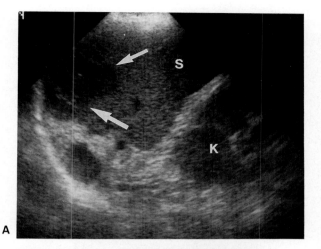

A

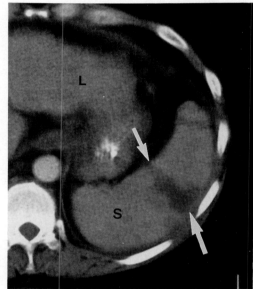

B

Figure 24-15. Splenic infarct. (A) A longitudinal left-upper-quadrant sonogram demonstrates a relatively hypoechoic, wedge-shaped mass (arrows) in the spleen (S). K = kidney. (B) Postcontrast CT confirms the presence of a wedge-shaped, low-attenuation splenic infarct (arrows). S = spleen; L = liver.

In the test image, a long lateral segment of the left lobe of the liver extended into the left upper quadrant, adjacent and lateral to the spleen. In normal patients, the liver is relatively hypoechoic compared with the spleen. With a limited field of view, and with only the spleen for comparison, the hypoechoic liver may simulate a fluid collection. The crescentic shape and location immediately adjacent to the spleen, as well as the low echogenicity, can mimic a subcapsular or perisplenic hematoma or fluid collection. However, with careful scanning, continuity between the "mass" and the remainder of the liver can be demonstrated. The correct

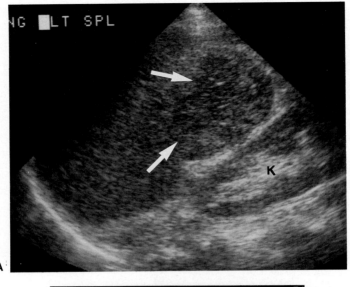

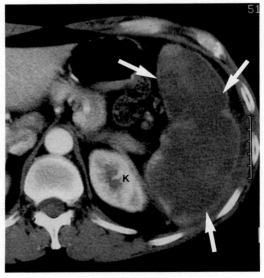

Figure 24-16. Splenic infarct. (A) A longitudinal sonogram of the left upper quadrant demonstrates heterogeneous echotexture in an area near the inferior margin of the spleen (arrows). This area is slightly hypoechoic compared with the remainder of the spleen. The abnormality appears limited to the inferior aspect of the spleen. (B) A postcontrast CT scan obtained 1 day later demonstrates a large low-attenuation, nonenhancing infarct involving nearly the entire spleen (arrows). Sonography underestimated the size of the lesion. K = kidney.

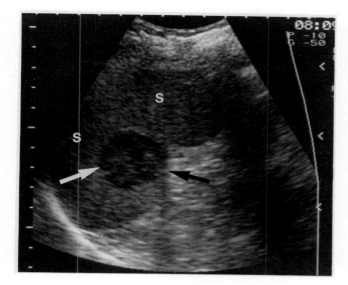

Figure 24-17. Non-Hodgkin's lymphoma. A longitudinal sonogram of the spleen (S) demonstrates a focal hypoechoic mass (arrows). Lymphoma can focally involve the spleen and create a hypoechoic mass that mimics other splenic lesions. Differential diagnosis relies on the detection of ancillary findings and history.

diagnosis of an elongated left hepatic lobe should be confirmed by the relative change in position of the "mass" in relation to the spleen with respiratory motion; the identification of blood vessels within the "mass," made easier by color Doppler sonography; and acoustic properties that are those of solid tissue rather than of fluid. Knowledge of this potential pitfall and careful observation during sonographic scanning should exclude the possibility of a left-upper-quadrant fluid collection in situations similar to that shown in the test case. If confusion persists, CT can be performed, but this should rarely be necessary.

The differential diagnosis of focal left-upper-quadrant pathologic processes can be difficult. As pointed out earlier in this discussion, it can be impossible to differentiate an abscess or hematoma from a pancreatic pseudocyst or to differentiate the multiple types of soft tissue neoplasms that can present in the left upper quadrant. In these cases CT, perhaps followed by fine-needle aspiration biopsy, is often necessary to confirm the diagnosis.

Thomas L. Lawson, M.D.

SUGGESTED READINGS

1. Arenson AM, McKee JD. Left upper quadrant pseudolesion secondary to normal variants in liver and spleen. JCU 1986; 14:558–561

2. Crivello MS, Peterson IM, Austin RM. Left lobe of the liver mimicking perisplenic collections. JCU 1986; 14:697–701
3. Dodds WJ, Taylor AJ, Erickson SJ, Stewart ET, Lawson TL. Radiologic imaging of splenic anomalies. AJR 1990; 155:805–810
4. Goerg C, Schwerk WB. Splenic infarction: sonographic patterns, diagnosis, follow-up, and complications. Radiology 1990; 174:803–807
5. Li DK, Cooperberg PL, Graham MF, Callen P. Pseudo perisplenic "fluid collections": a clue to normal liver and spleen echogenic texture. J Ultrasound Med 1986; 5:397–400
6. Middleton W. Sonography case of the day. Case 3: pseudosubcapsular splenic hematoma due to elongation of left hepatic lobe. AJR 1989; 152:1325–1326
7. Taylor AJ, Dodds WJ, Erickson SJ, Stewart ET. CT of acquired abnormalities of the spleen. AJR 1991; 157:1213–1219

Notes

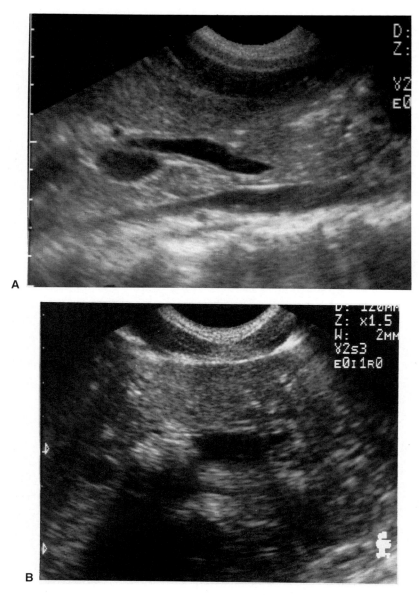

Figure 25-1. This 30-year-old man has abnormal liver function studies. You are shown a longitudinal sonogram of the porta hepatis (A) and two transverse sonograms of the liver (B and C).

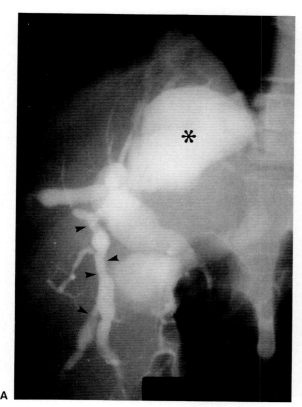

A

Figure 25-10. Primary sclerosing cholangitis. (A) A cholangiogram demonstrates cystic dilatation of one of the intrahepatic bile ducts (✽). Also note the characteristic focal strictures (arrowheads) of intrahepatic bile duct with intervening mild ductal dilatation. (B) A cholangiogram in another patient demonstrates strictures (arrowheads) and small ductal diverticula involving the CBD and common hepatic duct (arrows). Segmental intrahepatic bile duct strictures prevented complete filling of the intrahepatic bile ducts. The single intrahepatic duct that is filled demonstrates diffuse, irregular narrowing.

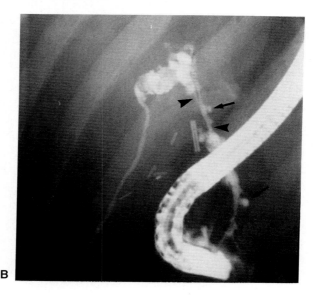

B

of ascending cholangitis, general malaise, and weight loss. However, the disease can be diagnosed in asymptomatic patients who simply present

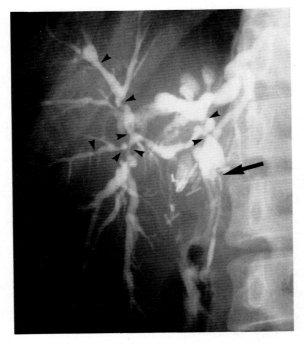

Figure 25-11. Cholangiocarcinoma superimposed on primary sclerosing cholangitis. A cholangiogram demonstrates the typical intra- and extrahepatic duct involvement with strictures (arrowheads) and intervening "skip" areas of mildly dilated bile ducts. There is a dominant stricture involving the proximal common hepatic duct (arrow) in the region of the porta hepatis. This stricture was caused by a cholangiocarcinoma.

with abnormally elevated serum alkaline phosphatase and bilirubin levels on routine screening serum chemistry studies.

The major complication of PSC is cirrhosis leading to portal hypertension with recurrent episodes of variceal hemorrhage and to liver failure. The disease is progressive, although the rate of progression and the severity of complications are variable. Some patients remain relatively asymptomatic for long periods, whereas others die of hepatic failure within a few months of diagnosis. Compared with the general population, there is no increased prevalence of choledocholithiasis **(Option (D) is false).**

The diagnosis of PSC is usually suspected from the combination of clinical presentation, abnormal liver function tests, and the typical cholangiographic findings. The differential diagnosis of PSC includes biliary strictures due to suppurative cholangitis, previous surgery, trauma, or intra-arterial hepatic chemotherapy and diseases, such as sarcoidosis, that can create an appearance mimicking PSC.

The cholangiographic findings of PSC are diffuse multifocal strictures involving both the intra- and extrahepatic bile ducts **(Option (E) is true).** Most commonly, both the intra- and extrahepatic bile ducts are involved by PSC. The intrahepatic bile ducts are almost always involved, sometimes more severely than the extrahepatic bile ducts. The disease rarely can be limited to the intrahepatic ducts. In the series of Majoie et al., both intra- and extrahepatic bile ducts were affected in 35 of 40 patients (88%); in 3 patients, only the extraheptic bile ducts were abnormal, and in 2 patients only the intrahepatic bile ducts were abnormal. The extraheptic bile ducts were involved in 100% of patients in the series of McCarty et al. and in 75% of patients in the series of Rohrmann et al.

On cholangiography, CBD strictures in patients with PSC have a variety of morphologic appearances and may be long, short, smooth, angular, or beaded. The extrahepatic ducts frequently demonstrate multiple small outpouchings characterized as diverticula (Figure 25-10). Intrahepatic duct involvement is usually characterized by smooth strictures alternating with areas of mild dilatation. There can be obliteration of the peripheral ducts (pruning). Diffuse dilatation of the intrahepatic ducts is rare. If diffuse dilatation is present with a dominant stricture in the region of the porta hepatis, cholangiocarcinoma should be strongly considered.

CT often demonstrates characteristic findings in patients with PSC. These findings include focal, irregular segments of intrahepatic bile duct dilatation (skip lesions) producing a beaded appearance (Figure 25-12). There can also be a lack of continuity of peripherally dilated ducts with the central ducts within the porta hepatis. In patients with longstanding PSC, cirrhosis with features of portal hypertension (splenomegaly and varices) can also be present. With high-resolution, contrast-enhanced CT, areas of mural nodularity, focal bile duct wall thickening, and mural enhancement can also be detected. It can be difficult or impossible to exclude the diagnosis of superimposed cholangiocarcinoma in these patients (Figure 25-13).

Ultrasonography can demonstrate thickening and irregularity of the CBD in patients with PSC. There can be focally dilated intrahepatic bile ducts, which mimic hepatic cysts. Careful scanning should be performed to identify a thin tubular structure, which represents a bile duct, entering such a "cystic" space. This observation should lead to the correct diagnosis of focal biliary ductal dilatation (Figure 25-14). A similar sonographic appearance could be present in patients with Caroli's disease, but the historical setting will be different, which should allow a correct diagnosis.

Patients with PSC can develop enlarged hyperplastic lymph nodes. Lymphadenopathy has been reported in 50 to 70% of patients with PSC. When the lymph nodes are large, adenopathy can be the dominant feature sonographically. The porta hepatis is the most common location, but benign lymphadenopathy has also been identified in the lesser omental lymph node group, around the head of the pancreas, and in the para-aortic chain. Lymphadenopathy can be identified by CT or by sonography

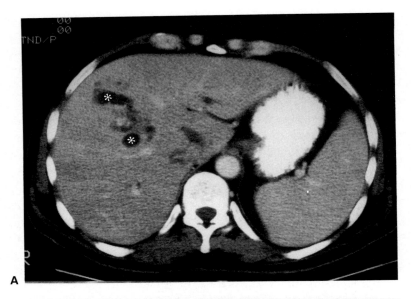

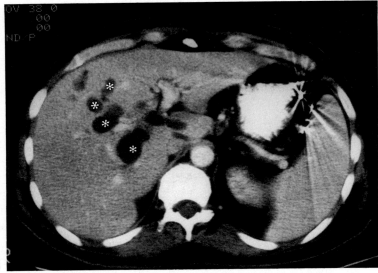

Figure 25-12. Primary sclerosing cholangitis. (A and B) Postcontrast CT scans demonstrate segmental intrahepatic bile duct dilatation (✱). The ducts have a beaded appearance as a result of the alternating areas of chronic inflammatory strictures and intervening uninvolved areas that are dilated.

(Figure 25-15) and can cause diagnostic confusion because enlarged porta hepatis lymph nodes are also visualized in patients with primary biliary cirrhosis and in those with cholangiocarcinoma.

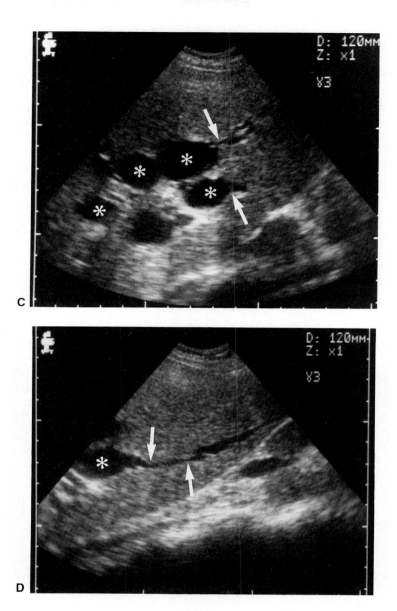

Figure 25-12 (Continued). Primary sclerosing cholangitis. Transverse (C) and longitudinal (D) sonograms through the right lobe of the liver demonstrate the focal ductal dilatation and beaded appearance of the bile ducts (✻) with intervening areas of irregularity and narrowing (arrows). (E) A longitudinal sonogram through the porta hepatis demonstrates the segmental areas of intrahepatic bile duct dilatation (✻). The extrahepatic CBD is narrow with a thick echogenic wall (arrowheads). PV = portal vein.

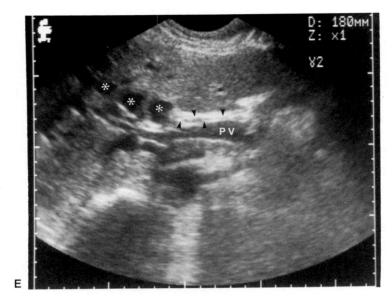

Figure 25-12 (Continued)

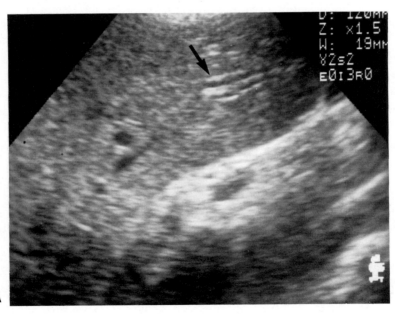

Figure 25-13. Primary sclerosing cholangitis with superimposed cholangiocarcinoma. (A) A longitudinal sonogram of the right lobe of the liver demonstrates focal segmental intrahepatic bile duct dilatation (arrow) manifested by a parallel-channel sign.

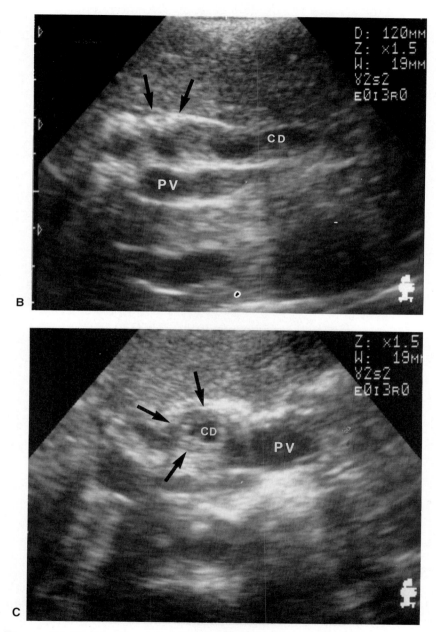

Figure 25-13 (Continued). Primary sclerosing cholangitis with super-imposed cholangiocarcinoma. Longitudinal (B) and transverse (C) sono-grams of the extrahepatic bile duct in the porta hepatis demonstrate a dominant focal, eccentric area of duct wall thickening (arrows). PV = por-tal vein; CD = common duct.

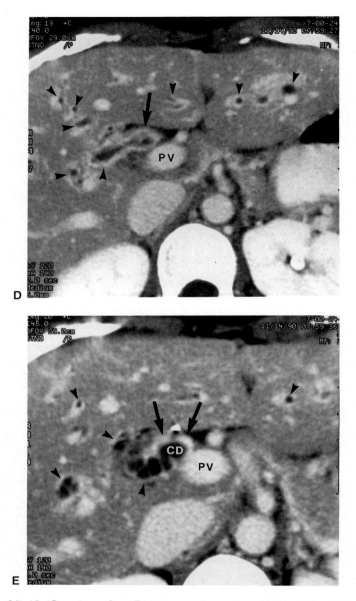

Figure 25-13 (Continued). Primary sclerosing cholangitis with superimposed cholangiocarcinoma. (D and E) Postcontrast CT scans demonstrate segmental intrahepatic bile duct dilatation (arrowheads) with enhancement of the bile duct walls centrally. There is focal thickening and enhancement of the bile duct wall in the region of the porta hepatis (arrows), corresponding in location to the abnormality seen sonographically. Cytologic sampling of this area revealed cholangiocarcinoma. PV = portal vein; CD = common duct.

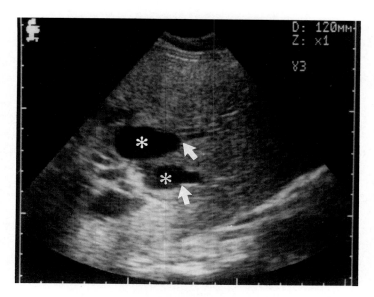

Figure 25-14. Primary sclerosing cholangitis. A transverse sonogram of the liver demonstrates focal cystic areas of bile duct dilatation (✳). Careful observation demonstrated minimally dilated bile ducts entering these cystic spaces (arrows) confirming the anatomic identity of the structure.

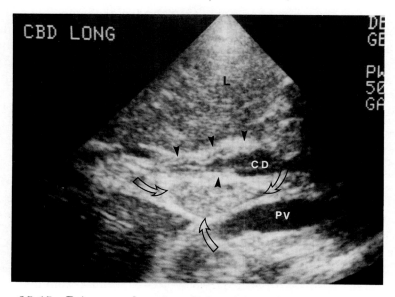

Figure 25-15. Primary sclerosing cholangitis with enlarged hyperplastic porta hepatis lymph node. A longitudinal sonogram demonstrates irregularity and thickening of the extrahepatic CBD wall (arrowheads). Note the enlarged hyperplastic lymph node in the porta hepatis (curved arrows). PV = portal vein; CD = common duct; L = liver. (Courtesy of William D. Middleton, M.D., Mallinckrodt Institute of Radiology, St. Louis, Mo.)

Question 112

Concerning Oriental cholangiohepatitis,

(A) its sonographic diagnosis requires identification of intrahepatic duct stones
(B) there is disproportionate dilatation of central intrahepatic bile ducts compared with peripheral ducts
(C) the bile duct stones have the same chemical composition as most gallstones
(D) it is commonly associated with cholangiocarcinoma
(E) on sonography, increased periportal echogenicity is typical

Oriental cholangiohepatitis (Oriental cholangitis, recurrent pyogenic cholangitis, intrahepatic pigmented stone disease) is characterized by the formation of pigment stones within dilated intrahepatic bile ducts (Figure 25-16). As reported by Lim, in virtually all patients sonography demonstrated stones within the bile ducts (98%) and bile duct dilatation (96%) **(Option (A) is true)**. While Oriental cholangiohepatitis is uncommon in North America, it is endemic to Asia and is one of the most common causes of intrahepatic bile duct stones in the Orient.

Both the intra- and extrahepatic bile ducts are dilated. Mild dilatation of the extrahepatic duct is present in almost all patients and is not related to the presence or location of the intraductal stones. When stones are present in the extrahepatic ducts, the ducts are significantly dilated both proximal to and distal to the stones. Dilatation of the intrahepatic ducts tends to be disproportionately central; the dilated ducts taper rapidly (Figure 25-17), so that the peripheral intrahepatic ducts are normal in caliber **(Option (B) is true)**.

The stones that form are soft pigment stones, which are described as muddy and claylike. They can be large and are often multiple, packing the central intra- and extrahepatic ducts with soft friable material (Figure 25-18). This material is composed primarily of bile pigment, unlike most gallstones, which are composed chiefly of cholesterol **(Option (C) is false)**. The relation of gallstones to Oriental cholangiohepatitis is unclear. However, patients with Oriental cholangiohepatitis do appear to have a higher prevalence of gallstones (40 to 70% of patients) than that in the general population.

The cause of Oriental cholangiohepatitis is unknown, but two theories linking the disease with parasitic infection, most commonly with *Clonorchis sinensis* and *Ascaris lumbricoides*, have been postulated. The first suggests that there may be chronic infestation of the biliary tree with parasites that induce ductal injury, leading to stone formation. The second theory suggests that the stones form around fragments of the parasites with secondary bile duct dilatation and pyogenic cholangitis.

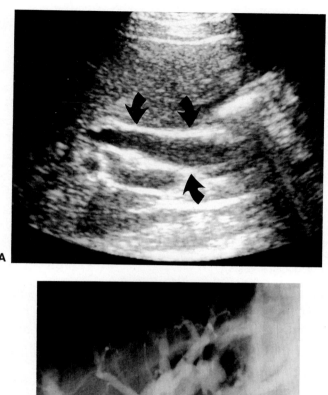

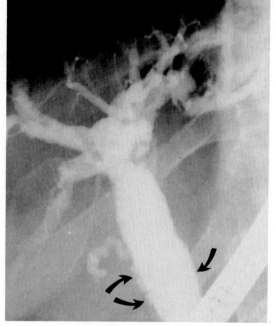

Figure 25-20. AIDS cholangitis. (A) A longitudinal sonogram of the extrahepatic bile duct demonstrates very subtle thickening and irregularity of the bile duct wall (arrow). The bile duct is dilated, measuring approximately 18 mm in internal diameter. (B) A cholangiogram demonstrates dilatation of the CBD with diffuse irregularity and nodularity (arrows) secondary to mucosal edema and inflammatory response. The intrahepatic ducts are also dilated. The abnormalities are more obvious on the cholangiogram than on the sonogram.

of the extrahepatic bile duct wall, are identified. There may be an abrupt transition between the deleted extrahepatic bile duct and the narrowed distal portion near the papilla of Vater. It may be impossible to differentiate these findings of AIDS cholangitis from a distal common duct stricture. Focal thickening or mass, which would be present with cholangiocarcinoma, or intraductal stones, as would be seen with choledocholithiasis, are not features of this disease. In sclerosing cholangitis, the luminal caliber of the extrahepatic bile duct is significantly smaller and the bile duct wall is significantly greater than is seen in AIDS cholangitis.

Question 114

Concerning choledocholithiasis,

(A) the absence of associated acoustic shadowing excludes the diagnosis
(B) the bile duct system is nearly always dilated
(C) the sonographic detection rate is about 85%
(D) it is commonly associated with cholangiocarcinoma
(E) a fatty meal stimulation test is usually positive with obstructing stones

In patients with an intact biliary system, stones in the bile ducts have usually migrated from the gallbladder (Figure 25-21). However, they can form primarily within both the intra- and extrahepatic ducts in patients with partial biliary obstruction and bile stasis consequent to biliary surgery, congenital abnormalities, traumatic or inflammatory strictures, or cholangitis (Figure 25-22). In about 25% of patients with extrahepatic duct stones, the calculi migrate upstream and lodge in the intrahepatic ducts. If these stones remain within the intrahepatic ducts, they can cause irreversible damage to the ducts and hepatic parenchyma.

Stones in the CBD can be silent but often cause partial or complete bile duct obstruction and cholangitis; they sometimes cause acute pancreatitis. The clinical syndrome usually consists of epigastric pain, jaundice, chills, and fever. There is no association of CBD stones with cholangiocarcinoma **(Option (D) is false).**

Calculi within the bile ducts can be identified by cross-sectional sonographic or CT imaging or, more accurately, by direct cholangiography (endoscopic retrograde cholangiopancreatography [ERCP] or percutaneous transhepatic cholangiography [PTC]). Sonographically, CBD stones classically appear as focal echogenic masses with sonic shadowing. When the CBD is dilated and the stone is surrounded by bile and not impacted distally, the diagnosis can be made confidently (Figure 25-23). However,

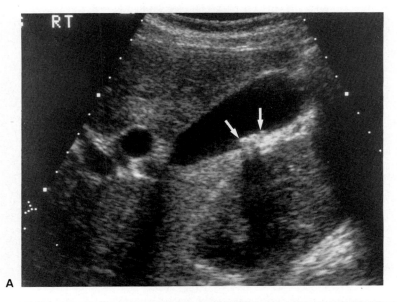

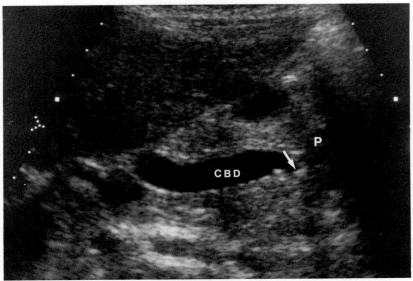

Figure 25-21. Cholelithiasis and choledocholithiasis. (A) A longitudinal sonogram of the gallbladder demonstrates several small gallstones in the dependent portion of the gallbladder (arrows). These stones cast sonic shadows. (B and C) Longitudinal sonograms of the CBD demonstrate dilatation of the CBD, which tapers rapidly in the region of the head of the pancreas. Careful observation demonstrates an echogenic focus (arrow) with subtle sonic shadowing. This represented an impacted distal CBD stone, which had probably migrated into the CBD from the gallbladder. P = area of head of pancreas.

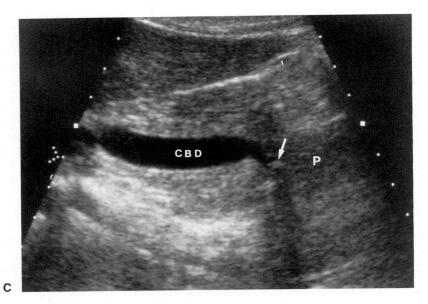

Figure 25-21 (Continued)

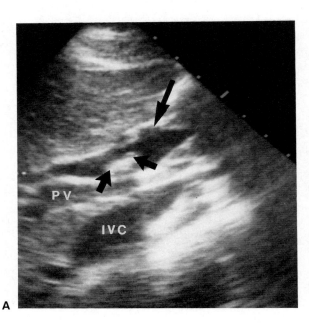

Figure 25-22. Chole-dochal cyst containing a gallstone. (A) A longitudinal sonogram of the CBD demonstrates focal fusiform dilatation of the midportion of the CBD (long arrow). Within the CBD is a large stone (short arrows). PV = portal vein; IVC = inferior vena cava.

if stones are small, distal, impacted, or partially obscured by gas-filled loops of bowel, making the diagnosis is difficult or impossible (Figure 25-24). In addition, 30 to 40% of patients with choledocholithiasis have a

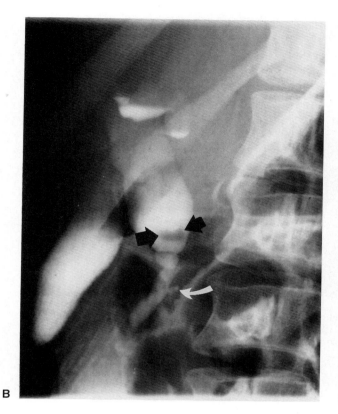

Figure 25-22 (Continued). Choledochal cyst containing a gallstone. (B) A cholangiogram demonstrates the segmental CBD dilatation and the anomalous high, right-angle insertion of the pancreatic duct (white arrow), which is a characteristic cholangiographic feature in patients with a choledochal cyst. The CBD calculus (black arrows) is identified within the choledochal cyst.

B

CBD of normal caliber. Small stones in these patients will probably not be detected sonographically. The expected sonic shadowing is obscured by the echoes from the surrounding soft tissues and technical artifacts. Therefore, the absence of associated acoustic shadowing does not exclude the diagnosis **(Option (A) is false).** The use of high-frequency transducers (5 MHz) focused at the depth of the CBD, scanning in multiple planes and patient positions, and constant manipulation of the gain, power, and signal processing is required to optimize the visualization of the sometimes very subtle sonic shadows caused by intraductal calculi.

As noted above, 30 to 40% of patients with acute obstruction have a normal-sized bile duct **(Option (B) is false).** In these cases, physiologic stimulation of bile flow within the bile duct with intermittent sonographic evaluation of duct size can be used to improve diagnostic accuracy. An oral fatty meal that releases cholecystokinin from the duodenum or a direct parenteral injection of cholecystokinin causes contraction of the gallbladder, relaxation of the sphincter of Oddi, and increased bile secretion. The diameter of the normal, nonobstructed duct will either

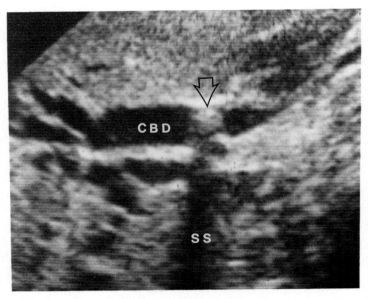

Figure 25-23. Choledocholithiasis. A longitudinal sonogram of the CBD demonstrates a prominent echogenic mass (arrow) within the CBD that casts a large sonic shadow (SS). A confident diagnosis of choledocholithiasis can be made.

decrease or show no change. The obstructed normal-caliber duct will increase in diameter, usually by 2 mm or more. The fatty meal stimulation test is positive if there is an obstructing stone, sphincter of Oddi, stricture or dysfunction. With this technique, Darweesh et al. reported a sensitivity of 74% and a specificity of 100% in detecting common duct obstruction **(Option (E) is true).** The etiology of the obstruction or the presence of stones may not be identified, but a positive test should lead to either PTC or ERCP, which are the most specific techniques for diagnosis of choledocholithiasis.

Overall, sonographic sensitivity in the detection of CBD stones ranges from approximately 30 to 70% in various reports in the literature. This wide range may relate to a number of factors, including patient selection and scanning techniques. Lower sensitivities for detection of choledocholithiasis can be expected if scanning is not performed meticulously in a variety of patient positions, including left posterior oblique, left lateral, and upright. Careful scanning with modern high-resolution equipment and the use of a variety of patient positions should result in an overall sensitivity for stone detection of approximately 50% **(Option (C) is false).**

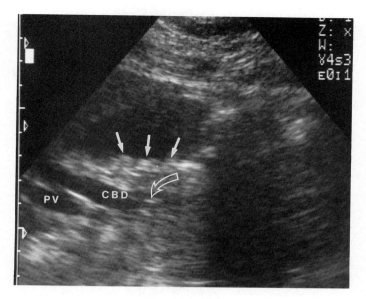

Figure 25-24. Cholelithiasis and choledocholithiasis. Numerous tiny gallstones are present within the gallbladder (straight arrows). The CBD is dilated. Very subtle echogenic foci (curved arrow) are seen at the distal end of the CBD with a suggestion of sonic shadowing. At the time of surgery, four small stones were recovered from the distal CBD. PV = portal vein.

CBD stones can be detected by CT in about 50 to 90% of patients. A stone is identified in the distal CBD as a focal area of high attenuation compared with the adjacent bile (Figure 25-25). When a stone is calcified, it is relatively easy to detect. However, approximately 80% of CBD stones are noncalcified and are composed of bilirubin and cholesterol crystals. These are more difficult to detect. They can be identified as focal intraluminal masses of soft tissue attenuation (with attenuation values higher than those of the adjacent bile). Sometimes a crescent or ring (target sign) created by the lower-attenuation bile surrounding or capping the stone can be seen, and this is a helpful diagnostic sign. In the series of Baron et al., 76% of CBD stones exhibited a target sign or appeared as a high-attenuation (calcified) mass.

Sonographically, the differential diagnosis of CBD stones includes adjacent metallic clips or focal collections of intraductal gas, which will create ring-down artifacts that might be confused with the focal sonic shadowing caused by a stone (Figure 25-26). However, unlike shadowing caused by a stone, the ring-down artifact is a focal zone of increased echogenicity (Figure 25-27). Other differential diagnostic possibilities

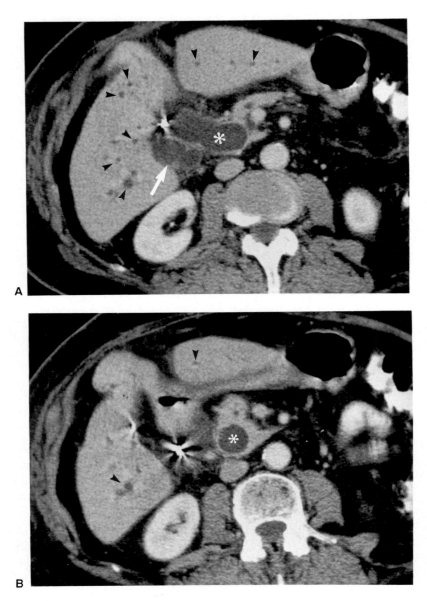

Figure 25-25. Choledocholithiasis. (A) A postcontrast CT scan in this patient with previous cholecystectomy demonstrates metal clips in the region of the porta hepatis. There is a large, dilated cystic duct remnant (arrow), a dilated common hepatic duct (✻), and dilated intrahepatic ducts (arrowheads). (B) A CT scan at the level of the head of the pancreas demonstrates mild dilatation of intrahepatic ducts (arrowheads) and a dilated CBD (✻). (C) A CT scan 2 cm lower than that in panel B demonstrates a crescent of low-attenuation bile (arrows) surrounding a higher-attenuation CBD stone impacted within the dilated CBD. Dilated intrahepatic ducts (arrowheads) are again noted.

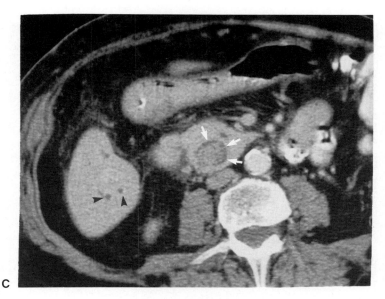

C

Figure 25-25 (Continued)

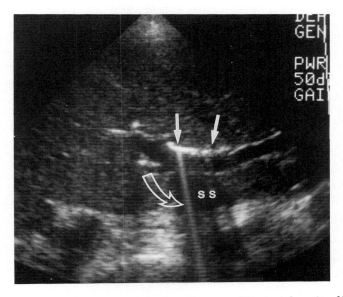

Figure 25-26. Pneumobilia with ring-down artifact. A longitudinal sonogram of the CBD demonstrates marked echogenicity at its superior portion (straight arrows). This is caused by intraluminal air. The air causes
both sonic shadows (SS) and a ring-down artifact (curved arrow). Sonic
shadows are caused by total sound reflection, and ring-down artifacts are
caused by focal reverberation of the acoustic energy with intermittent
return of the acoustic energy to the transducer. (Courtesy of William D.
Middleton, M.D.)

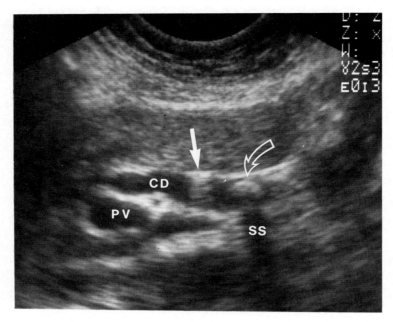

Figure 25-27. Sonic shadowing secondary to a stone and comet-tail artifact caused by metallic surgical clips. A longitudinal sonogram of the
CBD demonstrates an echogenic focus ventral to the CBD with deeper
echoes; this represents a comet-tail artifact (straight arrow) and is
caused by reverberation of the sonic energy within or between adjacent
metallic surgical clips with intermittent reflection of the sonic energy
back to the transducer. Adjacent to the comet-tail artifact there is a CBD
stone (curved arrow), which causes a typical sonic shadow (SS). CD =
common duct; PV = portal vein.

include polypoid cholangiocarcinomas; carcinoma of the pancreas that
involves the duct; foreign bodies, such as stents; or postoperative
sequelae (mucosal tags or polyps) (Figure 25-28).

Thomas L. Lawson, M.D.

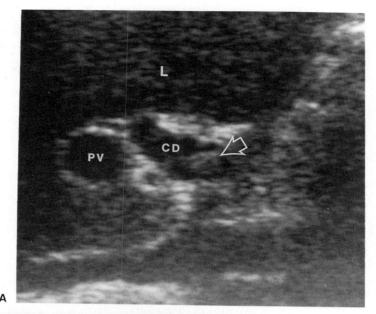

A

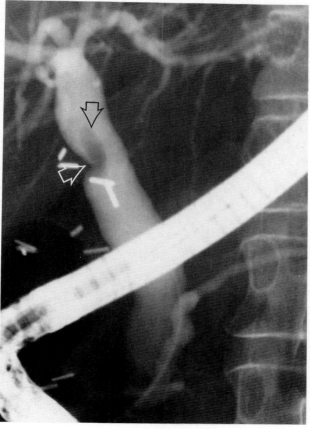

B

Figure 25-28. Post-operative mucosal tag. (A) A sonogram through the porta hepatis demonstrates an echogenic, ovoid soft tissue mass within the common duct (arrow). There is no associated sonic shadow. The patient had a history of a prior cholecystectomy. CD = common duct; PV = portal vein; L = liver. (B) A cholangiogram obtained after the sonogram demonstrates a redundant area of mucosa, a postoperative mucosal tag or polyp (arrows).

SUGGESTED READINGS

ORIENTAL CHOLANGIOHEPATITIS

1. Chan FL, Man SW, Leong LL, Fan ST. Evaluation of recurrent pyogenic cholangitis with CT: analysis of 50 patients. Radiology 1989; 170:165–169

2. Chau EM, Leong LL, Chan FL. Recurrent pyogenic cholangitis: ultrasound evaluation compared with endoscopic retrograde cholangiopancreatography. Clin Radiol 1987; 38:79–85

3. Lim JH. Oriental cholangiohepatitis: pathologic, clinical, and radiologic features. AJR 1991; 157:1–8

4. Lim JH, Ko YT, Lee DH, Hong KS. Oriental cholangiohepatitis: sonographic findings in 48 cases. AJR 1990; 155:511–514

5. Lim JH, Ko YT, Lee DH, Kim SY. *Clonorchiasis*: sonographic findings in 59 proved cases. AJR 1989; 152:761–764

6. Ong GB. A study of recurrent pyogenic cholangitis. Arch Surg 1962; 84:199–225

7. Ralls PW, Colletti PM, Quinn MF, Lapin SA, Morris UL, Halls J. Sonography in recurrent oriental pyogenic cholangitis. AJR 1981; 136:1010–1012

8. Schulman A. Non-western patterns of biliary stones and the role of ascariasis. Radiology 1987; 162:425–430

PRIMARY SCLEROSING CHOLANGITIS

9. Ament AE, Hagga JR, Wiedenmann SD, Barkmeier JD, Morrison SC. Primary sclerosing cholangitis: CT findings. J Comput Assist Tomogr 1983; 7:795–800

10. MacCarty RL, LaRusso NF, May GR, et al. Cholangiocarcinoma complicating primary sclerosing cholangitis: cholangiographic appearances. Radiology 1985; 156:43–46

11. MacCarty RL, LaRusso NF, Wiesner RH, Ludwig J. Primary sclerosing cholangitis: findings on cholangiography and pancreatography. Radiology 1983; 149:39–44

12. Majoie CB, Reeders JW, Sanders JB, Huibregtse K, Jansen PL. Primary sclerosing cholangitis: a modified classification of cholangiographic findings. AJR 1991; 157:495–497

13. Outwater E, Kaplan MM, Bankoff MS. Lymphadenopathy in sclerosing cholangitis: pitfall in the diagnosis of malignant biliary obstruction. Gastrointest Radiol 1992; 17:157–160

14. Rahn NH III, Koehler RE, Weyman PJ, Truss CD, Sagel SS, Stanley RJ. CT appearance of sclerosing cholangitis. AJR 1983; 141:549–552

15. Rohrmann CA Jr, Ansel HJ, Freeny PC, et al. Cholangiographic abnormalities in patients with inflammatory bowel disease. Radiology 1978; 127:635–641

16. Teefey SA, Baron RL, Rohrmann CA, Shuman WP, Freeny PC. Sclerosing cholangitis: CT findings. Radiology 1988; 169:635–639

AIDS

17. Da Silva F, Boudghene F, Lecomte I, Delage Y, Grange JD, Bigot JM. Sonography of AIDS-related cholangitis: prevalence and cause of an echogenic nodule in the distal end of the common bile duct. AJR 1993; 160:1205–1207

18. Defalque D, Menu Y, Girard PM, Coulaud JP. Sonographic diagnosis of cholangitis in AIDS patients. Gastrointest Radiol 1989; 14:143–147

19. Dolmatch BL, Laing FC, Federle MP, Jeffrey RB, Cello J. AIDS-related cholangitis: radiographic findings in nine patients. Radiology 1987; 163:313–316

20. McCarty M, Choudhri AH, Helbert M, Crofton ME. Radiological features of AIDS related cholangitis. Clin Radiol 1989; 40:582–585

21. Romano AJ, vanSonnenberg E, Casola G, et al. Gallbladder and bile duct abnormalities in AIDS: sonographic findings in eight patients. AJR 1988; 150:123–127

22. Teixidor HS, Godwin TA, Ramirez EA. Cryptosporidiosis of the biliary tract in AIDS. Radiology 1991; 180:51–56

23. Teixidor HS, Honig CL, Norsoph E, Albert S, Mouradian JA, Whalen JP. Cytomegalovirus infection of the alimentary canal: radiologic findings with pathologic correlation. Radiology 1987; 163:317–323

24. Vieco PT, Rochon L, Lisbona A. Multifocal cytomegalovirus-associated hepatic lesions simulating metastases in AIDS. Radiology 1990; 176:123–124

CHOLEDOCHOLITHIASIS

25. Baron RL, Stanley RJ, Lee JK, et al. A prospective comparison of the evaluation of biliary obstruction using computed tomography and ultrasonography. Radiology 1982; 145:91–98

26. Cronan JJ, Mueller PR, Simeone JF, et al. Prospective diagnosis of choledocholithiasis. Radiology 1983; 146:467–469

27. Darweesh RM, Dodds WJ, Hogan WJ, et al. Roscoe Miller award. Fatty-meal sonography for evaluating patients with suspected partial common duct obstruction. AJR 1988; 151:63–68

28. Gross BH, Harter LP, Gore RM, et al. Ultrasonic evaluation of common bile duct stones: prospective comparison with endoscopic retrograde cholangiopancreatography. Radiology 1983; 146:471–474

29. Jeffrey RB, Federle MP, Laing FC, Wall S, Rego J, Moss AA. Computed tomography of choledocholithiasis. AJR 1983; 140:1179–1183

30. Laing FC, Jeffrey RB, Wing VW. Improved visualization of choledocholithiasis by sonography. Radiology 1984; 143:949–952

31. Laing FC, Jeffrey RB Jr. Choledocholithiasis and cystic duct obstruction: difficult ultrasonographic diagnosis. Radiology 1983; 146:475–479

32. Mitchell SE, Clark RA. A comparison of computed tomography and sonography in choledocholithiasis. AJR 1984; 142:729–733

33. Pedrosa CS, Casanova R, Leszana AH, Fernandez MC. Computed tomography in obstructive jaundice. II. The cause of obstruction. Radiology 1981; 139:635–645

34. Simeone JF, Mueller PR, Ferrucci JT Jr, et al. Sonography of the bile duct after a fatty meal: an aid in detection of obstruction. Radiology 1982; 143:211–215

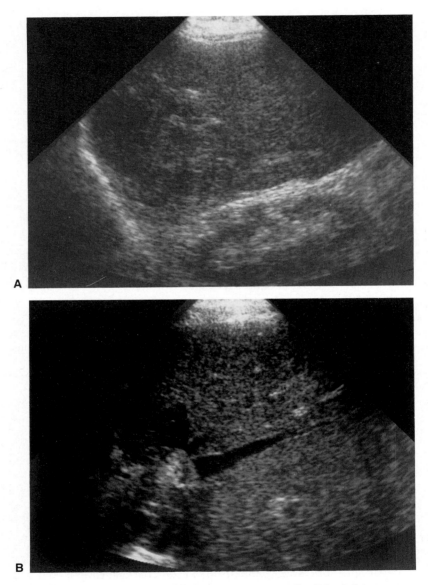

Figure 26-1. This 67-year-old woman presented with right upper quadrant pain. You are shown two longitudinal sonograms of the liver.

Case 26: Hepatocellular Carcinoma

Question 115

Which *one* of the following is the MOST likely diagnosis?

(A) Metastasis
(B) Abscess
(C) Echinococcosis
(D) Hepatic adenoma
(E) Hepatocellular carcinoma

Sonography is widely used in the initial evaluation of patients with upper abdominal complaints of uncertain etiology. It is recognized as a sensitive tool for detecting abnormalities of the gallbladder, biliary tract, liver, and kidneys. Figure 26-1A is a longitudinal scan through the right lobe of an enlarged liver. There is a heterogeneous, ill-defined mass (Figure 26-2A) that disrupts the normal echotexture of the posterior segment of the right lobe. Figure 26-1B is a longitudinal scan near the midline of the abdomen. It demonstrates an echogenic thrombus lodged in the junction of the hepatic veins with the inferior vena cava (Figure 26-2B).

Numerous sonographic patterns for hepatic metastasis (Option (A)) have been described. These include echogenicity greater than, less than, or equal to that of the normal hepatic parenchyma; echogenic calcified metastases; predominantly echo-free fluid-filled metastases (as a result of hemorrhage or necrosis); target or bull's-eye metastases composed of concentric hyperechoic and hypoechoic rings; and diffuse heterogeneity with disruption of the normal hepatic parenchyma (Figures 26-3 through 26-6). The very irregular margins and solid nature of the mass in the test images make primary or secondary malignancy the most likely diagnosis. Hepatic metastasis has been described as a cause of hepatic vein thrombosis and occlusion, but such cases are rare. Portal vein thrombosis, on the other hand, has been reported to occur in up to 8% of patients with multifocal or diffusely infiltrating liver metastases.

The clinical presentation of hepatic abscess (Option (B)) is variable. Common symptoms include fever, pain, diarrhea, nausea, and vomiting.

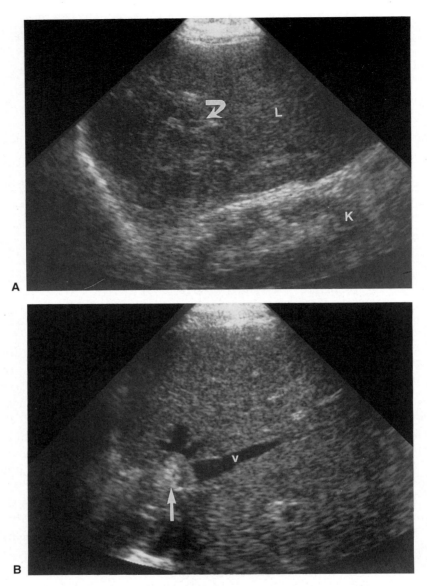

Figure 26-2 (Same as Figure 26-1). Hepatocellular carcinoma. (A) A longitudinal sonogram demonstrates an enlarged liver (L), which extends below the inferior margin of the kidney (K). There is a heterogeneous, ill-defined mass (arrow) within the posterior segment of the right lobe. (B) A longitudinal midline sonogram demonstrates an echogenic thrombus (arrow) at the confluence of the hepatic veins (V).

Many patients are elderly or immunocompromised. Common predisposing conditions include prior surgery, trauma, diverticulitis, appendicitis,

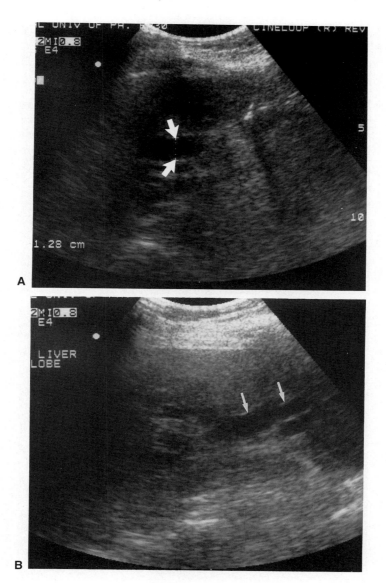

Figure 26-3. Metastatic breast carcinoma. This 55-year-old patient with a history of breast carcinoma presented with jaundice. (A) A transverse sonogram at the porta hepatis demonstrates a dilated common bile duct (arrows). (B) A transverse sonogram of the left lobe of the liver shows a massively dilated left intrahepatic duct (arrows).

and biliary and pancreatic disease. Abnormal liver function tests, leukocytosis, and anemia are common laboratory abnormalities. There may be single or multiple masses, with a spectrum of findings on sonography

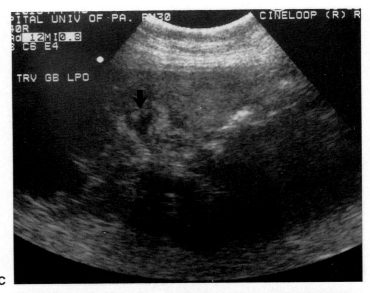

C

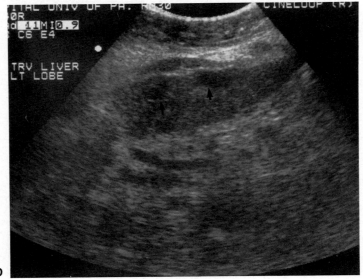

D

Figure 26-3 (Continued). Metastatic breast carcinoma. (C) A transverse left posterior oblique sonogram demonstrates a contracted, thick-walled gallbladder (arrow). (D) A transverse sonogram of the left hepatic lobe demonstrates several small hypoechoic masses (arrows) bulging the capsular surface.

(Figure 26-7). The right lobe is involved more commonly than the left. Acoustic enhancement, although variable in degree, has been described as a prominent feature of liver abscesses, occurring in approximately

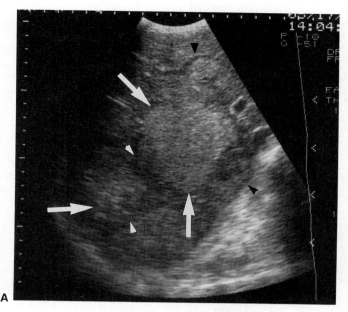

A

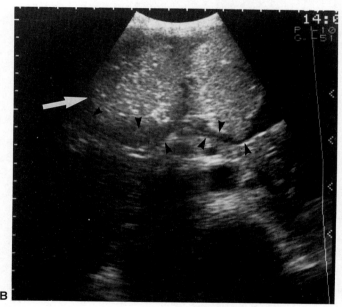

B

Figure 26-4. Metastatic islet cell carcinoma. This 63-year-old man complained of weight loss and abdominal distension. Physical examination revealed a firm, right upper quadrant mass and heme-positive stools. Sagittal (A) and transverse (B) sonograms of the liver demonstrate multiple hyperechoic masses (arrows) with hypoechoic halos (arrowheads). Metastatic islet cell carcinoma of the pancreas was diagnosed on fine-needle aspiration.

50% of cases (Figure 26-8). There are no reliable sonographic characteristics to differentiate abscesses from cystic neoplasms or complicated liver cysts. Needle aspiration biopsy is the only accurate method to make the diagnosis. The typical pyogenic abscess appears as a round or ovoid

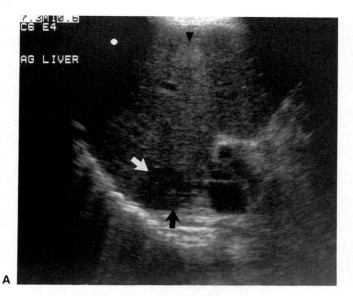

A

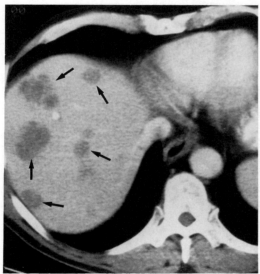

B

Figure 26-5. Metastatic esophageal carcinoma. This 66-year-old patient presented with a distal esophageal stricture, which was found to be secondary to adenocarcinoma of the gastroesophageal junction. (A) A sagittal sonogram of the liver demonstrates both hypoechoic (arrows) and hyperechoic (arrowhead) masses. (B and C) Postcontrast CT scans of the liver show both focal (arrows) and infiltrative (arrowheads) lesions within the liver, indicating more-extensive metastatic disease than was shown in the sonogram.

mass with a thickened, irregular wall (Figure 26-9). Internal characteristics include septations, nodular excrescences, and gas. The overall echotexture ranges from anechoic to hyperechoic. In the test patient, the clinical history and sonographic features make abscess an unlikely diagnosis.

Echinococcosis of the liver (Option (C)) generally produces single or multiple cystic masses that can be calcified, septated, or "solid" in

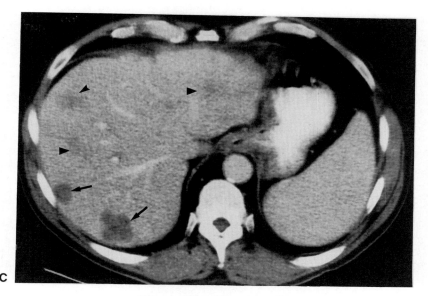

Figure 26-5 (Continued)

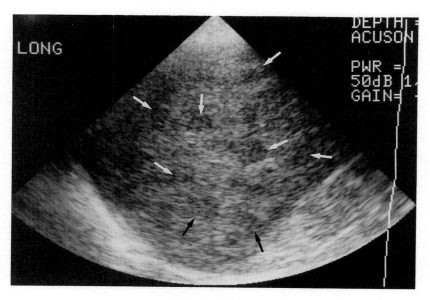

Figure 26-6. Mixed-cell lymphoma. A sagittal sonogram of the liver demonstrates a heterogeneous echotexture with poorly defined hypo-echoic zones (arrows) secondary to infiltrative involvement of the paren-chyma by mixed-cell lymphoma.

appearance (Figure 26-10). It has been postulated that secondary infec-tion can produce echogenic material that usually occupies the spaces

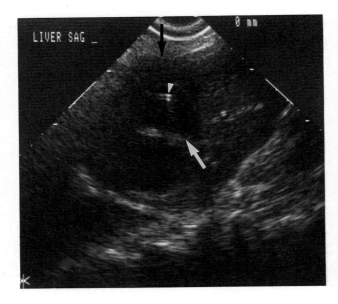

Figure 26-7. Hepatic abscess. This 80-year-old patient had persistent fever after splenectomy. A sagittal sonogram demonstrates a hypoechoic mass (arrows). Linear echogenic foci (arrowhead) denote a drainage catheter within the residual abscess cavity.

between daughter cysts, giving rise to the appearance of a solid mass. Hepatic alveolar echinococcosis can cause infiltrative lesions without well-defined borders, similar to the findings in Figure 26-1A. These masses can be extensive and are sometimes confused with malignant hepatic neoplasms because of associated stenosis of intrahepatic bile ducts and hepatic and portal veins. Hepatic venous thrombosis is not a feature of the more common form of echinococcosis but does occur infrequently in hepatic alveolar echinococcosis. The extensive thrombosis in the test patient makes echinococcal liver disease an unlikely consideration.

Hepatic adenoma (Option (D)) is usually a solitary, encapsulated, smoothly marginated mass (Figure 26-11). This benign neoplasm is composed almost entirely of normal or slightly atypical hepatocytes. Sonographically, the focal mass can appear hypo-, hyper-, or isoechoic relative to the normal hepatic parenchyma (Figure 26-12). Hemorrhage, necrosis, or areas of bile stasis can produce a heterogeneous echotexture. Hepatic adenomas are considered by some investigators to be premalignant lesions, and rapid growth has been described; however, invasion of hepatic vascular structures is not a recognized feature of this tumor.

On the other hand, invasion into and propagation along venous structures are well-recognized and common features of primary hepatocellular carcinoma (HCC) (Figure 26-13). An early diagnosis of vascular invasion is crucial in patients with HCC because involvement of the infe-

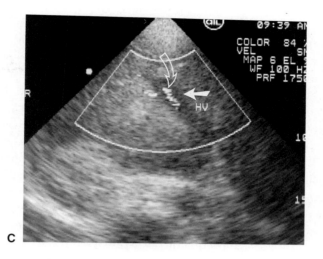

C

Question 116

Concerning echinococcosis,

    (A) no imaging technique can differentiate purely cystic hydatid lesions from simple hepatic cysts

    (B) suspected echinococcal disease is a contraindication to percutaneous aspiration

    (C) the brain is the second most frequently affected organ in humans

    (D) the sonographic features depend on the specific parasite

    (E) the presence of daughter cysts is pathognomonic

Hepatic echinococcosis or human hydatid disease refers to a parasitic infestation occurring in temperate climates, usually in sheep- or cattle-raising countries throughout the world. Areas in the United States where this disease is endemic include Arizona, Utah, the lower Mississippi Valley, and the Central Valley in California. Most patients become infected as children but often do not present with symptoms until adulthood. Increasing immigration is believed to be responsible for a rise in the prevalence of this disease in North America and Europe. The definitive hosts are usually carnivores, such as dogs or foxes. The intermediate hosts can be almost any animal but are usually herbivores, including sheep and moose. There are two modes of human infestation: direct, by contact with infected animals, and indirect, by intake of contaminated food or water.

    The process that leads to human infestation has been well documented. The adult tapeworm living in the jejunum of the definitive host lays eggs that are passed through feces into the environment. If these eggs are ingested, larvae are freed in the duodenum of an infected human and pass through the mucosa to enter portal vein branches within the liver. Over half of the reported cases of human infestation worldwide are associated with documented hepatic disease. Most of the eggs arrest in the hepatic capillaries, but some pass through the liver to the lungs and, less frequently, to other organs including the bones, brain, and pancreas **(Option (C) is false).** Larvae in these organs also lodge within capillaries and incite an inflammatory response composed mainly of mononuclear cells and eosinophils. Extrahepatic echinococcosis has many different appearances. Isolated peritoneal lesions or massive peritoneal spread can occur. Multiple lesions with the same characteristics as hepatic cysts are the most common findings in these other sites. Echinococcal cysts are composed of tissue derived in part from the parasite and in part from the host. The cysts are initially of microscopic size and grow larger over many years. The growth rate has been estimated to range from 0.25 to 1.0 cm per year. The true cyst wall is derived from the parasite and is composed of two layers: the regular outer layer, or ectocyst, and the thin germinal membrane, or endocyst. The endocyst is a nucleated, germinative layer, which gives rise to the brood capsules. The ectocyst has a very distinctive appearance, with innumerable delicate laminations like fine tissue paper. The pericyst, derived from host tissues, is composed of fibroblasts, giant cells, and mononuclear cell and eosinophilic infiltration. The intracystic fluid pressure tends to keep the ectocyst tightly adherent to the pericyst.

Echinococcosis in humans is caused primarily by two forms of the tapeworm: *Echinococcus granulosus* and *Echinococcus multilocularis*. *E. granulosus* infection is far more common than *E. multilocularis* infection. *E. granulosus* causes hepatic cystic disease, which has been classified by Gharbi et al. into five different sonographic types: Type I, round, simple cysts with well-defined borders; Type II, cysts with a detached membrane; Type III, multiseptated cysts with a honeycomb appearance; Type IV, hypoechoic, heterogeneous masses with peripheral or diffuse internal echoes; and Type V, cysts with calcified, thickened walls (Figure 26-10). The natural history of this disease tends to progress from simple fluid-filled cysts to more complex lesions. No imaging technique can differentiate purely cystic hydatid lesions from other simple hepatic cysts **(Option (A) is true).** Other complex predominantly cystic masses are occasionally confused with echinococcal disease (Figures 26-14 and 26-15).

The sonographic features of hepatic alveolar echinococcosis caused by *E. multilocularis* are quite different from those of disease caused by *E. granulosus* **(Option (D) is true).** In this relatively rare parasitic dis-

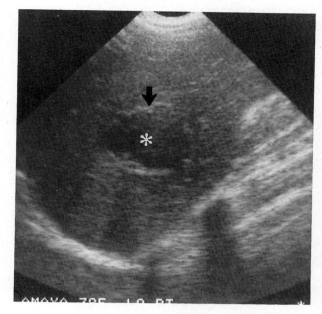

Figure 26-14 (left).
Amebic hepatic abscess simulating echinococcosis. A sagittal sonogram of the liver in a patient with a history of frequent travel to the Middle East demonstrates a hypoechoic mass (✽). Note the lobular contour and the calcified wall (arrow) of the amebic abscess.

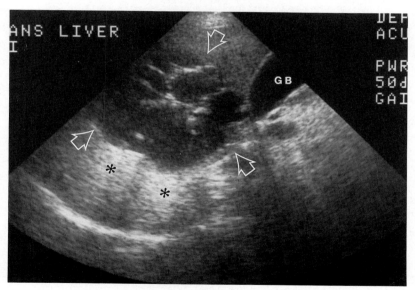

A

Figure 26-15. Mucinous cystadenoma simulating echinococcosis. This 59-year-old woman presented with a history of right upper quadrant pain and was evaluated to rule out gallstones. (A) A sagittal sonogram of the normal-appearing gallbladder (GB) reveals an adjacent complex mass (arrows) that contained multiple internal septations and areas of focal calcification. Acoustic enhancement (✽) confirms its primarily cystic nature.

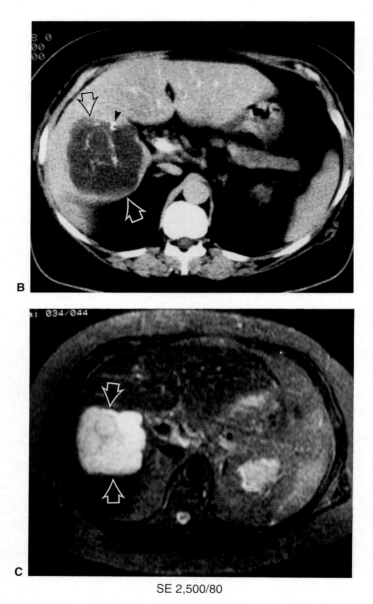

SE 2,500/80

Figure 26-15 (Continued). Mucinous cystadenoma simulating echinococcosis. (B) A postcontrast CT scan demonstrates the predominantly cystic
mass (arrows), as well as the thick septations and calcifications (arrowhead). (C) A T2-weighted MR image demonstrates high signal intensity
in the mass (arrows) as a result of its fluid nature.

ease, lesions are infiltrative without well-defined margins. Large areas of
the liver are often involved, especially the region of the porta hepatis.

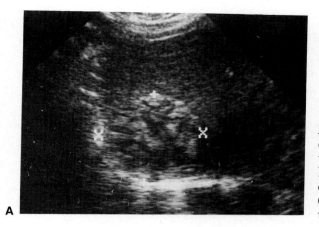

Figure 26-16. Echinococcal cyst. (A) A transverse sonogram of the liver demonstrates an echogenic solid mass (cursors) in the dome of the liver.

A

Encasement of the biliary radicles causes stenosis of the intrahepatic bile ducts and the hepatic and portal veins. Jaundice and portal hypertension are common sequelae. Necrosis can create large cavitary masses containing bile, debris, and sometimes pus. Didier et al., in a report of 24 cases, described echogenic, solid masses in 62%, biliary dilatation in 58%, calcifications in 54%, and irregular necrotic pseudocysts in 12%. The calcifications in hydatid cysts are commonly peripheral, not central. These cysts are typically round with well-defined walls and regular contours. The more-chronic cysts that have a solid pattern still maintain these wall characteristics (Figure 26-16).

There should be no difficulty in differentiating hepatic alveolar echinococcosis from the more common hydatid disease caused by *E. granulosus.* The morphologic appearance of the alveolar form of echinococcosis can mimic primary and secondary hepatic neoplasms. MRI, angiography, biopsy, and serologic complement fixation tests can be helpful for definitive diagnosis. Positive serologic tests narrow the differential diagnosis and virtually exclude other types of nonparasitic cysts. Similarly, differentiation of hydatid cysts from other liver masses is not difficult if a daughter cyst is found within the primary cyst. This is a pathognomonic sign of *E. granulosus* infestation **(Option (E) is true).**

Daughter cyst formation is part of the natural aging process. Daughter cysts replicate the structure of the mother cyst without the pericyst, a layer of compressed host tissues and chronic inflammatory cells (Figure 26-17). They can contain hydatid sand and granddaughter cysts. One maneuver when performing sonograms involves rolling the patient to disperse the sand, creating many tiny echogenic foci. This also helps in distinguishing these more complex echinococcal cysts from simple hepatic cysts. The daughter cysts arise from the inner, nucleated germi-

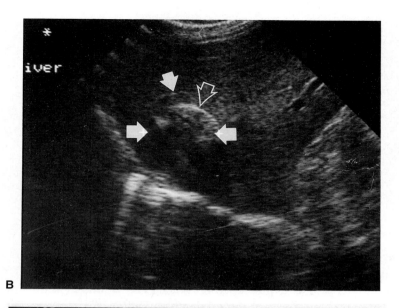

B

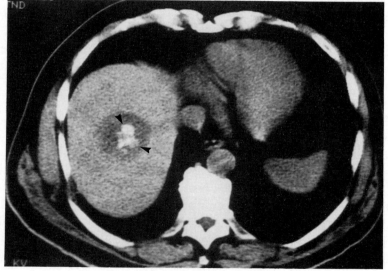

C

Figure 26-16 (Continued).   Echinococcal cyst. (B) A sagittal sonogram of the liver demonstrates a curvilinear echogenic band (open arrow) with acoustic shadowing secondary to calcifications within the mass (solid arrows). (C) A postcontrast CT scan confirmed calcifications (arrowheads) within the center of the low-attenuation mass. (D) A T2-weighted MR image demonstrates a high-intensity mass (arrow) containing curvilinear low-intensity areas suggestive of a collapsed membrane (arrowhead). The diagnosis of echinococcal liver disease was confirmed on fine-needle aspiration biopsy.

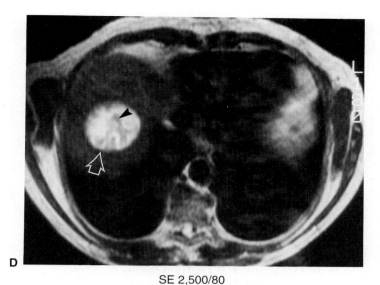

SE 2,500/80

Figure 26-16 (Continued)

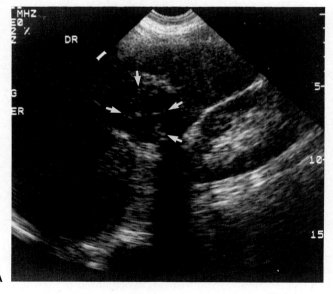

Figure 26-17. Echinococcal cyst and hepatocellular carcinoma. The patient is a middle-aged Greek American. (A) A sagittal hepatic sonogram demonstrates a complex mass with internal septations that represent daughter cysts (arrows).

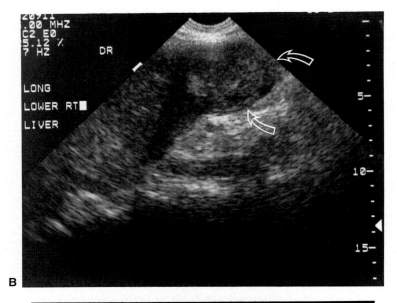

B

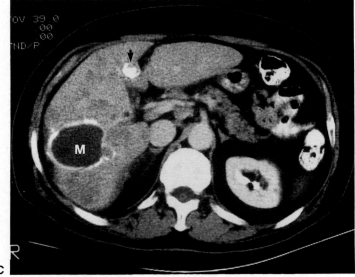

C

Figure 26-17 (Continued). (B) A sagittal sonogram of the right lobe of the liver shows heterogeneous parenchyma with a focal mass projecting from the inferior right lobe (curved arrows). (C) A postcontrast CT scan demonstrates diffuse heterogeneity of the right lobe of the liver with a focal calcified mass (M), which was found at surgery to be secondary to an echinococcal cyst. Note the calcified gallstones (arrow). (D) A CT scan of the caudal, inferior right lobe of the liver reveals a mass (M), which, at surgery, was found to be HCC.

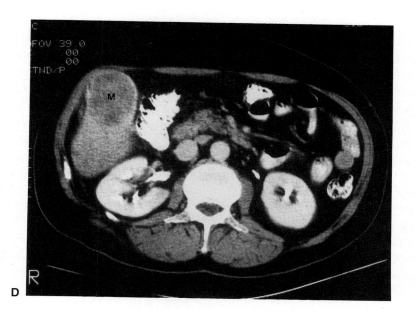

nal epithelium, and they can impinge upon blood vessels, causing vascular thrombosis and infarction. Cyst rupture can culminate in anaphylactic shock, peritoneal seeding and dissemination, and growth of secondary peritoneal cysts. Rupture can occur into the biliary tract, with resultant dilatation and cyst wall discontinuity. Fluid-fluid and air-fluid levels can be seen when the cyst ruptures and are not always indicative of infection. Hydatid cysts can become secondarily infected, changing the typical cystic pattern to a more solid echotexture. Another characteristic feature of *E. granulosus* disease is the "water lily sign." This results from the detachment and collapse of the germinal layer, which is seen on sonograms as an undulating linear collection of echoes lying in the most dependent portion of the cyst or floating in the cyst fluid. A sharply marginated, fluid-filled lesion with daughter cysts is most probably viable, whereas detachment of the membranes, capsular calcifications, and irregular borders are signs that the parasite is dying or nonviable. Complete cyst wall calcification usually indicates an inactive lesion; however, other viable noncalcified cysts can be present elsewhere within the liver.

Sonography has been used to monitor the response of echinococcal cysts to various treatment modalities. Drugs such as mebendazole and albendazole have been used in clinical trials; however, their efficacy in eradicating echinococcosis remains controversial. Sonograms in patients on drug therapy have documented a gradual reduction in cyst size; detachment of membranes; and development of a "pseudosolid" pattern with disappearance of the daughter cyst. Medical therapy has advantages, especially in patients with recurrent disease or in those for whom surgery is otherwise risky. Percutaneous puncture and aspiration of hydatid cysts were once considered contraindicated. However, there are now numerous reports of management of hydatid cysts with percutaneous aspiration, resulting in neither anaphylaxis nor peritoneal soilage **(Option (B) is false).** Khuroo et al. reported aspiration and irrigation with hypertonic saline of 21 hepatic hydatid cysts under sonographic guidance in 12 patients. One patient died of unrelated causes, and the remaining 11 patients experienced relief of symptoms and a decrease in liver size. Serial sonographic examination of the treated cysts revealed similar changes in all cases. The cavities were filled with high-level echoes consisting of cellular debris, dead scolices, hooklets, and membranes. Lack of further fluid secretion by the endocyst resulted in slow solidification, and the cyst developed the appearance of a pseudotumor. A combination of peritoneal drainage and drug therapy was proposed as preferential treatment in most patients. Surgery requires a longer hospitalization, and increased morbidity occurs in patients with multiple disseminated cysts, cysts in inaccessible sites, or cysts recurring after prior surgical procedures. Peritoneal spillage is known to occur at surgery, and deaths have been documented. Approximately 50% of all surviving patients continued to harbor echinococcal disease.

Question 117

Concerning hepatocellular carcinoma,

  (A) it is the most common neoplasm of the liver
  (B) measurement of the serum α-fetoprotein level is an accurate screening test
  (C) hepatic vein involvement is more common than portal vein involvement
  (D) calcification is most common in the fibrolamellar form
  (E) underlying cirrhosis limits the ability of both sonography and CT to assess the extent of the tumor

A wide histologic spectrum exists for primary liver neoplasms that arise from various epithelial and mesenchymal tissues (Figure 26-18). Hepatocellular carcinoma (HCC) is the most common primary liver malignancy and one of the most common malignancies in the world. However, it occurs much less frequently than metastases, which are estimated to be at least 20 times more common than primary liver tumors **(Option (A) is false).** Dissemination of metastatic cancer to the liver occurs via the portal veins, lymph channels, and hepatic arteries and, less frequently, by direct extension. Primary sites of origin in order of decreasing frequency include the colon, stomach, pancreas, breast, and

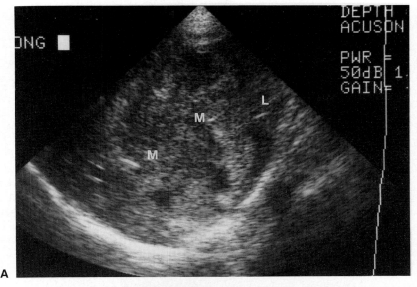

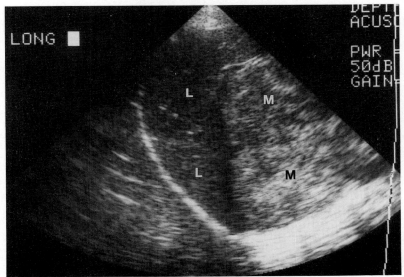

Figure 26-18. Primary embryonal cell sarcoma of the liver. Sagittal sonograms in a 15-year-old patient who presented with right upper quadrant pain. This large, predominantly hyperechoic, heterogeneous mass (M) has an echotexture distinctly different from that of the normal hepatic parenchyma (L).

lung (Figure 26-19). Metastases can be focal or diffuse and can cause hepatomegaly. The echogenicity of some primary and secondary malig-

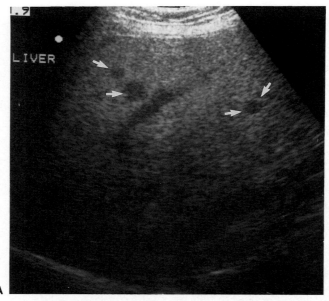

A

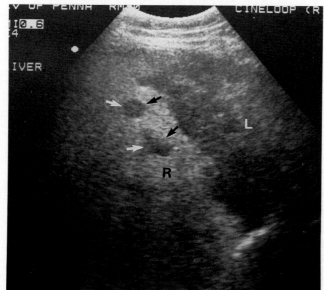

B

Figure 26-19.
Metastatic breast
carcinoma in fatty
liver. (A) A sagittal
sonogram demon-
strates multiple
small hypoechoic
masses (arrows),
which are second-
ary to metastatic
carcinoma. The
liver is echogenic
and was difficult
to penetrate sono-
graphically. This is
due to fatty in-
filtration. (B) A
transverse hepatic
sonogram dem-
onstrates diffuse
relative hypoecho-
genicity of the nor-
mal left lobe (L)
compared with the
echogenic fatty in-
filtration of the
right lobe (R).
Note the hypo-
echoic metastatic
deposits (arrows).

nancies can be so similar to that of uninvolved parenchyma in normal
and diseased livers that detection by sonography is impossible even in
advanced stages (Figures 26-20 and 26-21). Similarly, with current imaging technology it can also be difficult to differentiate a primary liver neoplasm from a metastasis prior to biopsy (Figure 26-22).

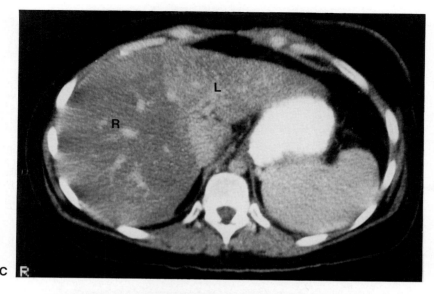

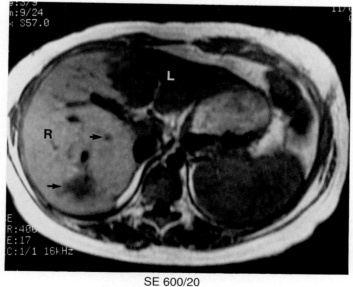

SE 600/20

Figure 26-19 (Continued). Metastatic breast carcinoma in fatty liver. (C) A postcontrast CT scan demonstrates homogeneous low attenuation in the right lobe (R). There is sparing of the left lobe (L) with a normal CT attenuation. (D) A T1-weighted MR image shows high signal intensity within the right lobe (R), with normal hypointensity in the left lobe (L). Small low-intensity defects (arrows) in the right lobe are metastatic deposits.

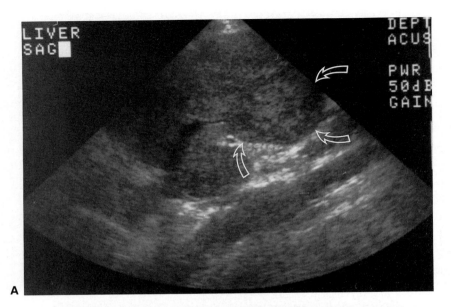

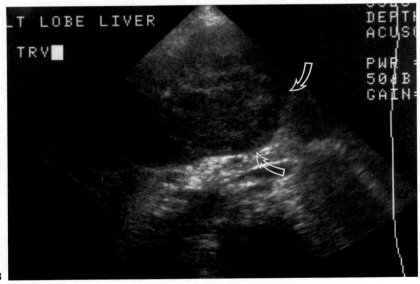

Figure 26-20. Diffuse infiltrative hepatocellular carcinoma. This 69-year-old obtunded patient presented with fever of unknown origin. Sagittal (A) and transverse (B) sonograms of the liver demonstrated diffuse heterogeneity with a rounded configuration to the left lobe (arrows). The findings are nonspecific but are incompatible with an abscess. Biopsy revealed infiltrating HCC.

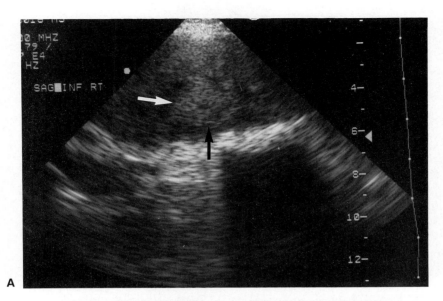

A

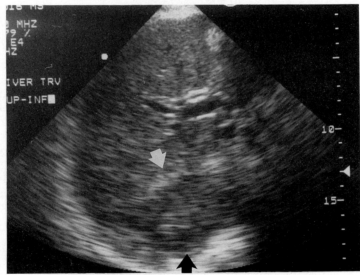

B

Figure 26-21. Hepatocellular carcinoma. This 77-year-old woman presented with abdominal pain, fever, and elevated liver function tests. (A) A sagittal sonogram of the inferior aspect of the right hepatic lobe demonstrates a vague hyperechoic mass (arrows). (B) A transverse sonogram shows distortion of the architecture in the posterior segment of the right lobe of the liver (arrows). These findings are nonspecific. Biopsy of this area revealed HCC.

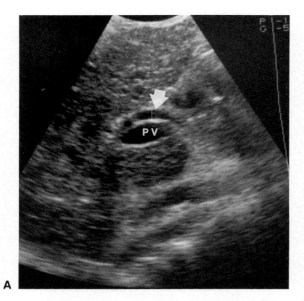

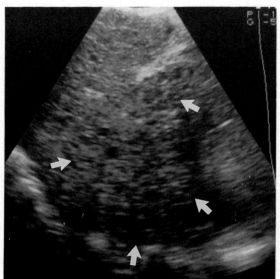

Figure 26-22. Partially necrotic hepatocellular carcinoma. This 60-year-old alcoholic man with increasing abdominal girth was referred to rule out ascites. (A) A sagittal sonogram of the porta hepatis demonstrates a normal common bile duct (arrow) but diffuse distortion of the liver architecture. PV = portal vein. (B) A sagittal sonogram of the right lobe of the liver demonstrates the coarse, heterogeneous echotexture of the hepatic parenchyma (arrows) as a result of the partially necrotic HCC.

One key to the diagnosis of HCC is a high degree of clinical suspicion. Liver function tests are rarely of any value because most of the abnormalities they detect can be ascribed to other diseases. α-Fetoprotein (AFP) has been reported to be a sensitive marker for HCC because it is synthesized by the neoplasm. However, AFP levels may not be elevated significantly when the carcinomas are small. In patients previously

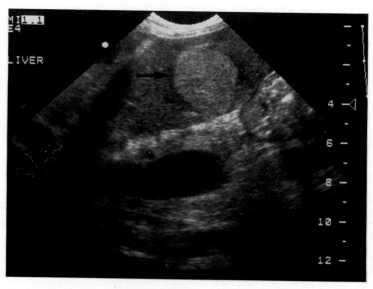

Figure 26-23. Hepatocellular carcinoma. (A) A sagittal sonogram of the liver in a 63-year-old woman with a long-standing history of sarcoidosis shows a large hyperechoic mass (arrow).

treated for HCC, elevations in the AFP level have been observed as a result of hepatic regeneration without evidence of proven recurrence of the cancer. Shibata et al. found a 39% sensitivity and 93% specificity for AFP levels in documenting the hepatic recurrence that had occurred in 31 of 75 patients who had undergone prior partial hepatectomy for HCC. The sensitivity of the AFP assay was significantly lower than that of sonography and CT **(Option (B) is false).** Others have reported variable sensitivities that range from 30 to 95%.

By sonography, HCC can appear hypoechoic, hyperechoic, or of mixed echogenicity relative to uninvolved normal hepatic parenchyma (Figure 26-23). At the time of initial detection, sonograms can demonstrate a small solitary mass, a large mass with smaller satellite lesions, a multi-centric nodular liver, or an infiltrative echo pattern with diffuse architectural distortion (Figure 26-24). In 1983, Tanaka et al. correlated the sonographic and histologic features of HCC in 20 patients. Hypoechoic lesions corresponded with solid tumor without necrosis. Hyperechoic lesions demonstrated two distinct changes, either fatty metamorphosis or marked sinusoidal dilatation. Complex lesions exhibited areas of liquefactive necrosis. Sheu et al., in a study of the sonographic evolution of HCC, reported that the echo pattern of these neoplasms varies somewhat over time. The major pathway involves small neoplasms less than 3

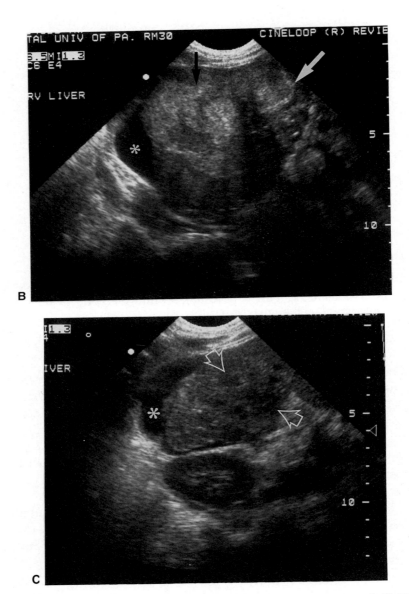

Figure 26-23 (Continued). Hepatocellular carcinoma. (B and C) Transverse hepatic sonograms demonstrate several smaller hyperechoic masses (black and white arrows) and diffusely heterogeneous echotexture in the inferior right lobe (open arrows). Ascites is present (✶). (D and E) Postcontrast CT scans demonstrate a large left-lobe mass (m). The right lobe (r) is atrophic, has an overall heterogeneous appearance, and contains multiple masses (m) inferiorly.

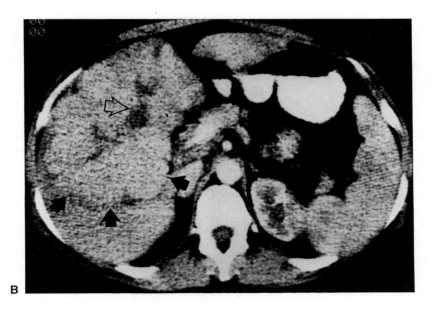

B

fication includes the micronodular form due to alcoholic liver disease and the macronodular form caused by viral hepatitis. The liver can be enlarged early on but becomes small and irregular as the disease progresses. Regenerating nodules are typically small, 5 to 15 mm, but they occasionally enlarge to 5 cm or greater, mimicking neoplasms. In addition, a strong association has been reported between regenerating nodules and synchronous or metachronous HCC. Histologic examination of some regenerating nodules has revealed deposits of HCC. Sonography is not a reliable screening technique for patients with cirrhosis who are at increased risk of developing primary liver malignancies. Dodd et al., in a prospective study of 200 patients undergoing liver transplantation, found sonography to be highly insensitive in the detection of malignant lesions in end-stage cirrhotic livers. The presence of underlying cirrhosis limits the ability of both sonography and CT to assess the extent of the tumor **(Option (E) is true).** MRI serves as a problem-solving tool because regenerative nodules are typically hypointense relative to the liver on spin-echo T2-weighted images, whereas malignancies are generally hyperintense.

Beverly G. Coleman, M.D.

SUGGESTED READINGS

HEPATOCELLULAR CARCINOMA

1. Cottone M, Marceño MP, Maringhini A, et al. Ultrasound in the diagnosis of hepatocellular carcinoma associated with cirrhosis. Radiology 1983; 147:517–519

2. Dodd GD III, Miller WJ, Baron RL, Skolnick ML, Campbell WL. Detection of malignant tumors in end-stage cirrhotic livers: efficacy of sonography as a screening technique. AJR 1992; 159:727–733

3. Friedman AC, Lichtenstein JE, Goodman Z, Fishman EK, Siegelman SS, Dachman AH. Fibrolamellar hepatocellular carcinoma. Radiology 1985; 157:583–587

4. Hayashi N, Yamamato K, Tamaki N, et al. Metastatic nodules of hepatocellular carcinoma: detection with angiography, CT, and US. Radiology 1987; 165:61–63

5. Kruskal JB, Kane RA. Correlative imaging of malignant liver tumors. Semin US CT MR 1992; 13:336–354

6. LaBerge JM, Laing FC, Federle MP, Jeffrey RB Jr, Lim RC Jr. Hepatocellular carcinoma: assessment of resectability by computed tomography and ultrasound. Radiology 1984; 152:485–490

7. Miller WJ, Federle MP, Campbell WL. Diagnosis and staging of hepatocellular carcinoma: comparison of CT and sonography in 36 liver transplantation patients. AJR 1991; 157:303–306

8. Sheu JC, Chen DS, Sung JL, et al. Hepatocellular carcinoma: US evolution in the early stage. Radiology 1985; 155:463–467

9. Shibata T, Kubo S, Itoh K, et al. Recurrent hepatocellular carcinoma: usefulness of ultrasonography compared with computed tomography and AFP assay. J Clin Ultrasound 1991; 19:463–469

10. Takashima T, Matsui O, Suzuki M, Ida M. Diagnosis and screening of small hepatocellular carcinomas. Comparison of radionuclide imaging, ultrasound, computed tomography, hepatic angiography, and alpha 1-fetoprotein assay. Radiology 1982; 145:635–638

11. Tanaka S, Kitamura T, Fujita M, Nakanishi K, Okuda S. Color Doppler flow imaging of liver tumors. AJR 1990; 154:509–514

12. Tanaka S, Kitamura T, Imaoka S, Sasaki Y, Taniguchi H, Ishiguro S. Heptocellular carcinoma: sonographic and histologic correlation. AJR 1983; 140:701–707

HEPATIC METASTASES

13. Atri M, deStempel J, Bret PM, Illescas FF. Incidence of portal vein thrombosis complicating liver metastases as detected by duplex ultrasound. J Ultrasound Med 1990; 9:285–289

14. Igawa S, Sakai K, Kinoshita H, Hirohashi K. Intraoperative sonography: clinical usefulness in liver surgery. Radiology 1985; 156:473–478

15. Wernecke K, Rummeny E, Bongartz G, et al. Detection of hepatic masses in patients with carcinoma: comparative sensitivities of sonography, CT, and MR imaging. AJR 1991; 157:731–739

HEPATIC ABSCESS

16. Juul N, Sztuk FJ, Torp-Pedersen S, Burcharth F. Ultrasonically guided percutaneous treatment of liver abscesses. Acta Radiol 1990; 31:275–277
17. Kuligowska E, Connors SK, Shapiro JH. Liver abscess: sonography in diagnosis and treatment. AJR 1982; 138:253–257
18. Oleszczuk-Raszke K, Cremin BJ, Fisher RM, Moore SW, Millar AJ. Ultrasonic features of pyogenic and amoebic hepatic abscesses. Pediatr Radiol 1989; 19:230–233
19. Ralls PW, Barnes PF, Radin DR, Colletti P, Halls J. Sonographic features of amebic and pyogenic liver abscesses: a blinded comparison. AJR 1987; 149:499–501

ECHINOCOCCOSIS

20. Acunas B, Rozanes I, Acunas G, Celik L, Alper A, Gökmen E. Hydatid cyst of the liver: identification of detached cyst lining on CT scans obtained after cyst puncture. AJR 1991; 156:751–752
21. Barriga P, Cruz F, Lepe V, Lathrop R. An ultrasonographically solid, tumor-like appearance of echinococcal cysts of the liver. J Ultrasound Med 1983; 2:123–125
22. Bezzi M, Teggi A, De Rosa F, et al. Abdominal hydatid disease: US findings during medical treatment. Radiology 1987; 162:91–95
23. Bret PM, Fond A, Bretagnolle M, et al. Percutaneous aspiration and drainage of hydatid cysts in the liver. Radiology 1988; 168:617–620
24. Didier D, Weiler S, Rohmer P, et al. Hepatic alveolar echinococcosis: correlative US and CT study. Radiology 1985; 154:179–186
25. Gharbi HA, Hassine W, Brauner MW, Dupuch K. Ultrasound examination of the hydatic liver. Radiology 1981; 139:459–463
26. Khuroo MS, Zargar SA, Mahajan R. *Echinococcus granulosus* cysts in the liver: management with percutaneous drainage. Radiology 1991; 180:141–145
27. Lewall DB, McCorkell SJ. Hepatic echinococcal cysts: sonographic appearance and classification. Radiology 1985; 155:773–775
28. Marti-Bonmati L, Menor Serrano F. Complications of hepatic hydatid cysts: ultrasound, computed tomography, and magnetic resonance diagnosis. Gastrointest Radiol 1990; 15:119–125

HEPATIC ADENOMA

29. Kerlin P, Davis GL, McGill DB, Weiland LH, Adson MA, Sheedy PF Jr. Hepatic adenoma and focal nodular hyperplasia: clinical, pathologic and radiologic features. Gastroenterology 1983; 84:994–1002
30. Welch TJ, Sheedy PF Jr, Johnson CM, et al. Focal nodular hyperplasia and hepatic adenoma: comparison of angiography, CT, US, and scintigraphy. Radiology 1985; 156:593–595

Index

Where there are multiple page references, **boldface** indicates the main discussion of a topic.

A

Abdominal radiographs
  appendicitis, 176
  emphysematous cholecystitis, 21
  intussusception, 193
  kidney stones, 575
  mucocele of the appendix, 190
Abortions. *See also* Selective feticide
  hemorrhage cause, 400
  missed abortion with degenerating prod-
    ucts of conception
    differential diagnosis
      ectopic pregnancy, 473–74
  placenta previa and, 392
  spontaneous, 496
  threatened, 496–97
Abruptio placentae
  degrees of separation, 401–3
  differential diagnosis
    hematomas, 403
    leiomyomas, 403
    nonpathologic placental fluid collec-
      tions, 403
    normal basal veins, 403
    placenta increta, 391
    uterine contractions, 403
    venous lakes, 403
  sonographic features, 402
Abscesses. *See also specific types of abscesses*
  by name
  differential diagnosis
    complex renal cysts, 108
    lymphoma of the kidney, 101
Acalculous cholecystitis
  AIDS and, 764
  causes, 7–8
Accessory placentas, 392
Acetazolamide, and renal tubular acidosis,
  567
Acetylcholinesterase assay, and Arnold-
  Chiari malformation, 44–45
ACN. *See* Acute cortical necrosis

Acquired cystic disease of the kidney, **371,
  373**
  differential diagnosis
    von Hippel-Lindau disease, 367
Acquired immunodeficiency syndrome. *See*
  AIDS
Acute cholecystitis, **7–9, 11–14.** *See also* Emphysematous cholecystitis; Gallstone-induced cholecystitis
  bacterial infection and, 7
  controversy over sonography and scintig-
    raphy use, 8–9
  differential diagnosis
    acute right upper quadrant pain, 7
    adenomyomatosis, 3
    gallbladder carcinoma, 334
  focal tenderness over gallbladder, 11–12
  gallbladder wall thickening and, 12–13,
    355
  gallstones and, 7, 11
  laparoscopic techniques, 8
  Mirizzi's syndrome, 8
  Murphy's sign, 11–12
  pericholecystic fluid collections, 13–14
  sonographic findings, 11–13
  treatment, 7
  wall-echo-shadow complex, 13–14
  without gallstones, 7–8
Acute cortical necrosis
  kidney failure cause, 567–68
Acute focal bacterial nephritis. *See* Acute focal pyelonephritis
Acute focal pyelonephritis
  differential diagnosis
    lymphoma of the kidney, 101
    renal cell carcinoma, 90, 92
Acute hepatitis
  sonographic features, 418–20
Acute pancreatitis. *See also* Chronic pancreatitis; Cystic pancreatic neoplasms;
  Pancreatitis
  differential diagnosis
    chronic pancreatitis, 303, 305–6

Arnold-Chiari malformation *(cont'd)*
  with lumbar myelomeningocele, 31
  neural tube defect, 44–45
  ventricle characterization, 47
Arnold II malformation. *See* Arnold-Chiari
    malformation
Arrhythmias, and ischemic colitis, 157
Arterioportal fistulas
  acquired arterioportal fistulas, 57, 59
  bruit and, 57–58
  differential diagnosis
    angiosarcoma, 57–58
    hepatic arterial aneurysms, 58–59
    hepatocellular carcinoma, 57–58
    recanalized paraumbilical vein, 58
Arteriovenous fistulas
  postcatheterization, 632–39
Ascaris lumbricoides
  oriental cholangiohepatitis cause, 756
Ascites
  portal hypertension diagnosis, 64
ASDs. *See* Atrial septal defects
Asphyxiating thoracic dystrophy. *See* Je-
    une's syndrome
Asplenia syndrome
  differential diagnosis
    congenital diaphragmatic hernia, 450–
      51
  situs inversus totalis and, 450–51
Atheromatous plaque, 640, 642, 654–56
Atherosclerosis, and hepatic artery aneu-
    rysms, 58–59
Atrial septal defects, 456
Atrioventricular septal defects, 457
Autosomal dominant polycystic disease
  differential diagnosis
    von Hippel-Lindau disease, 365
  seminal vesicle cysts and, 250
Autosomal recessive polycystic disease
  differential diagnosis
    duplication anomaly, 541
  sonographic features, 546–47
AVs. *See* Arteriovenous fistulas
AVSDs. *See* Atrioventricular septal defects
Azidothymidine, and *Pneumocystis carinii*
    infection, 431

B

Bacterial infections, and acute cholecystitis,
    7
Ball type brain appearance, 215
Banana sign, 31
Barium enema
  appendicitis, 176
  intussusception, 193–94
  ischemic colitis, 159
  mucocele of the appendix, 190

Beckwith-Wiedemann syndrome
  differential diagnosis
    trisomy 18, 594, 597
  omphalocele and, 604
Bell clapper deformity, and testicular tor-
    sion, 123
Benign prostatic hyperplasia
  clinical presentation, 246
  cysts associated with, 256–57
  definition, 245
  prostate cancer comparison, 245–49
  prostate-specific antigen and, 248
  types, 246–47
Bile ducts
  sonographic appearance, 737
Biliary calculi. *See* Choledocholithiasis
Biliary colic
  differential diagnosis
    adenomyomatosis, 20
Biliary obstruction, and gallbladder carcino-
    ma, 341
Biliary tract disease, and pancreatitis, 308,
    310
Bipartite placentas, 392
Bland thrombus
  tumor thrombus comparison, 79
Blighted ovum
  absence of normal living embryo and, 497
  first- and second-trimester bleeding
    cause, 400
Blind core biopsy
  peliosis hepatis, 417
Blood
  sonographic appearance, 708
Blood vessels
  communication in twin-twin transfusion
    syndrome, 518
Bochdalek's hernia. *See* Congenital dia-
    phragmatic hernia
BPH. *See* Benign prostatic hyperplasia
Bronchogenic cysts
  dextrocardia and, 447–48
  differential diagnosis
    congenital diaphragmatic hernia, 447–
      48
    cystic adenomatoid malformation, 445
Bruit, and
  arterioportal fistulas, 57–58
  arteriovenous fistulas, 633, 637–38
Budd-Chiari syndrome, **81–83**
  renal cell carcinoma and, 106
Bull's eye pattern
  hepatic abscesses, 351
Burns, and acalculous cholecystitis, 7–8

C

CAM. *See* Cystic adenomatoid malformation

Chronic cholecystitis, and
    gallbladder wall thickening, 355
    wall-echo-shadow complex, 13–14
Chronic hepatitis, 418–20
Chronic liver disease, and hepatocellular
    carcinoma, 329
Chronic pancreatitis, **308–10.** *See also* Acute
    pancreatitis; Cystic pancreatic neo-
    plasms
    differential diagnosis
        acute pancreatitis, 303, 305–6
Cirrhosis
    chronic Budd-Chiari syndrome and, 81
    detection of hepatic tumors, 674
    gallbladder wall thickening and, 357
    hepatocellular carcinoma and, 329–30,
        791, 814–15
    primary sclerosing cholangitis complica-
        tion, 748
Cisterna magna
    Arnold-Chiari malformation and, 31, 36,
        49
    Dandy-Walker variant and, 35
    prominent but normal cisterna magna
        differential diagnosis
            Dandy-Walker malformation, 42
Cleft brain, 204
Clonorchis sinensis
    oriental cholangiohepatitis cause, 756
Clostridium
    emphysematous cholecystitis cause, 21
Clubfoot, and spina bifida, 49
CMV. *See* Cytomegalovirus
Cocaine, and ischemic colitis, 157
Coiled spring appearance
    intussusception, 194, 196
Colon carcinoma. *See also* Carcinoma of the
        hepatic flexure of the colon
    liver metastasis and, 671
Comet-tail artifact, and
    adenomyomatosis, 3, 6, 17
    emphysematous cholecystitis, 21
Common bile duct. *See also* Bile ducts
    stricture of
        differential diagnosis
            oriental cholangiohepatitis, 737, 739
Common bile duct stones. *See* Choledoch-
        olithiasis
Complex renal cysts, **107–8, 110–13**
    differential diagnosis
        abscesses, 108
        lymphoma of the kidney, 101
        renal cell carcinoma, 92–93
        simple cysts, 107
    sonographic criteria, 92–93
Computed tomography
    AIDS cholangitis, 762
    AIDS-related lymphoma, 426–27

Computed tomography *(cont'd)*
    angiomyolipomas, 381–82
    appendicitis, 176
    calcified cyst criteria, 113
    choledocholithiasis, 766, 771
    chronic pancreatitis, 309
    cystic pancreatic neoplasms, 311–12
    endometriomas, 281
    endometriosis, 280
    hepatic abscesses, 345
    hepatocellular carcinoma, 815
    intussusception, 194
    Kaposi's sarcoma, 429
    kidney stones, 580
    liver metastasis, 678
    mucocele of the appendix, 190
    oncocytoma, 116
    oxalosis, 562–63
    pancreatic carcinoma, 316–17
    peliosis hepatis, 417
    Pneumocystis carinii infection, 433–34
    primary sclerosing cholangitis, 749
    pseudomyxoma peritonei, 192
    renal cell carcinoma screening, 373
    renal cell carcinoma staging, 106
    simple cysts criteria, 108
    splenic hematoma, 717
    splenic infarcts, 729–30
    von Hippel-Lindau disease, 370
    xanthogranulomatous   pyelonephritis,
        584–86
Concentric-ring pattern
    intussusception, 165, 169, 196–97
Congenital diaphragmatic hernia. *See also*
        Fetal diaphragmatic hernia
    associated anomalies, 454
    cardiovascular defects, 454
    chromosomal defects and, 454
    differential diagnosis
        asplenia syndrome, 450–51
        bronchogenic cyst, 447–48
        cystic adenomatoid malformation, 442–
            45, 447
        hydrothorax, 440, 442
    early prenatal detection, 454–55
    effects on fetal lung development, 461
    heart placement, 452–53
    polyhydramnios and, 455
    in utero surgical repair, 453
Congestive heart failure, and
    gallbladder wall thickening, 13
    hepatic hemodynamics, 72
Conjoined twins
    cause, 524
    risk of fetal mortality, 524
    union sites, 525

Constrictive pericarditis, and gallbladder wall thickening, 356
Cornual pregnancy, 486
Coronary vein enlargement, and portal hypertension, 65–66
Corpus luteum cysts, 407, 469, **499–501**
    early intrauterine gestation with hemorrhagic corpus luteum cyst
      differential diagnosis
        ectopic pregnancy, 472–73
Cremasteric response, and testicular torsion, 123
Crohn's disease
    differential diagnosis
      appendicitis, 187–89
      ischemic colitis, 169, 171
    sonographic findings, 169, 171
Cryptosporidium, and AIDS cholangitis, 762
Culdocentesis, and hemorrhagic ovarian cysts, 711
Cup type brain appearance, 215
Curettage. *See also* Dilation and curettage
    placenta previa and, 392
Currant jelly stool, and intussusception, 193
Cystadenocarcinomas, 283–85, 287–88, 290
Cystadenomas
    differential diagnosis
      hemorrhagic ovarian cysts, 709
Cystic adenomatoid malformation
    associated anomalies, 445
    differential diagnosis
      bronchogenic cyst, 445
      congenital diaphragmatic hernia, 442–45, 447
      mediastinal teratoma, 445
      neurenteric cyst, 447
      neuroblastoma, 447
      sequestration, 445
    types, 442–45, 447
Cystic fibrosis
    chronic pancreatitis and, 308
    differential diagnosis
      von Hippel-Lindau disease, 367
Cystic hygromas
    Down's syndrome and, 51
    lemon sign, 48
    MS-AFP level and, 607
Cystic pancreatic neoplasms, **311–12, 314–15**
    differential diagnosis
      acute pancreatitis, 306
Cystic renal dysplasia (Potter type IV), and posterior urethral valves, 537, 540
Cystic teratomas, **274–79**. *See also* Cysts; Teratomas
    differential diagnosis
      appendiceal abscesses, 270–71, 273
      chronic ectopic pregnancy, 263–65, 267–68

Cystic teratomas *(cont'd)*
    endometriomas, 268
      ovarian cystadenocarcinomas, 268, 270
    myelomeningocele and, 49
    sonographic appearance, 263
Cysts. *See also specific types of cysts by name*
    testicular, 136, 138
Cytomegalovirus, and
    AIDS cholangitis, 762
    AIDS patients, 422–23
    hydranencephaly, 211
    Pneumocystis carinii infection, 413

D

Dance's sign, and intussusception, 193
Dandy-Walker cysts
    differential diagnosis
      dorsal cyst of the fetal brain, 216
Dandy-Walker malformation, **40, 42**
    anterolateral splaying of the cerebellar hemispheres, 40
    central nervous system anomalies, 42
    Dandy-Walker variant, 40
    differential diagnosis
      prominent but normal cisterna magna, 42
      retrocerebellar arachnoid cyst, 42
      trisomy 18, 42
    hypoplasia or aplasia of the cerebellar vermis, 40
    lemon sign, 48
    spina bifida and, 49
Dandy-Walker variant
    differential diagnosis
      Arnold-Chiari malformation, 35
Dermoid cysts. *See* Cystic teratomas
Dermoid plugs, 263, 274, 278–79
Diabetes mellitus, and
    chronic pancreatitis, 310
    emphysematous pyelonephritis, 571
    ischemic colitis, 157
    prostatic abscesses, 257
Dialysis, and acquired cystic disease of the kidney, 367, 371, 373
Diaphragm. *See* Subphrenic fluid collection
Diaphragmatic hernia. *See also* Congenital diaphragmatic hernia
    lemon sign, 48
Diastematomyelia, and myelomeningocele, 49
Digital rectal examination
    prostate cancer screening, 247–49
Dilation and curettage
    hydatidiform mole, 406
Diverticulitis
    hepatic abscess and, 343, 780
    portal vein thrombosis cause, 75

Hydranencephaly *(cont'd)*
 hydrocephalus, 214
Hydrocephalus
 Arnold-Chiari malformation and, 35–36
 associated malformations, 222, 223
 Dandy-Walker malformation and, 42
 differential diagnosis
  hydranencephaly, 214
 hydranencephaly comparison, 212
 spina bifida and, 44, 46–47
Hydronephrosis. *See also* Fetal hydronephrosis
 differential diagnosis
  acute right upper quadrant pain, 7
Hydrops fetalis, 462, **621, 623**
 associated anomalies, 618, 620
 causes, 522–23
 polyhydramnios and, 523
 sonographic findings, 617–18
 twin gestations and, 509
Hydrothorax
 differential diagnosis
  congenital diaphragmatic hernia, 440,
   442
  liver, normal variant, 724
Hypercalcemia, and medullary nephrocalcinosis, 567
Hypercalciuria, and medullary nephrocalcinosis, 567
Hypercoagulable states, and ischemic colitis, 157
Hyperechogenic bowel, and Down's syndrome, 51
Hyperglobulinemias, and renal tubular acidosis, 567
Hypernephroma. *See* Renal cell carcinomas
Hyperparathyroidism, and
 chronic pancreatitis, 308
 medullary nephrocalcinosis, 567
Hyperplastic cholecystosis
 classification list, 17
Hypertension. *See* Portal hypertension
Hypervascular hepatocellular carcinoma
 differential diagnosis
  arterioportal fistula, 57–58
Hypoalbuminemia, and gallbladder wall
  thickening, 13
Hypovolemic conditions, and ischemic colitis, 157

I

Ileal resection, and oxalosis, 562
Immunocompromised patients, and hepatic
  abscesses, 343
Immunosuppressed patients, and emphyse-
  matous pyelonephritis, 571
Incidence. *See also* Prevalence
 Down's syndrome, 592

Incidence *(cont'd)*
 epididymitis, 129
 extrapulmonary *Pneumocystis carinii* infection, 431
 holoprosencephaly, 221
 Kaposi's sarcoma, 428
 spina bifida, 44
 testicular tumors, 135
 trisomy 18, 591
 Turner's syndrome, 597
Indefinite uterus sign
 pelvic inflammatory disease, 479
Inferior vena caval membranes
 Budd-Chiari syndrome cause, 81
Infertility, and varicoceles, 145–46
Inflammatory bowel disease
 portal vein thrombosis cause, 75
 primary sclerosing cholangitis and, 746
Inflammatory stricture
 differential diagnosis
  AIDS cholangitis, 764
Interhemispheric cysts
 differential diagnosis
  dorsal cyst of holoprosencephaly, 216
Internal carotid artery. *See also* Carotid
  stenosis
 Doppler waveforms, 629, 630–31, 640,
  653
 externalization of the common carotid
  waveform, 654
Intra-arterial hepatic chemotherapy
 primary sclerosing cholangitis and, 748
Intraductal pneumobilia, and emphysematous cholecystitis, 21
Intrahepatic pigmented stone disease. *See*
  Oriental cholangiohepatitis
Intrahepatic portal hypertension. *See* Cirrhosis
Intraspinal lipoma, and myelomeningocele,
  49
Intrauterine growth retardation, **519–21**
 causes, 522
 differential diagnosis
  twin-twin transfusion syndrome, 512–
   13
 single umbilical artery and, 553
 trisomy 18 and, 591
Intussusception, **192–97**
 differential diagnosis
  ischemic colitis, 163, 165, 169
Invasive mole. *See* Gestational trophoblastic
  disease
Ischemic colitis, **157, 159, 161**
 differential diagnosis
  Crohn's disease, 169, 171
  intussusception, 163, 165, 169
  mucocele of the appendix, 161, 163
  periappendiceal abscess, 161

IUGR. *See* Intrauterine growth retardation

J

Jaundice, and
  acute cholecystitis, 8
  echinococcosis, 797
  primary sclerosing cholangitis, 746
Jeune's syndrome, and fetal renal cystic disease, 547

K

Kaposi's sarcoma
  AIDS-related, **428–29, 431**
  differential diagnosis
    Pneumocystis carinii infection, 416–17
  risk factors, 424, 428
  subtypes, 428
Kasabach-Merritt syndrome, and cavernous hemangiomas of the liver, 679
Kawasaki's disease, and gallbladder wall thickening, 357–59
Kidney flexure
  differential diagnosis
    acute right upper quadrant pain, 7
Kidney stones, **574–81.** *See also* Choledocholithiasis
  xanthogranulomatous pyelonephritis and, 560, 582, 583, 584
Kidney transplantation, and
  acquired cystic disease of the kidney, 371
  emphysematous pyelonephritis, 571
Kidneys. *See also* Duplication anomaly; Fetal renal cystic disease; Fetal renal sonography
  normal appearance, 571–73
  normal fetal renal size, 549
  sonographic features in fetuses, 546
  tuberous sclerosis and, 374–75
  von Hippel-Lindau disease and, 368–69
Klebsiella
  acute cholecystitis cause, 7
  emphysematous pyelonephritis and, 571
KS. *See* Kaposi's sarcoma
Kwashiorkor, and chronic pancreatitis, 308

L

Laparoscopic cholecystectomy, 8
Laparotomy
  appendicitis diagnosis, 175
LBWC. *See* Limb-body wall complex
Left upper quadrant
  sonographic evaluation difficulties, 730–33

Leiomyomas
  differential diagnosis
    abruptio placenta, 403
Lemon sign
  differential diagnosis
    Arnold-Chiari malformation, 31, 35
  spina bifida and, 47–48
Leukemia, and gallbladder wall thickening, 357
Leydig cell tumors
  testicular, 135
LH. *See* Luteinizing hormone
Limb-body wall complex
  description, 604
  differential diagnosis
    trisomy 18, 597–98
Lipomas
  Dandy-Walker malformation, 42
Liver
  normal variant
    differential diagnosis
      left pleural effusions, 724
      left subphrenic fluid collection, 724–25, 727
      splenic infarct, 727, 729–30
      splenic subcapsular hematoma, 715–18, 720–21, 723
    sonographic findings, 715, 731, 733
Liver biopsy
  acquired arterioportal fistulas, 57
Liver dysfunction, and gallbladder wall thickening, 13
Liver metastasis, **671–74, 676–78**
  differential diagnosis
    fatty infiltration of the liver, 669–71
    hepatocellular carcinoma, 779
    lymphomas, 674
  gallbladder carcinoma, 341
  portal vein thrombosis and, 75
  route of dissemination, 802
Lobar holoprosencephaly
  brain appearance, 215
  description, 209, 211
Lobar nephritis. *See* Acute focal pyelonephritis
Lobar nephronia. *See* Acute focal pyelonephritis
Luteinizing hormone, and polycystic ovarian disease, 701
Lymph node metastasis
  gallbladder carcinoma, 341
Lymphadenopathy
  differential diagnosis
    acute pancreatitis, 301, 303
    primary sclerosing cholangitis and, 749–50
Lymphatic obstruction, and gallbladder wall thickening, 13

Lymphomas
    differential diagnosis
        liver metastasis, 674
        mucocele of the appendix, 190
        Pneumocystis carinii infection, 413, 415–16
        xanthogranulomatous pyelonephritis, 587
    gallbladder wall thickening and, 357
    of the kidney, **99–101, 103**
        differential diagnosis
            abscesses, 101
            acute focal pyelonephritis, 101
            complex renal cyst, 101
            renal adenoma, 101
            renal cell carcinoma, 89, 101
            sonographic appearance, 100–101, 103

M

Magnetic resonance imaging
    cavernous hemangiomas of the liver, 683
    endometriomas, 281
    endometriosis, 280
    hepatocellular carcinoma, 815
    liver metastasis, 678
    oncocytoma, 116
    peliosis hepatis, 417–18
    prostate cancer, 245
MAI. *See Mycobacterium avium-intracellulare*
Malacoplakia, 240, 241
Malignant melanoma, and gallbladder polyps, 24
Maternal serum α-fetoprotein
    Arnold-Chiari malformation, 44–45
    Down's syndrome, 50–51
    neural tube defect screening, 605
Measles, and intussusception, 192
Mebendazole
    echinococcosis treatment, 801
Meckel-Gruber syndrome, and
    fetal renal cystic disease, 547
    holoprosencephaly, 221
Medullary sponge kidney, and renal tubular acidosis, 567
Menstrual cycle, phases, 467, 469
Mental retardation, and holoprosencephaly, 221–22
Mesenteric adenitis with acute terminal ileitis
    differential diagnosis
        appendicitis, 186–87
Mesenteric artery
    occlusion of
        ischemic colitis and, 159

Mesenteric cysts
    differential diagnosis
        mucocele of the appendix, 190
Mesenteric hematomas
    differential diagnosis
        mucocele of the appendix, 190
Mesenteric tumors
    differential diagnosis
        mucocele of the appendix, 190
Metastatic disease to the liver. *See* Liver metastasis
Methotrexate
    malignant transformation of hydatidiform mole treatment, 407
Methoxyflurane anesthesia, and oxalosis, 562
Metronidazole
    hepatic amebic abscess treatment, 353
Mirizzi's syndrome, and cholangiography, 8
Molar pregnancy
    first- and second-trimester bleeding cause, 400
    hydatidiform mole and, 404
Monoamniotic twins
    anomalies risk, 524
    differential diagnosis
        twin-twin transfusion syndrome, 513
Monozygotic twins
    cleavage time, 523–24
    malformations risks, 525
    twin-twin transfusion syndrome and, 516
Mortality rates
    alobar holoprosencephaly, 221
    asplenia syndrome, 451
    congenital diaphragmatic hernia, 452–53
    conjoined twins, 524
    Dandy-Walker malformation, 42
    Down's syndrome, 592
    echinococcosis, 802
    emphysematous cholecystitis, 21–23
    emphysematous pyelonephritis, 571
    fetal renal cystic disease, 547
    gastroschisis, 601
    hydranencephaly, 214
    hydrops fetalis, 623
    limb-body wall complex, 597–98
    lobar holoprosencephaly, 221–22
    monoamniotic twins, 513
    omphalocele, 605
    oxalosis, 561
    semilobar holoprosencephaly, 221
    trisomy 18, 591
    twin-twin transfusion syndrome, 509
    velamentous cord insertion, 403
MS-AFP. *See* Maternal serum α-fetoprotein
Mucinous cystadenocarcinomas, 311
Mucinous cystadenomas, 311
Mucinous cystic neoplasms, 306, 311

Mucocele of the appendix, **189–92**
  differential diagnosis
    duplication cysts, 190
    ischemic colitis, 161, 163
    lymphoma, 190
    mesenteric cysts, 190
    mesenteric hematoma, 190
    mesenteric tumor, 190
    omental cysts, 190
    ovarian cysts, 190
    periappendiceal abscess, 190
    retroperitoneal masses, 190
Mucocutaneous lymph node syndrome. *See*
    Kawasaki's disease
Müllerian duct cysts, and genitourinary ab-
    normalities, 253
Müllerian ducts, embryologic development,
    249–50
Multicystic dysplastic kidney
  associated anomalies, 537
  differential diagnosis
    duplication anomaly, 537
  renal cystic disease and, 546
Murphy's sign
  acute cholecystitis, 11–12
Mycobacterium avium-intracellulare
    Pneumocystis carinii infection and, 413,
    434
  renal involvement, 568–69
Myelomeningoceles
  Arnold-Chiari malformation, 31, 46–47
  associated anomalies, 49
  hindbrain dysfunction, 49–50
  ventricular dilatation and, 224
Myomatosis. *See* Adenomyomatosis

N

Needle aspiration
  abscesses, 108
Needle aspiration biopsy
  hepatic abscesses, 783
Needle biopsy. *See also* Fine-needle aspira-
    tion biopsy
  oncocytoma, 115
  renal cell carcinoma, 107
Neisseria gonorrhoeae
  epididymitis cause, 129
  pelvic inflammatory disease cause, 475
Neoplasms
  Budd-Chiari syndrome cause, 81
Neoplastic disease of the liver
  differential diagnosis
    acute right upper quadrant pain, 7
Nephrocalcinosis, and renal tubular acido-
    sis, 563, 567–69
Nephrotic syndrome, and gallbladder wall
    thickening, 355–56

Neural tube defect
  Arnold-Chiari malformation and, 44–45
  MS-AFP and, 605
  risk factors, 44
Neurenteric cysts
  differential diagnosis
    cystic adenomatoid malformation, 447
Neuroblastomas
  differential diagnosis
    cystic adenomatoid malformation, 447
Neuromuscular anomalies, and spina bifida,
    49
NHL. *See* Non-Hodgkin's lymphoma
Non-Hodgkin's lymphoma
  AIDS and, 423, 424
  renal involvement, 89, 99–101
  target pattern, 673
Nonpathologic placental fluid collections
  differential diagnosis
    abruptio placenta, 403
Noonan's syndrome, 462
Normal basal veins
  differential diagnosis
    abruptio placenta, 403
Normal-variant lemon sign. *See* Lemon sign
NTD. *See* Neural tube defect
Nuchal fold thickening, and Down's syn-
    drome, 51, 53

O

Obstructing colorectal masses, and ischemic
    colitis, 157
Oligohydramnios
  effects on fetal lung development, 461
  fetal hydronephrosis and, 544, 546
  fetal renal sonography to detect, 549
  intrauterine growth retardation and, 522
  renal cystic disease and, 546, 547
  twin-twin transfusion syndrome and, 516
Omental cysts
  differential diagnosis
    mucocele of the appendix, 190
Omphalocele, 601, 603–4, 605, 607, 609–10
Oncocytoma, **114–17**
  differential diagnosis
    renal cell carcinoma, 93–94, 115
  sonographic appearance, 116
Oral cholecystography
  adenomyomatosis diagnosis, 17, 19, 20
Oral contraceptives, and
  hepatocellular carcinoma, 329
  ischemic colitis, 157
Orchitis, 132
Oriental cholangiohepatitis, **756, 758.** *See
    also* Acute hepatitis; Chronic hepati-
    tis; Viral hepatitis
  differential diagnosis

Oriental cholangiohepatitis *(cont'd)*
    AIDS cholangitis, 742–44
    choledocholithiasis, 744
    common bile duct stricture, 737, 739
    primary sclerosing cholangitis, 739,
        741–42
    sonographic findings, 737
Oriental cholangitis. *See* Oriental cholang-
    iohepatitis
Ovarian cystadenocarcinomas
    differential diagnosis
        cystic teratomas, 268, 270
Ovarian cysts. *See also* Hemorrhagic ovari-
    an cysts
    differential diagnosis
        endometriomas, 281
        mucocele of the appendix, 190
    simple versus hemorrhagic, 708, 709
Ovarian dermoids
    differential diagnosis
        ectopic pregnancy, 474–75
Ovarian torsion, **704–7**
    differential diagnosis
        appendicitis, 705
        endometriomas, 695, 698
        hemorrhagic ovarian cyst, 699
        polycystic ovarian disease, 695
        tubo-ovarian abscess, 698
    sonographic findings, 695
Ovaries, and pelvic inflammatory disease,
    476–77
Oxalates, and oxalosis, 562
Oxalosis, 561–63

P–Q

Pancake type brain appearance, 215
Pancreas
    cystic fibrosis and, 367
    description, 309–10
    von Hippel-Lindau disease and, 369
Pancreas flexure
    differential diagnosis
        acute right upper quadrant pain, 7
Pancreatic carcinoma, **316–18, 320**
    differential diagnosis
        choledocholithiasis, 774
Pancreatitis. *See also* Acute pancreatitis;
    Chronic pancreatitis
    gallbladder wall thickening and, 13, 357
    portal vein thrombosis cause, 75
Papillary necrosis
    differential diagnosis
        xanthogranulomatous pyelonephritis,
            587
Parallel-channel sign, and portal hyperten-
    sion, 62

Parasitic infections
    echinococcosis, 793–94, 796–97, 801–2
    oriental cholangiohepatitis and, 756, 758
Peliosis hepatis
    differential diagnosis
        Pneumocystis carinii infection, 417–18
    risk factors, 417
Pelvic inflammatory disease, **475–81**
    differential diagnosis
        acute right upper quadrant pain, 7
        appendiceal abscesses, 479–80
        chronic ectopic pregnancy, 265
        ectopic pregnancy, 473
Peptic ulcer disease
    differential diagnosis
        acute right upper quadrant pain, 7
        gallbladder wall thickening and, 13
Percutaneous aspiration
    echinococcosis, 802
Percutaneous drainage
    hepatic abscesses, 345, 350–51
Percutaneous needle biopsy
    hemangiomas, 683
    Kaposi's sarcoma, 429
    liver metastasis, 674, 676–77
Percutaneous transhepatic cholangiography
    choledocholithiasis, 766, 770
Percutaneous umbilical blood sampling
    twin-twin transfusion syndrome, 518
Perforated appendix, 175, 184–85, 270–71,
    273
Periappendiceal abscesses
    differential diagnosis
        ischemic colitis, 161
        mucocele of the appendix, 190
Pericholecystic fluid collections, 13
Pheochromocytomas, and von Hippel-Lin-
    dau disease, 369
PID. *See* Pelvic inflammatory disease
Pigment stones. *See* Oriental cholangiohep-
    atitis
Placenta accreta
    cesarean section and, 387
    definition, 387
    location, 396–97
    pathology, 403
    placenta previa and, 387
Placenta increta
    cesarean section and, 387
    definition, 387
    differential diagnosis
        abruptio placenta, 391, 403
        gestational trophoblastic disease, 390–
            91
        placenta previa, 389–90
        subchorionic hemorrhage, 390
    location, 396–97
    placenta previa and, 387

Prominent column of Bertin
  differential diagnosis
    renal cell carcinoma, 94–95
  sonographic appearance, 572
Prostate cancer, **236–45**
  benign prostatic hyperplasia comparison,
    245–49
  differential diagnosis
    prostatic utricle cysts, 229
  metastasis to testis, 136
  screening, 247–49
Prostate gland
  embryologic development, 249
  sonographic appearance, 238–39
  zonal anatomy, 237
Prostate-specific antigen
  prostate cancer screening, 247–49
Prostatic cysts, **249–53, 256–57, 259**
Prostatic utricle cysts
  differential diagnosis
    ejaculatory duct cyst, 229–30
    prostate cancer, 229
    retention cysts, 230, 233
    seminal vesicle cysts, 230
  genitourinary abnormalities and, 253
  sonographic findings, 229
Prostatitis, 239. *See also* Cavitary prostati-
    tis; Granulomatous prostatitis
Proteus, and
  acute cholecystitis, 7
  emphysematous pyelonephritis, 571
Proteus mirabilis
  epididymitis cause, 129
  kidney stones and, 574
  xanthogranulomatous   pyelonephritis
    and, 557, 581
Proteus vulgaris, and kidney stones, 574
Proximal tubular adenoma with oncocytic
    features. *See* Oncocytoma
Prune belly syndrome
  differential diagnosis
    duplication anomaly, 534–35, 537
    posterior urethral valves and, 540
PSA. *See* Prostate-specific antigen
PSC. *See* Primary sclerosing cholangitis
Pseudoaneurysms
  differential diagnosis
    adenopathy, 661
    hematoma, 661
    hernia, 661
  postcatheterization, **661–64**
Pseudogestational sac. *See* Ectopic pregnan-
    cy, pseudogestational sac
Pseudokidney pattern
  Crohn's disease, 171
  intussusception, 165, 195
Pseudomonas, and xanthogranulomatous
    pyelonephritis, 581

Pseudomyxoma peritonei, and
  cystadenocarcinomas, 283–84
  mucocele of the appendix, 190–92
PTC. *See* Percutaneous transhepatic cholan-
    giography
Pulmonary hypoplasia, and congenital dia-
    phragmatic hernia, 461
Pyelonephritis. *See* Acute focal pyelonephri-
    tis
Pyocolon
  ischemic colitis indication, 161
Pyogenic cholangitis
  differential diagnosis
    AIDS cholangitis, 764
Pyonephrosis
  differential diagnosis
    xanthogranulomatous   pyelonephritis,
      561
Pyridoxine deficiency, and oxalosis, 562

R

Recanalized paraumbilical vein
  differential diagnosis
    arterioportal fistula, 58
    portal hypertension and, 64–65
Recurrent pyogenic cholangitis. *See* Orien-
    tal cholangiohepatitis
Renal adenoma
  differential diagnosis
    lymphoma of the kidney, 101
Renal agenesis
  causes, 549–50
  fetal renal sonography to detect, 549
  multicystic dysplastic kidney and, 537
  renal cystic disease and, 546
Renal arcuate artery
  Doppler waveforms, 631
Renal carbuncle. *See* Acute focal pyelone-
    phritis
Renal cell carcinomas, **89–90**
  acquired cystic disease of the kidney and,
    371, 373
  detecting by sonography, 97–99, 104
  differential diagnosis
    acute focal pyelonephritis, 90, 92
    angiomyolipoma, 95–96
    complex renal cyst, 92–93
    lymphoma of the kidney, 89, 101
    oncocytoma, 93–94, 115
    prominent column of Bertin, 94–95
  evaluation of, 106–7
  features, 103–4, 106–7
  hyperdense cysts and, 103–4
  reversible hepatic dysfunction syndrome
    and, 581
  sonographic appearance, 581
  staging, 104, 106

Renal cell carcinomas *(cont'd)*
  von Hippel-Lindau disease and, 368–69
  xanthogranulomatous   pyelonephritis
    and, 582–83
Renal cellulitis. *See* Acute focal pyelonephri-
    tis
Renal cystic dysplasias
  fetal renal sonography to detect, 549
Renal cysts. *See also* Autosomal dominant
    polycystic disease; Complex renal
    cysts; Simple renal cysts
  acquired cystic disease of the kidney and,
    371
  autosomal dominant polycystic disease
    and, 365
  calcified, 112–13
  septations within, 110–12
  sonographic criteria, 92–93, 103–4
  tuberous sclerosis and, 375
  von Hippel-Lindau disease and, 368
Renal disease, and gallbladder wall thicken-
    ing, 13
Renal dysplasia, 546
Renal malformations, and Dandy-Walker
    malformation, 42
Renal neoplasms
  differential diagnosis
    xanthogranulomatous pyelonephritis,
      561
Renal phlegmon. *See* Acute focal pyelone-
    phritis
Renal stones. *See* Kidney stones
Renal tuberculosis
  differential diagnosis
    xanthogranulomatous pyelonephritis,
      561
Renal tubular acidosis, and medullary neph-
    rocalcinosis, 563, 567–69
Retained placenta, 392–93
Retention cysts
  benign prostatic hyperplasia and, 259
  description, 257, 259
  differential diagnosis
    prostatic utricle cysts, 230, 233
Retrocerebellar arachnoid cyst
  differential diagnosis
    Dandy-Walker malformation, 42
Retroperitoneal masses
  differential diagnosis
    mucocele of the appendix, 190
Reversible hepatic dysfunction syndrome,
    581–82
Rh disease, and hydrops fetalis, 621
Rhogam
  Rh disease treatment, 621
Right lower lobe pneumonia
  differential diagnosis
    acute right upper quadrant pain, 7

Right upper quadrant pain. *See* Acute right
    upper quadrant pain
Ring-down artifacts
  choledocholithiasis, 771
  similarity to comet-tail artifact, 3, 21
Ring of fire, 489
Rokitansky-Aschoff sinuses
  adenomyomatosis diagnosis, 5–6, 17, 19
Rokitansky nodules. *See* Dermoid plugs
RTA. *See* Renal tubular acidosis

S

Sacrococcygeal teratoma, 607
Salpingitis
  differential diagnosis
    appendicitis, 480
Sandwich pattern
  intussusception, 195
Sandwich pattern, and intussusception, 165
Sarcoiditis
  differential diagnosis
    primary sclerosing cholangitis, 748
SCH. *See* Subchorionic hemorrhage
Schizencephaly, 204
Scintigraphy
  cavernous hemangiomas of the liver, 683
  hepatobiliary, 8–9
  testicular torsion, 128–29
Sclerosing cholangitis
  differential diagnosis
    AIDS cholangitis, 764, 766
Scoliosis, and limb-body wall complex, 604
Scrotum
  vascular anatomy, **148–49, 151**
Selective feticide, and twin-twin transfusion
    syndrome, 510
Semilobar holoprosencephaly, **214–16, 218**
  description, 209, 211
  facial anomalies, 218–21
  sonographic findings, 203
Seminal vesicle cysts
  differential diagnosis
    prostatic utricle cysts, 230
  genitourinary abnormalities and, 250–51
Seminomas
  classic, 135
  testicular, 135, 140
Sepsis, and ischemic colitis, 157
Serous cystadenomas
  composition, 306, 311
Sertoli cell tumors
  testicular, 135
Shock, and ischemic colitis, 157
Simple appendicitis, 175
Simple renal cysts
  differential diagnosis
    complex renal cysts, 107
  sonographic criteria, 92–93

Single umbilical artery
associated malformations, 553
Situs inversus totalis
association with other anomalies, 448–51
Small bowel disease, and oxalosis, 561
SPECT imaging
cavernous hemangiomas of the liver, 683
Spermatic vein obstruction, 145
Spermatoceles, 136
Spermatocytic seminoma, 135
Sphincterotomy
biliary obstruction, 8
Spina bifida
associated anomalies, 49
fetal evaluation, 46
physical and intellectual disabilities of infants, 49
trisomy 18 and, 36
Spleen
imaging difficulties, 718, 720–21
sonographic findings, 715
Splenic fixture, and ischemic colitis, 159
Splenic infarct
differential diagnosis
liver, normal variant, 727, 729–30
Splenic subcapsular hematomas
differential diagnosis
liver, normal variant, 715–18, 720–21,
723
Splenic vein thrombosis, and venous enlargement, 65
Splenomegaly
portal hypertension diagnosis, 64
Spontaneous splenorenal shunts, and portal
hypertension, 65
Sporadic renal angiomyolipomas, **379–82**
Squamous cell carcinomas, and liver me-
tastasis, 671–72
Stab wounds
acquired arterioportal fistulas, 57
Staghorn calculi, 560, 574, 582, 583, 584
Standoff pads, 96–97
Staphylococcus, and xanthogranulomatous
pyelonephritis, 581
Starry sky liver, and hepatitis, 420
Steatorrhea, and chronic pancreatitis, 310
Stein-Leventhal syndrome, and polycystic
ovarian disease, 700
Strawberry gallbladder, 23
Streptococci
emphysematous cholecystitis cause, 21
Struvite calculi, 574
Stuck twin appearance, 509, 511–12, 518
SUA. *See* Single umbilical artery
Subchorionic hemorrhage
description, 401
differential diagnosis
placenta increta, 390
first- and second-trimester bleeding
cause, 400

Subclavian steal syndrome, 656, 660
Subphrenic fluid collection
differential diagnosis
liver, normal variant, 724–25, 727
Superficial femoral artery
Doppler waveforms, 631
Surgery
acalculous cholecystitis and, 7–8
angiomyolipomas, 382
appendicitis, 174
benign prostatic hyperplasia, 246
carotid stenosis, 653
choledocholithiasis and, 774
corpus luteum cysts, 501
cystic pancreatic neoplasms, 315
echinococcosis, 802
hepatic abscess and, 343, 780
hepatocellular carcinoma, 787, 813
hysterectomy for placenta accreta, 403
intraoperative ultrasonography for hepatic lesions, 678
ischemic colitis and, 157, 159
ovarian torsion, 704
pancreatic carcinoma, 320
primary sclerosing cholangitis and, 748
pseudoaneurysms, 664
testicular torsion, 123–24
in utero repair of diaphragmatic hernia,
453
von Hippel-Lindau disease, 370
Surgical trauma
acquired arterioportal fistulas, 57
Survival rates
congenital diaphragmatic hernia, 452,
455
cystic adenomatoid malformation, 443,
445
ovarian cystadenocarcinomas, 268
pancreatic carcinoma, 320
prostate cancer, 245
pseudomyxoma peritonei, 192
renal cell carcinoma, 106
vanishing twin and, 525
Swiss cheese appearance of the prostate
gland, 257

T

Tapeworm infestation. *See* Echinococcosis
Target pattern
Candida abscesses, 673
hepatic abscesses, 351
intussusception, 163, 165, 195, 196
ischemic colitis, 157
liver metastasis, 672–73
non-Hodgkin's lymphoma, 673

Temporal tap maneuver
  carotid arteries, 629, 653
Teratocarcinoma, 136
Teratomas. *See also* Cystic teratomas
  differential diagnosis
    hemorrhagic ovarian cysts, 709
  testicular, 135–36
Testicular arteries, 148
Testicular torsion, **122–25, 127–29**
  differential diagnosis
    epididymitis, 121–22, 130
Testicular tumors, 135–36, 138, 140–43
Testosterone levels, and prostate cancer, 236
Tethered cord, and myelomeningocele, 49
Tetralogy of Fallot, 457, 460
TGV. *See* Transposition of the great vessels
Thanatophoric dysplasia, 461
  lemon sign, 48
Theca lutein cysts, 407
Thrombocytosis, and renal cell carcinoma, 103
Thumbprinting
  ischemic colitis indication, 159
Tip of the iceberg sign
  cystic teratomas, 275
Toxoplasmosis, and hydranencephaly, 211
Transabdominal sonography
  cervical region, 393
  ectopic pregnancy, 486
  fetal abdomen, 604–5
  pelvic inflammatory disease, 479
Translabial sonography
  during pregnancy, 393
Transmediastinal arteries, 148
Transposition of the great vessels, 457, 460
Transrectal sonography
  endometriosis, 280
  prostate cancer screening, 247–49
  prostatic cysts, 249–53, 256–57, 259
Transvaginal sonography
  corpus luteum cysts, 499, 501
  cystic ovarian masses, 288, 290
  early intrauterine pregnancy, 497
  ectopic pregnancy, 467, 486, 488
  endometriosis, 280
  fetal abdomen, 604–5
  pelvic inflammatory disease, 479
  placenta previa and, 396
  during pregnancy, 393–94, 396
  pseudogestational sac of ectopic pregnancy, 484
Trauma
  acalculous cholecystitis and, 7–8
  Budd-Chiari syndrome cause, 81
  hepatic abscess and, 780
  hepatic abscesses and, 343
  pancreatitis and, 308, 310
  portal vein thrombosis cause, 75

Trauma *(cont'd)*
  primary sclerosing cholangitis and, 748
  splenic cystic lesions, 723
  testicular torsion and, 123
Treacherous calm of Dieulafoy, 175
Triploidy
  associated anomalies, 612, 615
  holoprosencephaly and, 221
  omphalocele and, 603
Trisomy 13
  associated anomalies, 612, 615
  fetal hydrops and, 620, 623
  fetal renal cystic disease and, 547
  heart defects and, 457
  holoprosencephaly and, 221
  omphalocele and, 603
Trisomy 18
  associated anomalies, 591–92, 612, 615
  choroid plexus cysts and, 611
  congenital diaphragmatic hernia and, 454
  differential diagnosis
    Arnold-Chiari malformation, 35–36
    Beckwith-Wiedemann syndrome, 594, 597
    Dandy-Walker malformation, 42
    Down's syndrome, 592–93
    limb-body wall complex, 597–98
    Turner's syndrome, 597
  fetal hydrops and, 620
  fetal renal cystic disease and, 547
  heart defects and, 457
  holoprosencephaly and, 221
  omphalocele and, 603
  single umbilical artery and, 553
  sonographic findings, 591
  spina bifida and, 36
Trisomy 21. *See* Down's syndrome
Truncus arteriosus, 457, 460
TTTS. *See* Twin-twin transfusion syndrome
Tubal or adnexal ring, 469–71, 487–89
Tuberculosis
  in AIDS patients, 413
  disseminated *Pneumocystis carinii* infection and, 434–35
Tuberous sclerosis, **374–75**
  angiomyolipoma and, 95
  differential diagnosis
    von Hippel-Lindau disease, 365, 367
  fetal renal cystic disease and, 547
Tubo-ovarian abscesses
  differential diagnosis
    hemorrhagic ovarian cysts, 709
    ovarian torsion, 698
Tubular ectasia of the rete testes, 138
Tumor thrombosis
  Budd-Chiari syndrome cause, 81
  portal vein thrombosis and, 79

X

Xanthogranulomatous pyelonephritis, **581–87**
  differential diagnosis
    lymphoma, 587
    papillary necrosis, 587
    pyonephrosis, 561
    renal neoplasms, 561
    renal tuberculosis, 561
  reversible hepatic dysfunction syndrome and, 581
  sonographic findings, 557, 560–61

XGP. *See* Xanthogranulomatous pyelonephritis

Y

Yersinia enterocolitica
  mesenteric adenitis cause, 186

Z

Zellweger (cerebro-hepato-renal) syndrome, and fetal renal cystic disease, 547